what people are saying

21st CENTURY SUPERHUMAN

Coming from a hungry generation of seekers, with innate sparks of desire for truth and awakening, I can say that **21st Century Superhuman** *is truly a powerful tool and masterpiece. A collection of wisdom, encouragement, information, and history. This book is a game changer. Information you may have already have is worded better then ever before, hitting home and resonating with you on every page. New essential information for the collective is presented, yet feels familiar to the soul.* **21st Century Superhuman** *is a great treasure for every home.*

Amber JoAnn Cook
Young Mom, Bright Light

The book **21st Century Super Human** *will be a huge key for the shift into multi-dimensional transformation and ascension of the individual, as well as for the Planet as a whole. As we move into living from the Heart and growing towards reaching our full potential,* **21st Century Superhuman** *gives you a jump-start into the process. No matter what age you are, young or old, or what point of the path you are on, this book needs to be on your shelf.*

Sam V. Meyering
Food Magician, Energy Worker

Love your book! There was only one copy left at the workshop and I got it! My friend borrowed it, and I can't wait to get it back! She is going to buy her own copy, yay!

So grateful you put this kind of a guidebook together. It contains so many far reaching correlations with the cutting edge, mindful teachings of so many respected others, Dr. Michael Ryce included. Truly a book who's time has come. My friend and I are considering using it as the "Master" text to teach a class.

Your book is a "strong spiritual backbone," covering the fact and the potential that now, there are really so many brain cells already in place in people's minds, ripe for further cultivation.... (Yay!) This is what we are ready to teach:

"Are we declaring, and faithfully applying what We Know, fearlessly, and powerfully? Are we Now stepping into actualization of our True Design LOVE? YES!"

Julie Matthews
Piano Instructor, Quantum Mentor

21st CENTURY SUPERHUMAN
Quantum Lifestyle

Live Your Potential NOW!

A Powerful Guide to Healthy Lifestyle and Quantum Well-Being

by Cary Ellis, DD
with Theodora Mulder, PhD
Front Cover Art by Franzi Talley

ALSO BY: Cary Ellis
Super Immunity Secrets -Fifty Vegan-Vegetarian Recipes & Immune Protective Herbs
Why Become a Vegetarian?
Benefits for Health and Longevity; Truth About Weight Loss

21st Century Superhuman, Quantum Lifestyle
Second Edition July 22, 2014
Protectrite Copyright 2013 © by Cary Ellis
ISBN-13: 978-0984171118 (Virtual Earth Village Publishing)
ISBN-10: 0984171118

PHOTO CREDIT: Rusty Albertson, Sharon Hall, Patty Tugas, Caroline Colie
PUBLISHER'S NOTE: dr. michael and jeanie ryce's names are in lower case by request honoring that they are a voice of Source; may many be blessed by their journey.

DISCLAIMER

VirtualEarthVillage.com

Virtual Earth Village Publishing
http://www.virtualearthvillage.com

To our Sisters and Brothers on
Planet Earth:

May We Live in a Way that
Aligns with our Greatest Potential,
Fortified by Nature's simple Wisdom
Grounded in Deep LOVE,
Compassion and Gratitude
Inspired to Infinite Possibilities.

And may we offer,
There is only one time
when it is essential to Awaken...

~ THAT TIME IS NOW ~

CONTENTS

READING: 21st Century Superhuman

Expand Your Brain-Power

Bold, italics, hyphens, commas, caps out of the ordinary suggest rich New meanings. When you bump into them, boldly expand use of your Mind into compelling New territories. Our explanation of Quantum physics is easy enough for a six year old to understand (as Einstein says), and it shifts us into tantalizing freedom of Mind-Body-Spirit that transcends limiting superstitions of former generations. Specially denoted words, phrasing and punctuation skyrocket understanding, to catch current waves of miraculous acceleration.

A mind stretched by new experience
can never go back to its old dimensions.

Oliver Wendell Holmes (1809-1894)
Progressive Physician, Author

Shift of the Ages, Shift
Field of Possibilities, Cloud of Possibilities, Field of Consciousness, Field, Divine Matrix, Web of
Life, Plenum, Vacuum
Essence, Effluvia
Conversational comments from Author and Contributor in italics
21st Century Superhumans, 21st Century Superhuman, Quantum Lifestyle,
Arc the Hologram, Arcing the Hologram
Yeshua-Jesus,
Mirror, Mirrored, Mirroring, Mind-Heart
LOVE, Not of LOVE, True Design LOVE, True Infinite Design LOVE
3-D 4-D 5-D (third, fourth and fifth dimensions)
All That Is, Ancient Aramaic, Ancient, Ancients, Ancestral Wisdom, Attention
Abundance, Being, Be, BE, Body-Mind-Heart, Breathe, Breathing
Conscious, Consciousness, Cosmos, Creator, Create
Evolutionary Leap, Leap, Freedom
Gamma, Great Master, Greater Mind
Heart, HUmanity -HUwomity
I Am, Journey, Life, Live, Living, Loving, Loved
Masters, New, Now
Observer-Creator, Oneness, Path, Planet
Quantum, Response-Ability
Smile, Smiling, Solar, Unity, Vibration
Vitality, Joy, Peace,
conscious-unconscious
dis-solve, dis-ease, dis-comfort, dis-integrate
in-formation, i-llnes
"reality," Response-Ability
space-time, time-space, timespace, spacetime
thought-emotion, we-llness, World

INTRODUCTION: *A Powerful Destiny*

Backed by science and chronicled by the Ancients, we are being irresistibly drawn into a surreal and empowering future, promising to carry us far beyond our wildest imaginings. We are Now riding the perfect wave into exciting new expressions of Health, Vitality, LOVE, Abundance and Co-Creation, as we merge with uncensored self-empowerment into a Newly Created *21st Century Superhuman* World.

> The possibility of stepping into a higher plane is quite real for everyone. It requires no force or effort or sacrifice. It involves little more than changing our ideas about what is normal.
>
> *Deepak Chopra MD*
> *Natural Physician, New Thought Author*

Grasp the magnitude of this: Celestial conjunctions that align only once every 26,000 years are activating our sense of Oneness with All Things. Earth's magnetics are lowest in 4,000 years, opening us to transformative shifts as *21st Century Superhumans*. Quantum physics, Now a frontrunner science, endorses the idea that magnetics, thought and emotion literally instantly reshape matter and events around us. The Heart is our most influential sending device (more powerful than the brain), and as we take a deep Breath, we realize the Ancients were right, the long prophesied *Shift of the Ages* is upon us...

What if this *Shift* predicted by the Ancients, rather than being a fearful cataclysm, guarantees answers to our most burning questions? What if New ways of thinking and Being turn painful health challenges, stressful economic struggles, fear, rage, sadness, corrupt banking, governments in turmoil, environment at risk into our *greatest triumph*?

This book is *the roadmap and breadcrumb trail* for this grand adventure! It *is the* Guidebook for our Now, to navigate looming personal and global crisis, launching us into the most thrilling Evolutionary Leap in human history, potentially as Life-changing as when humanity discovered language.

21st Century Superhuman is a potent manual with step-by-step instructions, that effortlessly changes everything. It answers compelling questions about *who we are, why we're here and where we're going...* Join author Cary and associate Teddi, as they Light the way with smiles, twinkling eyes, and a flair for making the outrageous fun, with what could be the script for a wild sci-fi movie or fantasy adventure, yet this is *as "real" as it gets!*

> ...I didn't come here to tell you how this is going to end. I came here to tell you how it's going to begin... I'm going to show these people what you don't want them to see. I'm going to show them a world...without rules and controls, without borders or boundaries; a world where anything is possible.
>
> *Neo*
> *The Matrix*

Same content Now published in both original 500 page version and 4 Parts for ease of reading.

PREFACE: *Collective Awakening to Health, Abundance and LOVE*

This is *THE* Guidebook for a powerful life-changing Journey, as we teeter on the brink of an Evolutionary Leap called the *Shift of the Ages*. Within these pages are essential tools for powerful thought Creation, healthy living, vitality, abundance, LOVE and to shine in the World as our True *Essence*, for we are about to be transformed.

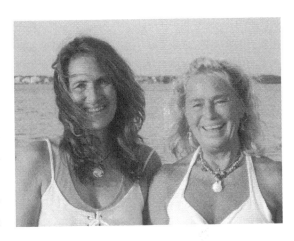

Breathe and Smile as you read, for there is much to absorb here, exposing a stunning New way of Being.

These are the four PARTS of the **21st Century Superhuman System:**

1. SHIFT OF THE AGES: Cosmic Light & Ancient Texts meet Quantum Physics

2. MIND: The BEST Secret Formula to Manifest LOVE, Health, Abundance

3. SPIRIT: Live Your Dreams: Success, Passion, Relationship, Community

4. BODY: Rejuvenation & Growing Younger - Healthy Eating, Cleanse & Detox

Each "PART" contains essential elements. Reading a little daily (whether you have the "big" book or four smaller ones) will provide deep integration of this essential material. Let your instincts lead. Your brain's capacity will increase, as expansive new insights become familiar. Mind-Heart-Body-Spirit adapt, as we put these concepts into practice in daily Life. As New brain cells and neurological pathways become activated, you may experience surges of vitality as well as the occasional need to rest more. Positive "rewiring" takes place, as we unravel old structures and beliefs. You will be amazed at what surprisingly fortunate doors miraculously open in your Life when you collapse old belief systems.

This book is a "download" from "Greater Mind" by Cary Ellis, primary Author. She and Teddi Mulder have collaborated for many years, so Teddi contributes her gift of telepathic "automatic writing - her energy graces the pages in italics. Stretch your Mind, let go old constructs; then move, walk, play, Breathe, Smile and come back for more. Read anywhere and you'll be in the very right place. As you read we promise, you will not be the same person you were yesterday! Quantum principles, Now a Global groundswell are generating a massive wave! Join literally millions around the Planet utilizing these powerful Keys to up-level the entire human Journey. *Don't miss out joining in on the fun!!*

We are often asked, "Would someone *please* explain Quantum physics to me, so that I can understand it?" As Einstein said, "Unless you can explain it to a six year old, you don't understand it well enough yourself." *This* is the launching pad, and it *is* a game-changer! *The Quantum journey requires opening the Mind to recognize that everything surrounding us emerges from thought. Wow!* This is a huge shift from thousands of years of thinking, "someone or something else is to blame." Pick up this book(s), read anywhere and you'll find the perfect input for " Now." Multiple readings activate more brain cells!

Transformation emerges from seeds planted; and soon you realize you are Jack or Jane climbing the Beanstalk into the clouds, looking back at the old Life far below, to which there will be no return, for the *treasure* lies ahead. We look forward to sharing this astounding journey with you, as we move together into brilliant expression far beyond what we've yet dreamed. As we escape the sleep-walk of millennia in this Collective Awakening, we discover greater expression of health, vitality, abundance and LOVE.

Physics isn't the most important thing - LOVE is.

Richard Feynman (1918-1988)
Nobel Prize Physics, Einstein Award

Welcome to what may appear more incredible than what you bargained for, yet once understood ultimately "the way." Join us to experience your Life transforming in mind-expanding and wonderful ways. Teetering on the brink of this ultimate Evolutionary Leap, we learn how to shed old self-destructive habits like water flying off a shaking dog.

Transformation of each Mind-Heart ignites this powerful change anew. Your participation is essential to the whole, so join with us on this adventure of a Lifetime, long called by prophets *Shift of the Ages*. Release old constructs; let them flow like molten lava into the archaeology of a distant past, freeing your spirit to soar in New ways!

Gather with others in this great collective Awakening, as with mutual inspiration you *"polish your shine."* As *we* build community spirit, *"where two or more are gathered"* miracles occur, and a rightly aligned Life reveals the clear path to Health, Abundance and LOVE.

We are grateful for extraordinary good fortune to share this amazing Journey; for as we step into expression of our True *Essence*, a new "reality" is born. We look forward to meeting you on the path, as shifting ourselves, we victoriously shift the entire Hologram!

LOVE and Blessings to All -

♥ *Cary & Teddi* ♥

Learning is finding out what you already know. Doing is demonstrating that you know it. Teaching is reminding others that they know just as well as you.
You are all learners, doers, and teachers.

Richard Bach
Illusions - Adventures of a Reluctant Messiah

FORWARD: *dr. michael ryce*

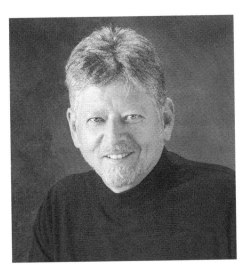

I have known Cary Ellis and Teddi Mulder for over 30 years, and have admired their commitment to growth and inquiry. I have encountered their minds researching and studying as I have myself over the years. Their approach offers essential keys to understanding, integrating and living a "whole" Life.

The adventure Cary and Teddi take us on is the path to elevating the entire being into wellness. Both Cary and her associate Teddi have lived and taught a true transformational healing journey for many years, and are about to share it with you. Prepare to enter an exceptional view from many levels of consciousness and well-being and be wowed! With 60 years plus of study between them, you will save yourself decades of reinventing the wheel. The years of research and wisdom each has tapped into in their lifework equals thousands.

On my path as a Naturopathic Physician I came to recognize that illness and aging were caused partially by our habits of everyday Life - yet even more so by the *root* of those habits in Mind and Heart. Whether our energy is freely flowing or inhibited by old unconscious thoughts and emotions of fear and hostility, plays a huge role in well-being.

Thoughts give rise to neuropeptides and chemical reactions, which produce physiological results...in the mind-body connection every change in the mental-emotional state causes a change in body physiology and...energy manifesting into physical matter. Feelings are chemical. They can kill or cure.

Candace Pert PhD
Brain Research Pioneer, "Molecules Of Emotion"

Perhaps the ancients who said, "Perfect LOVE casts out fear" and "The first Law [of health and human existence] is LOVE," knew exactly what they were saying. Beyond thousands of generations of history built on believing "someone else is at fault," we are beginning to look within. Many generations of human civilization built on this false premise, set up a foundation for chronic misery now playing itself out in the World.

I have had privilege of close association with translation of one of the oldest Ancient Aramaic documents, that recorded Jesus' (or in his own language of Aramaic, Yeshua's) actual teachings. Rather than a religious language, Aramaic is language of quantum physics. What Yeshua came to share with us is the most healing message on the planet today when rightly understood. *True Forgiveness* is not about letting someone else "off the hook" or pardoning. It is about removing anything within ourselves Not of LOVE that is resonating into form our current "reality." Once understood, shifting at this level is the wellspring of a Life of vitality, energy, creativity, joy and well-being.

> What controls the composition of your blood, and therefore the fate of your cells? ...signals from the environment...interpreted by the mind... The brain releases chemistry into the blood that controls cell behavior and genetic activity. If you change your belief and perception, you can change the chemistry of your blood and Create your own biology.
>
> Bruce Lipton, PhD
Biology of Belief

I have the highest respect for Cary and Teddi, whose lives are dedicated to living and teaching principles of practical everyday guidelines to awakening from the inside, while bringing Lifestyle practices into harmony with a path of Lightness and Well-Being.

This handbook is an amazing reference and guide for the home, family or individual seeking to refine Lifestyle with progressive mental and physical habits and tools. It addresses how we foundationally shift to the kind of true Life that flows from clear Mind, Heart and Soul, taking self-responsibility for our Creations to restore our True Design LOVE. The effort taken to adopt this New "enlightened" way of living will be well worth it, bearing fruit in greater Life and Vitality.

> The moment you change your perception is the moment
> you re-write the chemistry of your body.
>
> Bruce Lipton, PhD

And then, who knows what you will do with so much energy? Perhaps live the Life of your dreams... May you be blessed in your journey. We hold the space for every Mind, Heart and Being on the planet to live in radiance and well-being, flowing from returning to our *Essence - Pure LOVE.*

LOVE to You - You are LOVED.

♥ dr. michael ryce ♥

·"Why Is This Happening to Me... Again?!"
Landmark work with Khaburis Manuscript
Ancient Aramaic Forgiveness
WhyAgain dot org

ACKNOWLEDGMENT

Here we stand on the shoulders of giants...
by Cary Ellis DD with Theodora Mulder PhD

21st Century Superhuman, Quantum Lifestyle is a product of many productive years in the *Field.* Our wonderful teachers to whom credit is due, exposed us to vital truth founded in natural order and Universal Law. Much Gratitude goes out to those who guided us with their Presence through books, teachings and practical application. Many of these evolutionary Wisdom Keepers have now transitioned from this Life, after imparting timeless knowledge to us, to be passed on to you and *so the circle continues.*

We are honored to have been initiated into respected lineages that carried powerful truth forward. Notice when *you* are being blessed to participate in a Truth-carrying Lineage. Tony Robbins says, *"We Model Excellence by sitting at the feet of Masters;* duplicating their physiology and mental syntax we access the same part of our brain that they do."

The *Essence* of those who gifted us with their guidance continues today, with practical tools, systems and resources, transforming us and our World...

THOSE WHO HAVE GONE ON TO BE WITH US IN SPIRIT

Dr. Ann Wigmore, Founder, Hippocrates wheatgrass and living foods programs, honorary "grandmother" of today's raw food movement

Rev. Don Haughey, Founder, Creative Health Institute (formerly Hippocrates)

Dr. John Whitman Ray Founder Body Electronics: Health and the Human Mind, Body/Spinal/Cranial Electronics and associated Iridology

Dr. Max Gerson, Founder, Gerson Cancer Therapy, his daughter **Charlotte Gerson** (still living) and the ongoing work of Gerson Cancer Therapy Inst.

Bernard Jensen, DC, Iridology pioneer, body cleansing and detoxification

Dr. Christopher Hills, Founder Light Force Spirulina as a primary food source, enough food for all; University of the Trees; President, World Yoga Society

Dr. Hanna Kroeger, Master Herbalist

Sun Bear, Native American Shaman, Wisdom Teachings and Visionary

Jack White, Spiritual Educator, author *God's Game of Life*

Nellie and Ed Cain, Teachings on Universal Laws of the Kabbalah, author *Exploring the Mysteries of Life*

Drs. Marion and Mikele McCumber, Bishop of the Church of Tzaddi

Dr. Thomas Stone, Psychiatry, Environmental Medicine, pioneer in resolving brain disorders caused by environmental sensitivity and food allergies

Daniel Dieska, D.D.S. Holistic Dentistry

D.A. Versendaal, D.C., Educator, Innovator Applied Kinesiology, Contact Reflex Analysis CRA and Applied Trophology

James V. Goure Founder, United Research, Inc. & The Light Center. *"Mission:* To increase awareness of Oneness of All That Is by expanding Light, Peace & unconditional Love." Atomic Energy Commission 1947-75 which lead to healing the Planet w/prayers for Peace.

THOSE HERE DOING THEIR WONDERFUL WORK

Gregg Braden Author - *Divine Matrix, Awakening to Zero Point, Walking Between the Worlds,* and many more

Dr. Bruce Lipton *The Biology of Belief; Spontaneous Evolution* w/ Steve Bhaerman

dr. michael ryce Ancient Aramaic Forgiveness, *Why is this Happening to me Again?*

Dr. Richard Bartlett & Melissa Joy Matrix Energetics

Viktoras Kulvinskas *Survival into the 21st Century,* Co-Founder Hippocrates Health Inst.

Amrit Desai - Founder Kripalu Yoga

Anthony Robbins, Firewalking, Personal Power, NLP

John Davis, Coptics International TheCopticCenter dot org & SpiritualUnityofNations dot org, World Service Order

Dolphins, Whales, Animals, Earth Mother Gaia - ALL in our miraculous natural World

Additionally - Essene Gospels; Ram Dass; Parmahansa Yogananda; Garret John LoPorto; Roy Eugene Davis; Margaret Mead; Barbara Marx Hubbard; Jean Houston; Kryon; John Lennon; Drunvalo Melchizedek; Dieter Broers; David Wilcock; David Icke; Stephen Hawking; Barbara Marciniak; Ken Carey; Zecharia Sitchin; Peace Pilgrim; HeartMath Institute; Nassim Haramein; Michael Tellinger; Graham Hancock; Sacha Stone; Eckhart Tolle; John, Deo and Ocean Robbins; David Spangler; Peter and Eileen Caddy; Dean and Mary Hardy; Carl and Ortrun Franklin; Machalle Wright; Byron Katie; *Abraham Teachings* with Jerry and Esther Hicks; the family of HUmanity-HUwomity; Ascended Masters, Angels of Light, Great White & Rainbow Brotherhood, Beings of LIGHT and LOVE *in all dimensions.* We thank our families, LOVED ones, pets, friends and ancestors present and in Spirit from whose lives, passages and continuing presence we learn so much.

We are grateful to all gifted ones quoted here. Each showed up in an amazing way, as if to say, "I gave my life for freedom, enlightenment and empowerment of humanity, add me," as their perfect quote immediately appeared!

We grow daily as part of a Heart-centered *"Global Mastermind,"* Now transmitted with lightening-speed around the Planet. It is no longer possible to keep track of what ignites our inspiration. Excited to be part of this unfolding, millions are Now shifting Worldwide into an awakened state. The astounding News that that *only* way to change things on the outside is to shift ourselves on the inside to LOVE, is Now spreading like wildfire!!!

We are blessed, inspired and uplifted, to be moving into True Unity among humankind. Carl Johan Calleman, who left a prestigious scientific career to research the Mayan Calendar full time, offers its premise for our times:

> May we inspire You to feel like You
> are an integral part of the Universe.

~ *21st CENTURY SUPERHUMAN* ~

Breathe - Smile

Rest - Movement

Cleanse and Detox

Moderation in All Things

Purify with Water Inside and Out

Meditate - Merge with the *Field*

Nourish with High Frequency Foods

Align with Your True Design, LOVE

Mind & Emotion Marry in the Heart

There Is No 'Out There' Out There

Our Thoughts Create Our "Reality"

Compassion without Judgment

Clean Out the Unconscious

Cancel, Release, Let Go

Gratitude - Thank You

Mud Between the Toes

KNOW it IS [Done]

Be Your Prayers

Live Your Truth

Heart Coherence

Enjoy the Journey

Honor Others' Choices

Laugh, Smile, Dance and Play

Live Your Essence

Leap for Joy

BE at Peace

♥ LOVE ♥

www.21stCenturySuperhuman.com

Part 1
SHIFT OF THE AGES

Cosmic Light
& Ancient Texts
Meet Quantum Physics

Connect with your existence, connect within yourself, connect with this infinite beauty that you are made of.

And then express it in the World.

Make the World around you an expression of that beauty, of that power, of that consciousness.

~

Nassim Haramein
The Resonance Project
The Connected Universe

Part 1: SHIFT OF THE AGES - SECTION 1
COSMIC EVENTS

Knowledge... is not information. It's transformation.

Osho (1931-1990)
Indian Guru, Teacher Self-Inquiry

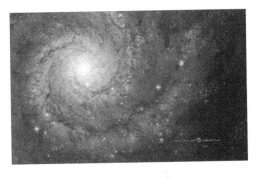

During millions of years of planetary history extreme events have periodically and dramatically affected all of Life on Earth. We are Now teetering on the brink of another such astounding transformational leap.

In the past, cataclysms such as devastating pole shifts, frightening land mass upheavals, brutal ice ages, widely destructive floods, and horrific wars stored fear deep inside the human psyche. Resulting prophecies about our "Now" steeped in superstition, based in realities little understood in context of the day. Fearful shadows were cast of Armageddon and apocalyptic judgement, misinterpreted, as apocalypse from Ancient Greek means to "uncover or reveal" the next phase.

We are Now precariously close to a tantalizingly long-awaited event historical cosmologists have called the *Shift of the Ages*. Despite fear embedded in the collective psyche, today's forward thinkers versed in astronomy and Quantum physics reveal to us that we are poised on the threshold of accessing knowledge about ourselves and our magnificence as a species far beyond anything yet imagined. This *Shift* Now dawning upon us, offers to be as dramatically Life-changing as adaptation to language was millennia ago.

The stage is set. The World is in deep crisis with severely outmoded socio-economic systems, misleading religions, failing institutions and governments in upheaval. Simultaneously, we have moved into intensified *Fields* of Light Now pouring to Earth, activating Mind-Heart to dramatically new levels. *Comprehension of who we are and how we operate in this World is mega-jumping.* Inventive ideas and new modes of Being required for a viable future, Now are pouring forth around the Globe. Millions dare to step forward, empowered with progressive ideals, birthing sensational action. With growing awareness, many have begun to put well-being of ALL first, and are honoring our Planetary Home.

Rather than "expected" cataclysm or apocalypse, *this Shift* is fueled by powerful Cosmic influences, activating an irresistible sense of Oneness within. We are about to discover, simple though it may seem, these faster moving Light photons are causing subtle but deep changes, impelling us to seek greater authenticity, creativity and connection.

Embracing Quantum physics' enlightened "reality," while moving further into this *Shift*, we are Being so affected by these evolutionary stimuli we will never be the same again.

The *only* Evolution is recognition of our ultimate *Oneness*.
If you don't understand this, it's business as usual.

Francis Lucille
Advaita Vedanta (non-duality)

Potential is emerging for global change that may have heretofore seemed unattainable. As suggested by Bruce Lipton and Steve Bhaerman in *Spontaneous Evolution*, as we wake up and move beyond imploding fear, materialism and its ensuing survivalism, we discover a wave of change utilizing this New awareness to shape an integrated, holistic future.

We are orbiting a place in space we only get to once every 26,000 years, where powerful Cosmic influences awaken Mind-Heart through stimulation of the pineal gland, activating heightened sense of Oneness with All things. Simultaneously, modern translation of Ancient texts dovetails with Quantum physics, advancing us into profound New awareness of how our World operates. There is potential for remarkable change to occur, uncommonly accessible during this Evolutionary Leap called the *Shift of the Ages*.

A Story

Once upon a time in the long, long ago, eternal crystals split into individualized light and dark patterns, forgetting they were intrinsic to the One. A holographic World spun into stars, galaxies, and Worlds within Worlds, as these individuations became intensely focused within. They transmitted thought to their offspring, gradually forgetting they were One with the ONE. As they became intent upon their own journey, they began to blame each other when something occurred, they sometimes even blamed Creator, the ONE. Thousands of generations fostered the idea that most things were "someone else's fault." Countries, boundaries and governments grew because of it. They built armies and had wars because of it. There was greed and many suffered because of it. They had pain and sickness because of it; they even had death...

Memory of their infinite powers of creativity diminished. They denied Response-Ability for anything appearing in their World. They had forgotten they were Innate Creators, and that their "realities" magnetized into Being through thought. As mis-belief settled in, they almost completely eclipsed connection with Source, their creative potential and their True Design LOVE.

An amazingly complex and brilliant civilization grew up with geopolitical and monetary systems founded in dogma based around, "hold onto what's ours," and "get what's theirs." Fixated on materialization and accumulation of goods, they had all but forgotten their most powerful asset under layers of fear and hostility. All it would take was one Moment of remembering their Oneness.

Cosmic forces were aligning to activate Remembering this amazing awareness that they were creative Beings made of LOVE. It was whispered from person to person throughout the land that once they had shed their old beliefs, they would easily emerge into a Free, Happy, Creative, Regenerative, Productive, Peaceful, Abundant Society. And so it was... ♥

Chapter 1

Great Change, Quantum "Reality"

May you live in interesting times...

Ancient Chinese

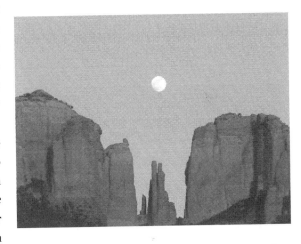

This Chinese saying about "interesting times," refers to those who live during great change, perhaps exciting for adventurous Souls who have learned to "let go," yet maybe unsettling for those attached to safety and security.

Great change propels us to release what holds us back, so we move into New dimensions of expression individually and Collectively. Everyone moves at their own pace, for "interesting times" are fraught with uncertainty for traditionalists, while containing greater creative possibility than any other point in history for those ready to shift.

Welcome to these "times of great change." We discover we are living on the brink of a powerful Evolutionary Leap promising to carry us beyond where we have ever been. Revolutionary insights offer great opportunity to restructure civilization for a viable future.

In the long ago, human culture focused on materialism, losing track of our True creative Design LOVE. This resulted in suffering: brutal wars, oppression, poverty, hunger and ignorance. We are Now activated by rare Cosmic Gamma rays and Light, exposing us to breathtaking New "realities," while Quantum physics and Ancient Texts reveal New ways to think, to birth a Civilization based in LOVE and creativity. Quantum tools at our fingertips, offer powerful methods to restructure Life and operate successfully within it.

Long ago with a good dose of "ignorance is bliss," we set off exploring the path of duality and materialism, based on getting "more for me." Duality means a "double existence" (more than One), having left behind original knowledge of our Innate Oneness where LOVE is the primary operating system. We forgot that we are *ONE* with ever-emerging Creation connecting us with All That Is, and we thought we were separate.

This took us into the murky waters of the "non-being" or separate mind, where we established Life around Not of LOVE philosophies and practices, and have remained there for thousands of years. We are Now entering what the Ancients called the *Shift of the Ages,* which promises to jog us out of *duality,* to remember our Oneness with All Things!

Our ancestors cultivated a "dominance" and "power over" culture based in control, judgment, blame, fear and hostility, protecting interests in the material World, forgetting their eternal nature. Fixed upon survival, early humans fought over food, shelter, resources, family, tribe, safety and security *(a pattern still going on today).*

This grand experiment has since played itself out Planet-wide, leaving us today with disintegrative and unsustainable systems. When early civilization discarded LOVE and Oneness as their primary "operating system," in exchange for blame-fear-hostility-judgment-control, it went something like this:

- keep what's ours
- take what's theirs if we need it
- attack them if they try to take what's ours
- escalate more lethal military technologies
- Create borders and boundaries to keep them out
- if we have something they want, increase the value
- false monetary systems become more and more inflated
- since we're smarter, stronger and more technical, enslave/indenture them
- take/do what we want without regard to how it affects the Earth and others

This brought diminishing returns, and they experienced themselves as separate rather than connected. They had forgotten they were an extension of the ONE, part of a giant holographic "reality" appearing individually, though intimately connected. As they faulted one another, playing power games they hurt themselves as well. They slipped into ignorance which hung like a dark mist, blocking the flow of Source energy and resulting in dis-ease, illness and death.

Such attitudes and habits perpetuated downward spirals of *energetic thought patterns Not of LOVE, creating unsustainable "realities,"* yet the entire civilization lived in *denial* of it. Today ruthless scenarios cascade globally in daily News, inciting revolt and rebellion. A crescendo of collapsing geopolitical and banking systems based on trillions of dollars of falsely perpetuated debt, is awakening awareness of deep need for change and futility of this way of life. Interplay of lethal war technologies where no one ever wins, robs billions of dollars of food from bowls of the hungry and education from the illiterate. Abusive eco-disasters foster ongoing species extinction, with volatile weather patterns inharmonious for all Life. Dissatisfaction and hopelessness leave many wondering "in quiet desperation," if this isn't potentially the fast track toward our own demise, wondering if there is anything we can do about it.

Is this the tailspin of the insanity of humanity? Possibly so, as Living outside of LOVE is a very real form of "in-sanity." As a highly intelligent race of beings, why are we still destroying ourselves and our Planetary home? Are we ready to wake up from a World established in the falsity of duality and separation (us vs. them)? As the "non-being" mind of materialism plays itself out with competition, our choice is to either continue toward imminent self-destruction, or change course to a New Civilization based in LOVE, by following this book: clearing out our old Not of LOVE thoughts, stories and attitudes, restoring our True Design LOVE. Are we ready to step onto the path of Remembering that we are all One, to live in Unity on Planet Earth, *"as if the God in all Life matters."*

A modern culture of "plenty" outrageously uses fossil fuel agriculture and transportation, while one billion out of seven are without sanitary sources of water. Even where basic survival needs of food, shelter, health and resources *are* met, modern civilization shows blatant signs of crumbling around us. According to Mazlow's "Hierarchy of Needs," as a global culture we are at the "peak of the pyramid," capable of responding to most situations with self-esteem, respect, creativity, morality, spontaneity and acceptance. Yet we currently default to less evolved practices, resulting in suffering and chronic stress from failing governments, corporate and economic monopolies and manipulative religions. Shall we inquire why we continue such self-destructive behaviors?

You cannot escape responsibility of tomorrow by evading it today.

Abraham Lincoln (1809-1865)
US President, Abolished Slavery, Preserved the Union

Extraordinary possibilities are afoot, offering insights for constructive change, renewal and redirection. Massive peaceful mainstream protests such as Occupy Movement and transparent news are Now bootlegged around the World to such a scale they are blatantly shifting our course. We are recognizing ourselves as connected Planetary and global citizens, with the same joys, pains, sorrows and triumphs! Our potential to Leap across the Evolutionary Spiral into a greater, kinder expression of who we are, is the greatest in human history! Expanding perception of how our existence operates and the power we have to change things, is awakening us to a New sense of who we are. Einstein's premise summarizes our emerging Quantum awareness:

If you think you're separate, you're living in an optical delusion.

This is a great "reframe." Einstein points out that we are not separate, and if you think we are you are deluded. This message has been preserved in spiritual traditions throughout the ages, though often distorted by self-serving dogma and politics. Quantum physics radically redefines "reality," bridging science and spirituality. It describes matter not as solid as we once thought, but ever-emerging from an *Infinite Field of Possibilities*.

Progressive Quantum physicist Nassim Haramein says, "What Nikola Tesla called "the aether" is the same fundamental Universal *Field* of energy called the Vacuum, Space, the

Zero Point *Field*, the Quantum Foam, the Source *Field*, God, the Plenum... call it what you like, we are made of and bathing in an infinite *Field* of Energy that we call "empty space."

> ...All attempts to explain the working of the universe [are futile] without recognizing the existence of the ether and the indispensable function it plays in the phenomena.... There is no energy in matter except that received from the environment.
>
> *Nikola Tesla*

This insight through Quantum physics, into how permeating the Presence of "Source" is, relaxes us into a more flowing existence. Nothing is as "solid or stuck" as it seems, and events and matter adjust as we shift our Attention! Everything from bank accounts to jobs, living conditions, health, relationships, pollution, wars and even compromised nuclear power plants can shift, as we move from fear into LOVE. *We are about to give you the "secret formula," so you know exactly how this moving of molecules works!*

Famous Quantum experiments demonstrated repeatedly over the last 100 years, that thoughts and emotions *magnetize* matter and events into Being with far greater certainty than we may have guessed. Once we play with this surreal potentiality, awareness about how we operate in this World changes *forever!* Like a wild sci-fi fantasy adventure, in this revolutionary approach what appear to be "obstacles" dissolve in an instant, when we *shift our thought patterns* to change our World! *Really? Really!*

This *is the real* future science. We will explore these sensational Quantum principles more intimately in coming chapters, exposing exactly how our *Attention* placed upon the *Field of Possibilities,* magnetizes matter and events into Being around us. Newton's Laws of Physics define matter as tangible, solid and mechanical. Quantum physics reveals amazing New evidence that matter and events move into new form *as readily as we shift our thoughts.* Fearlessly jumping in, to play with this idea that matter is mutable, opens us to amazing potentials within this New "reality." In fact *playing* with this idea is the best way to explore it. An incredible sense of Freedom floods us once we witness that we are the maker of our "reality," rather than at its effect!

Time and space are not as linear as once thought. Difficult as this may seem, to imagine, Quantum theory proposes there *may not be* time or space as we have known them. Time and space are defined by experience, rather than transiting a time or place. According to String Theory, Attention on an electron affects both its past and future. Time and space quite simply *mark the passage of consciousness! Whoa...* And yes, this does stretch the imagination to comprehend! We will get into this more in just a little bit! We have uncanny ability to *transcend* time and space. Experiment with putting away your watch, follow your intuition and "go with the flow" as Life allows. After all, who doesn't like to live in "timelessness" anyway? Cosmic influences stimulating our pineal gland are waking us up, drawing us into our flowing creative abilities, we may not have accessed since childhood.

Years ago Dr. John Whitman Ray introduced us to the then little known Quantum concept of the **"Ever Present Now,"** later popularized in Eckhart Tolle's book, *The Power of Now*. This potent, Life-changing Quantum awareness is shifting us to where past, present and future are flowing simultaneously! *Bend your mind around that!*

Physicists Now define time as a "medium for Quantum information transfers," also considering that multiple "realities" may initiate from the same point. Thought is magnetic and time is a magnetic field held together by thought. We will enter this more deeply as we move on in our *21st Century Superhuman* Journey. Meanwhile, let's play with expansion of thought *beyond time*. From this exciting vantage-point discover ability to "change all timelines." As we learn to interact with Creation from a place of LOVE, we move into where we can literally dissolve unhappy memories, as if they never happened, and set up a new resonance for past and future history.

This may mean accepting more of this kind of thought, that there is no such thing as death. If we are "missing" a Loved one, we can cultivate the ability to communicate with them in the "here and now," learning how there is no "separation," but a continual flow of Life, LOVE, Source and Creation. Teddi's friend Richard who passed suddenly a few years back, came to her in Spirit and said, "If you miss me, just pick up the cosmic telephone."

...the Newtonian idea of time as an absolute...flowing on its own is incorrect... time is a measure of the numerical order of change...Though we perceive events occurring in past, present, or future, these concepts may just be part of a psychological frame in which we experience material changes in space.

dailygalaxy.com April 26, 2011
Spacetime Has No Time Dimension

As we *21st Century Superhumans* play with transcending time and space, knowing our thoughts affect all Creation, we become aware of a Living Quantum "reality," far more malleable than once thought. Many Ancient indigenous tribes believe accessing our full Quantum potential requires shifting "out of time" and entering "dreams" of conscious Creation. We are going to learn how as we change magnetic vibration of thoughts-emotions, we also change history through time and space or "shifting timelines."

By 1949 Gödel had produced remarkable proof: 'In any Universe described by the theory of relativity time cannot exist.' Our research confirms Gödel's vision: time is not a physical dimension through which one could travel into past or future."

phys.org Apr 14, 2012 by Lisa Zyga
Physicists Work to Abolish Time as 4D of Space

That time and space do not exist as we have known them, stretches the Mind vastly into Quantum "reality." Here we enter past and future to change timelines, particularly once in our True resonance, LOVE. This moves us beyond cultural conditioning, into knowing ourselves as Living Breathing participants of Creation in the Ever Present Now. In our chapter on Meditation (Part 2: MIND) we share a powerful formula for dropping into the *Field* and inviting Creation to emerge in New ways. Soaring beyond time-space we learn to access our Innate creative *Essence,* immersing into the sensory-rich right brain World of the *Heart,* to restore it as our primary operating system, we hold positive vision for self, Loved Ones and Planetary Family.

Aligning with Heart and *Essence,* we learn to free ourselves from inhibiting old "unconscious programs" of doubt and fear, to Live in greater alignment with who we Truly Are. We enter an entirely New paradigm, founded in such things as "simple trust," knowing that "when one door closes another opens," when things don't go according to plan, "there is always a perfect plan unfolding," harmonizing with the "flow of Creation."

Learning to Live from *Essence* in this New ever-emerging Quantum "reality," is foundational to achieving our full potential in this World. Putting this into practice is the exciting adventure of the *21st Century Superhuman!* We suggest often, "Breathe and Smile," opening New neurological pathways to access True resonance of Mind and Heart, emanating from a radiant flow of LOVE, measurable with modern instrumentation.

Our natural navigation system has long been stymied, in a culture emphasizing productivity over creativity. The majority still act from this old paradigm, silencing the "inner voice." As *21st Century Superhumans* we are learning to restore our connection, to heed the True Source of our Being through the Heart.

Have you ever thought, "If I'd only heeded my 'inner prompting,' things would have been better?" Inner guidance is our *best* compass, with Heart being True North. Ask yourself these penetrating questions: "Am I expressing my *Essence* to the World? Do I Love my job or profession? Do I Love what I'm doing? If not, what even small changes can I make to align more with my True *Essence?*" *Students:* "Do I Love what I'm studying? Does it bring forth my True Talents? If not, how can I get more on track with *Me?*"

In Latin the root of conscience is "to know." Our conscience indicates the *knowing* within. Conditioned to ignore our inner guidance system, denial and disassociation have Created resistance to natural powerful flow of Life. Conforming to succeed or fit in, rather than following the Heart, is a residual of the blame-fear-hostility culture. When we deny True Self to comply with society (even if for "good reasons"), though we may not think so suppressing *Essence* shows on the face (worn), just as it did with Pinocchio (his nose grew).

Conformity impels us to fit in, avoiding "fear of punishment or rejection" and make money for security. Releasing these patterns can initially be terrifying, due to unconscious blockages from early childhood, environment and genetic programs. Letting go these old layers, we access renewed Vitality. Moving beyond such old programing is *key,* in our current Evolutionary Leap. Quantum "reality" *ONLY* Mirrors our Vibration, conscious and unconscious. "Reality" then becomes a "Mirror" for awareness of where to shift internally.

Whatever we observe in our World is a Mirroring of magnetic thought resonance in us. It may be based on old, forgotten, generational unconscious data, or it could be something we have judgement about. Either way, as we will learn in detail in upcoming *21st Century*

Superhuman chapters, *ALL that appears in our World is a Mirroring of that which is inside of us (both conscious & unconscious)!* Even we resisted the idea when we first heard it, yet we've had to shatter the illusion that someone "out there" is "doing it to us," and *it's an inside job.*

✗ If we don't like what's showing up in our "reality," it's up to us to shift on the *INSIDE* (*awesome tools for this ahead*). As we shift the outer will shift in response. The Truth of Our Being is reclaimed when we Live in the "Now," with True Guidance of the Heart, knowing every "Creation" is our own! Many are finding courage to walk away from what no longer serves them, to find new ways to Grow and be Happy, emerging into an entirely New paradigm. We will dig into the mechanics of this, learning how to Master our own Destiny.

Following the Heart and Living from *Essence* is *the* way to True Success. Releasing old patterns is required to access this level of connection with Self. Loving ourselves by expressing who we Truly Are, redirects the course of our existence, and profoundly affects All of Creation! Once on this path, we relink DNA codes and access Higher Mind and Heart, bringing forth the brilliance of our Being, unimagined from where we were. In the Truth of Who You Are is Your full Empowerment. This is *Quantum Lifestyle!*

Question: Why do you think the great God-Beingness of All there is gave us free will? Answer: ...so we would return to Oneness on our own...

Jack White (1934-1998)
God's Game of Life

Have things once entertaining lost their familiar appeal? Has the old "normal" become mundane? Do you ever find yourself wondering if "this" is *all Life is,* or if you will ever *do what you came here to do? If so, what that might be?* Such "Attention-getters" urge us to disengage from the old paradigm, for our "reality" changes as fast as we do, and we now have Quantum tools at our fingertips! Are you flowing, centered in your *Essence,* or are you white knuckled at the wheel? Perhaps you're already waking up, and as Abraham-Hicks says are ready to, "Pick up the oars and let the river carry you..." Are you expressing that unique spark of something special that only you have, that *no one else* can do? What is it, and how can you bring this forth as your way of Being in the World?"

We are living in thrilling "times of great change," that have rarely shown up in human history! Quantum physics is knocking at the door offering an entirely New paradigm of "reality." Our inner spirit feels "the call" of this wave, tugging at us to go beyond expectations of friends, society, family and associates. It doesn't necessarily mean we leave these people; yet we reach inward to Honor and represent more fully *who* We Are. Once we make this choice, we may move into "New frequencies" that require adjustments of the Life to continue. We may decide to leave *"Normal,"* such as "Working to pay for the car to drive to work at an uninspiring job, to get clothing we for job, to pay for the house we only get to sleep in at night." Is there a better way?

We are emerging beyond Ancient "programing" catalogued within self and humanity, of ancient "enslavement" patterns that dictated "punishment for disobedience." We will learn to remove such fear patterns from the unconscious in coming chapters, and pave the way to ultimate *Freedom, Creativity and Joy.* Groups are Now forming around the World on location and online, for participation in abundant, Creative Life expression, in cultivating a viable path to fully express our innate skills and talents.

Changes in the Cosmos Now impel us to open to the Heart, and move into holistic choices. Global Communities, "islands of the future" for Heart-centered living are Now emerging worldwide, stimulating an exodus of hundreds of thousands to move beyond old cultural norms, seeking Heart-based Living and Expression.

YOUR TRUEST ESSENCE - Make a list of your qualities of True *Essence.* Breathe, Smile and open to explore your True Potential, allowing awareness to flow. Make a list of your natural talents, abilities and what you LOVE doing, with any ideas that pop up as to how to merge these with steps toward productive, Joyful Life path. Collaborate with others Now *breaking Free,* to open doors to New possibilities, for *where two or more are gathered...*

> When you are ready to make that leap you will know. There will be no other choice. Suddenly you will realize that all your fears, all your problems, all your rational dilemmas, were just part of a dream, a fiction that you had been maintaining through your stubborn effort.
>
> *Ken Carey*
> *The Starseed Transmissions*

Things as we have known them *are* changing: the old is crumbling and the New is being born in these powerfully "times of great change." *21st Century Superhumans* around the Globe express Creativity and *Essence,* releasing Ancient Not of LOVE thought-emotional patterns that kept us from Being our best. New ways of Living, harmonious with Self and the Earth are emerging. No matter what it seems, things *are* unfolding perfectly.

> The Universe holds its Breath as we choose, instant by instant, which pathway to follow; for the Universe, the very essence of Life itself is highly conscious. Every act, thought, and choice adds to a permanent mosaic; our decisions ripple through the Universe of consciousness to affect the lives of all.
>
> Lest this idea be considered either merely mystical or fanciful, let's remember the fundamental tenet of the new theoretical physics: Everything in the Universe is connected with everything else.
>
> *David R. Hawkins, MD, PhD*
> *Power VS Force, The Hidden Determinants of Human Behavior*

Harmonizing our Lives with the dawning of a New Civilization on Planet Earth founded in LOVE, the answers we seek are carrying us forward into Quantum "reality." Together we are discovering revolutionary New ways to Be the dynamic amazing talented, Self-expressive Creator Beings we were born to be, as *21st Century Superhumans!* ♥

Chapter 2

Mayan Calendar Ends

Whether you call this Light, LOVE or Knowledge, its flame grows brighter each day. The Light reveals that civilization is in a birthing process as the old way of Life falls away and a new one emerges.

Bruce Lipton PhD and Steve Bhaerman
Spontaneous Evolution, Our Positive Future and A Way To Get There From Here

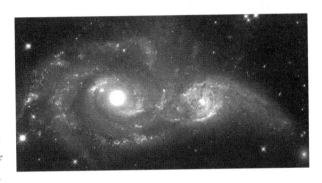

As many agonized over what would happen at "end of the Mayan Calendar" in December 2012, Mayan elders expressed concern that their cosmology was misinterpreted. It was not marking the end of the *World*, but the end of an *Age* (or the World as we knew it) *and beginning of a New era!* One of the most widely prophesied events in memorable human history, it has stirred controversial questions such as, "Will it be catastrophic?" "Is my life at risk?" "Is this the end of the World?" Implications of such questions still linger during this major transition in Planetary history.

Drunvalo Melchisedek, Founder of the *School of Remembering*, expert in Mayan cosmology and sacred geometry, tells us Dec. 12, 2012 was halfway point of the 26,000 year cycle known as Precession of the Equinoxes, where each astrological sign is on Earth's horizon at sunrise spring equinox for 2,000 years marking our transit through the Cosmos.

We are coming out of a cycle of karmic cleansing and imbalanced male dominance with Planet and human systems in widespread crisis. The good thing about crisis is, we can resolve it. The Feminine emerges to lead the way into a New paradigm, where Masculine-Feminine blends in perfect ecstatic balance. In serpentine-like movement through the Cosmos, we just completed a 13,000 year cycle of density, darkness and materialism, and though still feeling the pendulum swing of that old energy, we have moved into a new dynamic in the midst of this 26,000 year cycle noted by the Mayans. We have entered a grand cycle of our long orbit around our Galactic Center and Central Sun, crossing into *Fields* of intensified Light, entering a transformative New dispensation based in LOVE.

Excitingly, the 5th night of the Mayan Calendar of 2008 states we are entering the end of "manufactured lack." Cosmic energy shifts are Now activating a new *reference point* from where a "Community of Planetary Beings" is clearly emerging. From this point we access mutual co-Creation, Freedom and Support for the Individual and the Collective to express *who we Are* as creative Beings, birthing an entirely New Planetary paradigm for humanity.

Grasping Quantum theory and implications of how essential it is to clear unconscious thought-emotional patterns, we recognize that even Global crisis can shift easily, into an entirely New paradigm, as we clear our resonance to LOVE. We are about to learn that our "reality" is much more malleable than we've ever imagined and we can affect it instantly.

Carl Calleman left a prestigious career as a cancer researcher with the World Health Organization, dedicating full time to researching the Mayan Calendar following a Life-altering journey to Guatemala and Mexico in 1979. He let his Heart lead him into this New career and has shed revealing insights on the Mayan Calendar ever since. He offers that Mayan cosmology is based on the concept that we Live in a Universe guided by the Divine, and that the *Essence* of the Ninth Wave of the Mayan Calendar at the "end" of the age, is related to a body of ancient prophecies reflecting this essential wisdom:

This is the time of the "coming of age of humanity..."

Dr. Calleman proposes that this wave began October 28, 2011 (rather than December 21, 2012), represented by an important Mayan glyph, 13 Ahau. *"The glyph [13 Ahau] represents a Waterlily [Lotus?] symbol of beauty, abundance and growth, and the possibility of ascension out of the primordial soup of Creation. Out of the void, a spark of fire falls into the primordial ocean of possibilities and Creation spirals into life."* 13 Ahau also represents December 16, 2013, when the earthquake hit Japan, leaving disastrous cracks in the Fukushima Nuclear Plant, fast becoming a wakeup call for wise action and a catalyst for intelligent human change.

Dr. Calleman suspects linear time ends with this age. Because of the "high frequency of this wave" we are being naturally compelled to shift into a broader spectrum of harmonization with the Heart. As we align rightly within ourselves, things fall into place readily, because of the targeted frequency of this spontaneously emerging wave.

Mayan cosmology presents a series of nine waves built on simple physics, where each wave carries 20% higher frequency and intensity than the last. The Mayans say these waves are a buildup of consciousness, each one carrying us higher than the previous. All these waves are coming to an end simultaneously, when we will integrate what they have brought us. "Frontliners" around the World are catching and surfing this Ninth Wave of the Mayan Calendar, into New harmonious ways of Living on Planet Earth.

Fortunately, Dr. Carl Calleman tells us we will adapt step-by-step, as incoming shifts in consciousness arrive during peaks of the wave. Predictions include city-based Life gradually phasing out and evolving into exciting thriving connected villages, connected by permaculture and farm markets. The Mayan Calendar describes a simple process of adaptation to harmonious Earth ways to be actualized many places. Those aligned early with this change experience an emerging *Field* of Oneness, Freedom and Acceptance even Now. Dr. Calleman describes this in recent interview with *Lilou's Juicy Living Tour - YouTube:*

The Seventh wave that began in 1755 brought an "endarkened" unity consciousness to mankind. The Ninth wave also brings a unity consciousness, but one that is enlightened. We have already found a significant parallel between these two waves in that they began with huge Earthquakes, although those occurred at opposite sides of the Earth, in Lisbon and Japan respectively.

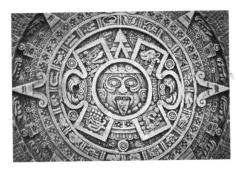

Another parallel is that the two waves started with revolutions to topple existing systems. The Seventh wave began with the American and French revolutions whose anti-monarchic nature gradually spread throughout the world. Revolutions of the Ninth wave have not only rejected monarchic rule, and are in the process of release from the phenomenon of dominance and rule over others as such.

Oneness field of consciousness carried by the Ninth wave won't allow systems where people give their power away to someone they have elected every few years. Deeper freedom based on sovereignty of all Souls is now being called for.

...The Oneness field of consciousness will not allow for an economic system where the power to print money determines what activities people spend their lives with...The driving force behind the world revolution of the ninth wave is the divine guidance that unity consciousness allows...

The chief point to realize is that ultimately this course of events, and the breakdown of dominance, is a result of a cosmic plan that has been described in the nine levels of the Mayan calendar...

Dr. Carl Johan Calleman, Seattle, WA
Ninth Wave Mayan Calendar: World Oneness Revolution

Solar activity, accelerating *Fields* of Light and alignment with the Great Central Sun of our Galaxy are activating us to recognize our Oneness with All Things, fast-forwarding us into to the unstoppable next phase of our Evolutionary journey. Ac Tah, Mayan Elder, travels, placing pyramids to ground these energies.

One of the things that my grandfather used to tell me was that people of my generation were going to live through a tremendous happening. This implied great responsibility from everyone because we were approaching the end of the era of unconsciousness and spiritual darkness.

The event would begin with a planetary alignment that would increase the Vibration of the Earth and diminish its magnetic field. The Earth would enter a new geological era; which would be a very auspicious moment for the return of our Mayan ancestors. He asked me to be ready to recognize *Hunab Ku, [astronomical event that marks the beginning of a new consciousness on Earth]*. He added that I would know what to do in due time because he had trained me for the task.

...*Maya*... [refers] to people who have reached a state of awareness where they understand the synchronicity of the Universe and the connections binding everything together, that one thing is not separate from the other. This Maya philosophy is summarized in their saying: "You are my other me."

Inlakesh - *You Are Another Myself.*

Ac Tah, The Man Who Talks
The Night of the Last Katün 2012 Maya

This Ancient Mayan philosophy is so simple, yet profoundly translucent with Quantum entanglement - as conveyed by Einstein's, "if you think you're separate..." you're living in an optical delusion... What we see in others is actually a Mirroring of ourself. Quantum physics wakes us up to this revolutionary "reality;" matter exists as an ever-emerging *Field of Possibilities* (of which we are part), and matter and events take shape based upon *our Attention upon the Field.*

In the beginning there were only probabilities. The Universe could only come into existence if someone observed it. It does not matter that the observers turned up several billion years later. The Universe exists because we are aware of it.

Martin Rees, Astronomer Royal
Astrophysicist 500+ papers, Albert Einstein Award

Thought and emotion are a Vibrational resonance within us, resulting in our "Attention on the *Field."* As we will learn in depth in upcoming chapters, our Quantum *Attention* calls "reality" into form. Bruce Lipton, epigeneticist, author of *The Biology of Belief* and co-author of *Spontaneous Evolution,* informs us that according to recent studies *only 5%* of thought is in the conscious mind, the other 95% is in the *unconscious,* carried as a residual from in utero, family and environment before age six, most of which we retain little cognitive memory.

We will also learn in upcoming chapters, how this Quantum principle dovetails with teachings of Jesus (Yeshua). His teachings, magnified through the lens of of Quantum theory thanks to modern translations of Ancient Aramaic teach us, rather than "letting someone else off the hook," original forgiveness in Aramaic meant to remove *our* unconscious content "creating" the situation (by our resonance on the *Field*).

The widely affirmed "Quantum Observer Effect," explains that Vibratory energy within us magnetizes "reality" into Being around us. In fact, the *Field* can only return to us or Mirror what we give it, as saying, "Be careful what you wish for, you just might get it."

Researchers...have now conducted a highly controlled experiment demonstrating how a beam of electrons is affected by the act of being observed. The experiment revealed that the greater the amount of "watching," the greater the observer's influence on what actually takes place.

sciencedaily.com
Nature (Vol. 391, pp. 871-874)

Quantum physics affirms Ancient Texts, as we sort out what all this means and none too soon, for early phases of what the Ancients called the *Shift of the Ages* is upon us. We either remain by the sidelines in our 3-D World, blaming outer circumstances for our fate, or embrace this *Shift* riding the wave to a New powerful phase of our Evolution, *where we are conscious creators of our "reality."* Chaos often precedes utopia, and so chaos is launching us into a future Utopian culture for "a thousand years of Peace *(just to get us going)!"*

In the past we have had brief glimpses of Golden Ages. They existed because great beings and avatars illuminated particular areas of the planet. Legends arose of mysterious realms such as Atlantis, Lemuria, Shamballa and Shangri-la. They are visions of utopian culture.

Brian de Flores
The Language of Light (Video)

Potent cycles occurring in the Cosmos are Now activating "wakeup-codes," built into our DNA long ago. Moving into greater Light *Fields* is activating hormones, triggering a stupendous shift in awareness. We have the knowledge and science to develop a peaceful, harmonious culture. The question is, will we access our deeper Wisdom and apply it in our Lives and our World? Will we activate our higher functioning DNA? As Quantum physics is Now revealing, this is up to us, and that we grasp this is critical to our viable future.

Internationally recognized authority, bridging science and spirit, leading voice in new biology and recipient of the 2009 Goi Peace Prize, Bruce Lipton tells us he *used* to teach that our genes carried instructions for our Lives. He Now realizes that our genes hold potentials like blank film, imprinted by the chemistry of our perceptions, beliefs and attitudes. *We write the story of our lives* from thought chemicals that bathe our cells and program our DNA. In these awakening times we realize the emerging choice of expression is up to us!

The Field is the sole governing agency of the particle.

Albert Einstein (1879-1955)

Our thought upon the *Field* determines movement of the *particle* into "reality." *Wow!* As Bruce Lipton tells us, thought Creates chemistry that defines our lives. Clearing out old conscious-unconscious thought launches us into a tantalizing New dynamic of Creation.

You hold the history of the Universe within your physical body....This time period was designed...to [restore] the original plan. Millions have been called to participate...because you understand that there is a...Divine plan...Sometimes you may wake up at night and literally feel...the restructuring of your DNA...

Barbara Marciniak
Bringers of the Dawn

This New Quantum paradigm jolts us to a shocking absolute "about face," exposing the astounding fact that *OUR thought and emotion calls forth everything we perceive as "reality."* (Are you sure it's not at least *partly* "their fault?" Nope). This is a gigantic leap in awareness from thousands of years of blame-fear-hostility culture believing "reality" comes from *outside of us,* a staggering misconception in a Quantum World.

On closer scrutiny, to be explored in-depth in upcoming chapters, we discover that according to Quantum physics, conscious-unconscious thought magnetics literally Create, instantly. Once understood this *IS THE GAME-CHANGER.* As Observer-Creators we call "reality" into being as we place our Attention (particularly unconsciously) upon the *Field.* This means we cannot blame *anyone else* for ANYTHING. *Seriously? Seriously.* The vibration of thought and emotion within us *magnetizes* our "reality" into Being.

ENTIRELY NEW APPROACH TO LIFE: Our thoughts Create (5% consciously - and "dangerous" 95% unconsciously). Put simply - our Words Create, our Thoughts Create, our Unconscious Thoughts Create. For anyone Now Waking Up, *it is urgently critical to become aware of every Thought and Word, and only use them to shape what you would like to call into Being around you.* We will also learn to clear the unconscious (coming up) so it does not sabotage us. Once we grasp this vital shift of perspective Life becomes a flowing river to which we contribute Positive Creation every moment.

We are overwhelmed with a deep sense of how powerful our thought is in shaping "reality." Shockingly, this brightly lights the path to *Ultimate Freedom. Everything* is up to *US! Our World is a biofeedback mechanism! The "Matrix" only Mirrors what we give it.* This mind-blowing science changes *OUR* Lives forever!

Many Now aware of these Quantum principles "hold the space with LOVE" for restructuring ALL on Planet Earth and beyond. Others will follow, for this is the backbone of the next phase of human Evolution. The Ninth wave of the Mayan Calendar urges us to Live with conscious intent, a wave Now being caught by many thousands Globally.

> Remember, we are all affecting the world every moment, whether we mean to or not. Our actions and states of mind matter, because we're so deeply interconnected with one another. Working on our own consciousness is the most important thing we do at any moment, and being LOVE is the supreme creative act.
>
> *Ram Dass*
> *Author, Be Here Now*

The "end of" the Mayan Calendar is neither doomsday nor the end of the World. It is the *end of an age* of Living in judgment-control-blame-fear-hostility. It is an Evolutionary Leap called the *Shift of the Ages,* launching us into Living from the Heart, according to our True Design LOVE. Are you on board? A peak of ascending consciousness is knocking at our door. Nudged irresistibly awake, we Now delight in exploring this adventure into expressing our *Essence,* as **21st Century Superhumans.** ♥

Chapter 3

Earth's Magnetics & Consciousness

For me, it is far better to grasp the Universe as it really is
than to persist in delusion, however satisfying and reassuring.

Carl Sagan (1934-1996)
Author - Contact, Cornell Professor, Advisor NASA, Cosmos TV

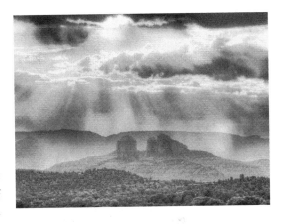

The Mayan Long-Count calendar, which began in 3114 B.C. describes precise tracking of our Galaxy's transit through space, identifying with uncanny accuracy exactly where we would be December 21, 2012. This end of the Mayan calendar links directly with influences to which we are currently being exposed.

During the last 30 years our Galactic orbit has carried us into massive *Fields* of accelerated Light photons, Gamma ray bursts and X-rays, while Earth's lowered magnetics and erratic Solar activity are activating us in extraordinary ways. Velikovsky foretold of the Van Allen Radiation Belt in the 1950s. He was little acknowledged at the time, though later it was discovered we entered yet another area called the Photon Belt, a doughnut shaped cloud, bombarding us with fast-moving particles of Light, that we will potentially be transiting for the next 2,000 years.

...not long after discovery of [Van Allen Belt] another...Photon Band was discovered in 1961. In conjunction others in the field of astronomy learned that our sun and solar system spiral through the Universe around 'something.' That 'something' is the central star of Pleiades, Alcyone... the central sun of our Galaxy.

As Alcyone and the Photon Band were studied, scientists recognized, like all things in our Universe, there is a cycle...best known as the Precession [of the Equinoxes] as we spiral toward and go through the Photon Band every 26,000 years. This coincides with the Mayan calendar, and what many have called the Grand Alignment of Earth to the central part of our Galaxy....

The 'Overlooked' Van Allen Belt & Its Relationship to the Photon Band
ImagineDoYou.com

In the mid-1980s Gregg Braden exposed radical views on our current Evolutionary potential, merging cutting edge modern science with Ancient tradition, to reveal great changes, Now potentially transforming us and the Earth. In his *Awakening to Zero Point* we catch a compelling glimpse of this extraordinary opportunity.

There is a process of unprecedented change unfolding within the earth. You are part of the change. Without...artificial boundaries of religion, science, or ancient mystic traditions, the change is characterized as dramatic shifts in the physical parameters of Earth accompanied by a rapid transformation in human understanding, perception, and experience. This time is historically referred to as *The Shift of the Ages.* As science witnesses events for which there are no reference points of comparison, ancient traditions say that the timetable is intact; the events of *The Shift* are happening now.

Gregg Braden
Awakening to Zero Point

A geologist, Gregg observed that Earth's geomagnetic record could be traced back eons in sedimentary layers. Astoundingly, he exposed that Earth's magnetics were plummeting to lowest in several thousand years, with pole movement on a regular basis! *NASA* explains the phenomenon of pole movement along with 10% reduction in our magnetic field:

At the moment [Earth's north magnetic pole is] in northern Canada. Scientists have long known that the magnetic pole moves...The pole [moved] during the 20th century...at an average speed of 10 km per year, *lately accelerating "to 40 km per year."* ...At this rate it is in North America and will reach Siberia in decades.

Earth's magnetic field is changing in other ways: Globally the magnetic field has weakened 10% since the 19th century... "[these changes are] mild compared to what Earth's magnetic field has done in the past."

...Sometimes the field completely flips. North and south poles swap places. Such reversals, recorded in magnetism of ancient rocks, are unpredictable. They come at irregular intervals averaging 300,000 years; the last was 780,000 years ago. Are we overdue for another? No one knows.

...Reversals take a few thousand years to complete, and during that time contrary to popular belief, the magnetic field does not vanish. "It just gets more complicated." ...[poles emerge in different places]. Weird. It's still a planetary magnetic field, it still protects us from space radiation and solar storms.

NASA Science
Science News 2003

We are living in *"interesting times."* Earth's poles are moving with magnetic field fluctuations which the World Center for Geomagnetism says began in the 1600s! This does not mean the end of Life as we know it, yet we *are in the midst of major Planetary changes.* Geologist, Gregg Braden correlated these geomagnetic findings with lives of Jesus and

Buddha, both on Earth during lowest magnetics of several thousand years; during such low magnetics human minds are most open. This history points to Now as having the potential for humanity to be open to such a shift prophesied as Christed or Buddhic consciousness. What a amazing opportunity during which to be here!

An exciting discovery by HeartMath® Institute, is we are intimately connected with the Earth; sensors show that Earth responds to our feelings. Her magnetic *Field* dropping may be a natural cycle, yet awareness of it we can consciously align *with* Earth Mother Gaia in a co-Evolutionary process, and support her with harmonious Joyful Living.

Earth's decreasing magnetic's generates a unique "softening" of mental constructs, resulting in less memory storage, less local field retrieval, and adjustments to our concept of time, all naturally opening us to flowing relationship with our existence. This explains how the "Collective Mind" may be more susceptible to absorbing New ideas during lower magnetic cycles. To our benefit, this increases our ability to gather and receive Creative inventive information from the Quantum *Field,* and find ways to Live naturally with Earth.

Leonardo Da Vinci, Albert Einstein, Thomas Edison and others took short "power naps." They awoke to their best ideas after the left brain had shut down, allowing them to more easily access the *Field of Possibilities, Unified Field or Divine Matrix.* Einstein would set himself up, pencil in hand, ready to jot down ideas immediately upon waking, as he was well aware of accessing Greater Mind. We can use this dynamic strategy to draw upon our ability to access Greater Potential, Solutions and Brilliance, beyond rational left brain.

Those who access Creative knowledge this way, report napping and polyphasic sleeping (4-5 hour blocks), clearing out "everyday mind" and capturing the surreal flow of ideas and solutions between short bursts of rest. Current planetary influences are triggering natural polyphasic sleep patterns. Many report waking with clarity of mind, capturing innovative creative concepts, supporting emerging visions for our Now.

CAPTURE YOUR DREAM STATE Keep electronic notes or pen and paper near where you sleep. Set your awareness for "Greater Mind" to expose creative solutions and wisdom while cognitive Mind sleeps. Jot down ideas and dreams immediately upon waking. Once cultivated, there will be sharper recall from REM dream states occurring in morning hours just before waking. Your creative ideas, are our World's solutions! As each person brings forth their brilliance, we birth a better World.

Celestial influences activating creative right brain in our current Evolutionary Leap, synthesize Feminine shamanic principle into perfect harmonious union with Masculine, as neither is complete alone. Beyond traditional roles, integrated Masculine and Feminine empower the individual and cultivate a complementary New paradigm, based in Balance, Creativity and LOVE. Men and women Now moving into gentle-strong Wisdom-Keeper roles integrate these two powerful polarities for a dynamic whole. Sacred Masculine and Feminine Now birth together an emerging New culture of Universal LOVE.

In *Spontaneous Evolution*, Bruce Lipton and Steve Bhaerman note contributions by the Iroquois Nation to the N. American constitutional system. The Iroquois exhibited respect for Feminine equality with a Council of Grandmothers keeping tribal balance, exposure to which strongly influenced Susan B. Anthony and Elizabeth Cady Stanton, early leaders of equality of women's rights. To our surprise Michael Tellinger even reports in bestselling *Slave Species of the Gods*, Native American Tribes recorded visitation around 2,000 years ago from a light skinned bearded man in white robes, who had ability to heal and graced them with teachings that became foundational to their wise and balanced cultural systems.

Physicist Nassim Haramein reminds us in *"Sacred Geometry and Unified Fields Part 2,"* that at its most basic the Masculine focuses on finite boundaries and the Feminine is open to all possibilities, the two merging finite with the infinite. These two polarities (which we each have within us and experience through interchange with one another), are essential to our existence and to Creation in our World. Exquisite energy emerges when these two aspects dance, with vital keys to equilibrium. One cannot exist without the other.

As we lighten left brain control, we shift into right brain Creative, non-linear thought, linked directly to the Heart. Masculine associates with left brain's practical, rational strategic functions, and Feminine with creative right brain. Men and women Now learning to collaborate in balanced roles, are flowing through the World with Greater Ease, Cooperation, Receptivity and Response. A New style of blending Feminine with Masculine is shaping dynamic New Earth interactions and paradigms.

In a 26,000 (25,920) year Galactic Precession of the Equinoxes, we have orbited to where we are receiving regular pulses from Alcyone, our Central Sun in the Pleiades. Intensified Light photons are activating our potential to turn the tide toward peace, natural prosperity, and restoration of balance on Mother Earth. Codons being switched on in our DNA expose and activate deep sense of "higher purpose" in this period of great change.

Holding-patterns around attachment to materialism are diminishing. Karmic relationships and old business structures respectfully find closure. Individuals and partners move on to vital roles they have come to play during this Planetary shift. *All hands* are being called *"on deck."* An exciting New creative human culture is emerging, where divine Masculine and Feminine are woven together with Mother Gaia, eliciting respect for *All Life*.

Those who "signed up" to play roles in emerging New frequencies are feeling an irresistible pull, magnetically drawn to others, Now appearing from Key Lifetimes. All skills are required. Many will come forward from all walks of Life, silently drawn as if by a homing device. *Simplify wherever you can and get ready to move forward.* It may become uncomfortable holding onto old ways, when we are being pushed to let go and flow into New ways of Being. Once accomplished, we adapt, discovering our New flow.

Powerful reunions are taking place among those last together in early Earth incarnations or knowing one another from the "stars," rejoining to bring forth unspoiled culture and community. Dynamic expressions set New energetic frameworks. Strongly individualized Souls join in Planetary healing, forging New timelines above and beyond antiquated social conditioning.

Many "undercover" Lightworkers may surprise even themselves, when their "purpose switches on," for they came into this Lifetime to help steer this ship a new direction. You will know who you are, though it may take some unwinding to untangle from the old, merge into the New, to expand into your entire Hologram. Honor self, play, use sunshine, laughter, Light foods and greens to support Mind-Spirit-Body, stepping fully onto the path.

Those who remain in more traditional families and partnerships are important sustainers within the transitional culture. They will cultivate New skills together as model families based in communication and LOVE in the family setting. In these homes natural Living and Healing practices will emerge, creative Lifework, and Education for children designed to bring forth Brilliance, rather than fitting them into the old limiting mold.

The rich Feminine aspect possesses innate capability to reveal Greater Mind. This skill has always been available, yet has been nearly eclipsed by left brain society's productive rewards for systematized obedience. Steve Jobs, Founder of Apple Computer, understood this, knowing his best people would produce better ideas when flowing naturally, so he cultivated a relaxed creative environment with couches, games, food and flexible schedules; this model is Now followed by Google and other progressive companies.

The art of Living predominantly in Greater Mind has been practiced extensively by tribal cultures, such as the Maori of New Zealand, whose views on "reality" go something like this: *"The conscious World is not the 'reality.' The spiritual dream World is the 'reality.' What we experience is merely the attempt of our minds to understand it."*

The *Field, the Matrix or the Dream World* is unlimited potential, waiting direction from our slightest thought to become matter and events. We are Now learning how to invite our existence into New form each moment and flow with it, while lowered Planetary magnetics voraciously nudge us into embracing this exhilarating Quantum experience.

QUANTUM HOLOGRAPHY: Accessing information intuitively and holographically from the greater *Field of Consciousness* is called Quantum Holography. Notice how information is accessed more quickly than ever before synchronistically from infinite sources, such as internet and cell phone. These are practical externalized examples of Holographic thinking.

Crucial awareness is how powerfully our thoughts affect events. Amazingly, bio-emotional energy Creates changes through time. In 2006 UNITEC conference Auckland, NZ, explored this intuitive connection with future events and how it can possibly work.

> ...intuitive perception of a future event is related to the degree of emotional significance of the event..both brain and heart are involved in processing a pre-stimulus emotional response to the future event... Focused emotional attention directed to the object of interest attunes...to the Quantum level of the object, which contains holographically encoded information about the object's future potential.

We stand at the threshold of a new era in scientific understanding of one of humankind's oldest and greatest enigmas: the perception of information about things far away in space or yet to happen in time... [and] intentional focus of bio-emotional energy to produce subtle but significant...effects on objects and events distant in space/time... [which] promises not only to profoundly change our understanding of the Universe and our connection to it in the deepest possible way, it will also affect how we view ourselves and our constructive influence on things distant or in the future.

Raymond Trevor Bradley with HeartMath® 2006
The Psychology of Intuition: A Quantum-Holographic Theory of Nonlocal Communication

At World Forum, international congress on *Geocataclysm* in 2011 with the Global Coherence Initiative, Dr. Rollin McCraty of HeartMath Institute offers that Global Consciousness actually affects the Earth during our current Planetary changes!

The compiled data indicated that our planet is going through a great transformation. Many scientists realized that the changes not only affect our weather and climate, but they also affect the lithosphere... the hydrosphere... the atmosphere and the magnetosphere...

...it is possible that we are seeing an effect of human consciousness acting on global weather?...Does the data correspond with uniting the emotions of many, allowing for more global peace and harmony?...So far we have taken an exploratory look at the possibility of global events being the catalyst for the kind of Coherence that we think of as a global consciousness.

Establishing the new Paradigm 2013 and Ongoing Global Earth Changes

Gregg Braden traveled to sacred sites around the World, searching records of Ancient civilizations that had experienced similar cycles to ours. Exposing secrets of monastic traditions he discovered *key instructions* to focusing in "Compassion without judgment" for "prayers to be answered." Research from HeartMath Institute corroborates that **focusing in Deep LOVE, Compassion and Gratitude produces Heart coherence, from which powerful Creation happens.** Entering this state opens the potential to activate more DNA strands in self and others, and brings forth our greatest potential based in our True Design LOVE.

Compassion refers to the arising in the heart
of the desire to relieve the suffering of all beings.

Ram Dass
Shift of the Ages

In the movie **Contact** (based on Carl Sagan novel), Jodie Foster plays a scientist who did not believe in God. Her experience of going into the "Cosmic All There Is," similar to Astronaut Ed Mitchell, flooded her with such incredible LOVE and Light that it utterly transformed her. She brings back her moving experience of Cosmic Awareness and the God-Force, where wide-eyed, she recognizes that she is One with Everything and Everything is One with her. Like others who doubt, she went from questioning her belief in

God to experiencing the God-Force completely, resulting in what we call, *"rewiring her DNA."* It is in restoring our True Design LOVE and in re-cognizing our *Oneness with ALL,* that we are truly set *FREE.* Following Astronaut Ed Mitchell's exposure to the mind-altering magnificence of Earth from space as a Living Being, and his radical comprehension of our *"Oneness with All That IS,"* Ed Mitchell founded IONS, Institute of Noetic Sciences, to research this all-encompassing state of "Consciousness."

Gregg Braden tells us in *God Code,* that when the *right switch* goes on, we go in an instant to having *more DNA strands activated,* as we enter LOVE, Compassion, Gratitude *(Heart Coherence) the ultimate state for which we are designed.* Jodie Foster's character like many, needed proof, though once she had this profound *experience* of Oneness, it was her proof.

Ascension is not about leaving the planet, getting rescued by off-world brethren or flying up into heaven. It is not about watching the Shift unfold online, or waiting for the external world to provide evidence of inner change. *Ascension is a Conscious choice to engage in Evolution.*

Sandra Walter
Creative Evolutions

This *is* **the** *Shift of the Ages: Merging into the Heart with an experience of Oneness, where individuality is transcended and an uplifting compelling desire to Live LOVE, Compassion & Gratitude takes over the Life.* Whether we call it God, Source or simply the Innate of All That Is, Quantum science Now tells us that we are individualized vortexes in a never ending *Field* of Conscious Intelligence, and our highest expression is LOVE. We explore the miracle of how this all operates more thoroughly in coming chapters, on our path to well-being.

Trust the dreams, for in them is hidden the gate to eternity!

Khalil Gibran (1883-1931)
The Prophet

Each individual who "gets" this, initiates significant potential for change on a Global scale. As this *journey* continues, we gain insight into how Deep LOVE, Gratitude and Compassion are Vital Keys to access our greatest capabilities as a species. **Quantum Lifestyle** removes all Not of LOVE resonance of thought-emotion (conscious-unconscious), so we flow from the Heart to resonate as a "tuning fork" of LOVE. As we clear conflicting energies to bring forth our capacity for LOVE, "reality" surrounding us shifts forever.

We are all here to cultivate the Heart of Compassion.

Ram Dass, Polishing the Mirror 2013

Deepening our understanding, we begin to comprehend how our "reality" is drawn into form from the *Field of Possibilities.* We focus with awareness on shifting thought-emotion. Wisdom Teachings of the last few millennia have always carried a thread of this expanded viewpoint, yet rarely understood by cultures of the day. Quantum theory tantalizingly correlates with these threads, nudging us to expand into a wave of Awakening that launches us Far Beyond where humanity has been before.

My decades of work exploring and applying the potentials to be found within both people and cultures, have convinced me that we have the ability to shift and move the obstructions of millennia. Consciousness has capacities that remain unused, except by the few, to remake both the world and time.

Dr. Jean Houston
A Midwife of Souls, by Tim Miejan, EdgeMagazine.Net

This anticipated Evolutionary Leap is impressive, as we wonder how we will let go 3-D *security,* find our focus and move forward into New dimensions of a brighter, freer experience of Life. As we release our grip on familiar programing, we daringly navigate a more fluid "reality" with powerful Quantum tools.

...we are living in the most complex times in human history. I realize other times in history thought they were it. They were wrong; this is it...in my travels around the world, which now are almost a quarter of a million miles, working in many cultures, in many, many domains of human experience -- I really discover that maybe we have ten or fifteen years of an open corridor to make a difference.

Many people, all over the world, are haunted by this. They wake up with a sense that they just cannot live out their lives as encapsulated bags of skin dragging around dreary little egos, and that all the walls are crashing down.

I mean, we are extraordinary -- the membranes have cracked through as cultures begin to flow into each other. We are on the verge of a true planetary culture, with high individuation of individual cultures...

Jean Houston Interview with Jeffrey Mishlove Ph.D.
Possible Human, Possible World Part I

One of our favorite movies, *What The Bleep Do We Know?* thrilled us with the Now Quantum buzzwords: ***"The question is, how far down the rabbit hole do you want to go?"*** And, as it was for Alice, we are now entering *"Wonderland...♥*

Dear Ones, Take no thought of the "past," it does not exist in the Realm of Spirit. Enter into Timelessness. It is your point of Power, for All is Known in the Now. Your Path has been one of letting go dawning realizations...to become the Master you were designed to Be.

Be assured you are watched over. Be assured we are by your side. Be assured "your Path" is being guided every step of the way. Empty your Mind... Fill your Heart...Listen to your Intuition, for it will Guide you...into Deep Listening...

Your Magnetic Field will draw unto you those people and situations to complete you. The Time is NOW to join with others to Assist your Planet into the next Dimension. Namasté.

Teddi's Guides ♥

Chapter 4

Pineal Gland & DMT *Spirit Molecule*

There are things known and there are things unknown,
and in between are the doors of perception.

Aldous Huxley (1894-1963)
Brave new World 1932

The pineal gland, near the center of the brain has been perceived by "advanced" cultures throughout history as an access point to higher consciousness; in Ancient Egypt we see it as the Eye of Horus. In our modern World the pineal gland is often calcified and atrophied by age eight, from indoor life, electronic exposure, TV, computer, phone, chemicals such as fluoride, any emotion below Joy and thought expression Not of LOVE.

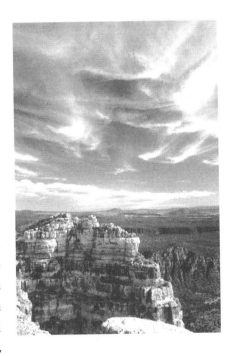

The pineal, master gland of the body, is most vital when we are in Joy and Enthusiasm and outdoors in natural daylight with eyes and skin uncovered. The pineal produces DMT, cousin to serotonin. Often called the "spirit molecule," DMT is a mechanism of our psycho-biological connection with "Source." Current Gamma rays and intensified *Fields* of Light stimulate increased DMT production, naturally awakening us to a sense of our Oneness with ALL things.

Historically sophisticated ceremonies and rituals for increasing DMT production by pineal and pituitary glands, have nourished and amplified the spiritual nature. Many such natural customs have been followed for tens of thousands of years in shamanic practices around the World. Yogic teachings and sophisticated Egyptian temple trainings for third eye, point to the pineal gland as our vehicle of en-Light-enment.

Natural exposure to Sun increases DMT production. Exposure to natural daylight is vitalizing, restorative and anti-aging, best done in moderation with eyes and skin uncovered. Our solar energy is bright due to diminished magnetic *Fields*; anything put on skin is found in the organs in 57 seconds, best to use edible oils such as olive or coconut for protection with natural vinegar for skin pH. Exposure to Solar energy increases vibrancy, vitality and stimulates healthy glandular function (increase gradually). Sun-gazers absorb nourishment from sunlight, with studies showing pineal-pituitary enlargement. One modern Sun-gazer claims to have gone 7-8 years without food, thriving on Solar energy alone. (*Caution: Sun-gazing should not be practiced without proper instruction or supervision*).

Vitamin D is normally manufactured in the body during solar exposure, so winter supplementation is important. Vitamin D3 with K2 produces excellent results, supporting mental and emotional well-being. Vitamin D3 is a hormone precursor, not actually a vitamin. It is manufactured by the body and is required for vitality and super-immunity.

Solar exposure has intensified with thinner magnetosphere and atmosphere, making moderation a good rule, although avoiding the Sun can leave us with deficiencies and low vitality. Find your balance. Who doesn't enjoy the beach, a walk, run, the garden or sitting outside? For the Sun-sensitive even getting outdoors in the shade allows us to take in natural daylight through the eyes, without glasses/sunglasses. John Ott (1909-2000) who filmed Disney's *Secrets of Life*, pioneered time-lapse photography and full spectrum lighting, demonstrated profound affect of sunlight on healthy pineal-pituitary function.

The pineal is the focal point of our built-in "antennae" that sends and receives magnetic waves of energy transmitted through our glandular system and into the World around us. The pituitary receives and decodes waves of information coming to us at extrasensory levels and sends energy from the Heart into our surroundings. Established by many traditions throughout the ages, a natural high is achieved with vibrant pineal-pituitary function. The pineal and pituitary glands attune us to current intensified Light frequencies and and are activated by highly Vibrational magnetic *Fields*.

Healthy pineal function enhances vitality, aids performance and slows aging. *Supermassive Galactic Plasma Ray* (YouTube) excerpted from *Solar (R)Evolution,* eye-opening book and documentary by German biophysicist Dieter Broers, offers profound insights into compelling current cosmological influences:

> On its journey through the Galaxy our Solar System routinely passes through areas known for their particularly intense Cosmic Activity. This activity affects our climate, and plays a significant role in the development of all affected Lifeforms...The state-of-the-art in earthquake prediction recently identified Gravitational waves and Gamma rays emerging from our Sun and from the Center of our Galaxy, which appear to have a correlation to recent global seismic activity....
>
> Radio waves in particular have an effect on biological systems, often underestimated. [An explosion predicted at Sagittarius A at the center of our Galaxy, is expected to send a surge of radio waves toward the Earth after mid-2013]. Our human DNA has a resonant frequency of 150 MHz. In this frequency range, even the slightest field strengths are enough to produce bio-

physical effects. They can cause mood changes and they trigger altered states of consciousness.

Reference measurements have shown that the 150 MHz high frequency wave in particular, activates production of our own psychoactive substances. One gland in the brain in particular the pituitary gland is one of the most powerful producers of such substances in the human body. The pineal gland is also hyper-sensitive when it comes to external magnetic fields and radio waves. It could for example act as an excellent transmitter and receiver of cosmic signals.

Dieter Broers
Supermassive Galactic Plasma Ray (Youtube)

Reminded by these natural influences to live according to our highest expression at this point in Earth and humanity's interconnected history, our capacity to express harmonic frequencies of LOVE is expanding. The pineal is a sending device, emanating our LOVING Vibration into the *Field* surrounding us, through the Heart.

The simple choice to Focus in LOVE or Compassion and clear all Not of LOVE from our being, has been a practice of Wisdom Traditions throughout the ages. Focusing on our inner "cleanup" has the potential to shift the collective toward a culture based in LOVE, Compassion and Gratitude, beyond were we have been, as noted in Mayan cosmology:

The Maya held that the pineal gland becomes more active after an astronomical event because solar radiation and moonlight both increase the brain's production of chemicals that alter human consciousness. The fact that we, as human beings, are more aware today than we were ten years ago, aware that everything in the cosmos is interconnected, that we are all one and the same, that we are whole and part simultaneously, is not a random event. The Maya knew that it was up to humans to care and do something about our future...

The *Maa yab* people made up the *Xook K'iinil* (calendar) not only to measure time, but also to measure solar winds, the Earth's warming and its influence on human's neuron activity (consciousness). The calendar's main function is to measure human perception and provide the signals that will determine the exact moment when we must become actively responsible for change. The Maya were aware that time is infinite and could be counted to infinity, however, they left us a calendar up to the year 2012 to leave it to our generation to commence a new count, in light of a new spiritual awareness.

Ac Tah, The Man Who Talks
The Night of the Last Katün 2012 Maya

As our pineal gland becomes more activated, producing more DMT, and limiting belief systems fall away, there is a natural adaptation of readily shifting into the Heart. In the blame-fear-hostility culture, *not* speaking and acting from the Truth of our being, whether to be polite, conform or protect ourselves has become a deeply ingrained societal pattern. None interested in participating in this phase of Evolutionary change can afford to continue such habits. It is highly self-limiting to operate outside of the Truth of who we are.

As we let go of these old paradigms, we begin to access greater knowledge of *Who we Are, Why We're here and Where We're going.* Activated by the Infinite flow of vitalizing Universal Light and LOVE, we Now express the Truth of our Being without reservation, flowing with breathtaking ease through Life as the Joyful Being of our Design!

Speak the truth quicker, have more fun per hour!

Leonard Orr
Founder, Rebirthing Breathwork

Leonard Orr radically taught that our true destiny is *immortality*, with a primary focus on Conscious Evolution. He met twelve immortal yogis including famed Haidakhan Babaji of the Himalayas. This was deeply transformative for him, inspiring him to teach that there is not a glitch between when we drop the body and when we awaken on the "other side."

Freeing the Breath is an essential tool to releasing unconscious content in order to restore our True Design LOVE. We teach a special type of **21st Century Superhuman** breakthrough Breathwork at our workshops. In these breathing sessions we learn to let go of old holding patterns, containing thought and emotion (conscious-unconscious) that inhibit the free flow of energy. We develop new breathing habits to easily release old thought-emotional content whenever it bubbles up. Cultivating such open breath habits powerfully supports us in entering the flow of New conscious Creation, while always being able to use the breath as a resource for clearing anything in the way. Using the breath in such a way activates our DNA and potential for long life and immortality.

A wonderful early teacher of Teddi's, Nellie Cain, who wrote *Exploring the Mysteries of Life,* told students when they walked through the door they would have the opportunity to transform their lives in a single evening. Nellie so powerfully held the *Field of LOVE,* that committed students alchemically shifted their entire approach to Life in just a few hours, aligning with Soul Purpose and absorbing the single greatest teaching of all, *LOVE.*

LOVE is the greatest power in the Universe. Without it there would be nothing. It is the creating, unifying, and sustaining Life principle by which all things have their existence.

Nellie Cain
Exploring the Mysteries of Life

As we *dive into this process,* committed to let go unconscious patterns when they show up, we will soon find ourselves look back asking, "Who is that person I was yesterday?"

Why, sometimes I've believed as many as
six impossible things before breakfast.

Lewis Carroll
Alice in Wonderland

In addition to accelerated particles of Light from the Photon Band, natural pineal gland activation is stimulated by Solar and Gamma ray activity coming from our Solar system and beyond. Infrared telescopes show a massive increase in Gamma ray bursts, recognized to stimulate increased production of the pineal-pituitary hormone DMT. Natural hormone DMT was discovered in 1972 by Nobel Prize winner Julius Axelrod which he demonstrated to have psychoactive and telepathic properties.

> N-Dimethyltryptamine (DMT)...a psychedelic compound...occurs in trace amounts in mammals, including humans, where it functions as a neurotransmitter and neuro-modulator...analogous to serotonin and melatonin...hypotheses suggest that DMT is produced in the brain...might be connected with visual dream phenomena. May be involved in creation of normal waking states of consciousness.
>
> *Wikipedia*

Natural hormone DMT is often referred to as the "spirit molecule," as it stimulates a sense of "Oneness with All things," connection with the Earth and All of Creation. Natural substances containing DMT have long been used for divinatory and healing ceremonies among Native Americans, South Americans and many traditions around the Globe.

Seekers take a "sacred journey" with a shaman, medicine man or medicine woman. Some traditional South American rites contain an Ayahuasca brew made of leaves and vines or San Pedro cactus; North American Southwestern tribes used Mescal and Peyote, while other plants around the World resonate similar qualities. These rites for expanding consciousness based on traditions going back millennia, draw many today. Some have used this to accelerate "waking up," always done with respect for body and the "sacred" process. *MEANWHILE...natural DMT activation* is coming directly to us from the Cosmos. Exposure to concentrated *Fields* of fast moving particles of Light promises to entice ALL on Planet Earth out of limiting structures and beliefs, to open naturally to LOVE and Oneness.

Beyond use of plants and herbs to activate the "spirit molecule," tremendously altered states are also achieved with dancing, drumming and rhythmic Breathing as used by tribal cultures around the World. Now integrated into modern shamanic practices, these along with meditation, lucid dreaming, fasting, prayer and pilgrimages to sacred sites also deepen this activated spiritual state. Consistent practice of such rituals can bring about deep change, healing and a sense of Oneness contributed to by elevated DMT, the "spirit molecule." By whatever method it becomes activated, increasing DMT triggers revelatory experiences and does much to connect us with expansion and greater expression of self.

Paul LaViolette, PH.D, president of Starburst Foundation, author *The Talk of the Galaxy, Earth Under Fire, Genesis of the Cosmos (Beyond the Big Bang)*, papers in physics, astronomy, climatology and systems theory, made predictions about interstellar dust in our Solar System ten years before its confirmation in 1993 with data from the Ulysses spacecraft and radar from New Zealand. This validates his awareness on current increasing ray activity:

> Dr. LaViolette predicted we would discover that high intensity volleys of cosmic ray particles travel directly to our planet from distant sources in our Galaxy, a phenomenon which is now confirmed by scientific data. He is also the first to

discover high concentrations of cosmic dust in Ice Age polar ice, indicating the occurrence of a global cosmic catastrophe in ancient times.

Dr. LaViolette connects predictions about Earth's potential for change with a central area in our Milky Way Galaxy called the galactic bulge. It is producing huge cosmic explosions that can affect major change in planetary and solar systems. He points out that this may be part of a 5,200 year cycle noted in the Mayan calendar.

Strong potential exists for global change as Solar activity increases and Cosmic waves and particles pour in from space, activating our DMT. Rather than reading these signs as a coming apocalypse, educated minds Now entertain the astonishing potential for humankind to move toward more en-Light-ened Living. As Oneness, Deep LOVE, Compassion and Gratitude are activated, societal change (even if a bit turbulent) is shifting our civilization to a New foundation, one based in kindness and betterment for ALL to Live in balance with our beautiful Earth Mother.

When you have a geomagnetic storm, you can change brain tissue itself. When you change structure, you change the entire species, in fact every living thing on this planet could be altered.

If you look historically you'll find massive global changes...often occur during certain times of geomagnetic activity...soon we will have a geomagnetic storm that will have the quality that will influence large numbers of individuals...

Modern science tends to feel somewhat uncomfortable when you make the assumption that all of us belong to the same species, and we're all exposed to the same environment, that global changes could affect us all simultaneously, and influence the direction of history. That takes away the sense of human control over our destiny...but I think the data indicates that it's probably correct.

...An increase in our consciousness sparked by this kind of grand celestial event, could provide us with a direct cognition of a hyper-real state of existence.

Supermassive Galactic Plasma Ray
Solar (R)Evolution excerpts, Dieter Broers (Youtube)

We are experiencing a wave of increased consciousness. Lowered Earth's magnetics provide a less protective "cocoon" thus we are receiving *more* activation from the Sun. Cosmic rays and Light particles are stimulating our pineal and pituitary glands and the body's magnetic system. Cosmic influences converging in and around us suggest the strong possibility that such an Evolutionary Leap has already quietly yet powerfully begun. The good news is, increased pineal activity slows aging and increases vitality!

EarthSky reported from Stanford News, Nov. 2013 on the largest Gamma ray burst ever recorded in history from the constellation Leo, which could lead to a rewrite on theories of how Gamma rays work. It was only half the distance from Earth as usual, with far more high energy photons than expected, affecting all nearby electromagnetic *Fields*.

Ours is a spiral galaxy. Most galaxies have a black hole at the center which ours does. Also at the center of our galaxy is one of the brightest stars known, called Alcyone of the Pleiades. At her website, Meg Benedictine of Mt. Shasta, author of *Soul Realized: Unlocking the Sacred Keys to Becoming a Divine Human* and Founder of *Unified Field Therapy* reported on these influences in early 2012:

> NASA has discovered the presence of an interstellar photon energy cloud extending from our galaxy's center toward the star Alcyone in the Pleiades.
>
> Using satellite data from telescopes on Voyager and IBEX, astrophysicists have documented our solar system's orbit entering the Photon Belt since 1972, when Pluto was briefly in the band. During the past decade, Earth spent short periods of time in the photon band - but has now entered it full time, starting in 2012 and lasting until 4320AD.
>
> NASA investigators say this photon band is turbulent and highly charged, triggering climate change, increasing solar storms and CMEs [coronal mass ejections]. Earth's changing atmosphere affects our natural environment, and significantly alters our human energy field as well. Recently NASA's Fermi Gamma-ray Space Telescope recorded two gamma-ray-emitting bubbles that extend 25,000 light-years north and south of our galactic center...
>
> No one can exactly predict the affects of prolonged intense photon energy to human biology, but clearly the harmonic DNA spiral is mutating within this environment. The infusion of Gamma photon light is transforming humanity at the molecular level.
>
> *Meg Benedictine*
> *Entering the Galactic Photon Belt*

In order to enjoy this adventure as **21st Century Superhumans** we are disentangling from 3-D commitments around city Life, pressured unfulfilling jobs, businesses or professions, inharmonious relationships, large isolated homes disconnected from the Earth and economic dissonance. It is essential to release and clear old "fear bubbles" and begin Living in New ways. Breathe, Smile and shift into resonating as "tuning forks" of LOVE, flowing from the eternal Source of Creation, shifting everything in our "reality" Now!

We learn to make choices aligned with our true Being, including reduced time commitments, living simply, growing a garden, joining with community and family, restoring Heart and Soul by expressing our *dharma* or creative service to contribute what we LOVE to society. By so doing, we awaken Ancient biological encoding dormant in our DNA, to emerge into full expression of our brilliance and genius as creative Beings.

Do you feel a little disoriented or upside-down lately? Many are experiencing emotional turbulence, physical symptoms such as spinning, dizziness or queasiness, a sense of pressure or not being able to keep up with shifting energies, buzzing, ringing in the ears or a sense that things are slowing down or speeding up. As New energies are activated in, around and through us, we shift, integrating these frequencies.

Our neurobiology adapts to altered states of consciousness, letting go of the old to make room for the New. We say daily, "I'm not the same person I was yesterday!" as Mind-Heart-Spirit-Body adjust. Breathing, Smiling, flowing in this transformation, we shed old layers and acclimatize to the New.

As old patterns of behavior and past emotional attachments are stripped away, our true essence is shining through the heavy layers of conditioning. Our intensive training as 'Warriors of Light' is breaking down ego resistance and false beliefs of Duality...honing and refining Core strength into resilient, unwavering integrity.

At times it felt like we had reached our breaking point, unable to continue forward...wondering how our body could endure another day of torturous purging! How could one being contain so much toxic, polarized energy inside? It boggles the mind! And yet, we can't turn back now...once we have tasted the presence of divine light, of unfettered freedom, of deep loving kindness...there is nothing to compare! Our only path is forward!

Meg Benedictine
Entering the Galactic Photon Belt

ALL Earth's inhabitants are receiving powerful Celestial transmissions Now, clearing and aligning our magnetics with Unity and Oneness, elevating DMT and initiating constructive DNA changes. This is very similar to upgrading computer software! The brain is neoplastic for adapting to these shifts. Such a feast of Cosmic influences have been at the root of Evolutionary shifts throughout the ages, nudging along even the unaware.

José Argüelles (1939-2011) organizer of 1987 Harmonic Convergence, reported on a Mayan prophecy about a powerful Galactic Synchronization Beam that would Create an enormous black hole or Hunab-Ku to influence and accelerate us during and post 2012. Such influences are bound to stimulate the pineal and up DMT levels, as well as advance or re-encode our DNA. After 15 years of studying current cosmology German Biophysicist Dieter Broers published his research in both book and documentary film Solar R-Evolution.

Human DNA exhibits a property that acts as an "antenna" for gamma radiation. Our DNA contains carbon crystals that react to radiation like a resonator. Moreover, all of the atomic elements of our DNA have the capacity to pick up electromagnetic energy like a radio antenna, whereas the carbon crystals amplify incoming electromagnetic signals, a mechanism we know from broadcasting technology.

Pretty much the same thing happens in our cells, whose structure enables them to receive electromagnetic signals from the cosmos...A beam of radiation, emitted from the center of the Milky Way, synchronized with solar cycles, could transform - in a sense, re-encode - the double helix of our DNA... Quantum physicist Brian Swimme became one of the first researchers [expressing agreement with José Argüelles' theories on Mayan prophecy]. In Quantum physics one could posit that an electrodynamic exchange occurs between solar electrons and human electrons...

[A potential] cataclysmic event concretely signaled numerous times in various aspects of Mayan culture...that the cyclical transition has a cathartic function: they speak in terms of "awakened human beings" who will carry out a "sacred mission" and will "cleanse the Earth" - and for whom a new consciousness and a new form of civilization will be ushered in once we pass through the initiatory threshold represented by December 12, 2012.

Dieter Broers
Solar Revolution

Recognizing these Cosmic activations, **21st Century Superhumans** are incorporating cleansing nutrition and regenerative *Quantum Lifestyle* habits, essential for clarity of Mind-Heart-Spirit-Body. Be sure to catch our guidelines in PART 4 to optimize your BODY on this journey. We are living in a miraculous, extended "Now," where Enlightenment results from integrating more *Light* into the Being. How we care for the BODY determines the Light-carrying capacity of cells, organs, brain and nervous system. Refining and harmonizing physical habits is an essential key to maximizing preparation for this Evolutionary Leap. Don't miss PART 4! (Get original 500 page version, or 4 separate books - same content).

Many now holding LOVE are raising frequencies for Mother Earth and all who dwell with her working within natural energy grids of the Planet. Literally millions are riding this wave, consciously connected with the *Field*, Globally. The single most powerful thing we do as **21st Century Superhumans**, is to shift into the Heart and put this Awareness into the *Field of Possibilities*. By so doing we shift our World to a Global culture based in LOVE!

You are more than your thoughts, your body or your feelings. You are a swirling vortex of limitless potential who is here to shake things up and Create something new that the Universe has never seen.

Dr. Richard Bartlett
Into the Matrix: Guides, Grace and the Field of the Heart

It takes a bit to release ourselves from 3-D entanglements that have prevented us from responding to Life from the Heart. Initially there may be fear of "letting go," and allowing ourselves to flow fully with our *Essence*. As we clear ourselves of residual constructs from the blame-fear-hostility culture, we find New ways to earn income, pay our bills, interact in relationship and communicate with others while aligning with our *Essence*.

We are not here to gain salvation from making a better world. We are here to awaken out of identification with form.

Eckhart Tolle

Be encouraged. Masters in the making throughout the ages have faced similar challenges from the Greatest to the least. Separating ourselves from illusionary purposes, to bring LOVE into every aspect of Life is the emerging New paradigm for our Now. Knowing our *True Purpose* as Individuals and aligning with our Oneness with All Things taps into our potential, to bring forth our gifts as a precious offering to a viable future.

This is a *HUGE* shift from a failing materialistic system, sustained through overgrown need for security, and producing little *real* emphasis on Heart centered Living. We unwind this by moving into the *Essence* of our Being. We may continue to enjoy home, clothing, hair style, vehicle, yet shift emphasis to the Heart and find what actually fulfills us. Connect with community, neighborhood, region, grow a garden, deepen relationships and find more meaningful ways to offer your talents to the World.

This is the wave for which we've been waiting. A thrilling, exciting Global Movement is afoot, with not just a few, but millions now responding to this wave of the Heart, carrying us forward into Evolutionary potential of our greatest dreams. As dramatic changes occur around the Globe, let us heed this Hopi Elders' prophecy:

The time of the lone wolf is over.
Gather yourselves! Banish the word 'struggle" from your attitude and your vocabulary. All that we do now must be done in a sacred manner and in celebration. We are the Ones we've been waiting for...

There is no turning back. Each who catches this "wave" assists the collective, by delighting in *BEING and LIVING* the Resonance of Vital Heart connection, thus shifting the entire Hologram. Many Now are Living more frugally, giving up unconscious pursuits in exchange for that which brings Joy to the Heart for betterment for Humankind. It may take a bit for such changes to advance, yet with current thrilling Cosmic influences, results are appearing in delightful ways, more easily than expected. The resonance of each who clears old unconscious, stuck patterns and programs makes choices to integrate greater self-expression and radically affects the entire Planet!

We are creating a collective planetary consciousness. This is hopeful; for a planet of 7 billion people, we all contribute equally. It doesn't matter how much money you make, what your station in Life is...what we're radiating into the global field environment counts the same.

Rollin McCraty
HeartMath Institute

21st Century Superhumans are ecstatically receiving activations in this metamorphosis of Awakening. A giant Evolutionary Leap for HUmanity-HUwomity, plants, children, animals, Earth Mother Gaia and All her creatures, is carrying us across the great Evolutionary Spiral into New Earth expression based in LOVE, Kindness, Charity and care for All Beings. That which has been established by Not of LOVE thinking is at its last crescendo and will ultimately dissolve as part of the illusion. Honor and be at Peace with your own and others' Journey, Trust that all is unfolding Perfectly, while holding coherent Heart space for Deep LOVE, Compassion and Gratitude. Breath and Smile. ♥

Chapter 5

Adapting to Solar Changes

A compelling case pointing to a wealth of scientific evidence, shows a remarkable correlation between increases in solar activity and advances in our creative, mental and spiritual abilities...

Dieter Broers, Biophysicist
Solar Revolution Documentary

Ancient societies understood that humanity is profoundly affected by the Sun. A Russian astrophysicist recently documented major human events over several centuries, showing that human affairs correlate directly with solar cycles and are even driven by solar events.

German biophysicist Dieter Broers' insights into current Cosmic influences, in his excellent book and documentary *Solar R(E)volution,* points out that Solar and Cosmic surges have tremendous potential to trigger

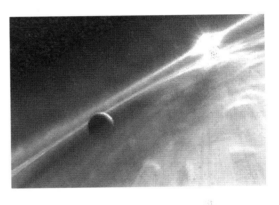

a hyper state of awareness. Such a shift is capable of advancing us into a new state of "waking consciousness," dovetailing with astounding Quantum principles that redefine how our existence operates, thus setting the stage for a very real Evolutionary Leap.

NASA reported our Sun going through a pole reversal late 2013, "The sun's polar magnetic *Fields* weaken, go to zero point, emerge again with opposite polarity. This is a regular part of the solar cycle," Stanford physicist Phil Scherrer explained, "This cycle was slower than usual, and if continues to be slow it could indicate a mini ice age coming."

When feeling out of sorts it may very well be due to Solar and Cosmic waves. Harmonize with this "reorganization" of your natural energy field. Rest when feeling the need, get out in nature, drink cleansing beverages, herbal teas or warm water, lemon water with cayenne or a pinch of baking soda, fresh juices, alchemical herbs and spices. Use essential oils to assist the body to adapt. Have bodywork or energy balancing done or do a hands-on exchange with a friend. Seek community with others of like-Mind, to dialogue about current changes. Breathe YOUR new level of Being. Breathe and Smile.

According to Quantum physicist Michael Konig, accessing hyperspace or dimensions beyond 3-D requires "phase-changes that access higher consciousness." He states, "This is the threshold at which humankind is now poised."

Aluna Joy Yaxk'in, brings us her message from *Star Elders* on integrating current intensified Solar activity. We connected with Aluna Joy in Mt. Shasta at the powerful turning of the Millennium in 2,000 and enjoy her ongoing insights on energies of our Now. Here is one of her Solar updates from summer of 2013.

Solar Flares Assist in Our Ascension

We have had four Class X solar flares in a couple of short days. These are very powerful flares. (for basics about solar flares google it or go to www.spaceweather.com) We feel solar flares just as they burst from the sun. Our technology feels the magnetic pulse about 48 hours after the solar explosion. This

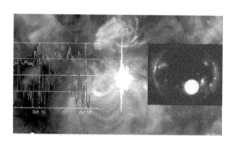

is so because humanity is connected to everyone and everything in the Universe, and our technology is not. As above, so below. Humanity is ONE.

Today my heart is racing, my head is aching, and I am writing this from my cozy, pillow-filled bed with my iPad. Many of you out there are having a huge range of odd symptoms, that by now I am sure you are all painfully aware of. But read on.... There is a reason for these events and our reactions to them. Remember . . . you are a spiritual being in an all too HUMAN body that is evolving and ascending.

The Star Elders say that these pulses of light (that we feel instantly), also infused with magnetic energy (that we feel 48 hours later), are part of the divine plan. With these multiple, layered flares, we are being infused and saturated with new light from a new paradigm. At least for now, we are not getting a break as this is the final stretch of a very long journey. These solar pulses stretch us beyond the form we are familiar or comfortable with. This is a part of the ascension process. When we can hold no more light, we feel like we are pushed to the very edge and feel like we could explode. These pulses of light are the framework for the new world we are building. Only then, the following magnetic pulse helps us release all that is not needed for our future. The magnetic pulses bring up to the surface everything that does not fit within the collective divine plan. We purge, detox, and let go and surrender from our body, mind and spirit. This purging Creates more space for more light.

Now the odd thing is that we are going through this ascension process all the while the outer world seems to be clicking along like business as usual. We didn't expect this. Yet inside our hearts, we feel like something big has changed within us, and the world feels very surreal. But if you look closely, you will see this shift in nearly everyone's eyes. You might see people with the subtle stunned look, with eyes like a deer caught in the headlights. Others will over-compensate by being overly happy and enthusiastic, because they can't admit they are feeling strange to say the least. Then there are those that are agitated and rushing around like they can outrun this wave of light. Then there are those that are still in full on denial. Don't worry . . . they will catch up quickly. And lastly there are the rare few that have already arrived at the finish line, and the rest are only a heartbeat behind them. The Star Elders say it does not matter what you do now. You can try out all of the avoidances above, but you cannot avoid, deny or out run this rush of light that we are in now.

At least for now, we have no space in between flares to ground ourselves and rebalance. We planned it this way, because we knew our body (that holds history

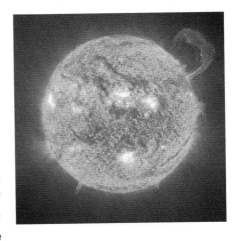

and memory) would run the other way like our Life depended on it. This is the old fight or flight memory that we will no longer need in the new world. Just when we have a bit of space to begin to face our purging shadow side, another pulse of light (solar flare) slams into us, thus not allowing us to retract back into a more comfortable and familiar territory.

How to deal with pulses... Simple... Let GO and let GOD emerge from inside of you. I laugh now as the Star Elders show me that old gory scene from the movie Aliens. Yeah... Their sense of humor keeps me going, along with the support of all of you out there. The world is pretty strange right now. We don't know which way is up and it's ok. We are being called back to basics, the core of spiritual truths and craving a return to a simple Life. And what we thought the ascension might be is not quite how it is showing up. The Star Elders have always told me that when we arrive, there are going to be some great surprises. Well... "Surprise!"

Just Breathe and know we are being protected and fiercely guarded by a divine plan set in action. Our star family is watching over us, as we transform quickly into something we can't even envision now. So Breathe, get yourself grounded as much as possible, and hang out with like frequency Soul family. We are going to survive, there is no doubt, and we will have the surprise of a Lifetime together.

Aluna Joy Yaxk'in, the Star Elders,
Solar Flares Assist in Our Ascension

As these powerful energies move through us, Breathe into your Heart center. Visualize and expand the Heart chakra as a spinning Torus field, that measures 8'-12' spherically around the body with a vortex at the center. This toroid form can be measured around the Heart with modern instrumentation. It is a powerful type of naturally occurring unlimited energy generator used in plasma physics, to Create electricity, water fusion, space stations, audio equipment and electrical transformers. It is a continually renewing flow of energy.

Learn more about the Torus field and view moving graphics in video online to better visualize. Thanks to HeartMath Institute Research Center for this Torus field image and for their extensive research on the power of Heart energy. They measure the Heart Center or

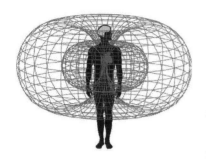

Heart Chakra as having the shape of a torus field just like this image. At the center of the torus field the Heart is in a vortex, fearlessly accessing unlimited energy from "Source." When we are "plugged in" to our unlimited power supply of our True Design LOVE, we find the backbone of everything we need for Life flows effortlessly.

In uterus when a sperm and egg join, 8 cells form, then the Heart takes shape at the center. At approximately day 21 the Heart begins to beat and a torus field takes shape, with the Heart as its center. It is an unsolved mystery exactly why. Physicist Nassim Haramein suggests the vortex at the center of the torus field, known in Quantum terms as a "black hole," is the magnetic energy that "holds the Universe together: LOVE."

Thrivemovement.com's film, *Thrive-Crop Circles are Clues to new Energy Technology!* describes that Crop Circle images focus on torus *Fields* as the foundation of Free energy, and they are now being researched as such. *It is said that one cubic foot of space contains enough energy to power all needs on Earth for the next 100 years!* This massively available energy, once harnessed, will power a future abundantly free to all, empowering us to Awaken to a Blissfully creative Heart-centered civilization.

Torus *Fields* are recorded in Ancient historical rock inscriptions as energy generators and to power UFOs. Some Quantum physicists believe all Creation is torus *Fields*, nested within torus *Fields*, within torus *Fields*. The Torus field is a 3-D expression of the Flower of Life of Sacred Geometry, describing fundamental polarities within the structure of Creation. These patterns are also found in the Kabbalah and I Ching.

As we offer our left brain more freedom to "relax and dance" with the right brain, we drop our thinking down into the torus field of the Heart, accessing the pure holism of our nature, through this powerful field generator. The right brain connects neurologically, directly with the Heart.

HeartMath Institute reveals that the Heart is 40-60 times electromagnetically stronger than the brain. *Wow!* **21st Century Superhumans** are learning to focus on thought-Creation through the Heart, sending Mind impulses of a pure, powerful resonance of LOVE, transmitted through the Heart into the World.

RE-Create MATTER - Play with imagining matter falling out of solid (particle) form and collapsing in waves into the *Field, to* Be "unmanifest." Invite your right brain into he *Field*, asking matter and events to emerge in New ways. Breathe and Smile. Notice that "reality" can shift, as readily as you open your Mind, allowing Creation to flow out of form and into new form through Attention of creative right brain and Heart on the *Field*.

> Your planet is poised on the brink of utter transformation. The form of this transformation has multiple expressions; it is you-the collective that will affect these outcomes to a greater or lesser degree...you have...the ability to change timelines and probabilities at the last moment of any event-whether personal or collective. [It] is as a matter of fact concerning your evolutionary potential...the path of the Initiate is to reach upward for the highest potential, regardless of what may or may not be happening around him/her.
>
> *Tom Kenyon*
> *The Hathors*

NASA's Voyager confirms that we have moved into a field of intensified photons of Light. They tell us that our Solar System is passing through an interstellar cloud that "should not exist," with potential to compress our atmosphere allowing more Cosmic rays to reach Earth. This portends to accelerate our Evolutionary Journey as predicted of old.

> "Using data from Voyager, we have discovered a strong magnetic field just outside the solar system," explains Merav Opher, of NASA... "This magnetic field holds the interstellar cloud together and solves a long-standing puzzle of how it can exist at all. There could be interesting times ahead!" says Opher.
>
> *Voyager Makes an Interstellar Discovery*
> *NASA Science News Dec.23, 2009*

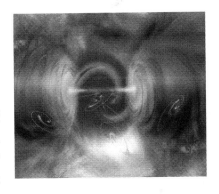

Space stations with precise instrumentation identify billions of Cosmic rays, confirming that there is more dark matter than Light in space as seen in this image of bubbles in the Milky Way, from NASA's Fermi Gamma-ray Space Telescope.

Nassim Haramein, Quantum physicist, author of *The Schwarzschild Proton Paper*, reports that "Standard physics identifies only 4% of our Universe, the other 96% is 'missing,' composed of 'dark matter' and 'dark energy.' What scientists have been ignoring is the incredible abundant energy found within space itself. They use *'renormalization'* in their formulas, then sweep the infinite density of the vacuum space under the rug mathematically." It is proposed that these dark field energies *are* the *Field*, the *Web of Life*, the *Divine Matrix*. Perhaps a critical mistake was made, when modern science decided to call space "empty," and we are Now reintegrating this Source *Field* in our understanding.

We are intimately connected with and affected by this "vacuum" *Field.* "Space" surrounding us, nourishes us with the Source of our Being. We are magnetically drawn to harmonize within the *Field,* to participate in the magnificence of "Creation" manifesting *through* us. This medium called "space" is a transmitter of *Fields* of energy, Light and Dark Light, photons, gamma rays, x-rays and more from our Sun and other Celestial bodies, continually flowing to and through us. A New level of relating to this expanded state of Being is stirring within us, thanks to Solar and Cosmic influences and Quantum awareness.

Open your eyes with awareness and you will notice we have entered intensified "technicolor" Light *Fields* where we are Now orbiting "space." This additional Light activates the pineal gland and through it the Heart, awakening an intelligent, self-aware ability to interact with the *Field* in unbroken connection with Source. Aware participants are "midwives" of our own awakening, assisting with birthing of our True potential as a phenomenal race of Divine Creative Beings.

As we free ourselves from Ancient self-limiting "programs," we launch into a New way of operating, on this tantalizing journey, engaging in our greatest Potential as *21st Century Superhuman*s. With dawning self-awareness that we are amazing individual expressions of an Infinite Whole, we are awakening far beyond the little "i" to recognize ourselves as the "We" of ever-flowing Creation.

We are now living in a time where a spontaneous awakening of a birthing process of awareness is manifesting for any Soul who desires it! Becoming aware that we are not our thinking minds, our emotions or our experiences is key. We are the awareness that lies behind the thinking mind that is becoming conscious of itself! This awareness cannot be pinned down or even grasped. It is beyond form! It can only be experienced! It is the truth of who we are and what connects us to everyone and everything!

The level of light coming into this planet and the level of help from physical and non physical beings has never been more fully at our disposal if we so choose to awaken! All we have to do is desire it and be willing to step back from our thinking minds and our emotions! All the intelligence of the universe is within us in this stillness. Profound peace, gratitude and compassion rest here in this awareness!

Stuart Royston
Citizen of the Earth

As Global citizens of our beautiful Planet and World community, we are awakening to our place within a magnificent Galactic community and beyond, where, in Quantum "reality" we are ALL ONE. Action taken to Live holistically Now, holds frequencies for others to move into. Space images from NASA and Hubble offer stupendous evidence, revealing an incredible Cosmos, of which we are part and we are One. Stepping forward into greater Wholeness, we activate full expression of Who We ARE, emerging into this miraculous, promising self-aware Evolutionary Leap, called the *Shift of the Ages.* ♥

Part 1: Shift Of The Ages - Section 2
How Quantum "Reality" Operates

Readers probably haven't heard much about it yet, but they will.
Quantum technology turns ordinary reality upside down.

Michael Crichton (1942-2008)
Bestselling Author, Producer, Screenwriter

Quantum physics is defiantly redefining "reality," so let's explore how it defines how our World operates. For thousands of years we've been thinking the World is "solid," that it runs by mechanical means, yet we are about to have our minds opened up and turned-on. Quantum Physics has been around for *over* 100 years and is Now getting exposure at the forefront of our culture, even showing up in such mainstream media as "Good Morning America."

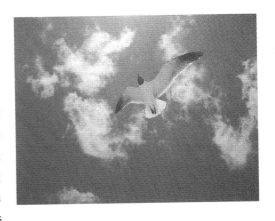

One of the first things that happens when you open up to Quantum principles is a plummeting "Oh no" feeling, *"please* don't tell me my "reality" is different than what I thought it is, I'm just getting used to this one!"

Nothing is solid. Nothing is fixed.
The Universal Substance is Wiggly.

Ian Lawton
Minister, Theology Inquiry

Once we allow Quantum theory to enter our World, a relentless "wiggly feeling" *does* set in. When we commit to embracing and integrating Quantum principles in our "reality," a lingering uneasy feeling queasily takes over while internal adjustments are sought, as if inquiring, "Are you *sure* this is correct?" And it does take a bit to realize this very natural "dizzy" feeling may be with us for a while...

If someone says that he can think or talk about Quantum physics without becoming dizzy, that shows only that he has not understood anything whatever about it.

Murray Gell-Mann
Nobel Prize in Physics 1969

Look at green sunlit leaves waving in the breeze on a summer's day, and imagine they are simply energy that has slowed itself down enough to appear to you as matter...*how can this be?* We present Quantum principles here in easy form to grasp, with the basics of *how* these new "rules" play themselves out in Life. We are learning together how to tumble into the equilibrium of rather than thinking "outside the box," it dawning upon us that "there is no box..." and so awakening to this New uncanny "reality" continues.

If Quantum mechanics hasn't profoundly shocked you,
you haven't understood it yet.

Niels Bohr
Nobel Prize in Physics 1922

Have you ever thought, "Would someone please explain Quantum Physics to me?" In even a micro-dose, Quantum physics changes how we relate to our World and our place in it. Our use of "reality" in quotes throughout the book is the first lesson in Quantum physics: *"reality"* is only as "real" as we make it. We will be exploring this in detail. Unusual capitalization infers a word carries Quantum meaning.

We are on the cutting edge of a new paradigm. We are excited to share the product of much thought-provoking study with you, distilled into an easy yet essential feast of Quantum theory spilling over into everything we do or aspire to: Health, Well-Being, Love, Abundance and more, thus our sub-title *Quantum Lifestyle*.

Quantum physics thus reveals a basic Oneness of the Universe.

Erwin Schrodinger
Nobel Prize in Physics, Max Planck Medal

The best way to experiment with Quantum theory is to simply *play with it* in familiar "reality," and have fun with it! Caution: don't get *too* serious, for as we are about to discover, Life is not quite as serious as we've worked so hard to make it. *Play* with these concepts and they will begin to make sense. We are about to overturn thousands of years of programming. Like it or not, we are Now *in a Quantum World... and it is a huge shift!*

When His Holiness won the Nobel Peace Prize, there was a Quantum leap. He is
not seen as solely a Tibetan anymore; he belongs to the World.

Richard Gere
Actor, Buddhist, Healing the Divide

At very worst, Quantum principles may be a bit uncomfortable as they access "forbidden" unlimited possibilities. At best they stupendously skyrocket our ability to enter shameless into potential as a species of Creator BEINGS, heroes of our own destiny rather than victims. Shall we follow this trail and reveal what is hidden ahead? ♥

Sci-fi has never really been my bag. But I do believe in a lot of weird things these
days, such as synchronicity. Quantum physics suggests it's possible, so why not?

John Cleese
Actor, Comedian, Writer, Film Producer

Chapter 6

When The World Was Flat & The Double Slit Experiment

Reality is merely an illusion, albeit a very persistent one.

Albert Einstein (1879-1955)
Theory of Relativity, Nobel Prize 1921

Around 550 B.C. Greek philosopher Pythagoras was one of the first to suggest the Earth was a sphere. He offered "reality" changing contributions to astrology, mathematics and music. He and his followers are believed to have been dedicated vegetarians. His uplifting and revolutionary principles of harmonious living, homeopathy and energy medicine are with us today.

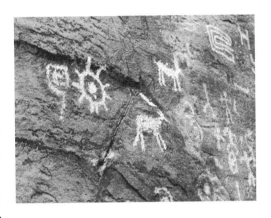

Many cultures held onto the strange notion that the World was flat into the Middle Ages, 500-1500 A.D. Even Columbus had to overcome this widespread prejudice in the 1400s, before he was victorious in getting support to sail to the "new World." Where would we be Now, if he hadn't pushed through ruthless limiting beliefs of his time and daringly sailed off "the edge of the known World!?"

It took 1,000 years for cultures globally including China, India and various Aboriginals, to move beyond deep-rooted and limiting belief that the World was flat. It requires quite the Leap Now to adapt to and integrate Quantum "reality" World-wide. Will we outdistance or parallel the "World is flat culture" in this next phase of self-aware Living? Confidentially, this coming change has all the possibilities of happening very quickly.

Awareness, filtered through the medium
of your beliefs generates your experience.

Dr. Richard Bartlett
The Physics of Miracles

Courageous thinkers risking Life and limb, changed the face of our World long ago. Copernicus asserted in 1530 Earth rotated on its axis daily and around the Sun in a year; he died in 1543 never knowing what a stir his work had caused. Inspired, Bruno suggested heretically in 1600 space was unlimited with more orbs beyond our Sun and Planets. He was tried in the Inquisition and brutally burned at the stake for blasphemy!

Under threat of deadly torture and death, Galileo again attempted to bring these concepts forward, resulting in imprisonment and later house arrest. However his progressive book, *Two New Sciences* survived. Galileo is considered early "father of modern physics." His statement that natural law is mathematical was highly praised by Einstein.

We are at a triumphant "jumping off place" ("interesting times - times of great change")... Quantum physics promises to launch us into *such* a different perspective of "reality," some may hold onto the secure "world is flat" philosophy forever, rather than venturing into the miraculous Quantum realm. Our wonderful teacher Dr. John Ray used to say, "If you're not ready for it, put the book on the shelf until you are. All things in good time, and 'when we're ready the teacher appears.'"

Quantum physics is redefining how we relate to our World, revealing radical New glimpses into the sensational awareness of *Who We Truly Are*. We may walk with "one foot in each World" while it's sinking in, so Relax, Breathe, Smile and Let Go, and let the *Field of Possibilities* emerge into form in exciting new ways around us.

Imagine the Universe beautiful and just and perfect.
Then be sure of one thing:
The *IS* has imagined it quite a bit better than you have.
The original sin is to limit the *IS*. Don't.

> *Richard Bach*
> *Illusions: The Messiah's Handbook*

Laws of physics established in the 1600s, were based on Newton's Laws of cause and effect operating in a 3-D World. His *Principia* formulated laws of motion and gravitation to dominate science's view of the physical Universe for the next 400 years. Quantum physics is Now introducing us to a World, far beyond Newtonian mechanical principles.

In 1913 Niels Bohr of Denmark, took the World by storm with the idea that atoms at rest do not exist as we were taught in school (like mini-solar systems). Instead he made the staggering announcement that atoms start out as *Clouds of Possibility,* as a wave or stream of particles! *They only form as atoms when Attention is placed upon them!* Are you ready to take a giant Leap into *this* Quantum "reality" that skyrocketed momentum of Quantum physics?

You take the blue pill, the story ends, you wake up in your bed and believe whatever you want to believe. You take the red pill, you stay in *Wonderland*, and I show you how deep the *rabbit hole* goes...

> *Morpheus*
> *The Matrix*

Lynne McTaggart's eye-opening investigative report *The Field, The Quest for the Secret Force of the Universe,* reports on experiments of the last 60 years in Quantum physics and consciousness. Her best-seller, well-described as "bridge between science and spirituality," verifies in detail the fascinating relationship between Quantum physics, prayer, thought and intention, exposing how this idea is shifting our *perception* of self and our World.

The word Quantum has to do with how a particle or electron takes up *space and energy (or not).* Where we discover pay-dirt is in the astounding awareness that the particle *only* moves into form *when our Attention is placed upon it.* Formulation of our "reality" has less to do with matter itself, and more to do with it being a product of Attention placed upon the *Field of Possibilities* by us, the "Observer."

Niels Bohr (1885-1962), modern "father of Quantum physics," daringly defined these New rules of electron behavior, still followed by physicists around the World today.

> ...an electron is not a precise entity, but exists as a potential, a superposition, or sum, of all probabilities until we observe or measure it, at which point the electron freezes into a particular state. Once we are through looking or measuring, the electron dissolves back into the ether of all possibilities.
>
> *Lynne McTaggart*
> *The Field*

If your jaw is not hanging open yet, you may need to read above again, or perhaps you already knew. The single most famous Quantum experiment, done literally thousands of times around the World, winning awards for being "the most beautiful experiment," is called the *Double Slit Experiment.* It was first performed in 1801(!) by British physicist Thomas Young, while exploring the wave-like nature of Light. Because he believed Light was made of waves, he had the audacity to hypothesize that interaction would happen when the light waves met. What he discovered was astounding then, and is even today!

To envision this experiment, imagine 2 screens one behind the other. Electrons shot through 2 slits in the first screen are expected to land in straight lines on the back screen. However, to our surprise they land in a splatter pattern, denoting they are in *wave form* (pre-matter) not particle form (matter). An unknowing Observer (mechanical or human) placed at the experiment, influences the electrons to become particles (simply by observing), the particles then land in a straight line on the screen behind as expected.

Whether human or mechanical, an Observer changes the results of the Double Slit Experiment. With Attention of an Observer, what *was* wave form changes into particles and lands in a straight line on the screen as expected, rather than the splatter pattern of the unobserved waves. It is worth reviewing *"Double Slit Experiment"* on Youtube (as we did:) to absorb it until understood, as this is foundational to everything that follows.

When Attention is placed upon the *Cloud or Field of Possibilities,* the "wave" collapses and takes shape as particles of matter. Thus it has been shown thousands of times over, that Attention placed upon the *Field* causes matter and events take form. Crazy as it seems, our *thought-emotion* is so powerful it actually directs how "reality" emerges around us. Stretch your Mind to comprehend this, though a Leap from our former perceptions, that yes, this means *ALL* "reality" appearing in our World is a product of our *Attention upon the Field.*

What appeared to put a halt to randomness was a living observer. One of the fundamental laws of Quantum physics says that an event in the subatomic world exists in all possible states until the act of observing or measuring it 'freezes' it, or pins it down, to a single state. This process is technically known as the collapse of the wave function, where 'wave function' means the state of all possibilities.

...according to Newton's version of "reality," a chair or even a planet was sitting there, whether or not we were looking at it. The world existed independently of us. But in the strange twilight of the Quantum World...a perfect hermetic world of pure potential, [it is] only made real and in a sense less perfect - when interrupted by an Observer.

Lynne McTaggart
The Field

Richard Feynman's Life (1918-1988), "No Ordinary Genius" (Youtube), explores his revolutionary thinking that changed the face of physics. He describes waves of the *Field*: It's as if there's an insect in the corner of the pond making waves when it moves; "reality" is multitudes of waves Mirrored by the *Field* (exampled by the pond) *for us to interpret as they come to us,* putting us in much different relationship to "reality" than we have been.

Feynman, 1965 Nobel Laureate in physics, is thought of as one of the ten greatest physicists of all time. He pioneered Quantum computing and nanotechnology, worked on the Manhattan Project and Challenger Space Shuttle disaster. *Wikipedia* reports:

Feynman was fond of saying that all Quantum mechanics can be gleaned from carefully thinking through the implications of this single experiment...The Double-Slit Experiment...which conducted with individual particles has become a classic thought experiment for its clarity in expressing the central puzzles of Quantum mechanics.

Richard Feynman called it "a phenomenon which is impossible ... to explain in any classical way, and which has in it the heart of Quantum mechanics. In reality, it contains the *only* mystery of Quantum Mechanics.

Richard Feynman
Nobel Prize Physics 1965

Quantum physics that emerged over the past 150 years is just Now going mainstream. Even in recent 20-30 years it was considered risky "science fiction." We are Now at a turning point when Quantum theory is becoming visible everywhere, even in kids cartoons! It is fascinating and exciting to view our "reality" as ever-emerging from thought. We will use the term "Observer-Creator" throughout this book, based on the Double Slit Experiment. Digging deeper into *21st Century Superhuman Quantum Lifestyle,* we're discovering sensational secrets to inviting each Newly Created moment into our World! ♥

Chapter 7

Quantum Threads in Ancient Tradition

Science is not only compatible with spirituality;
it is a profound source of spirituality.

Carl Sagan
The Demon-Haunted World: Science as a Candle in the Dark

Before we dive further into Quantum "reality" let's journey back into history, to examine Ancient cultures in which Quantum teachings were very much there, often concealed in wanton superstition and distorted understanding.

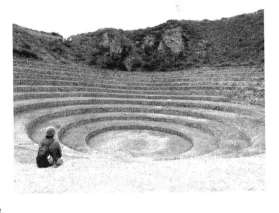

> You are a part of the largest story ever told...the evolution of the Universe. The Great Radiance is your Creator. Stars are your Ancestors. Your Life is a play within the Largest Play of All. All people and all things are part of your spiritual family.

Rev. Michael Dowd
Evolutionary Theologian

Graham Hancock's *Quest for the Lost Civilization* (Youtube) traces Ancient cultures collapsing and growing through Earth's cataclysms, purposefully passing knowledge on from one civilization to the next. He reports on monuments such as Ancient Egypt's Sphinx and Great Pyramids of Giza, Easter Island near Chile and Angkor Wat in Thailand, all built on the 30th parallel as perfect mirrors of constellations directly overhead *in 10,500 B.C.!*

He recounts "highly intelligent, bearded light-skinned people," traveling across the sea after surviving destruction of their continent Atlantis. Priest-scholars deposited science, astronomy, engineering, mathematics and spirituality in the Andes and Himalayas, where Earth's "kundalini" energy would be preserved, to carry this advanced knowledge to future generations. Energies of Light in the Himalayas, were carried forward by the Lamas of Tibet 12,000 years. The Aquarian Age dawned, this energy moved to the Andes in 2013.

> They knew wherever Light of the World settled, people of that region would become great spiritual teachers... It has always been that way, for this Light affected people who live near where it was coiled, and naturally brought them into a state of enlightenment depending upon their ability to receive it. The people of this new region would awaken and remember their intimate connection with all life everywhere and with God. Eventually they would remember the sacred place within their hearts where God resides, where all creation began. In remembering, they would become spiritual lights to the rest of humanity simply by their very being.
>
> *Drunvalao Melchezedek*
> *The Great White Pyramid of Tibet*

Plato wrote one of the few records of Atlantis in 360 B.C. He documented a story told by his father's 6th cousin Solon to a priest in Egypt, about a sudden destructive cataclysm with violent eruptions, floods and most likely an axis shift, sinking the fabled continent Atlantis around 9,500 B.C. Edgar Cayce, "sleeping prophet" included Atlantis in nearly 2/3 of his readings, some of which tell of severe floods that broke the continent into islands as far back as 28,000 B.C. Nearly 2,000 books written about Atlantis point to its survivors founding Egyptian, Sumerian, Indo-Aryan and South American civilizations with tools, language and mythos of a greater destiny.

Michael Tellinger exposes in *Temples of the African Gods,* a fascinating site now mapped in South Africa. Remains of settlements 3x the size of Los Angeles, contain millions of circular structures built to the Phi Ratio of da Vinci Man's perfect "Golden Mean." Stone devices hint at a sophisticated ancient civilization harnessing Earth's energy for power.

Computer simulations align a significant stone calendar at this site with Orion's Belt 200,000 years ago, correlating with records of off-Planet Anunnaki who came to Earth seeking gold. Late pre-historian Zecharia Sitchin documented this amazing story gleaned from 500,000+ Ancient Sumerian clay tablets in museum basements around the World.

These astounding detailed records reveal how the Anunnaki colonized Earth and genetically engineered slaves to mine gold. Buried in such genetic history likely lies the deep-rooted fear in the human psyche of punishment, that we are still freeing ourselves from today. Interpreting such findings with tools of modern science and recent archaeological digs of human bones dating back 200,000-400,000 years, opens doors to a staggering pre-history little yet imagined. Michael Tellinger's *Slave Species of the Gods* is a brilliant uncensored best-selling summary of this essential history.

Dresden Codex is thought to have been brought to Peru from Atlantis around 15,000 B.C., engineered by highly advanced race skilled with astronomy and computer technology. This eventually surfaced as precise Mayan calendar, containing the most accurate known system for tracking celestial cycles millions of years into past and future. It contains sophisticated forecasts of earth changes and warnings for our Now, correlating with Cosmic alignments and Celestial cycles we are just Now beginning to comprehend.

Mayan philosophy *Inlakesh: "I am another yourself,"* demonstrated knowledge*"we are One,"* dovetailing with *Quantum physics*. They preserved this teaching, easily understood by the simple, yet also the most intricately complex science of our existence.

Graham Hancock's *Quest for the Lost Civilization* reports Inca priests sacrificing living hearts of thousands of innocents, as in Mel Gibson's *Apocalypto*. Brutal Inca sacrifices had never made sense, yet now with awareness that the advanced civilization from long ago, must have told them, *"When HEART is with "Creator" you have immortality."* This was taken literally, overshadowing their entire culture with terror and insanity of brutal sacrifice.

What we understand *NOW* both in Quantum terms and through Ancient Aramaic teachings, is that we are designed to live through the *HEART* as Creator Beings in LOVE. Once understood, we connect with Source in an interrupted state of Being where there "is no death," with easy transition from one form to the next. Controlling religious dogma grew, cultivating fear rather than honoring our Oneness with ALL things and Source.

The advanced civilization of 15,000 B.C. *must* have conveyed this to the agrarian Pre-Columbian civilization. Inca, Aztec and Mayan cultures did not fully grasp the Quantum concepts, instead priests *literally* offered the "gods" physical living hearts to appease them throughout the Inca empire, even as recently as Chichen Itza in Mexico, 400 A.D. and the temple of Sun and Moon in Peru 1500 B.C. How often in history has higher truth been obscured by those unable to grasp its concepts?

> Avoidable human misery is more often caused not so much by stupidity as by ignorance, particularly our ignorance about ourselves.
>
> Carl Sagan
> *The Demon-Haunted World: Science as a Candle in the Dark*

The same documentary reveals the horror of children being sacrificed to the *constellations* to get *the sun and moon to stop*. Again, we might imagine they were also told by the "advanced race" that when we align with our True Design, which is *Eternal*, time and space *do not exist*. Thus they sacrificed children hoping it would make them *eternal*. Now with Quantum principles, in *awareness* of higher dimensions we discover *there is no time or space*. In that day literal interpretation was all that could be culturally grasped. The concept that time and space do not exist was beyond their comprehension; so they "appeased" the "gods" with human sacrifice to "stop time."

How many "sacrificial lambs" have there been, from crusades to crucifixions, witch hunts, dungeons and torture chambers, all conceived in thoughts of the blame-fear-hostility culture, eclipsing simple truth of our True Design LOVE and our Innate potential as Observer-Creators within an *Infinite Field of Possibilities?*

> Whenever our ethnic or national prejudices are aroused, in times of scarcity, during challenges to national self-esteem or nerve, when we agonize about our

diminished cosmic place and purpose, or when fanaticism bubbles up around us, then, habits of thought from ages past reach for the controls.

Carl Sagan
The Demon-Haunted World: Science as a Candle in the Dark

The "still small voice" of our True Being is *always* beckoning us to "wake up." At this Evolutionary Leap, all Not of LOVE thought, emotion, action must go!!! It is a "virus" in our "biocomputer." We will learn how easy it is to upgrade our "operating system."

According to Harvard studies we are carrying around 95% unconscious data, coloring our Creation from the *Field of Possibilities*. Upgrading our "operating system" to LOVE is essential, and we do it by clearing this unconscious content. Ancient threads actually carried this secret forward, which we Now have potential to understand for the first time in human history through Quantum physics and the Double Slit Experiment.

Yesterday we obeyed kings and bent our necks before emperors.
But today we kneel only to truth, follow only beauty, and obey only LOVE.

Kahlil Gibran

Cultural traditions *have* carried simple secrets of this True Source of Being in wisdom teachings, coded into ritual and language, held as sacred truths passed down through the ages, even if not fully understood in the culture of the day. In Jewish tradition the "Name of God" is not pronounceable. It is "HU," mouth Breath exhaled or inhaled - huuuuu: "The way to express the Sacred Name of God is to wonder, 'Are we alive in this World because we took in HUuuu the Breath of God? OR Have we left this World because we HUuuu let go the Breath of God?'" Considered so sacred to be unspeakable, the "Name of God," has been carried within this cultural tradition for many centuries, based on open breath.

Root HU is a reminder of continual delicious connection with Source through Breath opening us to Life. Often unaware Breath-holding Creates blockages in the body best to release and let go. When we "held points" Dr. John Whitman Ray used to say, *"Breathing is the opposite of resistance. Get that person breathing and they will free up the blockages!!!"*

Holding the breath when upset or in pain, establishes lifetime patterns of cutting off our supply from Source and storing painful thoughts-emotions *in the Body*. OPENING Breath is a major key to releasing these blockages. Approaching others with Open Breath fosters an innate knowing, that we are without hidden agendas.

Many Ancient Teachings include clarifying the Body with]Breath, such as Kundalini Yoga, Tibetan meditation and other traditions. In and out-Breath gives continual reminder of connection with Source, releasing "old data" carried in the Body. At deeper levels of meditation, in a state called Samadhi, Breathing and Heartbeat have been suspended for hours demonstrating eternal connection with Source beyond the physical 3-D realm.

Dr. ryce discovered, as moderator for translation of the Khaburis manuscript (one of the oldest know Aramaic codexes of the new Testament dated 160 AD), the Aramaic says, when Yeshua (Jesus) addressed a crowd he *"Breathed them,"* mis-translated by the Greeks as he "Breathed on them." Inspired by the modern translation, michael developed Stillpoint, an amazing process of merging with Source, to release fears, angers, anxieties, or whatever *holds the Breath* captive, in the illusion outside of LOVE, to merge again with Greater Self - "At-One with the ONE." Through this *Stillpoint* process, we use open Breath to release and let go all Not of LOVE thought-emotion.

Utilizing development of this process from the Aramaic, we teach open-mouth circular Breathing, with the Meditation [Part 2: MIND]. Our particular method opens channels through which we may have held resistance since childhood. By opening a passageway all through the body, a natural letting go takes place, freeing blockages and filters allowing unlimited energy to flow. Children may hold Breath when upset, a residual pattern often carried into adulthood. Learning to Free the Breath is a key *21st Century Superhuman* habit, to release vitality-lowering "old content."

Breath awareness was intrinsic to Indo-Aryan nomadic tribes, settling steppes of Central Asia, Europe and Turkey in 4,000-6,000 B.C. HU was interpreted by the Sufis as *There is no "reality" except God,* HUmanity exists *because of* continual flow of Source or "Breath of God." Freeing the Breath to reconnect with our True Design LOVE shifts our "reality," and thus the World around us. Hinduism's Vedic texts (one billion+ followers) teach Freeing self from duality or Illusion by focusing on inner *Essence* [LOVE], while freeing the Soul from its entanglement in matter.

Vedic texts identify what is called "Illusion" or *Maya*: I am light/dark, man/woman or my house/country/religion. Thus Soul caught in Illusion identifies with temporary body and elements Not of Source, such as gender, race, monetary system and religion. Under this *false-ego construct* one desires to control and enjoy matter. In so doing he-she serves lust, greed, fear and anger...falling deeper into the illusion... Only in *goodness* does the Soul develop wisdom, see things in real Light, find liberation and restore connectedness with All That Is... En-Light-Enment means moving from shadows of ignorance into a state of increased Light, nourishing Spiritual sustenance and Bliss.

Quantum principles expose eternal truth in Ancient threads, affirming our "reality" emerges continually from Attention upon the *Field*. With LOVE (and open breath) we produce a kind "Reality." Ancient anger, fear or hatred carried inside us also Mirror in our World. Gregg Braden reports in *Science of Miracles* (Youtube), according to Ancient Wisdom we are surrounded by the *Divine Matrix* or *Field*. Breathing, we take in this *Creative Field,* the very same molecules as did saints and sages throughout the ages. Shifting our focus to Compassion without judgment, we accesses the *Field* in the most productive way.

We *21st Century Superhuman*s are at an amazing crossroads in human history, accessing a revolutionary New perspective, to release millennia of misinterpretation. Whatever *stories* operated in our pre-history, whatever *beings and regimes* were here, our roots go back to the ONE. We are "creator-Beings" of LOVE.

Human aura images show our energy *Field* expands with Breath, Om, in interpersonal Love, and pristine natural settings. Learning to clear all Not of LOVE from Body-Mind-Heart, we experience our surrounding World as a living Mirror of what we carry inside. We elevate ourselves and the entire Vibration of humanity into this miraculous Journey, as we resonate True Peace and Freedom within, to all civilization on Earth and beyond. This is a thrilling Ever Present Now, when Quantum science and Ancient Wisdom Lovingly and brilliantly walk hand in hand, to show us the way...

> The cosmos is within us. We are made of star-stuff.
> We are a way for the Universe to know itself.
>
> *Carl Sagan*
> *Cosmos: A Personal Voyage (500 million viewers in over 60 countries)*

We are surrounded by a *Field* that responds to our Attention so perfectly it appears as our "reality!" We are still *learning* how all this works! As we clear old unconscious thought-emotion we learn how to shift toward a productive future, as Gregg Braden explains:

> We must *Become* the very things that we choose to experience in Life: the Peace, the Healing, the Compassion, the Cooperation, the LOVE, the Nurturing. We must Become these very Things, so the *Field* has something to Mirror back to us. This is the Way we will build a better world.

Our thoughts and emotions profoundly affect the very World in which we live. The *Shift of the Ages* is our Mind-Heart's Ability, Wisdom and Knowledge coming together in a miraculously orchestrated moment, showing us the way to shift within ourselves. Thus we consciously participate in changing our World. By shifting ourselves, everything around us changes. Gregg Braden shares in the video, *Secret Ancient Knowledge: The Divine Matrix*:

> Thought is the image of Quantum possibility. In the realm of all possibilities, every possibility already exists; our best scenario and our worst. With the power of our mind, by focusing either LOVE or fear on that possibility, we bring it into this world.

John Archibald Wheeler (1911-2008), known for coining wormhole, Quantum foam and black hole, later collaborator with Einstein, calls this a *"Participatory Universe."*

> You are not the doer, you are the door.
>
> *Dr. Richard Bartlett*
> *Matrix Energetics*

Let's dive into this thrilling New *Quantum "reality"* that has *always* been with us. Embarking on this grand adventure as **21st Century Superhumans,** we have literally mind-blowing tools at our fingertips, as we play a pivotal role in the dawning of an emerging New Culture for humanity as Creator-Beings, resonating through True *Essence,* LOVE. ♥

> This is my simple religion. There is no need for temples, no need for complicated philosophy. Our own brain, our own Heart is our Temple. The philosophy is Kindness.
>
> *His Holiness the Dalai Lama*

Chapter 8

The *"Field"* Awaits Our Command

"Reality" exists only where the mind Creates a focus.

Buddhist Mahayana Sutra

Once comprehended, the quote above changes our Lives forever. It reveals the key of focus, Quantum knowledge secreted in Ancient Traditions millennia ago, noticed by the few. Adapting to this profound Quantum awareness is a *huge* stretch for our belief system long considering matter solid in a 3-D Newtonian World.

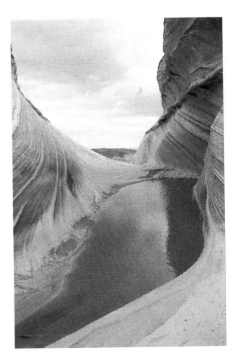

> So again, I remind you that when we measure something at the Quantum level, We change it. This is called the observer effect. So then, the question to ask ourselves is, "What lens of observation are we looking through?
>
> *Dr. Richard Bartlett*
> *The Physics of Miracles*

Are we really serious and ready to embrace that we are *Observer-Creators?* That Attention upon the *Field of Possibilities* through thought-emotion (conscious-unconscious) causes *ALL* matter and events to take shape around us as our "reality?" *Are we ready to embrace and integrate with this mind-blowing New way of experience our existence???*

Some Quantum physicists believe that "behind" us "reality" is un-manifest in wave form, only taking shape as particles, matter or events when we give it our Attention. Try it. Turn quick...see if you can catch matter in unmanifest wave form behind you! *Ha!*

Imagine making the internal shift to become this expansive! Quantum Awareness that we *are* Observer-Creators, offers us access to Ancient "codes" "programmed" to upgrade our "Operating System,." As we make this shift, we tap into our greatest capacity yet to be expressed, in this most powerful Evolutionary Leap in human history, the *Shift of the Ages.*

RESHAPING Quantum "REALITY" FROM THE FIELD: Become present with your Quantum Awareness each day. Relax into knowing that manifest and unmanifest existence is accessible to you. Experiment with interacting with the *Cloud of Possibilities.* Fall out of particle or material form, into wave form, and back into the *Cloud or Field of Possibilities.* Emerge with anticipation from the *Field* in new ways. Play with Quantum ideas: imagine your entire "reality" moving in and out of form in New, better ways. *Boundaries are imaginary - rules are made up - limits don't exist...*

Breathe, Smile, Focus Trust, Allow, Let Go...if noticing anything Not of LOVE such as stress, worry, sorrow, sadness, anger, hurt, fear, grief, blame give it to the *Cloud or Field of Possibilities* - toss it like a ball dissolving into the *Field - New will emerge.* **Smile. Breathe. LOVE.** German theoretical physicist Werner Heisenberg, developer of the Uncertainty Principle, awarded 1932 Nobel Prize in Physics for "Creation of Quantum Mechanics," sums it up this amazing New perception of "reality:"

> The atoms or elementary particles themselves are not real; they form a world of potentialities or possibilities rather than one of things or facts."
>
> *Werner Heisenberg (1901-1976)*
> *Nobel Prize in Physics in 1932, Creation of Quantum Mechanics*

We knew this in 1932 and are just Now catching on! What we used to think of as externalized "reality" or matter and events, is now a *"Field of Possibilities"* in Quantum terms? Even Einstein voiced discomfort with this when he said, "I like to think the moon is there even if I am not looking at it."

Everything in our "reality" is a result of our Attention upon the *Field.* This is a *HUGE* shift from perception that all is tangible as it appears! The tricky part we will be learning about is that this includes both conscious and unconscious thought. We will learn special tricks to untangle ourselves from our unconscious thoughts, otherwise they tend to "run the show."

Our "reality" is a Mirroring, a biofeedback of sorts, a gauge to let us know what is going on *inside of us,* whether we are aware of it or not. What is Mirrored in our "reality," is a mechanism showing us what we still have to clear to operate from LOVE.

NewsFlash! Creation changes as QUICKLY AS WE CHANGE OUR THOUGHTS!

Quantum science suggests the existence of many possible futures for each moment of our lives. Each future lies in a state of rest until it is awakened by choices made in the present.

> *Gregg Braden*
> *The Isaiah Effect*

QUESTIONING RELATIONSHIP TO "REALITY:" Playing with this concept, ask yourself:

- Why did *this* show up in my World today?
- What am I being shown about *myself?*
- What am I blaming someone else for, that is actually coming from me?

- If there is discomfort, I acknowledge it is my own, and give it Attention to clear it.
- What is being Mirrored, showing me where to shift internally?
- What can I remove from my internal thought (conscious-unconscious) that is out-pictured in my World as a Not of LOVE situation?

OBSERVE HOW LIFE SHOWS UP AROUND YOU: Suddenly Life becomes the *"messenger"* of our resonance, rather than happening *to us*. Notice what takes shape around you and honor it as your Creation. Whether feeling happy, sad, angry fearful, controlling or judgmental, none of this can be blamed on others. All is a Mirroring of our own *inner* landscape. People and circumstances are drawn by our Vibration who are a Vibrational match to us. Be patient with yourself, it takes a bit of adjustment from our old way of looking at things, and we will be learning great tools for refining this process.

If it seems like a "big leap," hang in there. **It is.** This is definitely a *level jump* to Quantum comprehension of our existence. It can be challenging to entertain this possibility, so radically different from how we've perceived our World until now, (when we thought that someone or something out there was always *doing it to us* or *outside us*), yet the more we entertain and play with this amazing Quantum science, the more it makes sense.

Research from fields as different as neuroscience and anthropology show that what you pay attention to shapes your brain and behavior in surprising ways that would have been hard to imagine even at the turn of this young century.

Whether you've paid rapt attention to classical music, like Joshua Bell, or compassion, like the Tibetan Monks, focused on the big picture like a Japanese, or the one big thing like an ancient Greek, perceived the world as a line like the American professor, or as a circle like his Chinese protégé - such differences have helped make you who you are.

The good News is that attention's ability to change your brain and transform your experience isn't limited to your childhood, but prevails throughout Life.

Winifred Gallagher
Rapt, Attention and the Focused Life, NYT Bestseller

We will be playing with these concepts throughout the book, so it will become more familiar and easy as we go along; repetition develops new synapses and neural pathways for the brain to integrate this New perception of "reality," a gift from Greater Mind-Heart.

How puzzling all these changes are!
I'm never sure what I'm going to be, from one minute to another.

(Alice) Lewis Carroll
Alice's Adventures in Wonderland

RECOGNIZE: I Am Observer-Creator. By Attention (conscious and unconscious) upon the *Field of Possibilities*, I Create *this* "reality." "Reality" magnetizes or resonates into form as a result of my Vibration. Experience yourself as a representative of Source, moving, Breathing, at One with the *Field of Possibilities*. Notice what happens internally as you enter into this awareness that your vibration is calling into Being or creating your "reality." Breathe, Smile and honor all of Life and Creation...

Our knowledge of Life and what makes us tick is surpassing where we have ever been in recorded history. Now we are learning we can actually shift our molecules *(that's right)* with thought *(how wild is this?)* beyond familiar laws of cause and effect. In Quantum theory matter, events and "reality" shift, based on our Attention placed upon them... Whether we feel we are, or feel we aren't putting Attention on the *Field, WE ARE.* Our new assignment is just to take it all in; Smile, Breathe and Be with how miraculous this all is...far beyond what we have yet imagined!

Continuing to upgrade everything we do,
is an important part of our ascension transition.

Bryan de Flores
LightQuest International

You may find some ideas presented here hard to believe, others may be quite surprising and some you may easily grasp. It doesn't matter. All we ask is that you allow yourself to be present, leave judgment aside, and if so inspired apply these principles gradually to your thinking and Life. Explore these New avenues of perceiving "reality," so the concepts develop meaning and you become open to absorbing New Truth.

We each - everyone on Earth - will sooner or later go through this process of ascension [awakening], whether we are ready for it this cycle or not.

Bill Ballard
The Great Awakening

Allowing mind and Heart to stretch in new directions, you do not need to believe or accept every idea. In fact you may find yourself actively resisting. This is okay. Resistance is a survival mechanism keeping us from old pain from Not of LOVE thought-emotion buried in the unconscious. We are now learning how to access our power as Observer-Creators to remove and change this content so it no longer holds resonance in our World.

Most of us encounter some level of resistance when we become aware of these Quantum principles, that all around us could actually be a product of our thought. However *it is true.* When we simply Breathe, Smile and Play along, we discover surprising inner shifts quietly taking place. *This is all that is required to shift internally.*

Are you ready to expand your awareness of what's possible, and as you do so, experience Life changing as you Live it? Venture with us into a World that may seem surreal, a journey connecting us with the very fabric of our existence. Put on your "adventurer hat," and get ready to explore Truth stranger than fiction, the New paradigm for attaining Life, Health, Vitality, Longevity, Success, Abundance and Well-Being!

Fasten your **21st Century Superhuman** seatbelt as we prepare for takeoff. Get ready for Self-Awareness, Joy, Immersion, Play, Willingness to Let Go and enjoy the process of REAL Living Now! *Wow....!* ♥

Chapter 9

Ready to Shake It Up?

You are more than your thoughts, your body or your feelings. You are a swirling vortex of limitless potential, who is here to shake things up and Create something new that the Universe has never seen.

Dr. Richard Bartlett
Matrix Energetics

How crazy is this, after Living in a 3-D World ruled by Newtonian mechanical physics: *There is no matter as such*, says Albert Einstein, *AND* we've known this since the early 1900s!

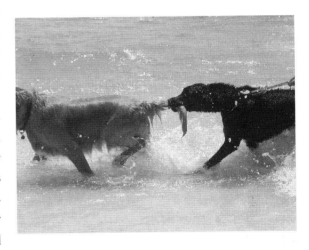

Let's imagine even with only a vague understanding of Quantum "reality," that an amazing treasure chest, *The Field of Infinite Possibilities*, is filled with unlimited creative potential, from which "reality" draws moment by moment. What we experience around us is a product of thought or Mind-energy acting on the *Field* (conscious-unconscious). As radical as we are willing to get, is how radically our World will shift!

> One day Alice came to a fork in the road and saw a Cheshire cat in a tree. "Which road do I take," she asked. "Where do you want to go?" was his response. "I don't know," Alice answered. "Then," he said, "it doesn't matter."

Lewis Carroll
Alice in Wonderland

Apply intention to where you are going, for possibilities are endless! Call it God, Source, Creator, *Divine Matrix* or the *Field*, where material "reality" flows in and out of being - a gigantic endless tidal ebb of sound, light, color, quarks, protons, electrons, energy and ether, constantly reshaping itself based on thought-emotion of its "Observer-Creators." Individual Attention, conscious and unconscious, plays a pivotal role in how "reality" takes shape. Declutter Now as Quantum particles are ready to jump at your command!

LET GO OF PUSHING AND WORRYING: Notice something you'd like to change or draw into your World. Notice how the "former you" might have pushed or worried to fulfill your wish. Now, "give it to the *Field*," and thank the *Field* for having more ways to take care of this than you could ask or think. Trust, relax and invite the *Field* to bring its waves into form in new Ways with LOVE. Breathe. Smile. Dance! Trust!

Make aware choices each moment, knowing that the *Field* is your playground from which "fluid Creation" emerges. Relax and let go control a little more than you have before. Our quality of *ATTENTION* shapes what returns from the *Field*. Holding onto a particular thought-emotion - such as worry reflects in what surrounds us. Relax your focus. Breathe and Smile. Invite Life to appear in New ways cleared to LOVE.

> Your loving Inner Being offers guidance in the form of emotion. Entertain a wanted or unwanted thought, and you feel a wanted or unwanted emotion. Choose to change the thought and you have changed the emotion and you have changed the creation. Make more choices in every day.
>
> *Abraham-Hicks*

Recognize the constant flux and change in "reality," as you ride the wave of creative energy from the *Field*. Now let go and free flow, trusting and allowing the *Field* to bring in something New, a slight shift or bigger, embracing wildly unlimited possibilities with LOVE, as your World begins to morph and shift, never going back to its original form.

SEND FEELINGS TO THE FIELD: Tap into good feelings you get as you connect with Life. Send these LOVING, peaceful, grateful, compassionate or content feelings to resonate in the *Field*; allow the *Field* to send back a Newly formed wave of possibility to your World. Where you feel less than good feelings, send those to the Field also, let them dismantle into the Field. Cancel all goals connected with them and let them go. Request all situations be reborn in new ways based in LOVE.

> The Collapse of the Wave Function
>
> After performing a weak collapse of the wave function, then you must allow grace to come in. I define grace as "that point where you erase your reliance upon external realities and allow for more of a perceptual process."
>
> *Dr. Richard Bartlett*
> *Matrix Energetics*

We will learn Ancient and modern techniques to refine our internal process, so our Attention calls forth what we truly desire from the *Field,* rather than Living by default. We are in the midst of reclaiming the most powerful elements ever available to humanity. As the Light of this Knowledge blazes through Mind and Heart, we launch into Alchemical *21st Century Superhuman* "reality" where Quantum transformation occurs. As we access this ability to shift ourselves, we also shift the entire "Hologram" of human existence. ♥

Part 1: Shift Of The Ages - Section 3
Making The Leap

Man's mind, once stretched by a new idea,
never regains its original dimensions.

Oliver Wendell Holmes Sr.
Poet, Writer, Physician (1809-1894)

Once upon a time we forgot our True Design LOVE, our Oneness with All Things and Quantum knowing that we are Observer-Creators whose "reality" emerges from thought... We are on a miraculous Journey to rediscover Living according to our True Design LOVE, with Cosmic energies showering upon us to activate this en-light-en-ing Evolutionary Leap called the *Shift of the Ages.*

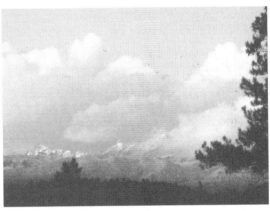

The day came when the risk to remain tight in the bud was more painful than the risk it took to bloom.

Anais Nin (1903-1977)
French-born American Author

At the University of Paris in 1982 it was found that electrons instantly communicated with one another at any distance. This remains one of the most profound findings of the twentieth century, exposing that electrons communicate with one another instantly no matter how far apart, negating Einstein's tenet that nothing travels faster than the speed of light. ***Thus physicist David Bohm (1917-1992) postulated that the Universe is a giant detailed Hologram, concluding that separateness is an illusion, and All is One.***

We are awakening to Greater Self in an Abundant Universe that is holding its arms open wide, for us to delight in the passion of our Hearts and irresistibly move into Living from *Essence.* Who knows what is about to be achieved as we make these juicy shifts, acting as a race of Quantum Holographic Beings, One with the *Web of Life?*

In a holographic Universe, time and space can no longer be viewed as fundamentals... At its deeper level reality is a super-Hologram in which past, present, and future exist simultaneously.... Our consciousness is the real us. Consciousness is everything and therefore nothing, as all is consciousness.

Paul Lenda, Guest Waking Times
Living in a Hologram, Our Holographic Reality

A "wiggly" feeling accompanies us as we dive into forbidden territory bridging science and consciousness, flowing in Quantum realms. It is not as solid as what we're used to, yet promises to launch us out of smug complacency on the precipice of this Evolutionary Leap into daring Greater Expression, as Quantum thought spins us into a New "reality."

At this time of Planetary awakening, we come to the realization that we're all connected and about to be born as Universal Humanity, where the evolutionary drivers we're facing are actually natural organic pressures to force our awakening.

Barbara Marx Hubbard
Communicator of Evolutionary Potential

Spontaneous Evolution by Bruce Lipton and Steve Bhaerman suggests that we are entering a positive evolutionary shift into **Holism**; Now moving beyond a dominant focus on materialism, science and physical laws into Consciousness, Compassion and Quantum principles. Rather than struggling for survival, they suggest we use our *best technology* to develop a sustainable future based on living in balance with Nature and the *Web of Life*. What a concept!

We are being forced into a situation wherein we either evolve or die. Which would you prefer? ...our personal preferences exert a lot more control over our reality than we have so far imagined. Consequently, what we choose to prefer might actually make a difference in the fate of humanity.

Bruce Lipton and Steve Bhaerman
Spontaneous Evolution, Our Positive Future and A Way to Get There From Here

As we travel this Adventure of a Lifetime, we **21st Century Superhumans** discover a surprising paradigm, that how and what we think and feel *does matter*. Integrating this foundational principle bridges a painfully apparent gap in emerging personal and Global agendas, encouraging us to respond in more clear, coherent, vital and LOVING ways. We are learning that progressive collaboration with one another with the spirit of conscious thought based in LOVE, is the only real bedrock for progressive viable solutions.

Everything is dependent on everything else.
We tend to forget that in our World.

Nassim Haramein
Transcendent 21st Century Physicist of the new Paradigm

We are about to discover how delicious movement into the Heart opens doors to what we consider thrilling 4th and 5th dimensional Living, opening us to greater creativity, flow and manifestation. Every moment holds the reminder to Breathe and Smile, releasing and letting go of old hypnotic shadows, restoring our Infinite True Design LOVE. Living in coherent frequencies of LOVE, Compassion, Gratitude *feeds* the *Web of Life,* delivering passion and commitment through the generative torus *Field* of the Heart, birthing an awe-inspiring New paradigm of continually creative, caring, thriving Human Civilization based in LOVE. ♥

Chapter 10

Beyond Time In 4 & 5-D

Courage Is a LOVE Affair with the Unknown.

Osho (1931-1990)
Indian Mystic, Teacher Self-Inquiry

Let's explore the concept of dimensions. A person acclimated to a flat dull 2-D World might find scintillating 3-D too much. Movie viewers pay big bucks for jump-off-the-screen in-your-face 3-D, rather than old-style 2-D. A thrilling World we can just about step into engages us with Blue-ray or 3-D glasses, entertaining and Life-like.

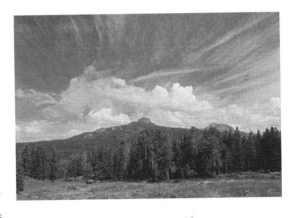

When Europeans came to the New World in sailing ships, Native Americans called the ships birds. There was nothing in their World that looked like sailing ships, so they had no way to recognize them, and translated the image into something familiar. This is why we don't generally see the 4th dimension or anything beyond it, because it's *so different* from what we're used to experiencing around us. Our adaptation to *recognizing* that other dimensions exist is the first step toward the possibility of experiencing them.

In 1915 Einstein's Theory of Special Relativity proposed that the Universe includes four dimensions. The first three we know of as "space" and the 4th is "spacetime," a dimension where time and space are inextricably linked. Einstein theorized time is inseparable from space. Sci-fi popularized timespace and spacetime into a familiar concept, also commonly accepted Now in physics circles. "Timespace refers to Spacetime, any mathematical model that combines space and time as a single continuum." (*Wikipedia*)

Physicists today are still exploring views of spacetime, considered an aspect of 3 and 4-D, yet nonexistent in higher realms. String Theory, also known as the *Field* or *Unified Field* recognizes 10-25 dimensions depending on the conversation. Quantum physicist John Hagelin, head of the TM® organization, describes the Super-String *Field* as like little wiggly rubber bands or effervescent ginger ale, photons constantly in motion, ready to respond to our Attention. String Theory explains our entire existence as a Hologram.

James Gates, Professor of Physics at the University of Maryland and Director of The Center for String & Particle Theory has made the astounding discovery, that below String Theory, describing the fundamental nature of the Universe is embedded computer code! These codes are digital data in the form of 1's and 0's, the same as what makes web browsers work, error-correction codes! Gates said, "We have no idea what these 'things' are doing there." Learn more in very interesting discussions on this discovery online.

Understanding our existence is more malleable than once thought, glimpses of transiting other dimensions come from those who report back. Penny Kelly shares about her experience of a vibrantly expanded state of being, after a full-blown kundalini experience in her book *Consciousness and Energy*.

> Let's assume that at the source level, there is only oneness - one mind/space filled with the exuberance of existence... Since I have personally experienced this primal state, I can say there is an unassailable awareness of an endless expanse of space, silence and stillness...What you can know in this primal state is...I Am - or the certainty that you exist...In this state everything seems to dissolve until there is only one simple awareness...

> Bliss is at best a poor description of the feeling this experience generates. You are a collection of tiny points of light in an ocean of what appears to be billions of points of light all filled with only one thing, the awareness of existence. This singular fact seems wedded to a boundless joy... Lack of experience with this state of original Mind is why it is difficult for most people to give credence to phenomena like clairvoyance, telepathy, or out-of-body experiences.

> *Penny Kelly, Consciousness and Energy*
> *Volume 1: Multi-Dimensionality and A Theory of Consciousness*

In 3-D or familiar "reality," noticing Light out of the corner of our eye, getting chills or goosebumps as we see, feel or hear something out of the ordinary is sensing the 4th dimension. We may experience an aura or living field such as those presented in energy field or Kirlian Photography, or we may get an intuitive "hit." Haven't you had the experience of thinking about someone just before they call, write, appear or you hear about them? This is a 4th dimensional experience. 4-D is the gateway to 5-D, where we access a "Lighter," more creative, flowing state of Being connected with the Heart.

We naturally access the 4th dimension in twilight states of sleeping, dreaming, meditating, or receiving extra-sensory messages. It is the realm of the paranormal where we experience expanded self, through telepathy, intuition, pre-cognizance, normal dream state, lucid dreaming, synchronicity and psychic phenomena. *In 5-D we enter full awareness of a higher Vibrational state, waking Presence interwoven with pure Awareness of our continual interchange with the Field.* As Penny Kelly relates, these perceptions are a window into a fuller experience of Oneness.

It has been demonstrated that telepathic ability is native to everyone, an Innate sixth sense that accesses information beyond ordinary 3-D. Our level of awareness depends upon exposure as well as internal encouragement to deepen. Allowing ourselves to notice what we sense, is a playful way to stick out our "big toe" to test the waters of the 4th dimension. Opening through the Heart we receive this information from other dimensions.

> It appears that the heart is involved in the processing and decoding of intuitive information. Once the prestimulus information is received in the psychophysiologic systems, it appears to be processed in the same way as conventional sensory input. This study presents compelling evidence that the body's perceptual apparatus is continuously scanning the future.
>
> *Rollin McCraty, HeartMath Institute*
> *PubMed.gov: Electrophysiological Evidence of Intuition:*
> *Part 1. The surprising role of the heart*

Some naturally see auras or Light *Fields* surrounding Living things. Others sense them, which is called clairsentience; still others access altered states with herbs or shamanic journeys. With a good teacher most can learn to access intuitive perception, including psychic ability, telepathy, clairvoyance and clairaudience as well as remote viewing and seeing auras and energy *Fields.* Life is then absorbed in a much broader way, including what is present around us and that what is being transmitted on other levels.

Quantum research offers much evidence that multi-dimensional experiences and forgotten natural traits of this 6th sense are accessible to all. The military consistently trains for remote viewing (ability to "see" things at a distance or in another part of the World), requiring no particular special ability, only *playfulness.* Quantum research demonstrates that literally everyone has intuitive capabilities, perhaps suppressed and dormant due to age-old superstition. All this is the realm of the 4th dimension.

> Puthoff and Targ [researchers] were turning into believers. Human beings, talented or otherwise, appeared to have latent ability to see anywhere across any distance...the inescapable conclusion of their experiments was that anyone had the ability to do this...even those highly skeptical of the entire notion. The most important ingredient appeared to be a relaxed, even playful atmosphere...that was all, other than a little practice.
>
> *Lynne McTaggart*
> *The Field: Quest for the Secret Force of the Universe*

Cultivating extrasensory perceptions, we notice what we sense naturally and build awareness of *playing* in this expanded self, getting familiar with how to identify our intuitive sense. As we get more comfortable with 4th dimensional perceptions, we open further to access the flowing experience of the 5th dimension beyond spacetime.

In 5th dimensional heightened awareness, we tune in to the process of Creation flowing *through* us, waves of thought (conscious and unconscious) revealing manifestation through the *Field,* settling into form as particles of matter and events. Root of the word manifest means, that which is "obvious." *Manifesting* brings "that which is" into form.

The popular idea of "manifesting" is a bit more complex than we think. "Imaging something" with conscious mind to "call it in," does not take into consideration powerful effect of our unconscious resonance. Wishing for a million dollars or the love of your life rarely happens instantly. Our 95% unconscious thought is a stronger Vibration in the *Field* than our 5% conscious thought. Thoughts and emotions are "tuning forks," holding resonance in the *Field,* naturally magnetizing Creation into form. For clear manifestation to, we must first clear our unconscious of conflicting data (more in upcoming chapters).

Clear the unconscious and invite New Creation based in LOVE. *NOTICE* the waves coming from the *Field* shaping matter and events according to your resonance in this Now. When you find yourself thinking old stuck thoughts again like layers of the onion, cultivate consistent practice of releasing and letting go. Breathing, smiling and honoring all experiences with LOVE helps release the old, forever. We will dig more deeply into eye-opening miraculous tools, to Master making these shifts easy, as we continue our journey.

Structured 3-D may become constricting as we play in this creative, flowing existence. Recognizing that what comes into form is a total product of our resonance, it becomes difficult to go back totally to settling for 3-D expectations that things "just are the way they are." Find balance between these Worlds, enjoying the transition, observing Life unfolding in new ways. Notice how you are shifting, more comfortable to yield when the Universe urges "go." Say YES! to juicy inclinations and express more *Essence...* Believe it or not, this *is* the 5-D experience. Old global systems are now reformulating old paradigms to Mirror, compliment and align with *Where We're Going and Who We're Becoming.*

MISHLOVE: Isn't there also a backlash going on?

HOUSTON: Of course there is. I mean, whenever you are on the verge of so much more, people say, "Oooohhh, uummm, I don't think so. No, no, back to basics. Back to fundamentalist fortresses of truth." Back to sanctifying of mediocrity. And also the incredible yearning for a pattern that makes sense, and we are in a time when literally all systems are in transition. Everything has shaken down into chaos. Everything is breaking down, standard-brand governments, politics, economics, religions, relationships. We are probably in the greatest shake up in human history.

What we are seeing is the sunset effect, you know, the sun gets brighter and blazes out before it goes down, the sunset effect of all the traditional ways of knowing, seeing, being, and a rising of fundamentalism. I don't think that's going to last very long, because the world is simply too complex.

Jean Houston with Jeffrey Mishlove Ph.D.
Possible Human, Possible World Part I

Many children have imaginary friends or creative experiences, important to be encouraged by caregivers. A nephew, like many children, had imaginary friends for the first few years of his Life called Zig-sig and Pig-wig. They had regular conversations and interactions (allowed by wise parents). Eventually on a family trip as he got older, these "imaginary friends" traveled on the airplane wing and did not return. 4-5 D visitations are a natural exploration of many dimensions of experience available to us, activating creative thought, imagination and broadening a child's idea of possibility.

Playing with imagination in 4-5-D strengthens use of right brain, to access Greater Mind for problem solving and envisioning. As our pineal and pituitary glands are activated by nature's current cosmic influences, we are accessing more multi-dimensional experiences. We naturally spend part of Life in 4th and 5th dimensions, during lucid-dreaming and dream states, where we naturally expand and activate creative authentic self-expression, whether aware or not. Neurologically, right brain connects directly with the Heart, and through the Heart we experience these inner-dimensional states of Being.

> When you truly realize you are Soul, and, on a greater level, a fragment of All That Is, you begin to desire to fill your physical form with more and more Divine Light. You find yourself on a path of Mastery, ascending back home.
>
> *Bill Ballard*
> *The Great Awakening - pearls2u Youtube*

Our "dear brother" Bill Ballard, sensitive to other dimensions and realms of knowing from early childhood, remembered early how to flow between them. He easily opened this state later in Life when he was drawn from the conventional World, to return to his natural path as a Lightworker, focusing on Ascension. He eloquently shares this growth process in his book *The Great Awakening* (see Bibliography for download link). His primary focus is in multiple dimensions beyond 3-D, holding frequencies in these Higher Realms.

> We are simultaneously students and teachers going through the process of increasing the Light in our own fields and vibrating ever higher. We find ourselves relearning or remembering many things we knew and have always known, hidden deep within our Soul. Being with others of same or similar Vibration, helps us remember and unlock codes of understanding that raise us into ever higher awareness and states of ever-expanding consciousness.
>
> *Bill Ballard*
> *The Great Awakening - pearls2u Youtube*

It can be beneficial to current awakening to keep a favorite picture from childhood (of self or another) that activates good memories, infusing openness into our Now.

CARY 4-5-D EXPERIENCE: I was so blessed to grow up in the country, with great parents and wonderful brothers, where I felt trees, grass and living things a montage of light and color, attuned to music of birds, crickets and silently falling snow. The "outer" 3-D World always seemed foreign and structured to me, something I had to "squeeze" myself into. Participating in what was "expected," always took effort to pull myself from the "real" World where I actually "lived," the

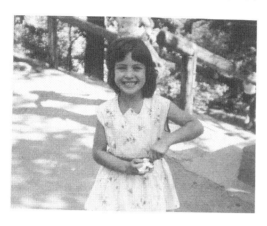

Inner Flowing Place where Nature and Spirit blended. It took years discover how to sustain this Mystical Connection from which I drew strength and my Deepest Creative Imagining.

Later connections with "Medicine Dogs" now with me in Spirit, BELOVED Maggie (woof woof! Gentle giant Anatolian-Black Lab), Daisy (Great Pyrenees-Golden Retriever), Hayduke (Golden Retriever) and Rama (Wolf-Malamute), Spirit (beautiful golden mutt) and several cats: Ninja, Stripe, Cassie and Wicket journeyed with me as "spirit guardians." Wilderness, snowboarding in deep powder, isolated mountains, remote river trips weeks on end, all sustained deep connection with finer dimensions. During coastal Ocean time with wild Dolphins at Dolphin Camp I co-developed, I swam with wild dolphins and consistently saw "Light not visible to the naked eye and heard celestial music." Being in diverse magnificent Wild Places, immersed in Mother Nature has always increased my sensitivity to staying present in other dimensions a thousandfold.

*A heightened sense of Sacred in all things goes everywhere with me Now. Sometimes I see things and often feel them. Einstein's statement, **Imagination is more powerful than knowledge** changed my Life forever. It helped me recognize the value of my Creative Mind, feelings and images left brain might have discounted. These days imagination and knowledge Dance. I am grateful for*

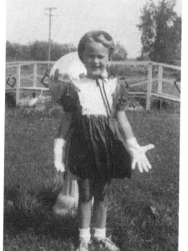

the blending of these two aspects that carry me through currents of Life! ♥ *Cary* ♥

TEDDI - 4-5-D EXPERIENCE: When I was small I saw energy around trees, animals, flowers and people. I told my mom, "That flower is really pretty. It has a sunshine around it." Mom would say, "I don't see it but I'm glad you do." It didn't seem like a gift it just seemed normal to me.

We wrote a book in school called the Voice of the River. We were instructed to sit by the river and let the river tell us a story. Each child listened to the river and reported back. We experienced Indians on the banks of the Grand River with birchbark canoes and lumber coming down for lumbermen to build our community. It seemed natural to me to be talking to our ancestors. We were fortunate as children to have such an insightful teacher who encouraged us to do such an exercise. Although she probably was not aware of it, she was teaching us to look into Life from 4-D.

Today I look back at the gift of being raised as an only child, and how fortunate I was to be born into a family supportive of childhood imaginings. It gave me opportunity to develop natural perceptions of other realms, that have continued to serve higher growth and development throughout my Life. ♥ *Teddi* ♥

Flowing between dimensions differs from what we're traditionally taught in school or the 3-D World. Trust your inner voice and respond from the Heart to intuitive messages. When a "bubble" Not of LOVE rises, Breathe, Smile, release, let go to restore the Presence of LOVE, perpetuating most Intuitive, Heart Centered Ways of BEING.

Insight is not a lightbulb that goes off inside our heads.
It is a flickering candle that can easily be snuffed out.

Malcom Gladwell
Blink: The Power Of Thinking Without Thinking,

It's an art to learn to heed our Intuition when it shows up, as its messages can be subtle particularly at first. Both men and women can learn to honor this receptive "Feminine" quality, expressing gentle inner strength and confidence to guide the Life. Mystery-suspense author Dean Koontz says, "Intuition is seeing with the Soul." Madeleine L'Engle, author of *A Wrinkle in Time* says, "Don't try to comprehend with your mind. Your mind is very limited. Use your intuition."

I believe in intuitions and inspirations...
I sometimes FEEL that I am right.
I do not KNOW that I am.

Albert Einstein (1879-1955)
Nobel Prize Physics, Max Planck Medal

It is a big leap to comprehend that how we focus within plays a key role in shaping what we experience around us. Letting go old layers to dwell in the Presence of LOVE, changes us forever to access Intuitive, expanded states of Being. How do we make this practical in our World? In order to enter into this flowing state how do we free ourselves from structures of time and space so dominant in our 3-D culture? Let's consider these questions and more.

Beyond the Myth of Time -
What would it be like to live beyond time?...The problem, in brief, is that time may not exist at the most fundamental level of physical "reality." If so, then what is time? And why is it so obviously and tyrannically omnipresent in our own experience?

June 2007 Discover Magazine
Newsflash: Time May Not Exist, Not to mention the question of which way it goes...

Imagine that in a surreal way, we like Alice in Wonderland are caught in a World that only *seems* very real. Waking up from this *dream*, we realize we've followed *clocks* to make every move, and they are not even tracking time, they are just counting ticks! Is there another way to live beyond time that is just now dawning upon us?

Once upon a "time," in the long, long ago, someone Created clocks, as a form of "reporting in." Earliest methods of marking time were sticks in the ground that eventually became sundials, tracking the movement of the sun through the sky and seasons. Earliest clocks as we know them were Created in the 1400's during the Middle Ages for reporting to work, family or military assignment, keeping the masses a well-managed workforce.

Newton believed time could be measured outside the Universe but this has been proven false. To our *great* surprise, according to modern Quantum views *time does not exist* apart from the Universe! *There is no clock ticking outside the cosmos.* Most of us have thought of time as Newton did: "Absolute, true and mathematical, time of itself and from its own nature flows equably without regard to anything external."

Einstein discovered instead, that time is part of the fabric of the Universe. Contrary to what Newton believed, our ordinary clocks do not measure something independent of the Universe. Clocks don't really measure time at all. They simply mark the ticks. *Wow!*

I recently went to the National Institute of Standards and Technology in Boulder, Colorado (government lab that houses atomic clock that standardizes time for the nation). I said something like, 'Your clocks measure time very accurately.' They told me, 'Our clocks do not measure time.' I thought, 'Wow, that's very humble of these guys.' But they said, 'No, time is defined to be what our clocks measure.' Which is true. They define the time standards for the globe: Time is defined by the number of clicks of their clocks.

June 2007 Discover Magazine
Newsflash: Time May Not Exist, Not to mention the question of which way it goes...

So, clocks do not actually measure time at all, they simply count the ticks. Do you just want to cry? Or laugh? Or do you wonder, "What have I been doing following a clock all these years?" Lewis Carroll's frenetic White Rabbit, taking his Watch out of his waistcoat pocket says, *"Oh dear, oh dear, I'll be late!"* and then pops down the large *rabbit hole* under the hedge with Alice tumbling after... Does his rant sound like anyone you know???

"I'm late, I'm late, for a very important date!
No time to lose, hello, goodbye,
I'm late, I'm late, I'm late!"

A century ago, Einstein's theory of relativity banished time as a Universal constant, presenting that past, present and future are not absolute. The Wheeler-DeWitt theory suggests integrating relativity and Quantum mechanics, with the idea that fundamentally the Universe must be timeless. Most physicists believe that ultimately a Universe where there is no time will be part of the blending of Relativity and Quantum Theories.

Brilliant German physicist Burkhard Heim (1925-2001) who could be regarded as a German Stephen Hawking, left the Max Planck Institute in 1954 due to an accident that took his sight, hearing and both hands, after which he worked in seclusion. He discovered the "unified mass formula," considered to be the *Holy Grail of natural science*.

Fellow physicist wrote in his memoriam, "Germany has lost one of its greatest thinkers and in terms of his scientific results, one of the most successful physicists after Heisenberg," (one of the key creators of Quantum mechanics). Biophysicist Dieter Broers' *highly* respected Heim, and shares in his book *Solar Revolution* a comprehensive overview of Burkhard Heim's *World model* describing *twelve* dimensions.

> Holistic unity of a conscious human being consists of the following [12 dimensions]: Terrestrial Space 1-3; Time 4; Structured Space 5-6; Information Space 7-8; Over space 9-12.

> The visible and measurable world...consists of...length, width, and height, plus time...for without time no change would occur. Time is also considered a physical dimension and...fourth dimension...is space-time...

> [These four dimensions are] in turn embedded in a more complex realm known as...Hyperspace, dimensions 5-6. What we refer to as matter is...controlled by the...mind, which...controls the material world.

This is far beyond where most of us are used to thinking or conceiving of our world, so it may take a bit to even absorb this. Even if you can grasp a bit of it, Heim's amazing observations give scientific perspective on experiencing our world much more expansively than we have commonly thought.

Heim through Broers goes on to explain that "matter is a product of the projection of Vibration into six-dimensional space, whose effects are felt in four-dimensional space... dimensions 5-6 serve as structuring space, dimensions 7-8 are information space [Akasha]. Dimensions 9-12 he labels God-space - from where Creation emerges. He associates the 'state of cosmic being' with dimensions 5-6, 7-8 and 9-12.

> Sentient beings continuously receive and transmit...information that is exchanged by these dimensions. The level of consciousness...determines the quality and potentiality of this information and access to it.

> *Dieter Broers*
> *Solar Revolution*

Broers states that the human mind extracts information from higher dimensions, and by observing the physicality Created, is able to gauge the quality of its mental projections. Another perspective of our Quantum model - observe what is showing up in the "reality" around us, and it will teach us how we need to shift and grow as it is a perfect Mirroring of the resonance within.

Ram Dass brought forth a perennial great philosophy of Living in *'No-Time'* in his 1971 book inspired by enlightened master Maharajji Neem Karoli Baba, from whom *"laughter, bliss and peace poured down on us..."*

Be Here Now...

Power of Now by Eckhart Tolle offers becoming an "observer" in Now, all else falls away, outside time and space. Simon Saunders, physics professor at University of Oxford says, "The meaning of time has become terribly problematic in contemporary physics. The possibility that time may not exist is recognized in physics as, *'The problem of time.'*"

The idea that the Universe is continuing to expand from the Big Bang Theory, may be the origin of what we think of as time, however there is no clock ticking outside the Cosmos making time absolute, and Einstein proved that time is part of the fabric of the Universe rather than a procession through it. It may come from the idea of entropy of a Universe ever-expanding that the endless march of time originated.

When Einstein's Lifelong friend Michele Besso died, he wrote a letter to the family that impacted the physics community forever. "Now he has departed from this strange World a little ahead of me. That means nothing. People like us, who believe in physics, know the distinction between past, present, and future is only a stubbornly persistent illusion."

Carlo Rovelli, French physicist at the University of Marseille and advocate of a timeless Universe, comments further on negligibility of time and space:

> We never really see time, we see only clocks...We say we measure time with clocks, but we see only the hands of the clocks, not time itself...
>
> In Quantum mechanics all particles of matter and energy can be described as waves. And waves have an unusual property: An infinite number of them can exist *in the same location.* If time and space are one day shown to consist of quanta, the quanta could all exist piled together in a single dimensionless point. Space and time in some sense melt in this picture. There is no space anymore. There are just quanta, kind of living on top of one another without being immersed in space.
>
> It is an issue that many theorists have puzzled about. It may be that the best way to think about Quantum "reality" is to give up the notion of time—that the fundamental description of the Universe must be timeless.

June 2007 Discover Magazine
Newsflash: Time May Not Exist, not to mention the question of which way it goes...

It is a strange feeling, how differently our Universe is made up than we've thought. How we've lived for thousands of years is dissolving before us... It's a huge Leap to move into this New paradigm, though Leaping we are! Live beyond time whenever you can! You may say, "I have 3-D commitments; I'm bound to time." We have lived so long with this view that we believe it to be true. Activate new brain cells, wrap your mind around 'No-Time,' let it flow through your Heart. Practice being in the 'No-Time' Continuum' and let it unfold... *Isn't this the reason we LOVE to go on Vacation? Of course, and it's quite Freeing!*

> ...the Eternal Now or Centre Point from which all time-zones radiate to infinity...is instantaneously in touch with all that any time zone embraces throughout eternity, having no beginning or end.

Murry Hope (1929-2012)
The Lion People

Discovering timelessness accelerates our **21st Century Superhuman** adventure. Free of time, creative Essence flows more generously, far beyond where it does in structured "reality." That we emerge as waves from the *Field* becomes more apparent, as we float through "mists of time" as did great seekers of the Grail Quest.

When we are in touch with our own essence, we break through the time barrier because this essence of our lives exceeds time and space concepts.

Chris Griscom
Time Is An Illusion

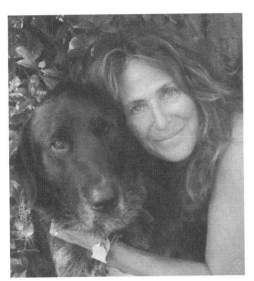

CARY - ON TIME - *Years ago a book called, "Time, Space and Beyond," explained Quantum physics in simple terms with cartoon graphics. That book was worn to shreds. It stretched my mind into new dimensions, that remain with me today. For years, I repeated to myself a principle revealed there, till it made sense, "There is no such thing as time or space and all things are happening concurrently." These days I find myself quite comfortable outside illusionary structures of time and space.*

Dr. John Ray used to tell us to be "In the Ever Present Now." Once this is accepted, we discover we are in parallel Universes at the same time...wow! It's one thing to hear it, and another to take it into our experience. I'm on the journey of integrating this level of Being. I have fun exploring it with Beloved four-leggeds, Maggie, Daisy, Rama and Hayduke, who walk with me Now in spirit.

Remember how it took 1,000 years for human culture to let go of the idea "that the World was flat?" We're on a faster track today, with internet and wireless communications creating a "global brain." It may take just one quick shift to fully embrace Quantum possibilities... and THAT'S what Quantum "reality" is all about!!! ♥ *Cary* ♥

TEDDI - ON TIME - *Time is an illusory concept of the 3-D World. It was constructed to keep order. Everyone can "jump-time..." Practice by Breathing deeply and trusting what you choose to experience.*

Many are Now recognizing that there is more to Life than just being physical or achieving success on societal levels. Many have come to know that the image they've presented to the 3-D World no longer fulfills them. They may feel restless inside long

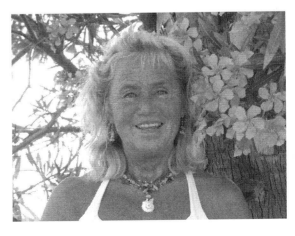

before they have answers for how to proceed into change. This stirring comes from their very Soul...asking to be "realized" deep inside... It comes as either a gentle awakening, or as such an intense feeling that they absolutely MUST change everything about their lives.

I have personally been through this "awakening process" as I reached levels in my own Life. Perceiving other dimensions and listening to intuition more deeply, I discovered how energies work to transform our World. Participating in multidimensional "realities" amplifies our choices and response to self and World.

*Chris Griscom writes in **Time Is An Illusion**, "When we are in touch with our own essence, we break through the time barrier, because this essence of our lives exceeds time and space concepts... At the onset we realize past and present are not separated. We discontinue using these purely linear concepts as a means of experiencing our reality."*

Once we have experientially accepted this new way of relating to "no-time," our Consciousness is transformed. We are no longer restricted to one-dimension, one-form, one-time. ♥ Teddi ♥

In the *'No - Time' Continuum* we are able to travel into the past and remove all Not of LOVE, by holding LOVE in that situation. We can Arc of Light and LOVE into the Future to Prepare the Way, and into the Past to clear the Past on all timelines! Operating outside time, "points of interest" may request restoration to the frequency of LOVE. By holding LOVE in past, present and future situations in 'No - Time,' we clear Not of LOVE events and *establish New timelines*. This is an entirely new perception of "reality" offered by Quantum physics.

Time is the moving image of eternity.

Plato (427 B.C.- 347 B.C.)
Founder of the Academy of Athens

Within this perspective we hold negative in one hand and positive in the other, with equal LOVE for both, thus altering timelines, history and possible futures, as we realign in this energy of Creation. Some experience it as past and future pouring into the Now, and as we hold LOVE in the Now, past and future are reborn. *21st Century Superhumans* are imbuing history with LOVE, shifting the Future NOW.

In her book, the *Intention Experiment*, Lynn McTaggart sites a prayer study done with 4,000 people in a fever epidemic. Among those prayed for there were less deaths; notably as well, those prayed for recovered in fewer days than those who weren't. Curiously enough, this prayer study took place **6-10 years *after*** the fever epidemic happened!

We invite you to practice until it is second nature to cast an Arc of LOVE to places, "times" and people you are guided to (like a lifeline). There are no accidents, only lessons, awareness and realizations. Timeless 5-D is a great way to Live in our Holographic World, as we "wake up" in this Evolutionary Leap. We can shift history with parents, grandparents, generations, wars, abuse and other events with LOVE. Think of a past event based in Not of LOVE, sickness or loss of a loved one. Focus LOVE to heal or clear that event or situation through timespace. This may take some practice as it is a New way of Being. As we familiarize ourselves with holding a *Field* of LOVE in all situations, we experience them shifting through "no-time." The biggest secret of all this is that the real place things shift is *inside us*. As we shift our vibration to LOVE, ALL "realities" change through timespace, which we are learning to traverse easily and quickly.

Dr. Wayne Dyer, psychotherapist, lecturer, and World–famous author says it well in his title, *You'll See It When You Believe It*. Essential Quantum understanding teaches us that rather than worrying about a news story or situation, we remove Attention from it. Then place Attention on what we choose to call into form with LOVE, as [if] it *IS* already [happening]. Practice with a situation you've been "concerned" about lately. As you completely let go of your concern and move into LOVE, the situation will fall out of form.

We Breathe, Smile and hold the *Field* with LOVE, knowing it is done, giving what we desire opportunity to flow into Creation. Nothing is good or bad it simply *is*, and is a biofeedback or Mirroring of what's inside us. As we shift our Attention on the *Field*, we call forth new frequency patterns that Arc the entire Hologram of our "reality."

> There is no matter as such. All matter originates and exists only by virtue of a force which brings the particle of an atom into vibration and holds this most minute solar system of the atom together. We must assume behind this force the existence of a conscious and intelligent mind. The mind is the matrix of all matter.
>
> *Max Planck (1858-1947)*
> *Originator of Quantum Theory, Nobel Prize Physics 1918*

The concept that thought or consciousness has the capability of "creating" everything in our "reality" is outrageous! Miracles occur as we practice this "technology" of *"asking"* in such a way that the *Field* fulfills our conscious request. Follow the steps in the Exercises below. **Arc the Hologram** by holding Attention on the *Field* with awareness, activating it with LOVE.

21ST CENTURY SUPERHUMAN ASSIGNMENT: *Be of Good Cheer. You are watched over, you are guided. You are LOVED dearly. Everything has unfolded perfectly, and now that you are waking up, you are able to change affects, intents and purposes. At the level of the Divine or Source, all that exists is LOVE. As we remove Attention from everything else it falls out of form, and only LOVE remains. Actualizing this is our "assignment" as* **21st Century Superhumans**.

> This awareness process can be compared to a stone falling into water, releasing concentric wave circles. Our consciousness and perceptions expand to experience amplified dimensions and scenarios, and by practicing perception and assimilation of these realities, time loses its influence on us.
>
> *Chris Griscom*
> *Time Is An Illusion*

ARCING THE Hologram: Okay, **21st Century Superhuman**s, enough theory. Shall we use our Newly-honed skills to make Quantum Shifts in our World? Let's "Arc the Hologram" Now with *"interdimensional potential of multidimensionality,"* as Chris Griscom says!

Affirm the following - Breathe and Smile...

- I ask without judgment or hidden motive
- I Now clear, cancel, release, let go all unconscious resonance
- I Am in touch with my *Essence*
- I Am a Being of *Pure LOVE, COMPASSION & GRATITUDE*
- Time is an illusionary ripple
- Dimensions exist concurrently at different frequencies (parallel Universes)

The list above contains clear steps for shifting our "reality." Use this list for reference until these skills become second nature. All emerges from a Hologram in the *'No-Time'* *Continuum.* Immerse each item below in the *Field* of Pure LOVE, following steps above. *Arc the Hologram,* transforming items on list below *with pure LOVE to change them Forever.*

World Wars • Holocaust of World War II • Decimation of Native Americans • Any and all genocides throughout history • Living Sacrifices Inca Empire • 9/11 • Current News Stories • Global Governments • World Banking, Natural Disasters • Weather • Fukushima • Earthquakes • Terrorist Activity • Poverty • Starvation, • Ignorance • Abuse • Environmental Dishonor • Factory Animal Farming • Personal Issues • Generational Issues • GMOs • You Fill in the Blank • Anything that bothers you past, present or future - **Enter the Hologram** with LOVE Now!

Settle into Deep LOVE, Compassion and Gratitude. Laugh, Breathe, Smile - dissolve the list above and all related illusions established in blame-fear-hostility-judgment-control. Shed the chrysalis and flap gentle wings into a New World defined and Created by LOVE.

Realizing there is no time "ticking away" as we have conceived it, we define it instead as a magnetic imprint of the movement of consciousness, that changes as we shift our perceptions. Global group, New Earth Nation has proposed a transitional plan for Zero Point Time, where the entire World follows one "marking of time," great new concept!

This Zero Point Time design will help humanity relate to the dynamics of spin and therefore have a better relationship to the fundamental laws of nature.

Nassim Haramein

They offer, *"Be the master of your time, not a slave to it.* We have disconnected from flow as a species with systems overlaid over natural cycles. Zero Point Time is a remedy; it has a single heartbeat at it's core, with rotation of the Earth beneath our feet, it is a primary connection to a wider Universe." We are literally moving out of linear time. It may take us a bit to grow into such revolutionary designations Planet-wide, yet as we do so, time-based "reality" mega-leaps into vibrant, scintillating New dimensions for us to play in. ♥

Chapter 11

Dimensional Doorways

They say: Think twice before you jump. I say:
Jump first and then think as much as you want!

Osho (1931-1990)
Indian Mystic, Teacher Self-Inquiry

Accelerated particles of Light in the Photon Belt, Solar flares, radio waves x and Gamma rays are Now bombarding us. This is speeding up molecules and naturally stimulating pineal-pituitary production of DMT the "spirit molecule," activating our Innate sense of *ONENESS with All that Is.*

Visionaries of these *interesting times,* describe this as a shift from 3rd into 4th and 5th dimensions and beyond. If it feels like things are accelerating, maybe they are. It's good to focus on what we desire, for in this intensified *Field* just a small shift of Attention puts us at a very different place on the shore.

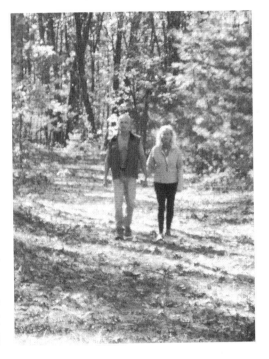

You must decide whether you are going to accept the inevitable in a state of LOVE and prepare yourself accordingly, or hold on in fear to the bitter end. Ultimately, these are the only two avenues of response. By the linear time this event takes place, humanity will be polarized according to these two adaptive patterns. All will be decidedly in one camp or the other.

Ken Carey
Starseed Transmissions

Clues in obscure pre-historical records suggest Ancient Puebloan, Mayan and other advanced cultures disappeared without a trace, possibly leaving via "dimensional doorways" into another plane of existence. We have little context to comprehend this in current views of "reality," yet this could be a very real possibility in the Quantum World, where parallel Universes are concurrent and timespace is shape-shifting!

Becoming more "awake" and moving our focus into the Heart is called the "Ascension" process. It does not necessarily mean we are going to rise up and disappear, although we could, and well may have at other times in history. According to prophecies, Now rather than leaving this dimension, we are transforming our entire existence into a higher Vibrational state. What exactly does this mean?

Accelerated particles of Light are activating us to shift into Living from Heart rather than the "head." Restoring LOVE as our primary operating system is key to the very nature of our existence becoming less dense and this "Ascension" process occurring. Knowing how our thoughts Create leverages us into more proactive creatorship. As our Vibration increases, perceptions shift, and we flow through a World that is transforming *as we are.*

> You incarnated here and now to experience rapid Soul growth via a duality learning process. Everyone knows something is "going on" at this time. It is no longer a secret... Everyone on Earth has a choice of Ascension...The one thing shared by this Universe with each individual fragment, is personal choice to experience as we choose. You can ascend - if that's what you choose - at your own pace.
>
> *Bill Ballard*
> *The Great Awakening*

Prophecies predicting a *New Earth* founded in Vibrational frequencies of LOVE permeate history. According to the Quantum model of parallel Universes, these realities could already potentially exist, without being visible to our current state of perception. This opens the door to explanation of how ancient cultures disappeared without a trace, with potential for similar to occur Now. Our ability to Live and Breathe LOVE imbues into our World particularly treasured frequency fields. Rather than such things being "supernatural," all "reality' is a direct result of the quality of our Attention on the *Field.*

> Ascension is going on in earnest. It cannot be stopped. Of course, as we activate at this dimensional level, we continue to play with balances within the duality. Individuals on the ascension path increasingly light up higher frequencies, while those in the lower fight to keep their powers and fourth dimensional control. This continues until the time of the dimensional shift, which is now guaranteed to occur.
>
> *Bill Ballard,*
> *The Great Awakening*

Adopting LOVE-Compassion-Gratitude as our "Laws of Living," freeing ourselves from blame-fear-hostility habits, we potentially Ascend into a higher frequency parallel Universe in 4-5 D *(and beyond),* described in Wisdom teachings throughout the ages as *New Earth.* We are thus response-able for a co-evolution process with our Earth Mother, Gaia or Pachamama (Earth as a Living Being). One author describes their breathtaking vision of Earth's ascension process this way:

The words you have will not describe the ecstatic explosion, nor can you imagine how you will all be in that time, when every atom and molecule on this planet and the whole planet herself will radiate with Divine Light. Such exquisite beauty is beyond imagining.

P'taah via Jani King, Act of Faith
spiritwritings.com

As we practice *Arcing the Hologram* (earlier chapter), we become aware of shifting to LOVE in all situations. Previously challenging circumstances fall away from consciousness as *we* make this dimensional shift. A Course In Miracles tells us that anything Not of LOVE is part of the Illusion, when focused clearly in LOVE all else will fall away.

Those with activated Heart chakras are now playing by 5th dimensional rules. Our creative powers are returning and our manifestation capabilities are almost instantaneous. We are above the levels of duality and are no longer being affected by those Vibrational events around us. We are in a 3-D / 4-D world, but not of it.

Bill Ballard
The Great Awakening

An easy way to access shifting dimensions (or dementias as we laughingly like to call it) and Ascension, is to simply notice when we experience various states of being, some dense, others more flowing. This post from Kelly La Sha offers valuable perspective on accessing such experiences.

Within the last few years, Ascension has become a very hot topic that has stirred up and brought forth many of our fears and self-doubts. To make matters worse, there are fear-based messages out there that suggest that you don't have what it takes to Ascend… unless you take a workshop or practice a complicated technique to prepare yourself.

Ascensions are not designed to be complicated for the ascenders. Ascensions are designed to assure that all imbalances are harmonized and all Souls are reconnected to Source and their sovereignty. God / We Created this project of chaos for Souls to experience separation from Source, and the Ascension is designed to reset the balance.

Anyone that tells you that it is more complicated than that has an agenda that doesn't include your highest good. The simplicity of the Ascension is the most beautiful and fulfilling part.. *It is our reconnection with Source."*

Kelly La Sha
Liquid Mirror Blog

As we awaken into this mysterious World lit by Quantum theory, grasping our Infinite power as Observer-Creators emerging in LOVE, old falls away like a baby chick hatching out of its egg or a butterfly emerging from the chrysalis. As we dedicate Body-Mind-Heart to Pure Conscious Creation, with thought-emotion based in LOVE, Miracles unfold in everyday Life. Once aligned with LOVE, all that is Not of LOVE falls away. With Heart as our "tuning fork," we reset our Vibration to LOVE. The Miraculous becomes a natural part of everyday Life. We expect Miracles and they automatically appear.

Miracles occur naturally as expressions of LOVE. The real miracle is the LOVE that inspires them. In this sense everything that comes from LOVE is a miracle.

Chapter 1:1-1.3 The Meaning of Miracles
A Course in Miracles® by the Foundation for Inner Peace

Everything that exists in our World comes from and is a Vibrational expression. The more we grow into recognizing this, the more we learn from the feedback of "reality" appearing around us. Lighter frequencies of LOVE in Mind and Heart elevate us beyond 3-D, and our molecules spin faster at these higher Frequencies. *Playing* with these seemingly outrageous concepts of Quantum physics helps integrate them.

As a Soul, you descend into the world of form, moving through its many phases and learning it's lessons. You then return into the ONENESS of ALL, bringing with you a completeness, a fulfillment, a knowingness, which could be gained no other way. Having come into the world of form, it is only through DESIRE and WILL that one raises him-herself back into the higher levels of consciousness...

It is only by Spiritual Desire and Will that the Earth plane is transcended and one moves into unfoldment in higher dimensions. Knowing this LAW, you begin to understand the operation of polarity in all dimensions.

Nellie B. Cain
Exploring the Mysteries of Life, 30 Years Research

Caught up in speedy beta-brain waves, a whirlpool of 3-D worry and concern, wondering how things will be taken care of, we call our doubt into form and limit ourselves from experiencing Greater possibilities. When we drop this chatter of Mind, and remove our ancient programing and filters, we open to the flow of *Infinite Possibilities of the Field, Greater Mind* and the *Divine Matrix*, conscious of how our resonance draws everything into our World. We enter 4-5D where desires, plans, hopes and dreams are fulfilled in miraculous ways, solutions appearing as if out of thin air.

Breathing, smiling, relaxing into *Essence*, trusting that our Hearts are One with Divine Flow, causes events take place at an entirely new level, with circumstances changing easily on our behalf. Realigning with Deep LOVE, Gratitude and Compassion, we resonate with harmonics or wavelengths of energy frequencies of 4th and 5th dimensions.

As we **21st Century Superhumans** enter this New Quantum World, Breathing and Smiling *literally* assist us to move between dimensions. Removing filters and limiting beliefs expands access to Greater Mind. As we easily and joyfully shift into Greater expression of self, soaring with the flow of Life, we enter New Dimensions, simply by entering higher Vibrational awareness of Mind and Heart. ♥

Chapter 12

Phase Shifting

...Creation is the product of synchronizing our energy with the Universe.
Once we experience the whole and recognize it, we become aware that we are
nothing but the Divine Creative Force...

Freydoon Rassouli
Visionary Artist -Fusionart, Bridging International Healing Art Project

Aligning with pure *Essence and* exploring 4-5 D can activate desire to make changes in relationships, job, home, location or whatever our lives are focused around. More Loving we remain through these inner shifts, the easier it is for those around us to adapt, and for us to make ecological, all inclusive Heart-based choices.

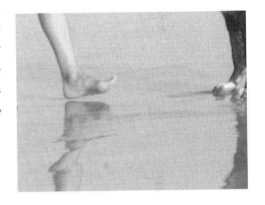

What lies before us and what lies behind us are small matters compared to what lies within us. And when we bring what is within out into the world, miracles happen.

Henry Stanley Haskins
Wall Street 1940

Moving into the Heart, and taking Response-Ability for all Creations in our "reality," letting go of blame-fear-hostility-judgement-control, helps us relate to others from the most Loving place possible. The more we dwell in our Hearts, continue to Breathe and Smile, knowing that all around us is a result of the Vibration carried within us, transitions are kindly and easily navigated, while sustaining Loving relationships. Operating from the Heart is the most profound shift we make, to maintain cooperative spirit, supporting better interactions with all. Releasing the idea of separateness we realize we we are All One.

A human being is a part of the whole called by us Universe, a part limited in time and space. He experiences himself, his thoughts and feeling as something separated from the rest, a kind of optical delusion of his consciousness.

Albert Einstein (1879-1955)
Nobel Prize Physics

Connecting with *Essence* refines focus, aligning our path with natural talents and abilities to bring forth our greatest gifts. In this newfound expression, moments we completely Ascend 3-D, absorbed in creative expression. Higher dimensional experiences are commonly accessed during right brain engagement, such as art, music, fishing, hiking, walking, running, playing, gardening, most athletic pursuits, drumming, dancing, sex and lucid dreaming. This brings about phase-shifting, where we move between expanded and contracted "reality" states, operating in multiple dimensions at once.

> Being in the 3-D & 4-D world but not of it, must be experienced to be understood. It requires ascending above fear-based patterning to realize you can be in the middle of the chaos and not be affected by it. Lower frequency manipulations continue to affect individuals vibrating at lower consciousness levels, while individuals resonating at higher levels, walk right through the chaos unscathed. It is a very interesting thing to experience.
>
> *Bill Ballard*
> *The Great Awakening*

J.J. Hurtak, Founder of Academy for Future Science, was transported through multiple myriad dimensions of "reality," and composed a complex but fascinating blueprint from coded information he was given, titled *The Book of Knowledge: The Keys of Enoch,* for the "quickening of the People of Light." Carol Matthews, professional ally wrote, "His work reflects extensive findings of astrophysics and promotion of cumulative understanding of all great religions. The Keys are musical keys of knowledge for the Soul."

> Quantum changes will affect every level of intelligence on the planet... We now have the opportunity to move collectively into another system of creation..
>
> *J. J. Hurtak*
> *Keys of Enoch*

In 3-D "reality" the World is "solid, secure, tangible, consistent" and feels "safe" because of familiarity, based in thousands of years of agreed upon collective thought. Quantum physics exposed tantalizing New perspectives on our World over 100 years ago! The Double Slit Experiment revealed how thoughts Create "reality," offering a clearly lit path to Living with focused intent. How do we leap from thinking "reality" emerges from "out there," when in truth it emerges from "in here?" Perception of self and World expands exponentially as we explore this way of Being. Extraordinary bliss of elevated Vibration awaits us, with courage to pursue our dreams rather than forfeiting *Essence* for status quo.

> I was exhilarated by the new realization that I could change the character of my Life by changing my beliefs. I was instantly energized because I realized that there was a science-based path that would take me from my job as a perennial "victim" to my new position as "co-creator" of my destiny.
>
> *Bruce H. Lipton*
> *Biology of Belief*

In *Solar Revolution,* biophysicist Dieter Broers reveals that our exposure highly intensified Solar and Cosmic activity is giving birth to a New age, "...boosting our brain capacity and expanding our minds in ways we never imagined possible." Major music and literary works were historically Created in presence of electromagnetic field disturbances. As Solar activity intensifies and Earth's atmosphere is exposed to unusually high amounts of Cosmic rays, signs increase that a spectacular Evolutionary Leap may be imminent.

> And so it's no surprise that most of us sense an accelerating planetary transition is underway. What this fateful epoch has in store for us is already plain for all to see. Virtually all of the unusual phenomena we are currently witnessing on Earth regarding climate, economy and the psyche is related to changes in electromagnetic fields, as well as to elevated levels of cosmic radiation. The speed and intensity of this process is set to increase in the near future.

> However, the extent to which these major changes pose a threat to us mainly hinges on the kind of knowledge we have at our disposal. If for example, we take at face value the shrill warnings of certain scientists and panderers to base (and baseless!) fears, we will be helpless and defenseless if the evidence they predict does indeed come to pass. But on the other hand, if we can grasp the principle that we are about to embark on a monumental process of transformation, we will be able to face what this process of quickening metamorphosis has in store for us calmly and without any anxiety or hysteria whatsoever...

> I've come to realize that the transition to a "next age" predicted by ancient cultures such as the Mayans will be marked by an evolutionary leap that will bring with it a new form of consciousness and harmony.

Dieter Broers, Biophysicist
Solar Revolution: Why Mankind is on the Cusp of an Evolutionary Leap

Moving into the Heart, Quantum fluidity elevates us beyond 3-D into 4th and 5th dimensions. This resonance shifts the Collective and amplifies LOVE, where critical mass tips the scales in phase shifts that accelerate change exponentially.

LET "Reality" FALL OUT OF FORM: Play with it. Go about your day and sense the molecules that make you up. Be aware that less than 1% of you is solid, the other 99.999% is *Space*. Breathe and Smile, notice that when you let go of what you are so attached to, it can fall out of form and emerge again in New Ways. Breathe and Smile. *Let Mind and Heart play!*

> A serious man cannot laugh, cannot dance, cannot play. He is always controlling himself, he has become a jailer to himself... Laughter brings your energy back to you... People who are happy, contented, are not the people to kill other people who have not done any harm to them... Have you ever watched in your own being — when you are happy, joyful, you want to Create something.

> This crisis gives a chance for courageous people to disconnect themselves from the past and start living in a new way — not modified, not continuous with the

past, not better than the past, but absolutely new. And it has to be done now – because the time is very short...

Osho
The Divine Sound That Is The Truth

Our Newly found awareness that we are all One, moves us to reflect Deep LOVE-Gratitude-Compassion for all situations. We Dance, Fly, Breathe, Smile, Laugh, Leap for Joy... Spinning, Playing, Rejoicing as we enter a Lighter state of Being...

At that moment, the rest of humanity will experience an instantaneous transformation of a proportion you cannot now conceive. At that time, the spell which was cast on your race thousands of years ago, when you plunged into the worlds of good and evil, will be shattered forever.

Ken Carey
Starseed Transmissions

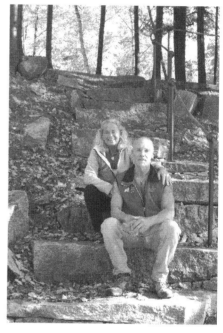

Upon meeting others, make smiling eye contact, Breathe and send them your Heart's radiance. There is a great likelihood they will return the smile, receive the feeling of honoring, acceptance and LOVE, relaying it wherever they go. This is such an easy and natural way to resonate Heart-connection into the World, a game of tag, "you're it," without it having to be intellectual or a thought process. Just such a simple practice can Create huge changes for us on the inside, as our gift to the World that will come back to us a thousandfold in the outer.

The dance goes from realizing that you're separate (which is the awakening), to then find your way back into the totality of which you are not only a part, but which you are.

Ram Dass
Be Here Now

Let go of blaming others, Living in ways that take Response-Ability for Creation of your experience! *How exciting is this!* Know that your life is a continual flow of your choice of thought-Mind energy. In a transformational flow of LOVE-Compassion-Gratitude, we dissipate any feeling of "separateness," to discover Joy in moments of continuous connection with self and others. This is phase-shifting between dimensions, when a natural sense of Oneness with All that Is flows in us, permeating our radiance in the World. ♥

Chapter 13

Change is Afoot

The measure of intelligence is our ability to change.
Creativity is intelligence having fun.

Albert Einstein (1879-1955)
Nobel Prize Physics (1921), Max Planck Medal (1929)

T he Mayan Calendar marks we are at the end of an "age," entering a new Cosmic cycle, transiting through a location in space we reach cyclically once in 26,000 years, and grander cycles of millions of years. Increased Gamma, x-rays and Light photons activate potential for powerful Awakening in this amazing Evolutionary Leap called by the Ancients the *Shift of the Ages*.

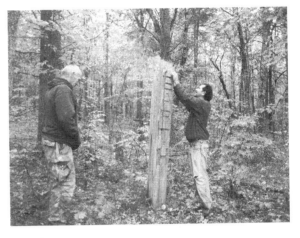

This amazing moment in Galactic history, whether we are aware of it or not, is playing a pivotal role in elevating our lives to New levels. At subtle levels we are atomically speeding up, and even tiniest choices can have a profound effect on the long term. Let go of being engrossed in moment-by-moment micro-demands of Life, to step up and notice most important reasons for our existence. Cultivate consistent prayerful thought as manifestation can be instant. Clear direction through Heart and Soul are available to us from Source. Call in guidance and you will receive. Current understanding gives us phenomenal opportunity to free ourselves from ancient debilitating programs, waking up with jaw-dropping awareness to *who we are, why we're here and where we're going.*

Remember the song, "It is the dawning of the *Age of Aquarius?*...peace will guide the planets, and LOVE will steer the stars... Harmony and understanding, sympathy and trust abound," written by the 5th Dimension! Uplifting and exciting, its lyrics project directly to where we are Now! We have entered the enlightened Age of Aquarius, with its futuristic and awakening influences on the horizon at spring equinox for the next 2,000 years.

The Aquarian Age is the beginning of the earth's transmutation, in which each Soul finds his/her True IDENTITY and purpose and then lives to be the Perfect Channel for the Expression of Divine Light and LOVE. Man will come to know himself to be an Eternal, ever progressing, Soul who is not limited to the earth's frequency, but is a Universal Being, who will find himself expressing throughout the ages upon an infinite number of planets and galaxies as he grows in consciousness and vibratory frequency.

Man is but an infant in the Cosmic Scale of Being, and he must traverse the many pathways of Life to reach his fulfillment. This can be a glorious and happy experience if it is approached with the spirit of adventure. But if one does not catch a glimpse of the Great Adventure, Life can be very dull and frustrating, and much time can be wasted in the mundane pursuit of materiality and satisfying the sensual nature.

Seek the Kingdom of Life and Light. Keep your feet steadfastly on the Pathway of Eternal Soul Unfoldment and be enraptured with the beauty of Life as it unfolds itself *in* you and reveals more of Itself *to* you!

Nellie B. Cain
Exploring the Mysteries of Life, 30 Years Research

Though she has "left the body" Nellie's wisdom inspires us today. We have entered an unprecedented opportunity to recognize ourselves as unlimited Eternal Creator Beings, with contact in higher dimensions and realms available to all.

Other influences linked with our 26,000 (25,920) year Galactic orbit offer insights on current status, issues and solutions. In Graham Hancock's documentary *Ancient Mysteries*, he reports the position of the three Giza Pyramids documents an exact astronomical period, identified in computer simulations as spring equinox 10,500 B.C. (approx. 6 precession cycles x 2150 years ago). Constellation Leo was on the horizon, the Nile River mirrored the Milky Way and the three Giza pyramids almost perfectly mirrored the Belt of Orion (by a few degrees). The Sphinx was built with a lion's head (before defaced), referencing Sirius and systems beyond from which came the fabled Lyran race. Murray Hope's the *Lion People: Intercosmic Messages from the Future* reveals arcane knowledge about this beneficent Ancestral Race, opening Minds to potentially great heritage of this epoch.

What is the relevance of this past? Did they know there would be Earth cataclysm 9,500 B.C. so extreme that all that would remain would be these megalithic forms of huge rocks? Ancient Ancestors, fabled Atlantean civilization, may be our Mirror, at the exact same place in Precession of the Equinoxes where we are today, as we enter into the next "golden age."

We are at a juncture in our survival as a species, awakening to *Greater* sense of who we are as Creator Beings of LOVE and how this awareness designs our future. Following *years* of intensive research, Graham Hancock believes this Lost Civilization left *essential clues* for us. (Incidentally, Hoover Dam was built to align with a star map, for this very reason, so it could be identified 10,000 years from now if we were not here).

Till recently traditional belief was that human civilization began only 6-7,000 years ago. Recent discoveries with current knowledge expose cycles of complex civilization as far back as several hundred-thousand years, proposing major redesign of our view on ancient history. A very advanced civilization (perhaps moreso than we) fabled Atlantis of 10,500 B.C. destroyed potentially by axis shift, plate movement, and melting polar ice caps, suffered mass destruction and global cataclysm up to and around 9,500 B.C.

According to Graham Hancock, this Ancient civilization pursued spiritual development and perfection of the Soul, before their World collapsed. They built these monuments attempting to bequeath advanced knowledge of Awakening, so we could continue where they left off rather than starting over. "It's as if we have *amnesia*," says Hancock, with little awareness of advanced wisdom that came before.

We consider mechanical solutions to problems, yet neglect our ability to use power of focused Mind, will and intent, which they developed to a high degree. Stories of ability to levitate huge rocks with sound peek at us from our past (such hidden knowledge echoes from Coral Castle, Florida). Sonar located chambers under the great Sphynx, predicted by Edgar Cayce in the 1940s, where records of advanced wisdom may be cached. Hancock suggests once this is released, we may find vital clues to creating a viable future for Earth.

Another advanced civilization of the last Golden Age, Gobekli Tepe in Turkey, had a highly refined civilization from 10,000 - 12,000 B.C. Their fantastic art and astronomy are completely rewriting antiquity. Robert Schoch PhD who re-dated the Great Sphinx to 7,000 B.C. as a tropical rainforest climate (first resisted then accepted by peer review 1991), reports recently found Gobekli Tepe culture Lived simply with few material goods, with deep focus on the Heart. Their culture was intentionally buried, leaving us their legacy.

We are Now capable of grasping clues left us from advanced cultures of this former Golden Age, while transiting the same region of space they did, certain to change our destiny with upside potential of activating a Golden Age. Astronomer Edmund Halley (1656-1742) identified Halley's Comet, and then recognized we were moving *toward* the Pleiades after noticing its 7 visible stars were in different positions than mapped by the Greeks. In 1961 Paul Otto Hesse corroborated these findings, also identifying the energy ring around the Pleiades 2000 light years wide, Now known as the Photon Belt. We entered these fast moving particles of Light in 1961 at the "Dawning if the Age of Aquarius," when Pisces and Aquarius overlapped in fifty year transition. Close constellations Orion, Sirius and Pleiades, play major roles in Earth's cosmological history and likely ET visitation.

Astronomer Jose Comas Sola (Barcelona 1868-1937) calculated we traverse the Photon Belt at the peak of our Galaxy's 26,000 year orbit. This peak coincides with Drunvalo's view that we are at the midpoint of 13,000 years. This is a huge region of space with intense electromagnetic radiation in the visible spectrum and beyond, with invisible light including x-rays, gamma rays, and a flow of magnetic Light profoundly affecting all Life on

Earth. This influence excites molecules, shifts atomic structure, and activates Living things to emanate their own Light. *Wow!* No one on Earth will escape this Awakening influence.

Another well-documented, radically provocative view that is a game-changer, is suggested by Walter Cruttenden of *Binary Research Institute*, that we orbit a binary or second star in our 26,000 year Galactic orbit. Surprisingly we learn that binary stars are the norm rather than the exception. He purports our binary star is Sirius, brightest star in the sky 8.6 light years away *near the constellation Orion.* This idea is gathering acceptance in progressive circles such as CPAK - *Conference on Precession and Ancient Knowledge.*

> The myth and folklore of ancestral peoples around the world hints at a vast cycle of time, with alternating Dark and Golden Ages. Plato called it the Great Year. Long believed to be a fairytale, there is now new astronomical evidence to show it has basis in fact. Moreover, because it is caused by acceleration of our Sun around another star, we learn that the Earth should soon be carried into a region of space that will have a beneficial affect on our atmosphere, nudging mankind into a higher age of consciousness.

> *Walter Cruttenden*
> *Lost Star of Myth and Time*

It is likely that current electrical systems based on Planetary magnetics may not work once we move further into this *Field.* Open Source groups Worldwide are Now developing essential free energy devices, drawing from the Unified *Field* surrounding us. Michael Tellinger documents advanced Ancient cultures using energy from sound resonated from Earth, quoting Nikola Tesla, *"Earth rings like a bell."* As we forge ahead in revolutionary directions, we emerge as an exciting *New civilization* fashioned by Evolution into Oneness.

> The *truth sometimes is so simple that we look past it*, ignore it and try to find a much more complicated answer, when all the time, it is there, staring us in the face, our passport out of the vortex into the future. When an anti-particle is formed, it comes into existence in a universe of ordinary particles, and it is only a matter of time.... a fraction of a second... before it meets and collides with an electron. The charges cancel, the total mass of the pair is converted into energy in the form of PHOTONS. This offers a new and unprecedented *powerful source of energy*. The PHOTON is about to become our way of life in the very near future.

> *The Photon Belt Story*
> *bibliotecapleyades.net*

"The Pleiades *encircled by this photon belt* 400 light years away, is part of a giant integrated system including our solar system, which orbits the Central Sun of the Pleiades, Alcyone." (*bibliotecapleyades.net*) Landmark book, *Hamlet's Mill* exposes Ancient astronomical knowledge operating on immense cycles carried forward in mythologies, documented in comprehensive detail. John Major Jenkins states in his preface, "Hamlet's Mill began a revolution in understanding the powerful sources of ancient myths. Although *Hamlet's Mill* tottered on the edge of oblivion for years, it has reemerged as fundamental text for progressive researchers who find the precession of the equinoxes lurking within most Ancient Creation myths around the World. "

As when human culture transitioned from thinking the World was flat, this New information about our Galaxy and Solar System connecting us with immense *Fields* of Light causes us to expand how we fit into Cosmic Cycles. Amazingly we have such ability to track our movement through space Now, as Dieter Broers calls it - "(R)Evolutionary."

Graham Hancock, author of *Fingerprints of the Gods* notes Ancient prophecies suggest entering this part of space, is a *signal*. Due to exposure to energies in this region we an Awakening is activated, where we are compelled to move beyond old destructive ways of thinking and Living. Humanity's capability to enter higher consciousness in this region of space, is a vital fulcrum point, on a legendary Galactic quest between Light and Dark, resolved only as we move out of duality or separation into Oneness. You may notice we are in visible, more intensified Light *Fields* Now, than most of us have seen in this Lifetime.

Some records show civilization "jump-started" around 6,500 B.C. moving Middle East, Egypt and India ahead, which may have been done by an advanced race from "elsewhere." Each predicting a Golden Age at certain points in our current cycle (potentially Now).

Sri Yukteswar, guru of Parmahansa Yogananda wrote *The Holy Science* in 1894 (pub. 1920) with revolutionary stance on the Yugas. He suggested that (rather than the Kali Yuga) we entered Dwapara Yuga 1700 A.D. an "electrical" age, and Now 400 years later are adept with electronic inventions. His calculations put us close to the Galactic Grand Center in the next few hundred years. Amazingly, he told of Universal magnetism as "Source *Field* for 5 electricities," identifying Einstein's Unified *Field*. Currently accelerated by photons of Light with Quantum focus, we know that by Attention on the *Field* we shift our "reality." *This is our "ticket" to the Golden Age.*

He describes what is coming as we move toward the "Grand Center:" we will Live telepathically, with clairvoyance common, in tune with animals, harmonious with Mother Earth. It may seem far from where we are right now, yet according to his Vedic projections, this is the cycle of the "demi-gods," where man realizes he is much more than his physical body. It results in a Golden Age, where consciousness has reached its zenith on Earth. Humanity no longer identifies itself in a physical body, we do amazing and wonderful things, achievable, as we align with *Essence*, the Heart, clear our unconscious and transform with Quantum understanding based in LOVE. Expanding into Greater capacities we move through evolutionary phases with Quantum level jumps, into full expression of higher consciousness during upcoming cycles.

The sun also has another motion by which it revolves round a grand center called Vishnu-Naabhi which is the seat of the creative power Brahma, the universal magnetism. Brahma regulates Dharma the mental virtues of the internal world. When the sun in its revolution round its dual comes to the place nearest this grand center, seat of Brahma, mental virtue becomes so developed that man can easily comprehend all, even the mysteries of Spirit.

Sri Yukteswar Giri (1865-1936)
The Holy Science

Once the Mind embraces this great overview of our spiral rotation through the Photon Belt of the Pleiades, around our Galactic Central Sun Alcyone, our Solar System's orbit around our Sun *with* binary star Sirius becomes familiar. Ancient historical symbols offer keys to this cosmology. It appears Earth has entered more "technicolor" ambient Light *Fields*, which may very well be the cool Light of Sirius, as we emerge into a regenerative highly advanced society with a culture built around Heart-based technology. *Exciting!*

NASA sent gyroscopes into space and ran tests to determine how fast our Solar System moves. Results of 436 km/sec. aligned perfectly with a 26,000 year orbit. As it was far from current thought they scrapped this experiment. However Ancient symbols contained this advanced understanding of our astronomy for over 6,000 years: Mayan cosmology's Hunab Ku, our spiral galaxy or Milky Way, and the Indus Valley's chariot that pulled the cosmos around a fixed center, the four direction and more that we are now interpreting. It is called the "mill" in the heavens reported in detail in *Hamlet's Mill*.

We are in a very special time, one that had never been before on this planet, or in this galaxy. As we align with the Galactic Center and the frequencies escalate beyond anything we have experienced in the human organism throughout all our incarnations, we will have many choices. As the Mayan's say, it is the end of time. But that statement can be interpreted many ways. What is happening is that many of the doorways of time, the other realities we have Created through our group consciousnesses, are coming together in a dissident song. The frequencies with which we align, will pull us into that doorway, that time track, that reality...

It is time for each human organism to, in gratitude and love, ask one's Divine or Higher Self to come into a greater alignment with the body. Then each person will become more aware of all creation, and of their power to Create. This is what is happening as we move to the new frequencies.

Each of us are unwinding coil of creation that is who we truly are. So, who will choose to move into this space of power, limitlessness, love and compassion? Who will prefer to keep walking in the shoes we have worn for the past 4,000 years?

"The Galactic Center, The Eye of Horus??"
davidicke.com

Amazing photo of the center of our Milky Way Galaxy displays prominent Sagittarius A, overlaid perfectly with the Eye of Horus from Ancient Egypt. Identified in Mayan cosmology as Hunab Ku, Source of Creation, astronomers believe this black hole has a mass millions of times that of our Sun, a large-scale electromagnetic field in the center of the Milky Way with amazing energetic potential. A blast of cosmic energy from Sagittarius A could activate the most powerful evolutionary leap in human history. Are we ready?

Ruins in South Africa used Earth's resonance with sacred geometry for power, and records from Ancient civilizations show sound harmonics used in ratios of the Eye of Horus for levitation of giant blocks of stone. Physicist John Hagelin suggests that as we get closer to the true Source of clean power emerging from the Unified *Field*, we move from large to smaller particles, beyond fossil fuel, electric generators and nuclear. Nassim Haramein relates these finer levels of energy flow freely in torus *Fields* and the "vacuum of space" or Unified *Field*.

As we move into a new paradigm, Michael Tellinger of South Africa proposes viable changes in economic, governing and energy systems that are ecological for all and Planet Earth based on the Ancient African Ubuntu philosophy, "I am because we are." From such ideas very real potential for a Golden Age is now emerging.

We've most likely been going through these cycles far longer than we imagine. Michael Cremo's *Forbidden Archaeology* reports on archaeological records dating fossilized human skulls to millions of years. Have we evolved to where we can carry our learning forward as was attempted in the last Golden Age? Perhaps we will yet access and decode messages they left, to assist us in our Evolutionary Leap and we'll move on to a New Level, leaving clues for our future selves.

Stimulated by accelerated *Fields* of Light and Quantum knowledge, change is afoot as we move into Oneness frequencies in this new energy matrix. In *Sacred Geometry and Unified Fields 6* (Youtube) physicist Nassim Haramein suggests with a smile, that Ascension may be our best choice; meaning restoring our True Design LOVE, lessening attachment to devolving materialism, moving into creative and fluid frequencies, becoming active co-creators of this New Paradigm.

In these Light-*Fields* a new kind of well-being, vitality, and enlightenment are naturally present. It is up to us to make the most of this incredible transit in human history from which we have the capability to launch into a a future far beyond where we have been. Have you noticed shifts within? Are old structures of "reality" less important or even meaningless? Do you find yourself smiling more often? Are you rocking like a ship at sea? Molecules are speeding up, with expanding awareness of how malleable our "reality" is.

> You and I are the force for transformation in the world. We are the consciousness that will define the nature of the "reality" we are moving into.
>
> *Ram Dass*
> *Author, Be Here Now; movie Fierce Grace*

Rather than seeing change as endings, recognize them as beginnings. Restructuring systems will match up with who we are becoming. We are moving toward awakening to our True Nature LOVE, Living harmoniously with one another, progressing forward as an intelligent, Wisdom-keeping civilization.

I've often said we're educated for a much earlier era, not for the immense complexity of who and what we are in human history. And people are discovering that the need, the yearning, that I find literally all over the world, to become what we can be -- and that's one of the main reasons why we find myth rising all over the world, because myth gives us the kind of coding, in the story of ourselves writ large, as the hero and heroine of a thousand faces. It gives us access to a much larger story, and all of us are on the verge of becoming citizens in a Universe larger than our aspiration and much more complex than all our dreams.

Jean Houston, Interview by Jeffrey Mishlove Ph.D.
Possible Human, Possible World Part I

We are Now cleaning out old "programming" as conscious Observer-Creators, to enter into full Potential of our True Design LOVE. As we each let go of illusionary purposes and follow Heart's *Essence,* human civilization is reborn. LOVE activates our DNA, expanding our capacity on this Evolutionary path. We transit this Spiral with naturally stimulated pineal activation connecting us powerfully with the Heart, to merge into Oneness. Our radiant Vibration flows into the collective, elevating joyful expression of the whole.

Everything is comprised of energy, Vibration and consciousness. When we explore a portion of the vast science of Quantum physics, we learn when something reaches critical mass, an UNSTOPPABLE SHIFT takes place. When an ELECTRON increases in Vibration, the moment it reaches critical mass, the entire electron is pulled up into the higher frequency, and nothing can stop that shift. CRITICAL MASS IS 51% of energy, Vibration and consciousness... When 51% of an electron is vibrating at a higher frequency, the remaining 49% is instantly ABSORBED into the new Vibration.

Patricia Cota-Robles
The Violet Flame

Each of us who accesses True *Essence,* holds space for Self and Others to evolve. Such rare opportunities are given us in human history when the Cosmos aligns just right, great Masters appear and Evolutionary Leaps occur. As we "hold the *Field"* together in prayer and Meditation, honoring Highest and best for ourselves and Pachamama - Mother Earth-Gaia, we literally put into motion vibrational frequencies that shift the entire matrix of Life, energy on Earth, events, circumstances, self and others. Our World responds to us!

As **21st Century Superhumans** we reshape our lives with Abundance of the Heart, Loving relationships and Well-Being from *Essence.* Activated by New energies, raising frequency of Mind-Body-Heart, veils lift and we restore Greater aspects of Who We ARE. ♥

To exit the world of chaos and confusion we have to die to our old stories and be reborn into a new Higher Story or Myth, a main theme of Cosmic History... This is something to deeply consider in light of your actual power to affect the entire holographic universe. There are no limitations when the whole of the cosmos is peering through your eyes.

1320 Frequency: Shift
Crossing the Bridge of Time by Red Queen

Chapter 14

There Is No 'Out There' Out There

This is the only radical thinking you need to do. But it is so radical, so difficult, because our tendency is that the world is already 'out there,' independent of my experience. It is not. Quantum Physics has been so clear about it.

Stephen Davis
Butterflies Are Free to Fly

Congratulations! For you who have made it this far, we're jumping in with "both feet." We trust you've integrated foundational principles of *21st Century Superhuman Quantum Lifestyle* and they are making sense. Are you playing with this on a daily basis, Breathing, Smiling and Being in your "reality" in new ways based on your True Design LOVE?

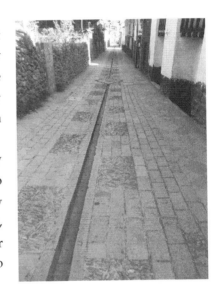

Are you noticing expanded perceptions about how You as Observer-Creator play a key role, calling into Being all you experience as "reality?" We are Now Activating more "brain cells" to comprehend this, removing old thought-emotional patterns left over from blame-fear-hostility-judgement-control culture to rewire our neurobiology with clarity from the Heart.

Thanks to impermanence, everything is possible.

Thich Nhat Hanh
Buddhist Monk

If anyone seems to be doing or saying something that makes your life more difficult, take a deep breath, step back and NOTICE - "there is no 'out there' out there." WHATEVER is occurring is a result of a resonance carried inside YOU!

This is Self-Mastery 101. As opposite as it is from how we've perceived things for millennia, welcome to how Quantum "reality" works. This is how *we* live our lives. Something feels uncomfortable that someone else does or says, we go inside and ask, "What am I feeling? What is the resonance inside of me? What goals do I have for this situation (ex: for the other person to be nicer...)? I cancel my goals for this situation and release it. I let go of the STORY. I Breathe, Smile and center in LOVE. I take Response-Ability. This is MY energy creating this "reality." I shift myself, I shift the entire situation.

We know this is a big leap. We may also need to evaluate our "nutritional soundness," if we've used food, sugar, caffeine, alcohol or drugs to numb ourselves, our Mind-Body may need nutritional support to hold these higher frequencies of thought. Our modern society is a "pancreas-adrenal" culture, meaning we use stimulus and suppression to manage stress and our hidden pain. To take charge of our Lives it's essential that we follow healthy nutritional habits to sustain high energy levels, and achieve New thought levels neuro-biologically (covered in Part 4: BODY and at our website).

We may consider blaming our genetics. For 100 years scientists thought DNA contained a blueprint for how our lives are structured. Yet Bruce Lipton, in the New field of epigenetics (above the genes) tells us what's emerging beyond genetic determinism.

Firstly, the new knowledge of how perception controls biology reveals that we are active participants in controlling the character of our health and behavior. Our ability to consciously control perceptions and environment has a profound influence on our lives, versus the old belief system where we are victims of forces outside our control. Secondly, when we live in the here and now, present all the time, and actively exercise our consciousness to run the show, we Create the Life we want, and it becomes heaven on earth.

Bruce Lipton, brucelipton.com
Danielle Graham, Genetics, Epigenetics and Destiny, superconsciousness.com

That "there is no 'out there' out there" comes from the Quantum concept that our "reality" is a product of our vibration. Although there *appears* to be an 'out there' it actually is a product of our "Attention," as the *Field* can only Mirror what we give it. Even among those who understand this, we discover more daily how this plays out in Life. Accepting Quantum understanding activates an ongoing process of inquiry, requiring compassion and patience for self and others. We will learn about this in greater detail in Part 2: MIND.

We live at the threshold of a universal recognition that the human being is not mere matter, but a potent, energetic field of consciousness. Modalities of the past millennium are quickly giving way to breakthrough technologies wherein we heal ourselves at *the level of all true healing, which is spirit.*

Michael Beckwith
New Thought Minister, Agape International Spiritual Center

Removing ourselves from victimhood we become aware that telling stories of how so-and-so did this or that to us, is a *denial* pattern. When we seek sympathy or empathy by telling our story of what someone else said or did, we avoid clear our own pain and content holding resonance. Memories stored in the unconscious from childhood or genetic memory from "defending our very life" take courage and focus to go into and clear.

In this New Light we become aware that anything carried in our unconscious as a "shadow," follows us Vibrationally into our "reality" *Mirrored in the Field.* Accepting this awareness, we recognize how conscious and unconscious thoughts have played a key role in our existence. This is one of the biggest "humps" to get over, as most of us have established masterful defenses to never have to go into this unconscious pain again.

Spiritual bypassing...has run rampant in both religious and non-religious circles. Spiritual bypassing is the act of using spiritual beliefs to avoid your unmet needs, deep pain and unresolved wounds. Spiritual bypassing is a form of avoidance. Because it's a form of avoidance it's a form of resistance. Spiritual bypassing is in fact the shadow side of spirituality.

The spiritual beliefs of any spiritual tradition, be it Christian, Hindu, Buddhist, New Age, Islamic or even self-help can provide ample justification for living in a state of inauthenticity. They can all provide justification for avoiding the unwanted aspects of one's own feelings and state of being in favor of what one considers to be a more enlightened state....

Authenticity is the highest state of being that the spiritual practitioner can achieve. In fact in the years to come, authenticity will become the replacement for enlightenment as the true goal of spiritual practice...

The journey of Life is not always a journey of bliss. Sometimes the journey through Life leaves you curled up on the floor in tears. This is the [heart] of transformation...think of a butterfly because our spiritual transformation is a lot like that. When a butterfly crawls itself into a space where it can cocoon...that butterfly will dissolve within that cocoon into a type of soup. That soup is nothing but pure genetic material. The butterfly had to break down completely in order to become a butterfly instead of the caterpillar. It's not like the caterpillar simply grew wings.

Teal Swan
Spiritual Bypassing (YouTube)

"Spiritual bypassing" is a societal epidemic established on thousands of years of blame-fear-judgment thinking, buried in collective and personal unconscious. Once faced head-on with tools we teach here, unwinding it is the release that brings True Freedom.

As we continue with the **21st Century Superhuman** journey we learn to courageously and effectively clear self-defense patterns residual from childhood punishment and Ancient genetic memory. As unconscious patterns are removed so is resonant "shadow creator" energy from the *Field,* and we move clearly into Creation from LOVE.

There is no escape from this New knowledge. We can go to work at our job, get coffee, sit at home, have dinner, watch TV with a beer or glass of wine to relax and settle for things "as they are," or we wake up to awesome awareness we cannot ignore. Every thought, every emotion plays an absolute role in every detail of *our* lives and in our surrounding World as well. Only as we make a pact with ourselves to release our deepest pain and express our greatest joy, do unspoken shadows dissolve and quit running our Lives.

If you awaken from this illusion and understand black implies white, self implies other, life implies death--or shall I say, death implies life--you can conceive yourself.

Alan Watts (1915-1973)
British Philosopher Higher Consciousness

We are intrinsic to the entire Hologram. Shift ourselves, we shift the Whole. The Universe is patient with our process; we each grow into and absorb these new things at our designated rate of speed. There is no right, wrong, good bad, or any judgment on our journey; we become as we become. The sooner we honor our "inner voice," and heed inner guidance, the more empowered and vital our Lives become. Living from our Truth reduces the learning curve, freeing us from many false pathways.

Every time you don't follow your inner guidance,
you feel a loss of energy, loss of power, a sense of spiritual deadness.

Shakti Gawain, Living in the Light

At this amazing Evolutionary Leap on Planet Earth, many shifts and changes are upon us. The more empowered our ability to Create through the Heart, the more easily we sail through all that is coming. Those awake are expanding into a New way of Life based on these principles, leading the way to a viable future.

Your DNA is a connective filament. What scientists are calling "junk" houses perceptions deep inside your body to allow you to become an entire perceiver, a fourth - fifth dimensional being. This awakening DNA allows you to change your eyesight, your hearing, increase Life-span, etc. This dormant part of your DNA that baffled the scientists is now coming to Life...

As DNA helixes come to full activation, there is an awakening of inner knowledge going beyond what the person has been taught. This inner knowledge is knowledge of self that says there is much more than this physical world. *Believe it. Know it. Understand it.*

Those of you who understand higher realms have felt very alone here upon the planet. There are now millions like you, forming a tremendous support group. You are beginning to meet and find one another, and you are beginning to thread your consciousness – one fine silk strand with other strands of consciousness. You will see a most beautiful creation come together without great effort because it is part of a plan and you are moved to do certain things.

You have complete control over everything. Until you discover that and believe it, you are subject to whatever anyone else wishes you to do in this free-will zone. And in your innocence, you have been exposed to things that have allowed your DNA, your intelligence and many things to be controlled. ...You are the one who controls your DNA...

Barbara Marciniak
Bringers of the Dawn

What is really up for us as a human race, is to know our Response-Ability as Creators of our Existence. What a magnificent and exciting opportunity. It is a giant Leap to let go of old ways of blaming something outside ourselves for our "reality." We may argue to hold on to it, yet ultimately as we shed this old skin we are born anew. We are now ready to release old stories, and Breathe New Creation into Being.

> The Shamanic Self plays and moves and heals within the stories. Even though the goal is when ready, to move beyond them.
>
> The Infinite Self operates from the place of SOURCE KNOWING beyond story and thus bypassing any need for micro-managing creation. You ARE the creator. Create a new story altogether. You are the dreamer. Dream yourself. In truth, this is happening all the time whether you know or not.
>
> Know thyself. There is only ONE MIND here. And it is yours.
>
> *Allen Smith*
> *Rainbow Didge Music*

For an immersion in Quantum "reality," and how it might be comprehended, read-listen to Stephen Davis' *Butterflies Are Free to Fly*, downloaded free at butterfliesfree.com. We are in similar transition to the World-changing shift in perception of 1400 A.D. when human culture realized the *World was Not Flat*, which took 1,000 years to be accepted around the globe. We trust our current shift is taking place quicker, resulting in current *Shift of the Ages*. Here is Stephen Davis' great explanation on this "confounding" topic in his chapter entitled, *THERE IS NO "OUT THERE" OUT THERE* which he encourages sharing:

> "If the holographic brain model is taken to its logical conclusions, it opens the door to possibility that objective reality – the world of coffee cups [and] mountain vistas- may not even exist….Is it possible that what is 'out there' is really a vast resonating symphony of wave forms, a 'frequency domain'...?" David Bohm said "the tangible reality of our everyday lives is really a kind of illusion, like a holographic image..."
>
> "If the concreteness of the world is but a secondary reality, and what is 'out there' is actually a holographic blur of frequencies...what becomes of objective reality? Put quite simply, it ceases to exist. Although we may think we are physical beings moving through a physical world, this is an illusion. We are really 'receivers' floating through a kaleidoscopic sea of frequency."
>
> ...Fred Alan Wolf and Lynne McTaggert both say, "there is no 'out there' out there, independent of what is going on 'in here.'" "What is 'out there,'" says Michael Talbot, "is a vast ocean of waves and frequencies, and reality looks concrete to us only because our brains are able to take this holographic blur and convert it into...familiar objects that make up our world.
>
> What this means is that there is no independent, objective reality "out there," but a wholly subjective reality Created totally dependent on what's "in here." In short, there is no "out there" out there...

In Quantum awareness our existence is emerging in wave form from the *Field*. We are in the midst of a *huge* transition to embrace this as science bridges Ancient Truth. Einstein says, *"Reality is merely an illusion, albeit a very persistent one."*

Material technology will emphasize the exploration of outer space, but the Light will come only to those who begin to explore inner space. Man-Woman must come to know themselves as divine beings, and let that manifest. This is a new concept for Man-Woman and it takes much time and energy of motion for them to come to this realization. But when they do, they will transform this world and reach new heights of Mastery over themselves and the material world.

When they know themselves to be a Divine Creation and Divine Creators they will bring untold wonders to pass. They will find the secret of CREATIVITY and nothing will be beyond their ability. The new man-woman will be MASTER Of THEIR FATES. He-She will WILL and produce their mental image into manifestation. And understanding of the Law of Vibration will give them a power over all matter. They will Create by MENTAL Vibration! They will Traverse the Universe by thought.

He-She will Heal by IMAGING, BUT BETTER STILL, IN TIME THEY WILL REQUIRE NO HEALING, for they will learn that *inharmony is their own Creation,* and they will learn to use CREATIVE LAW divinely for the good of all. This is hard to imagine; you will be amazed at the rapidity with which it will come, for the Earth is being prepared and the old order falls very quickly.

Nellie B. Cain
Exploring the Mysteries of Life (1972)

Know your own creative *Essence*, for no one but You is able to fulfill the Unique Purpose YOU came here to express. Commit to Living as the Being You Truly Are, beyond compromise for society or family. Vibrantly express your resonance in the World!

Speak the Truth quicker! Have more fun per hour!

Leonard Orr
Founder Rebirthing Breathwork Movement, Immortalist

Each individual who courageously leaves behind the old stories and enters the Heart to Living from *Essence* and LOVE, exponentially strengthens the New. Those who "hold the *Field* with LOVE," hold resonance for the New to come into form. Letting go resistance and blame, our Attention clears and shifts internally to LOVE, thus shifting the entire hologram. *There is no 'out there' out there...* Shift ourselves, shift the entire Hologram. ♥

..at higher levels of energy our fields of prayer act very quickly to bring us exactly what we expect. If we fear, it brings what we fear. If we hate, it brings more of what we hate...That is why you must monitor expectations carefully and set your field consciously.

James Redfield
The Secret of Shambhala

Chapter 15

What Is The Dream?

Remember that your perception of the world is a reflection of your state of consciousness. You are not separate from it, and there is no objective world out there. Every moment, your consciousness Creates the world that you inhabit.

Eckhart Tolle
The Power of Now

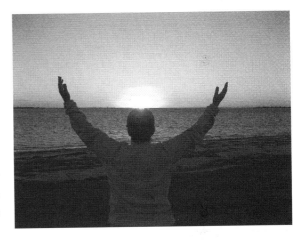

Let's accelerate our Journey with Quantum principles. If you strike a C tuning fork near another C tuning fork, the second will vibrate without being touched, because they are of the same frequency. Similarly with two guitar strings, strike one string and the same string across the room will Vibrate, yet if you strike a C tuning fork near an A tuning fork, nothing happens because they're different frequencies.

This is how our thoughts resonate our "reality" into form around us; they draw in matching frequencies. This is how our Hearts connect with those who are of a vibrational match. What we are resonating activates or draws in same resonance. Let's take a deeper look at how this works. Our "reality" offers a perfect biofeedback loop, presenting a reflection, or Mirroring of thoughts carried within us. *Wow!* As we learn to interpret this, we get better at noticing what is showing up in our World, how our thoughts are "creating," *and* we get better at removing inhibiting Not of LOVE thoughts.

It can be uncomfortable at first to accept that *everything* around us is a product of the resonance inside us; because then, we also have to accept that the World we've built around "it being someone else's fault" is *also* an illusion. Then it starts unravelling - *for example:* "why am I doing what I'm doing with my Life? because I thought someone else expected me to?" ...and then I realize it all came from inside me - my fears, my doubts, my dreams. Then I come back inside to search and find my *REAL* self, to figure out who I *really* am in the midst of all this, and how I choose to show up in the World - since it's all my Creation anyway. No more excuses that *anything* is "someone else's fault!"

So, whatever is "going on" in our lives, called "reality," *is* the result of a *signal* we're sending out, like a tuning fork or musical instrument; a resonance activating events, people and situations of matching resonance into Being in our World. *It's the simplest thing to understand how thoughts Create or resonate our "reality" into Being, yet we've been living outside it for so long, and constructed our World outside it, it may* **seem** *complicated.*

How do we wake up from this "Dream?" First, start noticing every day as your Life unfolds, that *this is your Creation.* When something goes great or not quite the way you'd like it, notice: "This came into being in response to resonance of *my* Mind-Heart." Remember the Double Slit Experiment? What's acting is our *Attention* on the *Field of Possibilities*, both consciously and *unconsciously.*

This can be a big leap to acknowledge that things in our lives we don't like, and things from the past that we didn't like, were all brought here by *lil' old us!* This is a complete re-write of our map of "reality." *Yes it is!* As it unwinds, priorities may change, friends, jobs, where we live, who we thought we were, who we realize we are - *and when the dust settles,* we will come out the other side with greater faith in our own Life than ever before. *As you free yourself by realizing you are creator of your Life, experiment with connecting with your own Heart and where it would like to go.*

As situations arise when we're feeling fear, anger, grief, sadness, guilt or blame we learn that it's our Creation, and it's up to us to shed the layers of thought-emotion Vibrationally calling this into being. As we do so, our ability to transform internally becomes more fluid. Physical cleansing, detox and Breath work can be helpful to move this energy, along with True Aramaic Forgiveness - clearing process which we will get to in upcoming chapters. As we "clean house" we begin to Create from *New thought.*

This *New thought* emerges from our deepening connection with our *Essence. A Course in Miracles* says, "When everything you retain is lovable [LOVE], there is no reason for fear to remain with you." As we become more clear and harmonize with LOVE, we discover that all true Creation is LOVE, and the "illusion" falls away.

> All aspects of fear are untrue because they do not exist at the creative level, and therefore do not exist at all. To whatever extent you are willing to submit your beliefs to this test, to that extent are your perceptions corrected. In sorting out the false from the true, the miracle proceeds along these lines:
>
> Perfect LOVE casts out fear.
> If fear exists, Then there is not perfect LOVE.
> But: Only perfect LOVE exists.
> If there is fear, It produces a state that does not exist.
> Believe this and you will be free.

A Course In Miracles
Electronic Version Chapter 1:IV:5-9

We are shifting into progressive concepts far beyond the old "world is flat" philosophy; a big change for us and our friends who've been galloping along in the same direction. These are "big horses" to rein in and change their course. As we absorb the realization that whatever we think of (even unconsciously) is going to come into being in some way, shape or form in our "reality," we access a learning curve to think about our Lives in new ways. It can be very helpful to seek out friends who are also choosing this way of clearing and Living to practice our skills, share our learning process, and solve and celebrate our trials and successes together!

♥ Together in LOVE ♥

As we live together, in LOVE, we change the World.
As we grow together in LOVE,
We release all old thought patterns and limiting beliefs.
As we share together in LOVE,
We change our personal history and
Interpretations of past and present circumstances.

We are connected deeply to the Universe,
To a Higher Consciousness and to Each Other.
We learn to stay centered, expand our awareness and
Trust our inner-voice, moment by moment.
By learning to listen, stilling our minds and
Setting our focus, we merge into Oneness.

We share the Vibration of LOVE and Wisdom within us...
And as we allow it to expand,
We remember what we have always known:
We are made of LOVE, we are uniquely special,
Our Light shines through any darkness and
We Create Miracles by being Together in LOVE.

Teddi Mulder & Nancy Dock
Natural Awakenings

Two years after landing on the moon, Edgar Mitchell founded Institute of Noetic Sciences IONS in 1973 to explore new physics and consciousness, as he had an overwhelming experience of the magnificence of Creation, for which nothing in life had prepared him; similar to Jodi Foster in the movie *Contact*. "He knew that the beautiful blue World to which he was returning is part of a living system, harmonious and whole - and that we all participate, as he expressed it later, 'in a Universe of consciousness.'" He knew that the uncharted territory of the human Mind was the next frontier, holding possibilities we had only yet to imagine.

Hologram is the name given to the hallmark discovery that the event history of all...matter is continuously...broadcast non-locally and is received by and interacts with other matter...through a subtle process of exchange of Quantum information. It brings the role of information in physical theories to the same level of importance as energy itself.

Ed Mitchell, Apollo Astronaut, 6th man on the moon
What is the Quantum Hologram

Ed Mitchell's dream has borne productive fruit toward cultural change. "Institute of Noetic Sciences (IONS) serves an emerging movement of globally conscious citizens dedicated to manifesting our highest capacities... Consciousness is essential to a paradigm shift leading to a more sustainable World. We encourage open-minded explorations of consciousness through a meeting of science and spirit."

Thanks to impermanence, everything is possible.

Thich Nhat Hahn
Buddhist Monk, Poet, Nobel Peace Prize Nominee

Ervin Laszlo reveals we *all* have access to what he calls *Akasha* or Greater Mind, the *Field of All In-formation*, which he encourages us to utilize, "The Quantum connection of our brain can serve us as a subtle but trustworthy compass, one long-known to traditional cultures yet largely ignored in the modern world."

Is your mind turned upside down? Yes, it may as well be, for we are changing 10,000 generations of thinking, and *out of chaos comes clarity*. We were challenged as well when we first integrated all this, as it is *such a departure* from blame-fear-hostility constructs that our culture has revolved around for so long. We are Now deeply immersed in and thoroughly enjoying *Quantum Lifestyle...*

Pull out all stops - play with it, sing with it, dance with it! Implement these new ways of Being and watch your life change around you. Dive in and be fully present. Clear, release let go what doesn't belong, immerse yourself in LOVE.

The Dream is Now. ♥

Don't worry that your life is turning upside down.
How do you know that the side you are used to
is better than the one to come?

Rumi
Thirteenth Century Mystic Poet

Chapter 16

A New Vision

When it comes to tsunami or shift in tectonic plates, if you...believe in consciousness even that you would say has a connection to turbulence in collective mind... You are part of nature...so if collective mind is turbulent nature is turbulent... When we settle down...nature will settle down.

Deepak Chopra MD
Natural Physician, New Thought Author

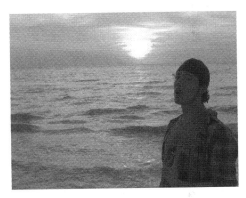

We are an amazing flow of Being emerging from the *Field of Possibilities* into wave form, coalescing around thought-emotional Vibration, causing our lives to take shape with particles we observe as matter and events. How we show up in the World, how the World shows up around us, what we say, think and do, who we connect with and all experiences magnetize into being as a result of our Vibrational *Essence*.

You have been submerged in a society...without light, and you have...vaguely remembered your light...so you could relate in that world. Now it is time for you to integrate into society the multidimensional world of Light and Spirit you represent so values and designs of this planet change completely.

Barbara Marciniak
Bringers of the Dawn

Stepping out of the old 3-D paradigm into Quantum "reality," where electrons wait in a *Cloud of Possibilities* and thoughts become things, where spacetime replaces time and space and parallel Universes operate feels a bit crazy and unknown. Relax. Our World changes as we change, the rest takes care of itself. In fact, our World *responds* as we change!

21st Century Superhumans are initiating a new expression for humanity coming from Creativity, Joy, Commitment to *Essence* and Living from the Heart, as our True Design LOVE. We are learning and implementing small shifts that grow bigger every day.

Every being is fluent in the language of light...it is the language of the Soul and of the spirit... The closest match to light language on Earth is Aramaic. ...if all of the current languages on this planet were blended together it would manifest as the original angelic language of light.

Brian de Flores
Language of Light Video

We are learning how the language of *resonance*, translates into Creation appearing as our "reality." True *Ancient Aramaic Forgiveness (not traditional forgiveness)* clears our own 95% unconscious content from our resonance. For thousands of years we've allowed blame-fear-hostility-judgment-control thought to resonate in our Lives, with the idea that "things are just as they are, and we are subject to them (victimhood)." Understanding Universal Laws and Quantum physics explains how our Universe actually works. Our creative resonance then becomes a *fulcrum point,* for expression of the Divine.

This New knowledge and wisdom prepares us for fulfillment of prophecies long carried forward in many cultures, a long heralded Golden Age of Enlightenment, where Universal Truths are expressed in an idealized society, where without our "corrupt data," all that remains is LOVE. Shift yourself, shift the Whole; *Arc the Hologram!* This is the *Shift of the Ages. Take along your tuning forks. Remember to clean off your Mirror!* ♥

21st Century Superhuman Vision

• We release, let go, cancel and clear all Not of LOVE thought-emotion.

• We Live from *Essence*, doing and expressing what brings us JOY!

• We are Smiling radiantly, Breathing openly; spiraling into LOVE.

• We resonate Wholeness and Well-Being in our Lives and on Planet Earth.

• Our DNA codons are "switching on" activating highest potentials.

• As Gandhi said, We Are " the Change we wish to see in the World." We "let the wind blow through us like wind through a screen door..."

• All on Earth Are educated, fed, comfortable and Joyful.

• Freedom while honoring others, is the birthright of All.

• Earth Mother Gaia (Pachamama) is honored and Radiant in her pristine beauty.

• Harmonizing, balanced Masculine-Feminine principles nourish our Creations.

• Every Creature is precious and honored, gifting us with Unconditional LOVE.

• All Children are playing- thriving; their joyous laughter floats on the wind.

• Natural Energy from the Unified Field freely runs our clean, technologically Wise Civilization with environmentally friendly power and transportation.

• We relate with Peace, Respect and Wisdom with all Beings in our Universe.

• Simple economic and governing systems supporting a united, collaborative, mutually beneficial Global community emerge from our True Design LOVE.

www.21stCenturySuperhuman.com

Chapter 17

Restoring Our True Design LOVE

Knowing has nothing to do with thinking,
but rather is a quality found in and through the heart.
So based on this theory, the less you try to think,
the more powerful your outcomes will be.

Dr. Richard Bartlett
Matrix Energetics

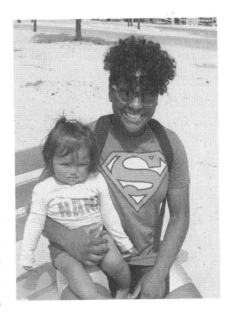

*T*he *Divine Matrix* or *Field* can only mirror to us what we give it it with resonance of our Attention (conscious and unconscious). Hence the Golden Rule, "Do unto others as you would have others do unto you." Our resonance returns in like-kind what appears as "reality." Rather than being a "rule" to punish or direct us, this is simply an explanation of how Creation operates.

As much as we'd like to squirm and say, "really, part of it has to come from someone or something else," the bottom line is, it all begins and ends with us. Our World is a giant biofeedback loop responsive to the "tuning fork" WE ARE. As we learn to hone thoughts-emotions (conscious and unconscious) to LOVE, our "reality" changes and so does our World.

> Never forget that you are not in the world; the world is in you... Creation is set up to bring you constant hints and clues about your role as co-creator. Your Soul is metabolizing experience as surely as your body is metabolizing food.

Deepak Chopra MD
The Book of Secrets: Unlocking the Hidden Dimensions of Your Life

When "reality" shows up around us, we Now say, "Very interesting what my Vibration drew in today. Is there anything to clear to bring my "reality" more into alignment with Heart?" Noticing what comes up with others or events of the day offers clues as to residue that may cling to our "crystal core of LOVE," to clear, cancel, release, let go, as it appears and surfaces. In coming chapters in this series are super-clearing tools for **21st Century Superhumans** to transform self and our World.

The more we practice these habits, the more natural it is to experience self in our own continually emerging Creation, and by response of our "reality" learn where we need to reset to LOVE. As we shed old layers of blame-fear-hostility-judgment-control, the Loving Radiance We ARE beams through and literally transforms "reality" showing up around us, as our True *Essence* shines in the World from the Heart.

The privilege of a Lifetime is being who you are.

Joseph Campbell (1984-1987)
Mythologist, Advisor to Stephen Spielberg on Star Wars Archetypes

The Jim Henson Movie, *Dark Crystal* (1987) contains great symbology for our Now. Jen, a Gelling on a quest to restore balance to his World, is returning a crystal shard broken off 1,000 years ago. *Mystics*, Masters of the Light, and *Skeksis*, Masters of the Dark suspenesfully journey to the chamber where the powerful Crystal resides. Jen and his friend Kira survive death-defying odds to barely get there by "Conjunction of 3 suns."

The Dark *Skeksis* prepare to receive uncensored immortality, obtainable only during this conjunction, if the Crystal is not restored. Jen risks his Life to valiantly return the shard to the Crystal, unifying it just as the *Mystics* plunge into the chamber! Our minds are blown as the *Mystics* and *Skeksis* merge into "One" as tall glowing Beings, they melodically resonate this as *we* realize Darkness and Light are part of the "same," neither bad or good.

Two polarities that hold duality in form have many representations: dark-light, day-night, yin-yang, positive-negative. Such opposites Create a charge holding Creation in form. Experiencing our own Darkness or shadows surfacing to merge with our Light, leads us toward wholeness, restoring our True Design LOVE. Even experiencing Darkness or that which we "don't want," is the perfect way to discover our Light. *"Without darkness how would we know what Light is?"* [Legend]

When something comes up, Smile, Breathe and say, "Ah-So," I did it again," notice, and return to LOVE. This is the Journey of En-light-enment or Awakening. Simple as it is, it's not about beating ourselves up because we're not perfect. Everything changes the instant we do. Creation is in a continual magnificent state of emergence based on Vibration.

There are only two ways to live your Life.
One is as though nothing is a miracle.
The other is as though everything is a miracle.

Albert Einstein (1879-1955)
Theory of Relativity and E=Mc2, Nobel Prize Physics

Our most native vibration is LOVE. All else is a natural response of Body-Mind-Spirit to notice what's in the way of this ever flowing current of Life. Whatever we think we see in others, is Mirrored back from us, including LOVE and ecstasy. As we let go of old "data" that has been running the show, things shift. New motivations from the Heart make us more awake and present. We are better, kinder, more thoughtful to others and are also truer to self. Offloading all thought-emotion Not of LOVE, we find better solutions, become more intuitive, and speak and live in Wisdom from the Heart. Good things come our way. We remove ourselves from chaos, and simply through shifting our resonance internally, become active participants in calling in a better World. *How simple is this?*

Old social and economic structures will crumble from their own decay, since they were not built upon spiritual foundations. Greed, lust, and power were their underpinnings, and they will fall into the dust of destruction before the new edifice be raised; the world MUST be transmuted!

The new cosmic Vibration of the earth will be greatly intensified and we Must raise our frequency in accordance. That which does not vibrate in harmony with the new Cosmic Vibration will simply disintegrate.The old order was built upon the premise that Man's strength gave him license to exploit his brother. The new Age will bring the realization that all are brothers-sisters in one spiritual community and must be equally respected and revered.

Some will panic as they find themselves involved in chaos where material possessions are stripped from their grasp. All who have been possessed by their possessions will find themselves stripped of possessions, but those who realize the possessions are loaned and to be used for the good of all will be able to have and use material goods.

Nellie B. Cain
Exploring the Mysteries of Life, 30 Years Research

We are unraveling insanity of corporate interests of the "strange culture of gold" at the crumbling foundation of governments, religions, nationalism and banking systems. It requires "shining the spotlight" *inward* to see what is *inside us* generating this frequency in our "reality." As we do so it becomes clear what old thoughts-emotions *we* need to let go of, to shift old paradigm thinking and our World to LOVE (more in coming chapters).

Ae change our cultural structure and dynamic *one person at a time.* As each of us "gets it" we make small changes that grow into bigger societal changes based on the Truth of Our Being, LOVE. To what extent we embrace this, is up to each of us. Some are ready before others to seek a flowing existence in harmony with self, one another and the Earth. There is more going on right now than changing our thinking; Cosmic influences are afoot and Quantum "reality" is shaking it up!

We need enlightenment, not just individually but collectively, to save the planet. We need to awaken ourselves. We need to practice mindfulness if we want to have a future, if we want to save ourselves and the planet.

Thich Nhat Hanh
Vietnamese Zen Buddhist Monk, Teacher, Author, Poet, Peace Activist

Shift of the Ages is about shedding outmoded thinking "off the mark" for thousands of generations, being replaced with thought compatible with our True Design LOVE. The Cosmos is focusing a perfect alchemical moment upon us like a tractor beam, triggering us naturally to "wake up," like kids' *Transformers* morph into an empowered and versatile state of Being and response to Life, moving beyond competition to mutual well-being.

> We are all becoming "universal humans," connected from within by the same process of creation, awakened to our heart's desire to give our greater gift to the world. This humanity is rising everywhere. Now we are connecting heart with heart and Soul with Soul to shift from fear to LOVE, rising as one planetary community.
>
> *Barbara Marx Hubbard*
> *Foundation for Conscious Evolution*

LET GO: All control-judgment-fear-blame-hostility. Laugh. Breathe. Smile! Let Life flows from the Heart, Joyful, Loving, *"no time,"* Creative, Smiling, Growing, Laughing, Playing, Blending...*(let go generational patterns, too)! What a revolution for all on Earth to do this!*

> Time is not measured in days and hours, as you know it, but according to the PLAN and it's outworking. It is hoped by the Hierarchy that much destruction can be averted, if man can be brought quickly enough to this new awareness. If humanity can be awakened and transmute their hates, greed, and intolerance, before the new planetary Vibrations are in full control, they can function in the new Vibration without experiencing the impact of it as a destructive force.
>
> These conditions are not being "visited" upon mankind as punishment, but are the natural consequence of planetary progression, which also brings a new Vibrational level, in which hate, animosity and material consciousness can have no place. The old falls of its own weight and those who are trapped in it will experience the chaos of it, but those who arise in LOVE and Light will know that it is The Great PLAN and they will let LOVE reign in the new order.
>
> *Nellie B. Cain*
> *Exploring the Mysteries of Life, 30 Years Research*

We offer you a map, and as Tony Robbins used to tell us, *"the map is not the territory."* The territory lies ahead, where we will learn practical skills for Living *Quantum Lifestyle,* activated by wonderful supernatural influences of our Now.

We are being molded and shaped, into what "Saints and Sages of Old" represented as they tread this path before us, showing the Way to Inner Peace, Trusting *All is well with the World*, Breathing and Smiling all the way... as we Now return to our True Design, LOVE. ♥

> For small creatures such as we,
> the vastness is bearable only through LOVE.
>
> *Carl Sagan (1934-1996)*
> *American Astronomer, Pulitzer Prize, Award-winning "Cosmos"*

Universal Laws

If you want to find the secrets of the Universe,
think in terms of energy, frequency and Vibration.

Nikola Tesla (1856-1943)
Serbian-American inventor, engineer, developed AC current

There has always a thread of higher truth conscientiously carried forward in Ancient cultures. One such thread was transmitted through Hermes Trismegistus of Ancient Egypt around 3,000 B.C., also known as Thoth who introduced astrology, alchemy and the Law of One. Essence of these Universal teachings has been carried forward into the modern World by the Hermetic Community, Gnostics, the Nag Hammadi Library and Kabbalah. In more recent years Drunvalo Melchisedek offers insights on this lineage.

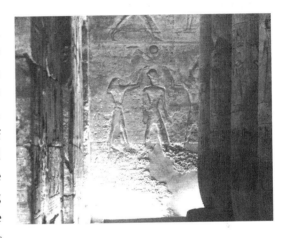

In 1908 a group anonymously called the Three Initiates wrote *The Kybalion,* carrying forward Hermetic philosophy of illumination from ancient Egypt, with instruction for modern Life. William Walker Atkinson wrote over 100 books under various pen names and is thought to be one of the authors, as *Kybalion* is very similar to his book *The Arcanum.* New Thought emerged, revolving around these "Universal Laws," intelligent immutable principles that govern our Universe. *The Kybalion* aligns with Quantum thought.

You are dwelling in the Infinite Mind of THE ALL, and your possibilities and opportunities are infinite, both in time and space.

The full *Kybalion* can be found in print with audio and text free online, containing Axioms and Uses for putting these Laws into practice. These seven Universal Laws reflect how Quantum physics operates in our World bridging modern science and Ancient texts. It is said when the seeker is ready they will find the Universal Laws. Here we are.

> Where fall the footsteps of the master,
> ears of those ready for his teachings open wide.

We are at an amazing evolutionary moment, where our minds are able to comprehend science meeting Universal Law. This offers opportunity for greater clarity, as we begin to move beyond cultural chaos. *The Kybalion* tells us we are "Masters of Creative Potential and Players in the Game" teetering at the *Shift of the Ages,* an unprecedented Evolutionary Leap, most prophesied in human history.

> The Principles of the Truth are Seven; he who knows these, understandingly possesses the Magic Key, before whose touch all the Doors of the Temple fly open.

> *The Kybalion*
> *Three Initiates*

The first 3 "IMMUTABLE" LAWS explain the science of how *all Creation* operates, aligning with Quantum physics, confirming how we participate as Observer-Creators.

Additional 4 "MUTABLE" LAWS define results of action within the first 3 and how to achieve balance, as Great Masters have in all ages.

The secret to obtaining anything we have dreamed of, comes from living according to these 7 Universal Laws, which are subject to LOVE and simply define how this dimension operates. Living accordingly with this Immutable Science of how the Universe functions, we discover the real path to success and flowering of our culture into a Golden Age,.

7 UNIVERSAL LAWS - That Govern the Universe

3 IMMUTABLE, ETERNAL Universal Laws

1. LAW OF MENTALISM *"The ALL is MIND, the Universe is Mental"* - Thought Creates. Thought Created all that is. In Aramaic John 1 says, "In the beginning was mind-energy, and by it were all things made that were made." Our thoughts Create. *Double Slit Experiment* - whatever Attention we put on the *Field* is Mirrored back to us (thought-emotion / conscious-unconscious).

> One of the old Hermetic Masters wrote long ago: "He who grasps the truth of the Mental Nature of the Universe is well advanced on the Path to Mastery." ...Without this Master Key, Mastery is impossible, and the student knocks in vain at the many doors of The Temple.

> *The Kybalion*

2. LAW OF CORRESPONDENCE *"As above, so below; as below, so above"* - The same pattern expresses on all planes of existence from the smallest electron to the largest star and vice versa. Fractals of Sacred Geometry: aspects of individuality manifest at any scale. We are part of a giant Hologram. Change yourself - change the whole. *ARC the Hologram!*

3.   LAW OF Vibration *"Nothing rests; everything moves; everything vibrates"* - Science endorses that everything in the Universe is pure energy vibrating at different frequencies. "......Quantum mechanics tells us that even in their ground zero state, all systems have fluctuations and have an associated zero-point energy as a consequence of their wave-like nature. Thus, even a particle cooled down to absolute zero will still exhibit some Vibrations." (Peter Baksa, *The Zero Point Field*, Huffington Post) The *Divine Matrix* - the *Infinite Field of Possibilities*

This Principle explains that differences between manifestations of Matter, Energy, Mind and Spirit, result largely from varying rates of Vibration...[this formula] enables Hermetic students to control their own mental Vibrations and those of others...'He who understands the Principle of Vibration, has grasped the sceptre of power.'

The Kybalion

4 TRANSITORY, MUTABLE Universal Laws

4.   LAW OF POLARITY "Everything is Dual; everything has poles; everything has its pair of opposites, like and unlike are the same. Opposites are identical in nature, but different in degree. Extremes meet. All truths are but half-truths, all paradoxes may be reconciled." Good and Evil, Dark and Light are simply two different Vibrations of the same. The Art of Polarization was a Hermetic teaching, that by changing our thought Vibration we shift and flow with form of a thing (e.g. from hate to LOVE, from pain to Joy). Transmutation.

5.   LAW OF RHYTHM "Everything flows, out and in. Everything has its tides. All things rise and fall. The pendulum-swing manifests in everything; the measure of the swing to the right is the measure of the swing to the left; rhythm compensates." A Master knows Creation has regularity, and does not become overly excited by one swing, or discouraged by the negative. If you feel yourself being pulled backward by a cycle, just keep your focus on your vision, and eventually the pull will release and you will again move forward.

6.   LAW OF CAUSE AND EFFECT "Every Cause has its Effect; every Effect has its Cause. Everything happens according to Law. Chance is but a name for Law not recognized. There are many planes of causation, but nothing escapes the Law." Every thought-emotion, word and action sets in motion an effect that materializes. Masters know that everything in their "reality" is a product of what has been set in motion by their Vibrational-thought energy. Once called the Law of *Karma*, there is no punishment - just results that come back from causes we put in motion.

7.   LAW OF GENDER "Gender is in everything; everything has its Masculine and Feminine Principles. Gender manifests on all planes." The *Kybalion* states that gender exists on all planes of existence (Physical, Mental, and Spiritual) with

different aspects on different planes. Everything and everyone contains these two elements. There must be balance between the two. Without the Feminine the Masculine is apt to act without restraint, order, or reason, resulting in chaos. The Feminine alone is apt to reflect and fail to actually do anything, resulting in stagnation. Masculine and Feminine together Create balance, productivity, success, fruitfulness. Depicted in Hindu philosophy as inseparable aspects of the ONE, Shiva the Masculine is the ocean and Shakti, the Feminine, the wave.

If a Law is not learned and applied,
then one has to go through the experience of the lesson.

The Kybalion
Three Initiates

Using the mutable Laws to discover equilibrium and transcend extremes is fundamental to changing circumstances of Life. Knowing the Universal Laws supports conscious Creation of intended "reality" and achievement of True Mastery. *Kybalion* offers insight into immutability of these Laws, and how all are subject to them.

We overcome lower laws, by applying still higher ones - in this way only. We cannot escape the Law or rise above it entirely. Nothing but THE ALL can escape the Law - because THE ALL is the LAW itself, from which all Laws emerge....Those Laws which THE ALL intends to be governing Laws are not to be defied or argued away. So long as the Universe endures, will they endure -- for the Universe exists by virtue of these Laws which form its framework and which hold it together. In THE ALL, indeed, do "we live and move and have our being." So, do not feel insecure or afraid --we are HELD FIRMLY IN THE INFINITE MIND OF THE ALL.

The Kybalion
Three Initiates

The *Kybalion* teaches that those who use these principles achieve a level of Mastery in this World. By obeying causation of higher planes they can rule on their own plane. They become "movers instead of pawns;" they are "players in the game of life" rather than influenced by suggestions, wills and desires of others, heredity and environment.

Any individuals who have attained any degree of Self-Mastery do this to a certain degree, more or less unconsciously, but the Master does this consciously, by the use of his Will, and attains a degree of Poise and Mental Firmness almost impossible of belief on part of the masses who are swung backward and forward like a pendulum. They (the Masters) cannot annul the Principle, or cause it to cease, yet they have learned how to escape its effects upon themselves, depending upon the Mastery of the Principle. They have learned how to USE it, instead of being USED BY it.

The Kybalion
Three Initiates

We may wonder about the meaning of "Law," "Is it a Law that can be broken or is it a Law to control me?" Universal Law is a description or explanation of how the substance of our Universe operates. It is called Immutable because it simply IS. One of Teddi's early teachers, Nellie Cain author of *Exploring the Mysteries of Life* offers an excellent discussion in her book and spent six months teaching her students Universal Laws.

Teddi says at first it was difficult to grasp, because they were so abstract, but once Nellie interpreted them and they discussed examples and how they are at work all the time, it became easy to see practical application in everyday Life. Teddi discovered how essential it was to understand the Universal Laws in our journey on the Earth-Plane. Earth is a school and these are the "Laws" that run it. Do you want to make your life easy? Learn about the Universal Laws. (Look for video upcoming at our website).

Adopting these principles may seem difficult, yet it becomes natural as we integrate them into Quantum awareness. (1) How thought Creates our "reality," (2) Change ourselves, change the Hologram (3) The *Field* is constantly vibrating - waiting for our thought upon it to magnetize into Creation. These first 3 Universal Laws, equate to Quantum principles. The four Mutable Laws refine our interaction with the first three.

We can call these the seven Universal Laws, *OR* they are the description of how things operate in our Quantum World. Once understood they shape how we relate to Life for more effective, productive, abundant, healthful, successful and intelligent ways of Being. Don't like something? Use the Law of Polarity to moderate your response. Play with one until you get good at it, and then include the next. You'll find yourself a Master soon!

We notice current events on Planet Earth and many things crumbling around us, because they were founded on blame-fear-hostility-judgement-control thought, ignorant of Universal Law. Suddenly, we understand how Quantum physics and these 7 Universal Laws change our Lives, because we *Know* that redirection of our *Mind-Energy* or *Thoughts* is required to change the whole. *Seriously. Change our thoughts, change the World.*

Behind every atom of this world hides an infinite universe.

Rumi
13th Century Persian Poet, Sufi Mystic

Many (millions) are starting to "get it" around the globe. It's not always easy, it is a transition; our entire civilization was established on the belief for a very long time (a blink of an eye in timespace), that most things are the fault of something or someone else "out there." "*Come on now, this particular situation can't be my fault?*" Yes. It can. Remember, "All is Mind." *Universal Laws remind us that we are part of Universal Mind.*

Divine Matrix provides a neutral surface that simply reflects what's projected onto it. The question is whether we understand its language... Do we recognize the messages we're sending to ourselves as the Divine Matrix?

Gregg Braden
The Divine Matrix, Bridging Space, Time and Miracles

BUDDY SYSTEM - CHANGING THOUGHT: Changes of thought and perception require deeper levels of integration. Cultivate a "buddy system" with friends, family, community becoming Awake. Support each other to Free the logjam of old thought-emotional content running the show. Help each other reframe these kinds of thought "stories:"

- Those *@!%&s in another country, or that government or...
- GMOs, pesticides or radiation is ruining our food supply
- What someone else is doing is bothering me
- I wish that dog would stop barking
- Spousal blowups, withholds, or ignoring
- Why is my kid doing this?
- I don't like the way my body, skin, face, hair looks
- I'm bummed about my economic - work situation
- Oh great, winter is coming again

Mind-Energy is creating all this. *Your* Mind-Energy. *My* Mind-Energy. It's *difficult* to understand how *(just about impossible at first)*, and it *is a a big thing* to get, yet once we get it, Life changes! *Yeah!* How about turning each item on the list above (or *your* list) around, recognizing that *resonance* begins with you and turn it into LOVE?

Let's face it. We're doing "double-time." First of all, we're canceling, releasing, letting go of everything in our *unconscious container* Not of LOVE, *from our entire Life AND bloodline.* There is a lot to this, because this *Vibrational resonance* has been running the show almost "forever," and these old ways of thinking are very ingrained. In fact layers of fear of punishment and old stored inside us *resonate* whenever we make a choice to do things differently. *Let's throw those layers to the wind.*

Our human forms are composed of and surrounded by an infinite myriad of forms, all in constant motion, from the subatomic to the cosmic in scale. This is...the enchanted dance of existence, the divine interplay of consciousness and energy. Amid this divine play we seek fulfillment, perfection, flow, freedom, enlightenment, Oneness..

Ram Dass
American Spiritual Teacher, Author 1971 classic Be Here Now

Undo generational conditioning established in ignorance of Universal Law. Restore awareness and harmonize with Source. Clear your *unconscious* container and outmoded *defense patterns* such as: "run away, clam up, yell, rage, cry, eat, don't eat, get stressed, depressed, worry, fret, drink, smoke" or whatever denial patterns have been hanging around to keep us unconscious. Wake up and clear, releasing need for these.

Clearing and establishing good patterns, turning this energy around, with practices such as meditation, running, singing, Breathing, cycling, yoga, get out in nature, play with kids, dogs, etc., awesome! Be sure to clean out "old data" from the unconscious container of early history and family conditioning with upcoming *Freedom Tools* in Part 2 - MIND.

It impacts us in so many ways that we can feel it's an impossible-to-be-free-of aspect of our lives. Bid this one goodbye. Just because you've been infected with a traditional **meme**, *[a belief that gets passed from one person to another or culturally],* and programmed to repeat and pass it on to future generations, doesn't mean you're unable to disinfect yourself and reprogram your inner world.

These funny little non-things called memes are thoughts you allow to become your master - and make no mistake, every excuse you've ever used is really a meme disguised as an explanation. Yet you can deprogram yourself from these mind viruses. A virus isn't concerned with whether it's contributing to your well-being or your ill being because it only wants to penetrate, replicate, and spread.

You don't have to be a victim of anything that was transferred from another mind to yours. Your beliefs have made these memes seem like second nature to you. While excuses are just thoughts or beliefs, you are the decider of what you ultimately store away as your guide to Life.

Dr. Wayne W. Dyer
Excuses Be Gone, How to Change Lifelong, Self Defeating Thinking Habits

We feed ourselves with LOVE or Fear. Each is a different polarity, bringing its own *resonance* into form. We resonate in fear producing chaos, or we nourish ourselves with LOVE and cooperation. The choice is up to us, our Mind-Energy determines results. Where we focus Attention shapes what is Mirrored back from the *Field*. It *Is* simple. This is a new way of perceiving our World with greater precision than ever before.

We are Now experiencing consciousness peaking waves, building on one another from the Cosmos moving through Earth's energy grid. Unity Consciousness and Universal Law are being restored in all dimensions. We are at an amazing historical fulcrum point, with *capability to understand these scientific principles and apply them to taking charge of our Lives. There will be a resulting end to greed, separation, and actions against humanity and the Earth based in the "strange culture of gold,"* as systems outside of Universal Law crumble.

UNIVERSAL LAWS SUMMARY: The first 3 IMMUTABLE Universal Laws tell us: (1) Intelligence or Universal Mind is the basis of Creation; (2) We're part of a giant Hologram - when we change ourselves we change the whole; (3) The unified *Field* is full of energy, constantly moving like effervescent ginger ale - waiting to be qualified with Vibration to come into form. It is that simple. Add to this the 4 MUTABLE Universal Laws we use for equilibrium: (1) Polarity - dark and light, (2) Rhythms and cycles, (3) Cause and effect, and (4) Gender. When we respect and use these principles, we discover the power of the first 3 Laws defining how All Creation emerges from LOVE.

Whenever reality cannot be explained,
a certain niche is opened within consciousness....

Barbara Marciniak
Bringers of the Dawn

MASTERY NOTES - 7 Universal Laws

1. I and my "reality" are emerging from my Thoughts (conscious-unconscious)

2. I Am Aware that as I shift within myself, the entire Hologram shifts. We are One - as we are many reflections of a Unity of Consciousness.

3. I offer the *Infinite Field Of Possibilities* of continually moving creative essence Vibrationally clear Attention. I practice skills and tools supporting me in continually refining my resonance, clearing to LOVE.

4. Based on the Law of Polarity, I can say Gandhi and Stalin in the same sentence without judgment, knowing they are two different Vibrations at opposite poles of the spectrum, and by changing *my thought* to LOVE, I change their form.

5. I Breathe, center myself and "go general," knowing that based on the Law of Rhythm, all extremes will return; I remain focused on my Vision.

6. Based on the Law of Cause and Effect, my every thought-emotion, word and action sets in motion an effect that materializes, aware of choosing well that which I focus upon.

7. I honor and acknowledge both Masculine and Feminine, bringing them to balance within me and my World. Unbridled Masculine results in chaos, Feminine alone stagnation; merging the two brings balance, harmonization and productivity.

AWARENESS IS IN-FORMATION: Potential within us empowers us to embrace destiny by design rather than default. These Universal Laws describe how our Universe works, and how to operate within it. There is no punishment. They are simply guides offering us guidance to refine our actions in this World to be more effective, now explained in modern terms in Quantum physics!

21st Century Superhumans are waking up. We are Grateful for these guideposts along the way. We are patient with self, learning to take in many new things during this *Shift of the Ages*, shifting ourselves to shift the whole. Cosmic and Planetary activation (called in by our vibrational desire to evolve) Now stimulates this Evolutionary Leap, bringing forth greater expression of *Who We Are, Why We're Here and Where We're Going* - humanity-huwomity expressing as our True Design LOVE.

NEXT: **PART 2: MIND**
The BEST Secret Formula to Manifest LOVE, Health, and Abundance

Part 2 MIND

*The BEST
Secret Formula to
Manifest LOVE,
Health, Abundance*

What affects one part of Life affects all Life.
In other words,
as I Am lifted up in consciousness
ALL Life is lifted up with me.
Instead of polarizing against everything
we disagree with,
we need to Create a New reality,
a reality that reflects our Oneness
and makes the concept of separation obsolete.

Patricia Diane Cota-Robles
Who Am I? Why Am I Here?
EraOfPeace dot org

Part 2: Mind - Section 1
21st Century Superhuman
A New Frontier

Yes, you are creating your reality AND reality is creating you.

Nassim Haramein
Transformational Physicist, Founder, The Resonance Project

So, Hello, what brought You here?

Are you just curious about who or what the *21st Century Superhuman* is?

Or would you secretly like to Be *One?*

What if - we have super-powers to Create anything we choose?

What if - we are well, fit, radiant, full of vitality?

What if - we extend traditional Life-span?

What if - LOVE transforms ALL, in our ongoing Journey as "Observer-Creators?"

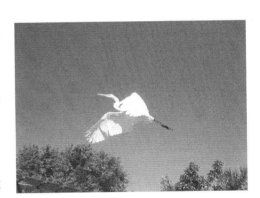

What if - we so Align with our Hearts and our *Essence* that we change the course of Civilization Forever?

What we are looking for is what is looking [for us]...

St. Francis of Assisi (1182-1226)
Order of St. Francis, Order of St.Clare

Are you ready for *"Mission Possible?"* Are you ready to be your own kind of ninja? *21st Century Superhuman, Quantum Lifestyle IS* about Living in such a way to reclaim and actualize our True Design LOVE, to be amazingly Alive, Healthy, Joyful and Abundant every moment! As you journey with us on this path we trust you'll discover Inner Peace as we have, reclaim Vitality, Energy, Tools and Resources to do whatever you Dream!

To some this may seem like a fairy tale... if you're still walking on good old' Planet Earth, and you've entered the realm of Quantum "reality" you're discovering we are Now embracing capabilities far beyond what we've yet imagined. Being a *21st Century Superhuman* is the adventure of a Lifetime, actualizing unlimited potential with secrets of *Quantum Lifestyle...*

Outstanding thought leaders point the way, offering insight to a better future for *21st Century Superhumans*. Ervin Laszlo's bio reads like Who's Who of brilliant minds; proponent of "new Thinking," twice nominated for Nobel Prize, 2001 Goi Peace Award, author of 89+ books in nineteen languages, 400+ articles, Sorbonne, University of Paris, coveted Artist Franz Liszt Academy of Budapest, research grants Yale, Princeton, more.

Laszlo concurs with physicist David Bohm, that the substance of the Cosmos is a *Field* of *in-formation that by its presence "forms" the recipient.* He uses the Ancient term *Akasha* (containing past, present and future). *Huffington Post* blog *Akashic Think...* offers "16 Hallmarks of Laszlo's Akasha Paradigm" - summarized below. *(Link in Bibliography).*

ERVIN Laszlo'S AKASHA PARADIGM "GUIDE FOR A new World" *(summary)*

The Akasha Paradigm tells us that we live in an interconnected, intrinsically non-local world. Everything happening in one place also happens in another, and in some sense everywhere.

I am part of the world. The world is not outside of me. I am part of nature, I am part of society, and society is part of me. I am a self-sustaining, self-evolving dynamic system arising, persisting and evolving in interaction with everything around me. I am one of the highest, most evolved manifestations of the drive toward Coherence and wholeness in the Universe.

There are no absolute boundaries or divisions in this world, only transition points where one set of relations yields to another. Separate identity I attach to other humans and things facilitates my interaction with them. There are no "others" in the world: We are all living systems, part of each other.

I cannot preserve my own Life and wholeness by damaging that whole, even if damaging part of it seems to bring me short-term advantage. When I harm you or anyone else around me, I harm myself. Collaboration, not competition, is the royal road to the wholeness that hallmarks healthy systems in the world. Self-defense/ national defense needs to be rethought. Comprehension, conciliation and forgiveness are are signs of courage.

Wealth, in money or in any material resource, is means for maintaining myself in my environment...it commandeers resources all things need to share if they are to live and thrive. Exclusive wealth is a threat to all in the human community. Beyond the sacred whole we recognize the world in its totality. Material things and energies and substances they harbor or generate, have value only if and insofar they contribute to Life and wellbeing with the web of Life on this Earth.

True measure of my accomplishment and excellence is my readiness to give. Every healthy person has pleasure in giving, a higher pleasure than having. The share-society is the norm for all communities of Life on the Planet; the have-society is typical only of modern-day humanity, it is an aberration.

I recognize the aberration of modern-day humanity from the universal norm of Coherence in the world, acknowledge my role in having perpetrated it, and pledge my commitment to restoring wholeness and Coherence by becoming whole myself: whole in my thinking and acting -- in my consciousness.

Ervin Laszlo's Team
Akasha Think... Huffington Post, What Is Akasha Consciousness -- For You?

Laszlo describes why evolution is an informed, not random, process, where potential for sustainable development through popular movement is turning tide from global breakdown to global breakthrough. He sees 2012-2020 as a critical period to change course of geopolitical crisis. As Chancellor of *Global Shift University*, he offers change accelerators, defined as coalescing agents for social action and cultural awareness, a great model.

Giordano Bruno Globalshift University is an online global institution, committed to Create informed and ethical agents of change to bring new consciousness, fresh voice, up-to-date thinking... transforming obsolete paradigms and empowering co-creation of an equitable, responsible and sustainable world.

"What if" of Planetary change and emerging new paradigms:

•*What if*-Ervin Laszlo hadn't tapped into Greater Mind, to offer his brilliant paradigm changing views and action?

•*What if* - Gregg Braden hadn't brought our Attention to Cosmic cycles and the importance of "remembering" how to communicate with the *Field*?

•*What if* - Lynn McTaggart hadn't written her comprehensive documentaries on Quantum research and how it defines consciousness and "reality?"

•*What if* - Jean Houston had not traveled the World these last many years tying together threads of continuity?

•*What if* - Steve Jobs had not persistently followed his dream to make Apple Computers and devices super-user-friendly for the everyday person?

• *What if* - Nassim Haramein hadn't pioneered physics beyond existing paradigms?

• *What if* - Dieter Broers had not had tragedy that lead him to share *Solar Revolution*?

•*What if* - Nellie Cain, Jack White, Sun Bear, John Whitman Ray, Godfrey Ray King, Max Gerson, Ann Wigmore, Bruce Lipton, Yogananda, michael ryce, Tony Robbins and **all the rest** had not stepped forward and passed their batons to *us*?

Children of the future *do not care* if you own a business with debt/income ratios, if you are enslaved in job security, if you owe on college loans, if you're retired and living on a fixed income. They do care that you are lost in the swale of a dying culture; they are praying back through time, that you will step up to the plate and participate with *YOUR Brilliance* in a culture being reborn in LOVE, Heart and *Essence*.

Children of the future care that we step away from the meaningless, and start Living for the meaningful. They care that *You* Wake Up to Remember Your *Essence*, what Lives inside *You* as Your Greatest Gift to Humanity, that *You* Start Giving it. That *Your* Mind, Heart, Talents, become part of the Collective Shift, changing Humanity's future FOREVER.

Consciousness is a vast ocean, and thinking is the waves and ripples on the surface of the ocean. Every wave and ripple has a very short lived Life - it is very fleeting do not identify with your thoughts.

Eckhart Tolle
Power of Now, A new Earth

Bringing forth ALL we are, we let go of meaningless scattered thoughts and learn to resonate from our deepest state of "Being-At-One" with ALL that Is. Are you ready to let go of things that don't matter any more, and commit to those that do? To make changes to attain different results by accessing *Essence*, Heart and Soul?

As we open ourselves to the realization of the in-formed Universe, this shift in our collective awareness heralds a resolution in schisms that have divided us for so long – both among and within us. It is this cosmic odyssey that the ancients often portrayed in their myths and legends and their adepts described as the sundering of the One to its ultimate reunion with itself.

Ervin Laszlo, ervinLaszlo.com
Systems Philosopher, Founder GlobalShift University

"Akasha" in Sanskrit means "the space," element of higher perceptional senses, where there is a record of our past, present, future Creations. Such reflection may inspire us to enter a New Frontier as **21st Century Superhumans**, with New awareness of our Creation.

War, starvation, our own and global suffering, push us to wake up beyond unconscious action. Exiting outer "chaos" where we have perpetuated "a separate sense of self" built on blame-fear-hostility "stories" we enter inner sanctum "space" to peace beyond suffering. We allow what "is" in the Now as Eckhart Tolle says. We recognize we are creator-Beings. Letting go identification with "stories" New clear thoughts and words are born as our conscious Attention on the *Field*. Breathing and Smiling we resonate "reality" into Being from a New place of formless, timeless *Essence* flowing through the Heart as LOVE.

Go instead where there is no path and leave a trail...

Ralph Waldo Emerson (1803-1882)
American essayist, Transcendentalist Leader

The **21st Century Superhuman** awakens, sits or lies still, Breathing, Smiling, connecting with the *Field*, the ONE, Source of All that IS. Entering Heart-space we hold resonance of Deep LOVE, Compassion and Gratitude in the Field. We cancel "goals," offering them to the *Field* to emerge as a Newly formed "reality" based in LOVE. We naturally contribute our Gifts to the Collective for the Greater Good of ALL, Intrinsically Connected as ONE. ♥
"You are not a drop in the ocean. You are the entire ocean in a drop." Rumi

A Sioux Story: The Creator gathered all of Creation and said : "I want to hide something from the humans until they are ready for it. It is the realization that they Create their own reality." The eagle said, "Give it to me, I will take it to the moon." The Creator said, "No. One day they will go there and find it." The salmon said, "I will bury it on the bottom of the ocean." "No. They will go there too." The buffalo said, "I will bury it on the Great Plains." The Creator said, "They will cut into the skin of the Earth and find it even there." Grandmother Mole, who lives in the breast of Mother Earth, and who has no physical eyes but sees with spiritual eyes, said, "Put it inside of them." And the Creator said, "It is done."

Part 2: MIND

Chapter 1

Meditation & Inner Stillness

Yesterday is gone. Tomorrow has not yet come.
We have only today. Let us begin.

Mother Teresa (1910-1997)
Missionaries of Charity, 1979 Nobel Peace Prize

Wise spiritual teachers through the ages have taught us to be in the World yet not of it, because much of the modern World has been established around the illusion of materialism without LOVE at its foundation. Many Ancient teachings offered a path to Free us from the "maya" of illusion. Inner Stillness and Mediation are keys carried forward from Ancient tradition around the World, a rich path to accessing Greater Self, Higher Intelligence, Pure Creativity and merging with our Oneness with Source.

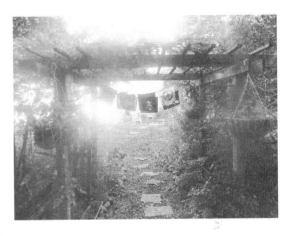

In the *Field* of knowledge is all possibility.

Maharishi Mahesh Yogi (1918-2008)
Founder Transcendental Meditation worldwide movement

Until recently most scientists made the mistake of believing space was empty, though the complete opposite has Now been shown to be true. It is says Quantum Atom Theory (Youtube), "teeming with pairs of virtual particles constantly coming in and out of existence....The particles have positive and negative charges, called matter and antimatter." This creative energy *Field* of "dark matter" makes up 94% of what surrounds us, with "dark energy" making up another 5%, *leaving only 1% for what we perceive as matter!*

"Virtual particles only manifest when something such as our Attention disturbs the Quantum vacuum." The closer we observe an electron, "the more of a beehive of activity Quantum space becomes, creating a perfect Mirror." Physicist Nassim Haramein in *Science behind the Unified Field* (YouTube with Lilou Mace) explains the 99.99% space we are made of as well as that between stars, galaxies, atoms and even inside the atom is not *empty*, it is full. We are bathing in a fundamental energy, and it *is* the Source of all of Creation.

Knowledge of Ancient Wisdom around the World lost to modern science, is now being replayed in Quantum theory. Nassim Haramein says, "When measured we found it [space] was infinitely dense with energy. My theories are showing this is the Source of everything, the Source of the material World. "It is the medium that connects all things. "When I analyzed how much energy is in a proton, it is as much energy as in the Universe; it is a Hologram, showing that all is interconnected." This Universal space with its Creative potential is called the "vacuum." Nassim smiles and says, *"May the vacuum be with you!"*

Decide what you want; don't think of intermediary conditions. When Nature works for us, we should want what we want and Nature will work it out for us.

Maharishi Mahesh Yogi (1918-2008)
Transcendental Meditation Worldwide

Lynn McTaggart calls it the *Field*. Accessing this *Quantum Unified Field* through stillness and going inward, brings forth our Greatest Potential, combining what is deep within the Source *Field* around us, and immersing us in active Creation. We (Cary & Teddi) both are Grateful to have been introduced to meditation early, first Transcendental Meditation or TM® with Sanskrit mantra, and later mindful and Vipassana meditations.

We recognize tremendous value of meditation as an essential *21st Century Superhuman* technique, to enhance clarity, focus and connection with Source. Literally within three weeks of beginning meditation (15 minutes 2x/day), electrodes read a dramatic shift from limited brain coherence to dynamic whole brain integration. Regular transcendent meditation increases performance, ability to actualize visions and dreams and integrates ever deepening productive states as a natural part of one's Life.

Nature is favorable to our effort when human awareness is established more and more in pure consciousness.

Maharishi Mahesh Yogi (1918-2008)

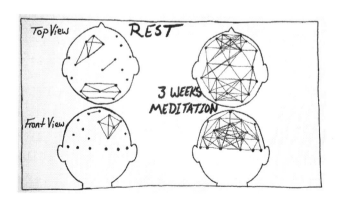

The image above represents electrodes measuring brain coherence, graphically showing that Meditation increases intelligence and all capabilities. Meditation won modern culture's Heart during the last 150 years. It is no longer a "mystery," it is Now a science with centers, groups and learning available everywhere. Meditation turns outward direction powerfully inward, to explore quieter and deeper levels of Mind and more powerful levels of intelligence. Regular meditation has an effect on us similar to reducing the resistance in an electrical wire, improving connection with our True "Power Supply." **Meditation is like strengthening muscles with exercise, developing skill at centering our Lives in the well of Infinite Creation, by going within.**

Even World events are ultimately susceptible to our state of Mind. Over 600 studies documented by the Transcendental Meditation (TM®) community have shown consistently, numbers of meditators focused on any particular situation radically change it. TM® studies demonstrated war activity in Israel and crime in Washington D.C. radically reduced in direct proportion to meditators' focus, with consistent duplicatable results.

IONS founded by Astronaut Ed Mitchell has a Meditation Bibliography with nearly 6,000 published scientific studies, (most comprehensive listing in the World) demonstrating powerful results of meditation for health, intelligence, productivity and success, also affecting events and weather. Meditation is historically a rich philosophical tradition.

Today's contemplative practices extract the science of modifying everyday states of consciousness by disengaging from normal distracting thought. Various forms of meditation extracted from spiritual practice offer Benefits of enhanced precognition, telepathy, synchronistic experiences and access to Greater Mind.

Transcendental Meditation opens the awareness to the infinite reservoir of energy, creativity, and intelligence that lies deep within everyone.

Maharishi Mahesh Yogi (1918-2008)
Transcendental Meditation Worldwide

Anyone can learn to Meditate. Two common and easy types of Meditation are:

1. *Transcendent Meditation:* uses a mantra or repeated word each time a thought arises, to gently *entice or invite* the mind back to its inward focus. Choose your own mantra "LOVE," "Gratitude," "Compassion," "Peace," or Sanskrit can be obtained through a TM® teacher, with additional advanced practices offered at tm dot org.

2. *Mindful Meditation* - brings the mind inward when noticing it is following a thought (Zen practice). Vipassana, taught and practiced by Buddha, purifies the mind and brings peace. (Advanced forms access fractals or self-similar patterns in Creation).

QUANTUM LIFESTYLE TOOL - MEDITATION - HOW TO MEDITATE: Sit comfortably upright on chair or couch or can be done lying in comfortable position. Use clock until 15-20 minutes becomes natural and easy 1-2x/day. For a busy person upon waking may be easiest, lying or sitting quietly in bed or chair, with same before sleep. Cultivate your own method, blending this into your *Quantum Lifestyle*, gently making room for your practices behind the scenes among family and daily routines.

> At last I found the banks of eternity and there I sat, musing, to plunge, swim, and melt in that ocean of immortality. Melting myself within Myself , I became the ocean of luminous light. All dream waves of many incarnations have melted into the sea of one flame.

> *Parmahansa Yogananda (1893-1952)*
> *Self-Realization Fellowship, Autobiography of a Yogi*

When beginning if you would like to, say or think a short prayer or vision of Consciousness. Become still, breathe gently. When aware that a thought arises, simply repeat your mantra or bring mind back to center. When first starting busy "monkey mind is common, though soon you will find yourself falling deeper and deeper into the silence and peace of inner realms. When complete, gently reintegrate with the outer. If you are the only one in your household Meditating, it will bring a peaceful air. Invite others to join you.

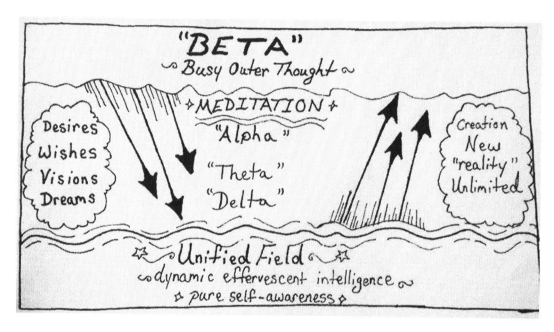

FAVORITE CLEARING MEDITATION: Sit comfortably feet uncrossed or lie down. Center. Light candle and/or incense if you wish. Call in Higher Realms according to your personal way of connecting: Christed consciousness, Buddhic consciousness, Ascended Masters, Angels, Great White-Rainbow Brotherhood, Beings of Light and LOVE in all dimensions of timespace, Guides and Teachers, departed Loved Ones, Pachamama or Earth Mother Gaia and her Elementals.

• Cancel all goals. Be specific. Then cancel goals conscious, unconscious, subconscious and incomplete.

• Invite assistance of Aramaic Rookha d'Koodsha (Part 2: MIND) to clear your unconscious of "old unconscious data."

• Give your goals to the *Field*. Trust. Let Go.

• Invite Perceptions and Intentions of LOVE.

• Open Mouth circular Breath to release holding patterns in Body

• Drop down into the *Field* through brain wave frequencies: Beta, Alpha, Theta, Delta.

• Carry with you whatever is currently "up" for you: hopes, dreams, visions, worries, cares. Specifically take those things with you that you cancelled goals for above.

• Dive into the *Field* of "effervescent gingerale," let ALL go into wave form and then dissolve out of form into the *Field, including YOU!*

• Invite Source to bring forth Creation in New ways, in a wave of LOVE. TRUST SOURCE. Give up figuring it out. Let the Infinite take over. Watch your Life change.

• This process can be practiced separately or combined with mantra or mindful Meditation. Continue to Breathe with open mouth. Bring closure with GRATITUDE.

HOW MEDITATION WORKS: Physicist John Hagelin presented similar image at Science and Nonduality SAND conference with his talk, "Is Consciousness the Unified *Field*?" He revealed how transcendent meditation takes us beyond thought, visualization, cognitive presence, contemplation and data to *PURE BEING*, to abstract awareness, at the foundation of mind and basis of all matter. Awareness usually sharply bound by focus, relaxes, expands and becomes infinite, identifying with the Universal *Field* at the basis of the Universe. Meditation gently *invites and entices* us into complete quiet, in bliss, where mind quiets and global coherence envelopes the brain.

Hagelin appeared in "The Secret" and "What the Bleep," and is a Quantum physicist forwarding progressive ideas on Unified *Field* Theory, integrating cutting edge concepts on where we are headed in our understanding of ourselves and our place in the Cosmos.

Spokesperson for Transcendental Meditation, Hagelin has pioneered the use of unified field–based meditation technologies proven to reduce crime, violence, terrorism, and war and to promote peace throughout society-derived from ancient Vedic science of consciousness. He has published groundbreaking research establishing existence of long-range "field effects" of consciousness generated through collective meditation, and has shown that large meditating groups can effectively...provide a practical foundation for permanent World peace...

sourcewatch.org

Is it best to release doubts, fears, daily challenges, thoughts about our own and global issues such as GMOs, positioning between countries, economic challenges, and system reformation. Rather than worry, we have greater effect by clearing our unconscious, centering in Alpha-Theta brain waves, holding our vision and calling it in from the *Field*. For instance rather than focusing on eco-damage, focus on the wholeness of Mother Earth, rather than being fearful about our bank account see it filled with abundance.

Put your hand on your heart and ask yourself what kind of world
do I want to live in? And now ask yourself, how can I make this happen?

Deepak Chopra MD
Natural Physician, New Thought Author

We play an active, vital, participatory, positive creative role by clearing our unconscious "data." "Never think of failure, for what we think will come about." (Maharishi Mahesh Yogi)

Consciousness is the basis of all life and the field of all possibilities. Its nature is to expand and unfold its full potential. The impulse to evolve is thus inherent in the very nature of life.

Maharishi Mahesh Yogi (1918-2008)
Founder Transcendental Meditation Worldwide

The *Longevity gene* goes up an astounding 30% in two months of meditation, discovered by Elizabeth Blackburn, who received 2001 Nobel Prize for demonstrating effects of this anti-aging enzyme! With meditation we enter Greater Mind, carrying us beyond limited thought. Restoring our True Design LOVE through goal canceling is our Master-Key to effective shifting of all timelines and "realities." Meditation is one of the best tools available for expanding our capacity for Health, Longevity, Success and solving Global issues.

Upon a completely still calm ocean appears the shape of a wave.
That shapeless is taking a form - actually in neither of them is there a difference.

Swami Brahmananda Saraswati (1868-1953)
Guru of Maharishi Mahesh Yogi

We are participants in the dynamics of the Universe. Thought Creates ripples in the fabric of timespace, of which 5% is conscious or we default to 95% unconscious (Harvard). Entering into creative consciousness with LOVE, unprecedented change occurs beyond what the rational mind has conceived. Inner Stillness, Meditation and LOVE tap into our *most powerful* creative potential, activating Conscious Creation through meditative Attention that invites the *Field* to flow into form at our "command."

New light photons, oscillations, or Vibrations continuously come into existence relative to our thought, a continual flow of cause and effect. Wave particle duality of light forms an interactive process, continuously forming a blank canvas that we can interact with, turning the possible into the actual.

Quantum Atom Theory (Youtube)

Moving beyond limiting concepts established in "the World is flat" culture, we learn that Life and what we call death (transition from one state to another) continuously interchange with the living Quantum *Field*. Learning to trust the Eternal Flow of existence begins to free us from limiting beliefs, to enter into joyful participation in Creation of our "reality." Gratitude and peace activated through Inner Stillness, turn energy expressed into a cognitive moving force, shifting past, present and future "realities" through timespace.

Quantum Atom Theory tells us, "In the continuous process of Creation we see time imprinted on the *Field*. At every point in space and time we can interact with the *Field*, to turn the possible into the actual, shifting past-present-future "realities!" Time is not a continual progress forward," it is where past and future have expressed themselves through consciousness. Consider it! Quantum wave particles are unformed and forming, based on our Attention upon continuous uncertainty of the *Field*

...the whole atomic structure is currently profoundly reshaped at the most fundamental Quantum level and at the subatomic Quantum level, before elementary particles appear in this 3D and 4D holographic reality.

Georgi Stankov
General Theory of the Universal Law

Experiencing Life as a malleable process, designed by the resonance within us, we learn that our thoughts profoundly shape "reality." Bruce Lipton reminds us in *Science & Theory behind the Tapping World Summit,* of one of the most critical details to come to Light to date, also a key teaching of Yeshua/Jesus in properly translated Ancient Aramaic: 5% of our thoughts are conscious, the other whopping 95% is UNCONSCIOUS, leaving us spiritually bankrupt unless removed. We are a bio-computer in need of an owner's manual. For us to really get what we *Desire*, requires canceling goals to clear ALL Not of LOVE "data." This cleans out the virus and installs a New program. Meditation daily for clarity and renewal also offers access to vital tools, little used in modern culture.

In our **21st Century Superhuman** Journey, *LOVE defines our Perfect Design*, it is the *Essence* of the *energy* of which we are made. It operates our core level as Aware Creative Beings, expressing through our capacity for Pure Positive Creation.

LOVE is a state of being, a higher Vibrational reality...few beings who have achieved this transcendent level of consciousness positively and permanently impact the entire world...with Kindness, compassion, caring and positive attitudes...one chooses moment by moment the path of kindness and compassion.

Lifeoncue.com
The Power of LOVE
A Spiritual Definition of LOVE

Our True Presence LOVE as a Vibration *elevates All*, infusing the Greatest Joy into the human experience, permeating our World with generative Creative flow from the *Field*.

It is wrong to think LOVE comes from long companionship and persevering courtship. LOVE is the offspring of spiritual affinity and unless that affinity is Created in a moment, it will not be Created in years or even generations.

Kahlil Gibran (1883-1931)
The Prophet

Higher Dimensional LOVE for which we are capacitors, transmits *through* us into the World, amplifying through the Heart as our Compassion grows. Mother Teresa's mission transcended illusions of this World. She unites us around a selfless all encompassing *Divine* LOVE, a healing balm for humanity, the embodiment of Compassion.

There are two kinds of poverty, material poverty where people are hungry for a loaf of bread. But there is much deeper, much greater hunger, and that is the hunger for LOVE; that terrible loneliness... LOVE begins at home... We will be able to overcome the world with LOVE.

Mother Teresa (1910-1997)
Missionaries of Charity, 1979 Nobel Peace Prize

Even in personal relationships we can learn to transmit all our connecting through this deep, universal LOVE. Our simple *Essence* founded in LOVE, flows through us into the World. This is how true positive change happens *one person at a time.* **Stepping into Heart-based Living from Essence with LOVE is how we shift the course of human destiny.**

We must be willing to let go of the Life we planned
so as to have the Life that is waiting for us.

Joseph Campbell (1904-1987)
American Mythologist, "Follow Your Bliss"

Synchronicities, people, things and events appear miraculously, as we Live from *Essence* in the current of Divine expression of the One, of which we Are and Are Part.

Everything passes, nothing remains.
Understand this, loosen your grip and find serenity...

Lama Surya Das
American born Tibetan Buddhist and Spiritual Activist

The more we Live from our True *Essence,* we shed old layers as they surface. They clear less traumatically than before, because we realize we are better off without them. Practicing **21st Century Superhuman Quantum Lifestyle** skills, we find Freedom in the Heart, from which we now respond to Life, and our "reality" is born *anew* each Now Moment.

Every time you are tempted to react in the same old way, ask if you want to be a
prisoner of the past or a pioneer of the future.

Deepak Chopra MD
Natural Physician, New Thought Author

We are at the Perfect place in our Now. If we experience another being upset "at us" or feeling upset, even in the distance "road rage" or someone irritated at the supermarket, we ask ourselves, "Is this bubbling up for me to clear, to bless, or is it a test to see if I'm still reactive to this issue?" Whatever resonance appears in our "reality" near or far, gives us clues there is something to clear to deepen to LOVE. Refocus. Breathe. Smile.

If you think you're free and
you don't know you are in prison - you can't escape.

Gurdjeff (1866-1949)
Fourth Way, Enneagram

Rejoice, as you enter this New State of Being. Breathe. Smile. Bless others with your presence. When a stressful situation comes up, it's good to notice we may be clearing a generational dynamic. Use *goal canceling* processes in upcoming chapters to restore the Presence of LOVE. Enter Inner Stillness and the well of Creation through our Meditation. Incorporate when issues come up to transition into continual renewal.

If we allow our thoughts to arise and dissolve by themselves, they will pass through
our mind as a bird flies through the sky, without leaving a trace.

His Holiness Dilgo Khyentse Rinpoche (1910-1991)
Revered teacher of the 14th Dalai Lama

On the radio on a recent trip it was interesting to note call-in shows offered palliative solutions to relieve pain, encouraging the individual to "move away from the situation or speak up." Yet without the understanding that thoughts Create our "reality," solutions were palliative at best. Taking Response-Ability for our "reality" as our thought-Creation, offers a clear path to shift any situation being addressed in Life. Cultivating the Meditation habit will develop consistency and a deep sense of inner peace.

When you think everything is someone else's fault, you will suffer. When you
realize everything springs only from yourself you will learn peace and joy.

Dalai Lama
His Holiness the 14th Dalai Lama

"Programs" or repeated patterns from family, environment and generations are stored in the unconscious. When uncomfortable situations come up, they are generally an echoing of these. Clearing out these old Vibrations helps release these echoes. Tools from the Ancient Aramaic (coming up in next few chapters) are powerfully freeing on this Quantum path as *21st Century Superhumans!*

Your intentions have Created an upward trend in your Life. New opportunities are coming your way, your inner and outer self radiate this positive growth...enjoy the present and the process. Trust each moment is taking care of itself...stay focused on now, let go of worry...enjoy these gifts.

Doreen Virtue
Angels Oracle Cards

Progressive physicist Nassim Haramein's unification theory, known as the *Haramein-Rauscher* metric, "a new solution to Einstein's *Field Equations*," and his last published paper

The *Schwarzschild Proton*, offer a fundamental change in our current understanding of physics, consciousness and Quantum entanglement.

HOW WE CAN CHANGE TIMELINES: Nassim tells us that from a Quantum entanglement perspective, there is a "string" from us to our imprint in space-time of a particular experience and thought. We can go "along that string" in our mind and modify the information including our thoughts-memories-emotion about it, changing the influence of the experience. When another is involved, their string crosses yours, so when you clear within yourself, you also shift entanglement with them, shifting the entire "Hologram."

This is why upcoming Ancient Aramaic "goal canceling" is so effective from a Quantum standpoint. Nassim says *"as we change the information on the structure of spacetime... it impacts our future and past, because we make different decisions from that moment on."* Your specific state is recorded on the structure of spacetime as you move through it in this dimension. It can be changed at any time, showing how our choices affect the Whole. *Shift yourself, shift the entire Hologram with LOVE.*

Transcending "material illusion" for that which is "eternal," is the spiritual quest of outstanding great traditions. We have the opportunity today to bypass confines of religion, bringing together science, cosmology and Ancient texts and teachings to enter more deeply into the *Essence* of our being. Quantum physics overlights our comprehension in a simple explicit way, of the power behind changing our internal content to change our "reality."

The Field is the sole governing agency of the particle -
the invisible energy fields around us govern matter

Albert Einstein (1879-1955)
Theory of Relativity, Nobel Prize 1921, Max Planck Medal 1929

Imagine a World with ALL thriving naturally and harmoniously on Mother Earth, simple needs met with creativity and play, an attainable cultural ideal for humanity / huwomity and our birthright. Current 3-D "reality" based around materialism is a collective cultural thought Vibration held in form by an electromagnetic charge, because so many agree on its Newtonian form. This 3-D "reality" is based upon what the five senses perceive, and may be constructed because of our loss of connection with our eternalness. As we experience ourselves as ever emerging energy beyond matter, Breathing, Smiling and aligning with our True Design LOVE, we move into higher knowledge of our reason for Being, able to follow intuition in 4-5 D, where Pure Creation continually flows through the Heart.

This Universe of ours, what is it really? Here we are, centers of consciousness, surrounded by buzzing confusion, which we try to understand. But we are of the selfsame stuff of the Universe -- perhaps ultimately a cloud of energy interacting with other clouds of energy... What we experience is not external reality per se but our interaction with it, in a very real sense -- we are constructing our Universe from ourselves.

Dennis Elwell
Cosmic Loom

Seeming unhappy circumstances are often doorways to a more fulfilling Life; as through the "dark night of the Soul" Truth of Mind-Heart is exposed. Wakeup calls compel us to delve deeper into the resonance deep within for our purpose, when lost in the external we hunger for our True Reason for Being.

> ...deep or sudden and unexpected change challenges the meaning and understanding we've Created, to "make sense of Life." We've developed meanings as "road maps of reality... Change often takes us into new territory where old maps are no longer sufficient.
>
> A triggering event can be the death of parent or child, divorce, serious illness, financial disaster, or anything unexpected... Every change *is* a type of death to an old way of living or being. Yet, ironically, change, dying to the old, is one a defining characteristic of growth. To live is to grow; to grow is to change; to change is to die to the old. Many changes open us to an accelerated pattern of growth..."
>
> Yet we fear death, and this very fear of death, the fear of change, is also our fear of Life itself. To be fully alive, we must be willing to be changed, to surrender into the moment without resistance; we must be willing to "die daily," even moment by moment. To resist these "deaths" is to resist Life.

Robert Brumet, Unity Minister
Finding Yourself in Transition,
Using Life's Changes for Spiritual Awakening

From a *dark night of the Soul* and *near death experience* came a life-changing epiphany for filmmaker Tom Shadyak, in powerful documentary, *"I Am"* made after a years coma from a cycling accident. He discovered that in some native cultures gross materialism is equated with insanity, so he began following St. Augustine's, *"Determine what God has given you, take from it what you need; the remainder is needed by others."* His proceeds support non-profits, to usher in a loving, kind, compassionate, equitable World activated by union with the Heart.

Many are Now escaping the inertia of the old to break Free, focusing the life from Inner Stillness to that which is meaningful to Heart and *Essence*. A societal trend is afoot to Live such concepts as: Small is Beautiful, Downsizing, Growing a Garden, Going Organic, Yards to Gardens, Farm to Table, Follow Your Bliss, Sacred Sexuality, Live Your Dreams, Urban Change, Co-Housing Communities, Shop Local-Eat Local, We are One, Toxic-Free Fashion, Karma Free Food, Animal Rescue Groups, Education, Women's Co-ops, programs to relieve Hunger, Water, Sanitation and Orphanages.

The Occupy movement has been a great opportunity for many join together, get "outside the box" and be a Voice. As some take the leap, others discover courage and community to follow. Taking the risk to beyond old boundaries "opens doors where there were only walls before." Finding ways to make *small changes* right where you are, is a huge step to accessing Heart-centered Living.

> Gently resist the temptation to chase your dreams into the world; pursue them in your heart until they disappear into the Self, and leave them there.

> *Maharishi Mahesh Yogi (1918-2008)*
> *Founder Transcendental Meditation Worldwide movement*

It can be as simple as asking ourselves at any given moment, *"Am I Focusing, Breathing, Smiling and Coming from My Heart?"* Is my direction coming from old "corrupt data" or "New" Heart alignment? Am I functioning from LOVE or from Fear? Am I releasing what doesn't belong? Am I holding on too tight? Am I accessing "Stillness and Meditation" for solutions? Feelings can help us identify what motivates us, and what we need to let go of.

> The cave you fear to enter
> holds the treasure that you seek.

> *Joseph Campbell (1984-1987)*
> *Mythologist, Author*
> *Advised Stephen Spielberg on Star Wars Archetypes*

Inner Stillness and Meditation are tools to break Free from Mind-chatter. Regular practice gives us a fresh start on how our Attention is placed upon the *Field,* thus making a Vibrational match to draw in what we desire rather than what we don't. Once we enter this coherent state, we attract others resonating similarly. You may suddenly discover you and those around you are at ease, because of the *place of deepening peace within you.*

> Rising incidence and intensity of gamma radiation over the last decade has been precisely documented...Our cell nuclei, approximately 97% dormant DNA just waiting to be activated, could potentially endow us with completely new traits.

> *Biophysicist Dieter Broers*
> *Solar REvolution*

We are ALL being nudged into the Heart by Cosmic influences. Each of us is essential to the Whole. Clear our old "data" and cultivate friendship with others on the path, to accelerate transformation by growing together. Join with self-affirming gatherings, or initiate your own Sacred Space Community. Give to projects for which you feel compassion - local and Global. Have fun, play, laugh, share with others, let your authentic self be expressed, and enjoy the LOVE YOU ARE. Find a way to Serve. Find a way to Play. Uniting with others eases the *Shift.* ***Know it to Be So in Inner Stillness, and so It Is...*** ♥

Part 2: MIND
Chapter 2
BEING Prayer

BE the change you wish to see in the World.

Mahatma Gandhi (1869-1948)
Autobiography: Story of My Experiments with Truth

We are a "tuning fork" holding our own tone or resonance in the World. We are "movie projectors" of the *Field*. Waves of Creation pass through *us* to bring "reality" into being based our resonance! *We get to choose* how "reality" bears witness to the Vibration within us.

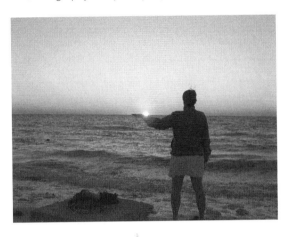

Like a drop of water in the ocean with many other drops, we ride waves of which we are part, materializing into sensational form, from individual and collective thought. Our natural "tuning fork" resonates LOVE at the center of our Being, and as we "clean it up," it resonates more and more with our Heart's Truest Desires.

We are Now Freeing our Minds from blame-fear-hostility-judgment-control thinking, that reduced flow of LOVE in our "realities." Every resonance in us sends ripples into and is Mirrored back from the *Field*. The **21st Century Superhumans** *Quest* is to clean out lower Vibrations from our conscious and unconscious thought-emotion, to fully access True *Power of Mind and Heart.*

> Don't be fooled into believing that what you see is what is real. Your focus upon what you are wanting is indeed causing the Universe around you to shift and line up with what you are expecting.
>
> *Abraham-Hicks*
> *The Communion of Light*

Gregg Braden, geologist and Nassim Haramein, Quantum physicist, both reveal that during their scientific education they were taught *space was empty.* Quantum physics recognizes "space" as the *Field of Possibilities* or *Divine Matrix*, a continually creating rich and full generative *Essence* surrounding us, from which we emerge within the *Web of Life.*

Traditional cultures recognized and honored the *Web of Life*, as vital to ALL in their ultimate Earth Wisdom.

The one thing that connects all things is SPACE. Perhaps the greatest error in the standard model of physics is the fact that they ignore...that the vacuum of space is not empty - it's actually completely full with energy! ...we see that it is highly energized with..."vacuum fluctuations" known as aether, plenum, zero point field, Quantum foam, space and the vacuum...

Nassim Haramein
The Resonance Project

Quantum research has exposed the amazing truth, that the *brain* does not *contain* information rather it *accesses* information through the Mind from the *Field,* which is then filtered by the brain based upon our beliefs and capacity. Holonomic Brain Theory *actually* defines our brain as a "holographic projector." This theory was originated in 1987 by psychologist Karl Pribram with David Bohm, who developed the Implicate Order in physics. Previously, electrons were perceived as separate. Pribram and Bohm found them to be wave-forms existing in multiple locations simultaneously. *Okay -wow! Is this how we are ALL One?*

...subatomic particles are entangled...because at a deeper level of "reality" these particles are not individual but actually extensions or emanations of the same wave-forms.

Memories, or prior experiences, are stored in holographic-like form and retrieved through cognition, in order to activate...thought into "reality."

Pribram and Bohm agreed that some sort of "super Hologram" contains all the information about past, present, and future, like a compact disc containing spatial information that can be read, or decoded, by a laser beam.

Wikipedia

Such a concept takes us into an entirely new realm and mindset, to grasp this idea of how the brain accesses Greater Mind. Higher intelligence comes from our ability to let down our guard enough to go into the *Field of Possibilities* to access unlimited information. Einstein trained himself to fall asleep, pencil in hand, so immediately upon awaking he would write down details of what he had picked up in the *Field* during sleep.

We are also told that consciousness is a *quality* of the *Field,* and that our consciousness does not come from inside us, rather when we relax through practices such as Meditation, Prayer, Chanting and Movement we open ourselves to consciousness flowing in the *Field.*

Looking for Consciousness in the Brain is like
looking inside the Radio for the Announcer.

Nassim Haramein
Resonance Project, Connected Universe

Such a wild theory gradually makes more sense, as we assimilate Quantum principles and expand our perception of "reality." The *secret* of the Hologram is that if you chop up a holographic image (such as that found on a credit card) into tiniest pieces, in every fragment of the Hologram *(under magnification)* is contained a complete image of the original picture. When we change our internal resonance as **21st Century Superhumans** we shift the entire Hologram of existence surrounding us. This is what we call, **Arcing the Hologram** like an arc-welder making a weld.

According to Gregg Braden in the video "Secret Ancient Knowledge, Gregg Braden, The Divine Matrix" (YouTube) this is how nature makes changes quickly on a grand scale, through *The Divine Matrix*. We are just Now absorbing the astounding fact, that we are part of this Universal Hologram of Life. Change within us reflects as a shift in the *Whole*.

> When we form Heart-centered beliefs... in the language of physics we're creating the electrical and magnetic expression of them as waves of energy... So clearly we're "speaking" to the world around us in each moment of every day through a language that has no words: the belief-waves of our Hearts.
>
> *Gregg Braden*
> *Spontaneous Healing of Belief*

In an experiment with 2 photons (fast-moving tiniest particles of Light), when a change is made with the first photon not only does the second miles away follow it exactly, *EVEN MORE AMAZING* is that often the second photon moves *before* the first photon. Numerous Quantum physics experiments demonstrate messages are not sent *through* the *Field, they exist as part of the Field. Wow!*

Several studies Now measure resonance of human consciousness at some 40 places on Earth. During globally noticed events, this resonance naturally increases. What is more amazing is that when a highly visible unexpected event occurs such as 9/11, *24 hours previous on 9/10 the resonance spiked!* This allows these scientists to know an event is going to happen *before* it does, further demonstrating that consciousness supersedes time.

It is emerging from these studies, that we are part of the *Field of Possibilities*, the *Web of Life*, the *Divine Matrix* existing all around us and of which we are part. Key to shifting events through the *Field* is to operate from the Heart with LOVE, pineal activation under current Cosmic influences is enhancing this function. Our consciousness is one with Earth.

> All things are feeding information to the vacuum and the vacuum is feeding it back. The amount that you are able to feed into the system, is related directly to your amount of resistance, as to how much information can come in.
>
> *Nassim Haramein*
> *Resonance Project,*

Thousands of years of judgment-control-blame-fear-hostility we've inherited from our generations, has encouraged conformity rather than expansive thinking, subservience rather than creativity, fear rather than LOVE - all of which we might call "resistance." As a result we use only 5% of our Mind-power consciously. 95% is sequestered in the unconscious as "shadow" thought-emotion, waiting for us to release it and let it go. *Are we ready to sweep out and Leap beyond our shadows?* This Ever-Present-Now offers the greatest opportunity in millennia to become aware of of denial of our unconscious pain and patterns, and remove them to access full Power of Mind-Heart. (More in coming chapters).

> We encourage all of you to dig deeper into your center of your own sphere, to find the knowledge that exists within and is reflected by each one of us. Together as a team, we on this planet can attain increased levels of understanding that Create coherency and resonance... a unified field.
>
> *Nassim Haramein*
> *Resonance Project*

As we launch into this Leap across the Evolutionary Spiral, we break Free from old paradigms, discovering our creative brilliance and embracing our World in New ways. Be patient with yourself and stay with it, as it is a "dance" of agility in the Quantum arena to move through releasing old patterns when they come up and shifting into LOVE. As we we leave behind *World is flat* constructs, our World changes inside and out. Breathe and Smile.

When you change the way you look at things,
the things you look at change.

Whatever we think it is, it is. Life is either full of good things and good people or bad things and bad people. When we are fixed on an idea or expectation, we are sure to get it. This continues until we "wake up," change our consciousness and our Creation.

PLAYING IN THE HOLOGRAM: Let go of all thought-emotional expectations of any other person, event or experience. Let "reality" fall "out of form," into the *Field*. Imagine how you would like the Hologram to reshape itself, such as global peace, money in your bank account, relationship, healing new job. Offer *playful details* in your mind of *how you ARE once this has already happened,* such as throwing money up in air, dancing in the dark, Loving going to your job-home-relationship, leaping for joy with new vitality.

> ...we may think of the heart as a belief-to-matter translator. It converts perceptions of our experiences, beliefs, and imagination into the coded language of waves that communicate with the world beyond our bodies...
>
> *Gregg Braden*
> *Spontaneous Healing of Belief*

Gregg Braden relates his intent search for clues in Ancient Wisdom teachings, for the *language of how to communicate with* the *Field or Divine Matrix*. He journeys far into Tibet where Ancient Tradition is little touched by the modern World. In a remote monastery he asked an elderly monk why he played gongs, bowls and chanted for hours before praying.

The monk explained that playing gongs and chanting was to get into a particular feeling, to be able put his prayers out and have them answered, *a feeling beyond all judgment.* When Gregg asked him what the feeling was, the translator explained it was Compassion. The translator also told him that when the monk Breathes in the *Divine Matrix* surrounding him, it is the same as the feeling of "Compassion without judgment." "This Compassion and Divine Matrix are the same. Our science is now showing that when rightly understood, our feeling has the capacity to change the molecules of our World."

Asking with the voice is not enough. We must speak to the Field in the voice that it recognizes. It recognizes the power of our Heart, going out in electrical and magnetic waves. When you Create the feeling in your Heart as if your prayer is already answered, that Creates the electrical and magnetic waves that bring the answer to you.

Gregg Braden
The Divine Matrix (video)

Gregg discovered a second vital key on how to communicate with the *Field* or *Divine Matrix* in records in Ancient Texts preserved at Nag Hammadi and Coptic Libraries. Some of these important texts were removed from Judaeo-Christian *Bibles* around 350 AD.

Whatsoever ye ask the Father in my name He will give it to you. Hitherto ye have asked nothing in my name. Ask and ye shall receive that your joy may be full

John 16:24 (traditional verse)

Here are lines that were removed telling HOW to ask, from the original Aramaic:

All things that you ask straightly, directly from inside my name you will be given. So far you have not done this.

Ask without hidden motive [such as judgment-control] ask from Heart
be surrounded by your answer [feel as if it has happened]

Be enveloped by what you desire [it has already happened]

that your gladness be full

When you **make the two one** [Mind-Heart]

If the two **make peace with each other in this temple** [us]

They will say to the mountain, "Move away!"

And it will move away.

Gregg's finding of these keys from Ancient Texts and Teachings, is a critical piece of exact instruction on how to communicate effectively with the *Field*, which we might also call effective prayer. This knowledge carefully carried forward for centuries aligns perfectly with principles of Quantum physics and how our thoughts Create our "reality."

When you marry your thought and emotion into one single potent force you have the ability to speak to the [*Field*]; and we must *feel* that our prayer has already been answered.

Gregg Braden, The Divine Matrix (video)

Bringing thought down from *Mind* in upper 3 chakras to meet feeling from the lower 3 chakras in the *Heart*, send out powerful magnetic signals of combined thought-emotion through the Heart. This is the language that the *Field* recognizes, and to which it responds.

Gregg tells two stories about praying for rain that we will share here, because understanding this is so critical to how we move forward as conscious creators in our World. One prayer brought rain to new Mexico during a drought and the other brought torrential rain, to desperately dry Australia.

Gregg's Native American friend took him along out to the mesa, to "pray rain" in dry New Mexico. Then his friend got up and said, "Let's go to dinner." Gregg said, "Wait, I thought you were going to pray for rain. I didn't hear or see you do anything." His friend said, "If I pray *for* rain, it would never happen. As soon as you pray *for* something you have just acknowledged it is not here. When we say, 'Please let there be peace, healing, relationship' we acknowledge it's not here."

So Gregg asked him, "What did you do when you closed your eyes?" His friend told him he *felt the feeling* as if the rain has *already happened* - his naked feet in the mud, so much rain there is *"mud between the toes,"* running through *Fields* of corn and the corn is high because there has been so much rain; smelling the rain in the flowers and seeing it pouring down the pueblo; then he gave thanks for the rain that had *already happened.*

This is *SO IMPORTANT FOR US TO GET.* ..somehow long ago we gave away our power, and forgot how to pray by holding in Mind-Heart that it has already happened as co-creative Beings, One with All Things and the *Field of Infinite Potential.* Restoring Ancient memories, we bring into our prayer experience that what we ask for already *IS.*

1. Ask without judgment, control or expectation
2. Be "surrounded by our answer" - feel it as already happened
3. Be enveloped by what we desire - experience that it already *IS*
4. Breathe the *Field* - Compassion - Deep LOVE - Gratitude

Gregg also shares a woman with an inoperable 3.5" cancerous bladder tumor being treated at a medicine-free clinic in China, where we actually watch (YouTube) the tumor disappear with ultrasound in 3 minutes. They work on her "...without judgment; they did not say 'bad cancer go away' or 'we're going to use radiation.' They said 'now we're going to choose a new reality,' as if she was already healed. Their chant, 'Wasa,' means 'already done,' 'may may may,' meaning NOW! Her body responded; physical reality must respond to the language it understands."

Nassim Haramein champions essential link between physics and consciousness. He has been playing with Quantum theory since age nine, is Founder of the Resonance Project whose mission is "to further *understanding* of the connections between human beings (energetic, physical, and intuitive) and larger forces leading to *right action* in the World." His latest paper, *The Schwarzschild Proton,* passed peer review, marking a new paradigm in the World of Quantum theory, describing nuclei of an atom as a mini black hole where protons are attracted by gravitation." He hints this gravitation at center of black holes could be LOVE. View trailer "The Connected Universe" at http://www.resonance.is

Nassim "meditates daily to keep my Heart open" while playing with revolutionary physics theories and surfing in Hawaii. He tells us that "Infinite Nature" is present in every atom, meaning we're exchanging information with "ALL Things in the Universe ALL the time." His YouTube videos reveal an eye-opening understanding of current Quantum theory on a practical basis.

> ...you are an active participant in the Universe creation, right now! [This] is the ultimate understanding, the ultimate massage of this new energy technology. That is, the energy, the technology and you are one.
>
> *Nassim Haramein*

We apply this knowledge beyond the personal to affect global change. To do so we *remove ourselves from fighting* things we don't want, *because wishing for something not to happen, simply holds it in Creation.* Instead, we focus our Attention on what we desire by feeling, through the Heart without judgment, what we desire, as it's already happened (mud between the toes).

Studies demonstrated in the 1970s that with groups Meditating, Coherence occurred in society, crime rates went down and Life improved. There has been a global movement toward *Praying Peace* which has proven very effective. To achieve ongoing change on a global scale, it is revealed that a number of people **consistently holding the "experience" of peace, with feeling through the Heart, without judgment, as it already IS, calls forth the World we desire.**

NUMBERS to = that THE World IS CHANGED

Studies show it takes the square root of 1% of a population "being" peace, for it to shift.
1 million people x .01 (1%) = 10,000
Square root of 10,000 is 100 people! (to shift 1 million people)
Earth's population is around 7 billion
1% is 70 million
Square root of 70 million is 8366
8,366 people HOLD Peace, LOVE, Balance, Healing, Enough for All
shifts our entire World!!! *How easy is this?* Let Peace begin on Earth, and Let it Begin with ME...pass it on!

WE ARE THE ONES WE'VE BEEN WAITING FOR: With over a billion people now on the internet growing numbers are learning to envision positive solutions for global issues, and groups around the World are "holding peace" and visions of well-being and wholeness. As we hold peace, LOVE, plenty, balance, well-being, *ALWAYS IN THE EVER PRESENT NOW*...it is a shift away from trying to "fix" things, from being stressed, from worrying about what might happen, shifting into our **Heart's Desire and IT IS SO.**

As a reminder - most of us still carry unconscious data, old patterns Not of LOVE holding resonance in the *Field* (when groups quit praying peace, things somewhat go back to the way they were). In upcoming chapters, we find removing this content from self is essential to shifting the collective consciousness, resulting in lasting Global change.

ARC THE Hologram Now!
LOVE · COMPASSION · GRATITUDE

As Quantum Experience deepens, we become aware that all things, situations, people and events are *emerging anew from the Field of Possibilities Constantly.* What we have thought of as matter and form is an Eternal state of flux and flow. What appears as sameness comes from static patterns of thinking held *within us.* The more we embrace Quantum living, thinking, being, the more our Existence flows in new and miraculous ways. Breathe. Smile.

You get there by realizing you are already there.

Eckhart Tolle
The Power of Now

BEING PRAYER: *HOLD HAND OVER HEART,* bring Mind down into Heart, bring feelings up into Heart, Breathe through Heart. Smile. Connect with Mother Earth (Pachamama). Feel her energy run through you from her core, all the way up through your chakras and out to our Central Sun Alcyone and back. Feel yourself flowing as One with Earth, the Stars and ALL of Creation. Enter the vortex at the center of your Heart's energy field. Send LOVE through your Heart spinning out miles beyond your body into the Web of Life. Intensify feelings, knowing and connection, creating a coherent signal of Deep LOVE, Compassion and Gratitude for what is now being reshaped in the *Field.* Release yourself and your VISION of what already "IS" into the *Field* to be brought forth New form. Breathe. Smile. Give thanks. LOVE.

- Mind and Feeling Are ONE.
- Bring feeling up to Heart & Mind down to Heart. Marry them in Heart.
- I Breathe the *Field* from a *feeling-state* of Compassion without judgment
- I am surrounded by - *feel* - my answer - smell the rain
- I am joyfully enveloped by my desire - *It Is So (mud between the toes)*
- I say to the mountain, "Mountain move!" And it moves.

With practice our Quantum ability to access Power of Mind and Heart to shift "reality" becomes our new "norm" as **21st Century Superhumans**. Most exciting, as we tune up our inner resonance of thought-emotion to our True Design LOVE, we remember an entirely New-old paradigm where Life unfolds in an ongoing process of shifting the entire Hologram within with LOVE. ♥

Chapter 3

Response-Ability

Placing the blame or judgment on someone else leaves you powerless to change your experience; taking responsibility for your beliefs and judgments gives you the power to change them.

Byron Katie
Loving What Is

What is True Response-Ability? It is our Ability to Respond. It is our Ability to Recognize that our thoughts and emotions hold resonance in the World, that our "reality" is simply a Mirror of this. We Respond by clearing our own internal content Not of LOVE. This is Response-Ability.

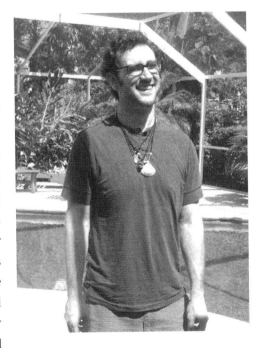

"SOUND VIBRATES SAND:" Search for these fascinating videos on YouTube, with visual demonstration of sand moving into complex forms simply with sound. This is very much how thought and emotion resonate in our World. Thoughts go out as frequency patterns Vibrating matter and events into being (like sound). Watch particles move into beautiful patterns as a result of Vibration. Similarly Vibration of thought-emotion causes matter and events to take shape from our Attention upon the *Field*. This is the first Universal Law - ALL is Mind: thought Creates.

Our thoughts-emotions are like "tuning forks," creating Vibrational energetic patterns that shape *potential* (waves and particles) into form around us. Taking Response-Ability means stepping into an empowered role, releasing the idea that anyone or anything else is at cause in our World, Responding to our own Creation.

WHO IS TO BLAME? Think of someone in your Life who you relate with on a regular basis. Consider an "issue" you notice with them; someone close such as primary partner, former partner, parent, child, sibling, employer, friend. *Okay, have someone in mind?* Notice what you feel the issue is with this person and just be with it. Can you look inside yourself and find that same resonance (or judgment of it) inside you? Or Are you thinking, *"Oh no, I don't have that in me. They do!"* Well, the truth is, the *Matrix or Field* can only brings us a *match to our resonance.* Those with matching "puzzle pieces" to ours are a vibrational match.

Remember how a C tuning for will make another C tuning for ring across the room, but not a G? We can only "magnetize" in those with matching resonance or "tuning forks" to our own. The sooner we can acknowledge this the sooner we attain clarity in our Lives. You may just find yourself laughing once realized how obvious it is that those who are drawn to you are those with matching energy frequencies. The quickest and best way to clear these things is to clear OURSELVES!

Think of what bothers you the most through interaction with them. Now notice your hostility, judgment, fear, grief, criticism, or resistance to the situation. Take note of what comes up for you, also notice whether it "rings a bell" from other relationships or situations. Most likely this is not the first time you've experienced this in your Life in interaction with another. These things are like "layers of the onion" and tend to come up over and over again, just with different names and faces. As our friend dr. michael ryce says, "If this has happened 85 times with 50 different people, who was there every time? You." At first it may seem difficult to identify what's inside us, when we are used to blaming others for our discomfort. *Enjoy this process; look inside self to get clear.*

OUR PERCEPTION: In Quantum "reality," "there is no out there, out there," so what appears as our perception of another is coming from a resonance within us, received through our filters. Noticing what is Mirrored by this other person, we have the opportunity to remove our old thought-emotional patterns showing up in this situation.

According to Harvard studies 95% thought-emotion is stored in our unconscious, 5% in our conscious. So it is a residual Vibration from something that most likely happened long long ago, very likely not even to US! As it may very well be a genetic resonance. This "tuning fork" will keep "ringing" in our World until we remove it from our own unconscious. Until we become aware of this Quantum patterning, it's easy to remain in "denial" about it, because it was very likely "life threatening" when stored.

Byron Katie's workshops and groundbreaking book, *Loving What Is* offer tremendous introduction to the realization that no one else is to blame and there are no victims. We will be learning to clear this unconscious data, a "rewiring" from cultural norms.

> As long as you think that the cause of your problem is "out there"—as long as you think that anyone or anything is responsible for your suffering—the situation is hopeless. It means you are forever in role of victim and you're suffering in paradise.
>
> *Byron Katie*
> *Loving What Is: Four Questions That Can Change Your Life*

RESPONSIBILITY - PARTNER TO BLAME: Responsibility definition: "called to account as the primary cause, motive or agent." This definition is a residual of the blame-fear-hostility culture, where one takes "responsibility" so they don't get punished! We only blame another for being at "cause" if we've forgotten we're a "creator." Once we *know* everything in our World comes from resonance in us, self becomes accountable for what shows up in our "reality," so there is no one responsible.

Aw we Wake Up, we become Response-Able or Able to Respond to all situations as our own Creation, for *anything* appearing in our "reality" with LOVE. We will learn the exciting news of how this operates in greater depth, on our *21st Century Superhuman* adventure!

CORRECT TRANSLATION OF FORGIVENESS: The word "forgive" in Ancient *Aramaic* (the language of Jesus or Yeshua) was translated by the Greeks as "pardon," for in their culture the only comprehension they had is that others were to blame or accountable. This "power-over" culture of the day had no brain cells to understand that we "Create our reality," so they mis-translated Yeshua's (Jesus') teaching on "forgiveness" to mean pardon or let off the hook. This has carried over into our modern-day "forgiveness," that I'll let you "off the hook" for what you "did to me."

Now we as Quantum Beings already understand that no one else is to blame for our "reality," and there is no one to let off the hook - because whatever "reality" we are experiencing, was Created from resonance inside of us! *Right?* Yeshua or Jesus's teachings of "forgiveness" were QUANTUM - he understood Quantum physics. He knew we Created our own "reality" with our Vibration (conscious-unconscious), so True Aramaic Forgiveness was "to remove our own unconscious content resonating in the situation!"

BLAME = DENIAL: Blame comes from the blame-fear-hostility culture that forgot its ability to Create. Blaming someone else keeps us from having to look inward to deal with and remove our own Ancient pain, buried in the unconscious. Blame "takes the pressure off me" and makes you responsible, so I can stay in denial about my old painful data. Let's clear ghosts and shadows out of the closet holding frequency in our "reality."

I fundamentally don't believe in evil. I believe that there is just confusion.

Nassim Haramein
The Resonance Project

Let's say for example we're angry at our "stepmother." She took all the money and as a result we're angry at, resentful of and blaming her, as we consider her "responsible" we make sure she is "punished" by our thoughts, words, actions.

In the Quantum World the stepmother shows up in our World, as a Mirror of Vibrational content inside of us. We magnetically draw each other in (like 2 tuning forks of the same note) so we become aware of what we need to clean out of our unconscious "Not of LOVE." So guess what our job is, instead of blaming her, that's right, look inside ourselves to remove the ancient Not of LOVE resonance inside ourselves. *Seriously? Yup!*

She is not "responsible" and no forgiveness required. She is Mirroring what we need clear away, which may be our fear that our money will be taken, or really it could be any of thousands of things, that will be discovered as we go through upcoming worksheet processes.

> Our parents, our children, our spouses, and our friends will continue to press every button we have, until we realize what it is that we don't want to know about ourselves, yet. They will point us to our freedom every time.
>
> *Byron Katie*
> *Loving What Is*

Interestingly enough Jesus, Buddha (500 B.C.) and Zoroaster (1500 B.C.) all spoke derivatives of Ancient Aramaic, focusing teachings according to *modern translation,* on self Response-Ability for our "Creation." Reflected in this instruction given 2,000 years ago it is obvious all three were teaching about Quantum "reality." Humanity-huwomity had just not yet quite developed the "brain cells" to get it and were stuck in old blame patterns.

> Do not judge, or you too will be judged. [Judging is holding our creative Attention upon the *Field* - holding in form what we are judging].
>
> For in the same way you judge others, you will be judged, and with the measure you use, it will be measured to you. [Whatever resonance you hold in the *Field* will be perfectly Mirrored back with matching resonance]
>
> Why do you look at the speck of sawdust in your brother's eye and pay no attention to the plank in your own eye? [Thought-emotion Not of LOVE]
>
> How can you say to your brother, 'Let me take the speck out of your eye,' when all the time there is a plank in your own eye? ...first take the plank out of your own eye, and then you will see clearly to remove the speck from your brother's eye. [Take Response-Ability, remove YOUR Not of LOVE thought-emotion, conscious-unconscious calling this "reality" into Being, rather than blaming others]
>
> *Matthew 7:1-5*
> *Biblegateway.com*

Judgment *is* our Attention on the *Field,* which will then Mirroring this unconscious content in the "reality" surrounding us. Yeshua (Jesus) spoke parables in Ancient Aramaic containing these Quantum principles, not broadly understand by the culture of the day. The "splinter" and "beam" are the unconscious content each carries, resonating as our Vibration in the *Field.* As we "judge" or blame, our Attention on the *Field* magnetically attracts similar resonance, to show us what we're in denial about. Yes we know, we resisted too when we first heard this - *"Really? It has to be at least a little their fault?"* No. It's all us!!!

> You are your only hope, because we're not changing until you do. Our job is to keep coming at you, as hard as we can, with everything that angers, upsets, or repulses you, until you understand. We LOVE you that much, whether we're aware of it or not. The whole world is about you.
>
> *Byron Katie*
> *Loving What Is*

Blame allows us to stay in denial of something that was hidden away because it was so painful. Such content (in our unconscious) is always based in "survival experiences" we or our generations faced in the blame-fear-hostility culture. It seems confusing at first because we are so conditioned with blame thinking. It does become easier with practice. The operative word here is practice. Once we shift from thinking it's someone *"out there"* to knowing *"it's all an inside job,"* we move away from blame, to take Response-Ability for what our "resonance" is creating in *all* situations. Thus every situation, every person, every event becomes a *GIFT,* showing us what is blocking our True Design LOVE. As we progress forward in this new way of thinking, it becomes easier and more familiar to keep clearing.

THE CURE: Take "true" Response-Ability when something appears in your World Not of LOVE, by clearing your own unconscious content. It can take a while to unravel our old paradigm thinking, and let go of *feeling responsible* to others' expectations. As we grasp this at deeper levels that each person is response-able for "reality" as they experience it, we relate from a New perspective, where each person knows they can change at any moment, and to never to be "sorry." This becomes clearer the deeper we go in these principles.

It's exciting to live from our Hearts, taking Response-Ability for any "reality" emerging from Not of LOVE within us. We clear it, Breathe, Smile and step into a greater flow of LOVE. The more we get excited about and deepen our desire to express fully who we are, the faster this change occurs.

> When we stop opposing reality, action becomes
> simple, fluid, kind and fearless.
>
> *Byron Katie*
> *Loving What Is*

THE GIFT OF ESSENCE: Response-Ability is speaking, living, Being the Truth; bringing our Gifts into the World rather than what we "think" someone else expects. As we release ourselves from "fear of punishment" and "need to comply" that has held us in its spell so long, we begin to Breathe the *REAL AIR OF FREEDOM.* We Breathe and Smile more. Our neurobiology frees up. We do things for reasons of the Heart rather than obligation. As we step into True Being, synchronicities open doors. Once we enter this Aligned state, we entrain with True *Essence* and Life naturally flows.

Cultivating Quantum understanding we shift from "responsible" to Response-Able. Knowing our thoughts-emotions resonate "reality" into being around us, we cultivate Ability to Respond immediately upon noticing what is Mirrored in our World, taking action to remove anything Not of LOVE holding resonance.

HOW YOU FEEL RESPONSIBLE AND WHY: Think of the many ways you feel responsible to others or situations and for what reasons. Make a list and after each situation note how to shift internally to come more into *Essence.* Continue until you have cleared out all sense of responsibility based in fear, judgment, expectations of others, and have replaced it with

Response-Ability from *Essence* of Heart. *Notice throughout your day whether you respond from your Heart or out of traditional "responsibility."*

This is an unwinding, be patient with yourself. We change inner constructs by allowing our process to integrate. Learning to live as who we Truly Are is the mission of the **21st Century Superhuman**. Think of your talents and special qualities. Reflect on these and imagine expressing them Free of old limiting beliefs. Breathe and Smile. LOVE.

Response-Ability vs responsibility Quiz

- WHAT Situation am I feeling *responsible* to?
- HOW - Do I express *responsibility?*
- WHAT IS THE FEELING OR THOUGHT making me *respond* this way?
- WHO is acting as my Mirror?
- WHAT IS IN MY HEART When I listen to my Heart - what is being asked of me that I've chosen to override, due to sense of hidden "responsibility" to outer expectations? *Dig deep - as may be buried under layers of cultural conditioning.*
- WHAT ACTIONS to take... to move into Response-Ability, clear my own content and get back on track with my True *Essence* or Heart?
- Breathe, Smile...open new neurological pathways!

Exchanging "responsibility" for Response-Ability, restores "power" of Heart. Blame, a sense of responsibility and outer expectations, all cut off flow of Life Force, resulting in pain, unhappiness, dis-ease, dis-comfort, dis-harmony and despair, rampant in our World. As we return to *Essence,* we open up to flow of Life from Source, and *our World changes!*

We may experience pain, sadness, fear or anger, when we reflect on what we've "lost" or what has been "taken from us" as we've given in to the demands others. As we dig deeper, we discover *even this* is a result of our own thought-emotional content to be cleared.

We need more Light about each other. Light Creates understanding,
Understanding Creates LOVE, LOVE Creates Patience, Patience Creates Unity.

Malcolm X (1928-1965)
Muslim Minister and Human Rights Activist

False "responsibility" ties into ancestral thought patterns, passed down the line in family traditions, as guilt, fear, rage and punishment, producing some of the deepest darkest stories and shadows in human history. As we *release, clear and let go, we restore resonance* to out True Infinite Design LOVE! We are stardust! We are golden!

For too long man has encased himself in a shell of misunderstanding and fear... [like] the shell of a turtle. Man has pulled himself into this shell thinking he would be protected by it. In "reality" it has only impeded his spiritual progress...There is little progress as long as we are content to be encased in fear, misunderstanding,

168

falsity, hatred, intolerance, or any encumbering shell. Only as we burst out of these shells will we be free.

...They must come to recognize that the True Man [Woman] is the spiritual one. He/she has qualities of consciousness and understanding far beyond the limitations of earth. When this is realized, we will come out of our shell and move forward...into a new world of experience and expression...

Nellie B. Cain
Exploring the Mysteries of Life

Restoring our True Design LOVE and our fullest Expression as Creative Joyful Beings, Breathing and Smiling, is the Journey of the **21st Century Superhuman.** Unraveling shadows that have weighed us down is essential to taking this Evolutionary Leap. It may feel like we're letting go of part of self, as we release shells of fear that have kept us **responsible** to something outside *Essence* for so long, yet we enthusiastically get through it!

Once we release this misplaced sense of "responsibility," it also becomes easier to let go of suppressive habits that keep us from feeling our pain of loss of self, such as alcohol, smoking, excessive TV, excessive or heavy foods, drugs and distractions, such as our "story" about how it is someone or something else's fault. Let each one walk their path without trying to save, rescue, push or cajole. The more we align with LOVE, we Create a New magnetic resonance and "reality" around us, which Hearts naturally follow.

People have a hard time letting go of their suffering. Out of a fear of the unknown,
they prefer suffering that is familiar.

Thich Nhat Hanh
Buddhist Monk, Author, Peace Activist

We access more Authentic Self as our shell of fear falls away. We clear our *own* content resonating our "reality" into being. We become truthful and express from the *Heart*. We Smile and Breathe, we Jump for Joy as we free ourselves, from antiquated beliefs that our Life is bound to the expectations of others. We renew commitment to Live from *Essence*.

So universal is the habit of blaming circumstances or other people for the troubles of our own lives - the fact that the source of all trouble lies entirely within us meets with contradiction and resentment... It takes courage to look to one's self entirely for pain which seems to be caused by others, but if once we do it, and are thoroughly clean-cut about it in every thought and word and action, the release from bondage seems almost miraculous.

Annie Payson Call (1853-1940)
How to live Quietly 1914

In Blink Malcom Gladwell tells the story of a woman auditioning for role of principal French horn at the Met. No women were in the horn section as they were considered "not as good" as men. When this woman was declared winner she stepped from behind the try-out screen, and a gasp went up from the judges' panel as they saw it was a woman. They knew of her as a horn player substitute with no idea she was this "good."

When the screen Created a pure Blink moment, a small miracle happened, the king of miracles is always possible when we take charge of the first two seconds: they saw her for who she truly was. The key to good decision making is not knowledge. It is understanding. We are swimming in the former. We are desperately lacking in the latter.

Malcom Gladwell
Blink: the Power of Thinking without Thinking

Others may actually *like us better,* once we recover True Self Expression - at least *we'll like ourselves better!* All Vibrational energy we experience in our World begins within and is Mirrored back by matching frequencies. It is an endless loop! How about making it LOVE? Clearing conditioned and ancestral patterns, then Breathing into the Truth of Who We Are frees us to access our own Higher State of Being. Our clearing process is easier, quicker and we don't take things so personally, because we know they are simply reflecting back to us our own resonance. The more we align with self, the more authentic our Life becomes!

In my experience, we don't *make* thoughts appear, they just appear. One day, I noticed that their appearance just wasn't personal. Noticing that really makes it simpler to inquire.

Byron Katie
Loving What Is

CURRENT UNDERSTANDING OF QUANTUM THOUGHT:

- The *Field, Divine Matrix* or *Web of Life* surrounds us and we are of it
- Our "Reality" emerges from the *Divine Matrix* or *Field of Possibilities*
- Our *Attention* upon the *Field,* calls "reality" into being
- *There is no 'out there,' out there.*
- I Am a Response-Able Observer-Creator
- We clear *all* within ourselves Not of LOVE Mirrored in our "reality"
- The *Field* responds instantaneously to messages of Mind-Heart
- Heart Coherence is Deep LOVE, Compassion and Gratitude
- Focusing through Heart without judgment, it IS (mud between toes), marrying Mind-Heart we shift the whole. *Arc the Hologram with LOVE.*

21st Century Superhumans clear all Not of LOVE thought-emotion Mirrored in our "reality" from self. We let go of *responsibility,* and instead act with Response-Ability, shifting our internal Vibration to align with LOVE through the Heart.

We honor and are patient with self and others, recognizing it may be a bit of a process to get this fully integrated. We find others with whom we can apply these principles and learn together. As we keep at it, it becomes our New "norm." We resonate like a bell from the Heart into the World conscious of how we are calling "reality," into Being, Response-Able for our "reality" Living more and more from *Essence. Yeah!* ♥

Chapter 4

Effluvia: Letting Go Our "Story"

Who put the bop in the bop shoo bop,
who put the ram in the rama rama ding dong?

Barry Mann & Gerry Goffin - The Platters
Who Put The Bomp 1961 (Lyrics)

Patricia Cota-Robles, Founder of Studies for Humanity's Purpose, reminds us we're moving through thousands of years of human *Effluvia*, holding this third dimension in form as a direct result of density of excessive negative thinking.

> Millions of people are so buried in the Effluvia of their negative belief systems that they cannot raise their heads above the chaos and confusion effectively enough to reunite with their [Higher] Selves.

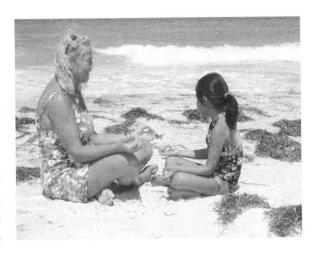

Patricia Cota-Robles
Violet Flame

The word *Effluvia* describes *stories* perpetuating blame, and has brought much laughter to us since discovering it. *Effluvia* describes chronic stories blaming someone or something for what is going on in our World. Once we know how our thoughts Create our "reality," any conversation blaming others, reflecting the News or World at large becomes pointless. In fact, we may politely excusing ourselves from such conversations and social interactions focused around *Effluvia*, simply holding negative images in form.

> There is a way between voice and presence where information flows.
> In disciplined silence it opens. With wandering talk it closes.

Rumi
13th Century Persian Poet, Sufi Mystic

Effluvia is a culturally accepted *numbing mechanism*; to keep mind and mouth busy with blame-judgment Attention outside ourselves, to avoid dis-comfort of removing *our own disassociated content* from Mind-Heart that holds Vibration in our World. We learn to let go these "stories" as we become aware. *Farlex* Dictionary online offers this on *Effluvia*:

A usually invisible emanation or exhalation, as of vapor or gas. A byproduct or residue; waste. The odorous fumes given off by waste or decaying matter.

How much of our Life focuses around "story," based in unproductive thought or conversation? "What does so and so think? Did you hear what happened? How am I going to get this done? I don't have enough time, money, energy. *This* is going on in the World. It's their fault that..." *Effluvia* conversation or thought that goes on and on...gossip, observation of others Not of LOVE, or just telling stories over and over again must go.

Reflective Meditative traditions call this "monkey mind." Letting go of "monkey mind" or *Effluvia* of scattered Mind-energy is best sent packing, despite the fact that we may argue we are "solving" problems or figuring things out. *Effluvia* accesses layers of "corrupt data" in our subconscious like a computer virus that must be cleared away to operate well, and for us to make the shift from continuing to hold these things in Creation in our World.

There is a place where all things begin, a location of pure energy that simply "is." In this Quantum incubator for reality, all things are possible. From our personal success, abundance, and healing to our failure, lack and dis-ease...everything from our greatest fear to our deepest desire begins in this "soup" of potential.

Through reality makers of imagination, expectation, judgment, passion and prayer, we galvanize each possibility into existence. In our beliefs about who we are, what we have and don't have, and what should and shouldn't be, we Breathe Life into our greatest joys as well as our darkest moments.

The key to mastering this place of pure energy is to know that it exists, to understand how it works, and finally to speak the language that it recognizes. All things become available to us as the architects of reality in this place where the world begins: the pure space of the Divine Matrix.

Gregg Braden
The Divine Matrix

Any Vibration within us resonates the *Field*, sending out waves like ripples in the pond of our "reality." When *Effluvia* thoughts come up, learn to step out of *STORY*. Focus the mind around what is desired in LOVE, and remove *your own content* causing this "story" being Mirrored back to us. In upcoming chapters we will learn how to "cancel and clear" with instructions from the Ancient Aramaic, given us by Yeshua (Jesus) for clearing the resonance of our 95% unconscious content that expresses as stories or *Effluvia*.

In our Collective we have founded and perpetuated blame-fear-hostility beliefs. Most are secreted away in the unconscious where 95% of our resonance is carried. It's essential to "take out the garbage" or "clean house" to cancel, release, let go this content, that shows up to let us know it's there to be removed. Coaching or partnering with others who are doing this work can be of great assistance to Create consistency, to keep moving through our old "stuff" and back to LOVE. Sadness, grief, rage and fear expressed in *Effluvial* stories, resonate deep unconscious pain. Compassion without judgment, for both self and others restores LOVE through Heart Coherence.

Supporting, encouraging and inspiring one another to move out of "story" and its *Effluvia* is accomplished by clearing what is holding the issue in resonance at the unconscious level. Participating with parents, friends, relatives, partners, former partners, children we may experience our "story" or *Effluvia*; yet even in these situations, we can share how thoughts Create "reality" and find new ways to be together. Shifting habituated conversations becomes easier with practice.

> It is important to expect nothing, to take every experience,
> including the negative ones as merely steps on the path, and to proceed.
>
> *Ram Dass, Be Here Now*

Remove yourself kindly from conversations with others replaying "stories" of blame, fear, hostility, guilt, shame, victim mentality and "poor me." Do your own clearing, knowing that this is a *gift*, reflecting the resonance *you* need to clear. You may have already cleared it, yet still have *judgment or want control*; or perhaps it is simply a space to *hold LOVE and Compassion without judgment.*

> The significant problems we have cannot be solved
> at the same level of thinking with which we Created them.
>
> *Albert Einstein (1879-1955)*
> *Nobel Prize Physics, Time Person of Century*

As we grow on this path, we learn to use our deepening Compassion to share what we know in a kind way, with clarity and empathy, allowing each person their journey of Awakening. The best place to Create change is within ourselves - as this effects the entire *Field*; we will see others change around us as we shift and clear within.

> ...a small alteration in one place can permanently shift an entire paradigm. Visionary and philosopher Ervin Laszlo describes the reason this is so: "All that happens in one place happens also in other places; all that happened at one time happens also at times after that.' Nothing is 'local,' limited to where and when it is happening." As the great spiritual teachers such as Mahatma Gandhi and Mother Teresa demonstrated so eloquently, the nonlocal holographic principle is an immense force - a "David" to the "Goliath" of change in the Quantum world.
>
> *Gregg Braden, The Divine Matrix*

When we desire positive Creation to surround us, *Effluvia's* interrupting frequencies reduce clarity. Get rid of the chatter holding Not of LOVE Creation in form. Our chapters on cleansing and detox address the important subject of toxins, crystalizing "negative" thought in the body, from excess food waste to silver-mercury fillings. Cleaning up our physical vehicle can help a great deal to detoxify even our conversations.

I do not understand the mystery of grace,
only that it meets us where we are and does not leave us where it found us.

Anne Lamott
New York Times Bestseller - Grace

Stories are addicting, a habituated denial mechanism, buffering us from clearing *our own* deepest pain Vibrating this situation into Being, terrifyingly hidden in the shadows of our unconscious. As long as we remain addicted to "story," we tend to tell our "stories" to others, carrying on the drama of self-perpetuating misery. To truly free ourselves from *Effluvia* or "stories," requires clearing *our* "old data." Mind-chatter is a log-jam in our "river" of pure positive creative potential. Shifting out of *Effluvia* or "story," into peace and clarity changes our "reality" and that of the Whole, so vitality and energy can flow.

7 Keys to Effluvia Busting!

1. I release ALL "Stories" and opt out of participating in others' stories of blame

2. I release all beliefs that I am a victim

3. I recognize my "reality" is a Mirror of what I'm carrying inside.

4. My conversation reflects me taking Response-Ability for my "reality."

5. I regularly remove, cancel, clear all thought Vibration "Not of LOVE."

6. I find a way to hold LOVE, Compassion or Gratitude in all situations

7. I Breathe and Smile, KNOWING I am an Observer-Creator, that what I experience in my "reality" comes from that which is contained within me.

How powerful is it to recognize we are *Quantum CREATORS?* We no longer perpetuate pain and suffering by carrying Not of LOVE thought in our conversation. We release it back to the *Field* to become a "butterfly" or something beautiful. Breathe, Smile, Focus in Pure LOVE, Compassion, Gratitude, clear our old 'data.' *The rest is Effluvia!*

EXAMPLES OF EFFLUVIA We most likely have engaged in *Effluvia* or "story." Think of ways you've participated in conversations that contained *Effluvia*: criticizing, judging, blaming, complaining, worry, manipulation, control, thinking its our job to "fix it" for someone else. Know that we are now letting go of *Effluvia. And let's not judge even ourselves!* We are learning-growing. Breathe and Smile. *Yeah!*

Nothing in the world can bother you as much as your own mind, I tell you. In fact,
others seem to be bothering you, but it's not others, it's your own mind.

Sri Sri Ravi Shankar
Founder Art of Living Foundation

Connected with our True Design, we resonate through Pure LOVE into our World. "Effluvia Busters" are now disengaging from Not of LOVE chatter, consciously switching into Truth of Being and clarity of their energy of Mind and Heart.

It's Time To Walk Our Talk! More than just theory, Quantum activism is the moral compass of Quantum physics, that helps us actually transform our lives and society. So let's walk our talk, and make brain circuits of positive emotions. We just do it. We practice. Let some of us be good, do good. Be with God some of the time, be in the ego some of the time, and let the dance generate creative acts of transformation. With this resolution, with this objective in mind, I invite you to become 'Quantum Activists.'

Amit Goswami
Theoretical Quantum Physicist, What the Bleep

Every moment contains the opportunity to choose - do we wake up and explore this New territory? Or do we remain asleep? Grace is the gift of patience and kindness to ourselves. Bono's U2 Lyrics *"Grace: She travels outside the karma karma... Grace finds goodness in everything."* Creation is waiting for us to step fully into our capability. It is a leap from where we have been, yet doable with Quantum principles, releasing, letting go that which does not serve, ushering in what does.

Grace is within you. Grace is your self. Grace is not something to be acquired from others. All that is necessary is to know its existence is in you. You are never out of its operation.

Ramana Maharshi (1879-1950)
Outstanding Guru Self-Inquiry

We are immersed in a *Field* of fast-moving energy continuously reshaping itself. The *Field* yields electrons to our thought. The instant we change, matter and events change too.

Maybe we should quit paying so much attention to the 1% that makes up matter, and instead focus on the other 99.999% that is space. Instead of matter defining space, space defines matter. This is a fundamental change in consciousness. First of all to understand that you are mostly space, and then that the space defines you instead of you defining it.

Nassim Haramein
Sacred Geometry & Unified Fields Part 2 (YouTube)

As we dissipate our "stories'" *Effluvia*, we open the way for the ultimate Creation we are capable of Being, Receiving, Living and Giving. As we merge with our connectedness with Source; our Life becomes an ever-flowing blessing of Creation and manifestation. *Breathe in Freedom to BE and Create moment by moment from LOVE!*

~ where Attention goes energy flows ~

A side effect of letting go of *Effluvia* may lead us to simplify: perhaps sell a large home and move into a small cottage, community or neighborhood, discover joy in simplicity of less material possessions, share meals, gardens and sacred space flowing between homes.

Many are arriving at the conclusion that excessive possessions are also *Effluvia*. End Stories! Be an "*Effluvia* buster!" When you find yourself in a cloud of *Effluvia*, shake it off and move into Breathing, Smiling and Focusing on conscious creative waves of Being.

EFFLUVIA: STORIES, GOSSIP, BLAME - Any thought, internal dialogue, external dialogue or conversation based on thinking outside of LOVE, Compassion and Gratitude.

> 1. Our "reality" comes from thought-emotion inside us (conscious-unconscious)
> 2. Experiencing anything we "don't like" in our World, we clear it from *self*
> 3. We consciously express through *Essence* from the Heart
> 4. *I Am* Compassion, Gratitude and LOVE. Breathe. Smile.

EFFLUVIA BUSTERS' CODE

• I NOW RELEASE ALL STORIES, GOSSIP, BLAME

• Anything that Appears in my "reality" conversation or experience Not of LOVE, is a *gift*. I look *inside myself* for thought-emotion, conscious-unconscious, genetic-experiential holding resonance in this situation. I Am "Response-Able," by clearing this content from *my* Mind-Body continuum Now.

• I Breathe, Smile and Allow...

• I Trust All is Unfolding for the Highest Good of All Concerned, and release any thought-feeling of it being my job to "fix it" for others.

• I Am a Being of Deep LOVE, Compassion and Gratitude

• I Recognize the Cosmos is now Awakening me to my True Design

• I Focus, Breathe, Smile, Experiencing the Presence of LOVE flowing through me

• I Am Aware Daily that my "reality" is called into form by my Quantum Resonance

• I Now Commit to being an *Effluvia* Buster. All Thoughts, Conversation and Internal Dialog are based in Pure LOVE Creation! If I find myself in a conversation or situation Not of LOVE, I kindly shift the conversation or excuse myself because "I have somewhere else to BE," or I kindly share Truth that we are "Observer-Creators" and we are now shifting our "reality" with LOVE.

• Shift ourselves. Shift the entire Hologram! Of course with LOVE!

> The inspiration you seek is already within you.
> Be silent and listen.

> *Rumi*
> *13th Century Persian Poet, Sufi Mystic*

21st Century Superhumans Now releasing *ALL STORIES* with LOVE! ♥

Part 2: MIND - SECTION 2
OUR TRUE DESIGN LOVE

LOVE is the most fundamental force of creation.

Nassim Haramein
Resonance Project

The purpose of our journey is to awaken to Living from *Essence,* the Heart and our True Design LOVE. You'll find here a "trail of breadcrumbs," for *how* to accomplish this easily and well in these *interesting times of great change.*

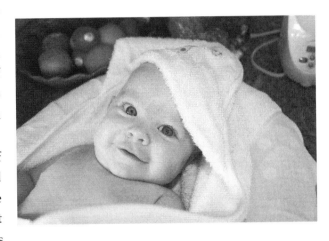

LOVE is an amazing series of harmonious octaves toned to call forth resonance of Pure Positive Creation. LOVE is Sound Current vibrating Life into Form. LOVE is an ever-flowing *Field* of Source Energy, giving itself to us, ebbing and flowing with whatever energies we place upon it. LOVE is seen by some as radiant Light. LOVE is experienced by many as a deep feeling of peace and comfort.

Holding a Newborn gives us a miraculous experience of this LOVE, a precious representation of True Humanity-Huwomity, where purity, essence, sweetness, and the radiance of new Life shine forth. What is this LOVE we are made of? We gather from Quantum physics that a *Living Field* surrounds and permeates us, described in many ways.

- *Cloud* or *Field of Possibilities, Plenum, Vacuum, Source Field*
- 94% Dark *Field & 5% Light Field* surrounds us in "space" (NASA)
- *Divine Matrix* (Gregg Braden) - The Zero Point *Field*
- Akasha - past present future (Ervin Laszlo) "The Space" Sanskrit
- In-formation that "forms" the recipient (David Bohm)
- Electromagnetic field of the Heart 5,000x more powerful than the brain
- Source energy that flows more fully through us, as we free ourselves from blockages
- Andean Shamans carry Ancient Star wisdom that speaks to the Smallest Particles
- Consciousness or *Field* of Intelligence, permeating everything
- Flow of Consciousness like a river - containing whirlpools (us)
- Open BREATH - HU-in HU-out; SMILE - merging with Source

• *Field* surrounding us - Compassion without Judgment (Tibetan Monks)

Science explains the unexplainable, as a *Living Field* that we emerge from, that we are sustained in, that we return to, that we call LOVE. A quality or *Essence* within us, of God, Source, Creator, Great Spirit, Shiva, Buddha, Christ, Divinity, the ONE and more. This *Field* through which we express in Creation is a pure flow of what we call LOVE.

Truth is One, Paths are many.

Swami Satchidananda (1914-2002)
Founder Yogaville® Integral Yoga® International

Out of the *Field* flows the great river of LOVE, the basis of our Being. Our thought and self is like a whirlpool in the river, expressing our individuation. J. Krishnamurti in conversation with David Bohm (YouTube) tells us "'me' is the movement which thought has brought about." Our "operating system" is LOVE or consciousness, our software is thought "calling in" Life, through the "computer" of our existence.

When a computer has a virus or corrupt files, they need to be removed for the computer to run well, metaphoric for us removing our "corrupt data." Gregg Braden describes our operating system here as consciousness, which we will call Universal LOVE. Our experience of Loving - connects us directly with Universal LOVE.

When we want to see our computer do something different, we don't change the operating system – we change the commands that go into it. The reason why this is so important is that consciousness appears to work in precisely the same way.

If we think the entire Universe is a massive consciousness computer, then consciousness itself is the operating system, and "reality" is the output. Just as a computer's operating system is fixed and changes must come from the programs that speak to it, in order to change our world, we must alter the programs that make sense to reality: feelings, emotions, prayers, and beliefs.

Gregg Braden
The Divine Matrix, Bridging Time, Space, Miracles and Belief

Human energy *Fields* are measured to be strongest and most vibrant when expressing LOVE. HeartMath Institute's research has shown that Coherence of Mind, Heart and Body occurs when we experience Deep LOVE, Compassion and Gratitude. They have developed a finger sensor, with which one can integrate coherent emotions in just a few weeks, supporting vitality, well-being and productive Life.

Are you ready to rearrange what you've always thought about your Life? To be reborn into the being of LOVE you were designed to BE? We are stepping out of the World of illusion, and into resonance with the Truth of our BEING. *21st Century Superhuman Quantum Lifestyle* is about realigning our Vibration with the LOVE flowing from deep within us, and clearing out everything in its way, so this river can flow!

Nassim Haramein, transformational physicist tells us, *"LOVE is the most fundamental force of Creation."* ♥

Part 2: MIND

Chapter 5

Loving

We're all just walking each other home.

Ram Dass
Be Here Now

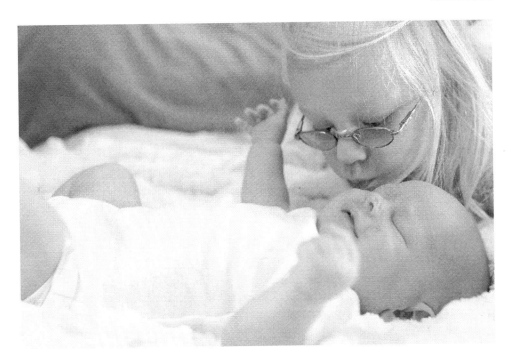

Can our Soul help but be touched by this Beautiful Image? This is HUmanity-HUwomity at its best. We are about to learn how to restore our Human Life by removing what's inside us that has limited us from this miraculous Essence, to restore our True Design LOVE.

Loving introduces us to the single most Miraculous State of Being to which we are irresistibly and magnetically drawn, because it leads us to remember and embrace our True Design. Loving and being Loved are ultimate experiences of Body, Mind, Emotion and Spirit in this World, directing us in subtle and not so subtle paths toward immersion in a sea of ever-flowing Divine LOVE, from which we emerge and are designed to Live, Flow and have our BEING eternally.

Loving produces a highly alchemical state, replete with serotonin, opiates, happy hormones and neuropeptides. Our receptor sites are designed to have LOVE molecules attach to them like puzzle pieces or a key in a lock, communicating a sense of well-being to Mind-Body and World. If we are meant to enjoy a natural drug or high, this is it! In fact, many get "drunk" on Love or the idea of Loving, and never wake up from the "dream," to connect with the *Greater LOVE we ARE*. We are about to learn *this is an "inside job!"*

In the movie *"What the Bleep do we know..."* animation of neuropeptides connecting with receptor sites *(worth seeing)*, depicts how we become addicted to substitutes through this perfect Body mechanism. When instead of LOVE, fear, hostility, stress or grief connect with neuroreceptors, Life force is reduced and gradually wears us out.

The Love we experience and express to, for and with others is one of the most profound experiences we will ever have in this Lifetime, because it Mirrors the LOVE we

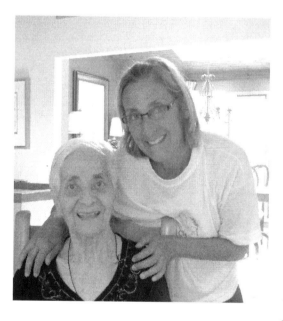

are designed to *be nourished by*. Conversely, being without Love or letting it go is one of the most difficult, crushing, devastating experiences of Life. There is no greater joy in this World, than Loving: our Newborn, Child, Parent, Lover, Spouse, Sibling, Friend: falling in Love, puppy Love, Loving a mentor, self-Love, expressing Love with a pet or Love for Mother Earth and all of her Creation.

Loving is the act of God Loving through us. And the Truth is this LOVE can never be taken away. These experiences of externalized LOVE are to teach us about the eternal LOVE that flows through us. We can think of those we Love as being our "angels," for they teach us more about ourselves than we will learn anywhere else.

Loving activates the wonderful, health producing "LOVE chemical," oxytocin, supporting good health and long Life. This is why those who participate with extended family, marriage and companionship Live longer. When we find our Loved ones unattractive, it is *our* fear and hostility taking over. As we clean out *our thought content*, to realign with LOVE, we restore and maintain balance and well-being with our Loved ones.

Joan Ocean, wild dolphin communicator shares that when a dolphin is faced with something they have to make an adjustment for, they stay within themselves and go through a process of shaking it off, then they go back to playing, enjoying the delight of shared Life with other pod members. We would do well to take a lesson from them; clear ourselves when something comes up and *return to Joy!*

Touching, Hugging, Embracing, Looking into another's Eyes, sharing Intimacy, Breathing, Playing and Laughing together, are all Sacred Expressions of LOVE, intrinsic to our very Nature; as we are creative Beings of LOVE. These activities all stimulate oxytocin, the LOVE hormone, which lets us feel safe, at peace and content.

The LOVE we Are, is a Noun not a Verb. It is a state-of-Being. It is like the 2x4 structure of a house, with "skin" around it. We can get lost in the outer sensory experience of the "skin," which the Mayans called maya or illusion of the 3-D World; yet Loving leads us to Remembering, Knowing and connecting with our True Design LOVE and reason for Being.

> The most important aspect of Love is not in giving or the receiving: it's in the Being. When I need Love from others, or need to give LOVE to others, I'm caught in an unstable situation. Being *in* Love, rather than giving or taking Love, is the only thing that provides stability. Being *in* Love means seeing the Beloved all around me.
>
> *Ram Dass, American Spiritual Teacher*
> *Be Here Now (1971), Polishing the Mirror (2013)*

"Loving" takes us by the hand, and shows us the way to LOVE. It offers us the *gift* in this World that lights the path to return to our True destiny and Oneness with All. In unaware stages of relationship we can get caught in "projections" on the "other," such as them not meeting or not meeting our expectations, being or not being Loving, being unavailable, Mirroring rejection, or other issues that color the experience of Loving.

We are about to learn more about how these projections come from *inside us* and how to remove them forever. Aware Loving relationship offers profoundly safe, supportive Sacred Space;. When issues come up they are addressed together to Lovingly take Response-Ability and clear. We will learn how to remove *from within us*, what takes us away from LOVE, so our neuroreceptors can run on the premium fuel for which they were designed.

We will be learning "Ancient Aramaic Forgiveness," which dr. michael ryce has spent close to thirty years bringing forth from the original Aramaic Texts with a team of scholars. Here is his description to get us started learning the true intended meaning of Forgiveness.

> Most of us are familiar with the popularized form of forgiveness, where we think everything in Life is everyone else's fault, and if we forgive them everything will be okay. This is the Greek act of pardoning, substituted to let the other person "off the hook," and has nothing to do with Forgiveness. With pardoning I can disconnect what's happening in me from you, when in your presence I don't experience it so it may improve our relationship. Yet it doesn't remove what's happening inside of me.
>
> The true Aramaic Forgiveness process is when you go inside yourself, and change the content of your mind. If your mind is producing hostility or fear in any of its forms, and obliterating your Humanity [your True Design LOVE], then the work to be done is the work of Forgiveness - the work of removing all hostilities and fears that have been structured into your mind, holding you out of the truth of who

you are. The truth of who you are is the awesome presence of LOVE - as is everyone else on the Planet. If it has been obliterated by war, pain, guilt, grief, trauma of cultures we live in, then our work is to take Response-Ability to become the kind of individual that chooses to function as a True Human Being as this Awesome Presence of LOVE.

dr. michael ryce
Mindshifter Radio Show, whyagain.org

This is the path each of us will tread as we awaken to the Quantum fact, that resonance inside us Creates our "reality." In upcoming processes, we will uncover layers of unconscious content "driving our boat."

By living their wisdom, compassion, trust, and LOVE, visionaries of our past challenged "software" of belief that spoke to the "operating system" of consciousness. As seeds of new possibilities, they "upgraded" our reality.

Today we have the same opportunity... We *know* that with knowledge to upgrade what we say to the *Divine Matrix*, relatively few people can make a big difference. So what do we do with such knowledge? What happens if one person decides on a new response to an old and hurtful pattern?

What occurs if someone chooses to respond to "betrayal" or "violated trust," for example, with something other than hurt and anger? What takes place when one [family] member begins to watch the 6 o'clock News without feeling the need for revenge or to get even with those who have wronged and violated others? What happens is this: That single individual becomes a living bridge – both the pioneer and midwife – for every other person with the courage to choose the same path.

Gregg Braden
The Divine Matrix, Bridging Time, Space, Miracles and Belief

Everything we experience even in our most Loving relationships, emerges from *our* thoughts and what is *within us*. We grasp essential Quantum principle that Jesus taught, though it was little understood by the culture of 2,000 years ago. As each of us chooses to step forward into our greater *Essence*, Being and Living from the Heart with LOVE, we become a "living bridge," "holding frequency" and opening the way for others to choose.

We *21st Century Superhumans* are embarking on an adventure that will change our Lives, Minds and Hearts forever...increasing our capacity for LOVE, Abundance, Vitality and Well-Being. Are you ready to go beyond limiting beliefs held by human culture for thousands of years and transform yourself miraculously into magnificent expression of Who and What You came here to BE? Let's Breathe, Smile and shout a resounding, YES!!! ♥

Out beyond ideas of wrongdoing and rightdoing,
there is a field. I'll meet you there.

Rumi
13th Century Sufi Mystic Poet

Chapter 6

Our True Power Supply

Concerning matter, we have been all wrong. What we have heretofore called matter is energy, whose Vibration has been so lowered as to be perceptible to the senses. There is no matter as such.

Albert Einstein
Nobel Prize Physics

Ask a Quantum physicist if we are "solid matter" and they will tell you that we are an "energy vehicle." It's a stretch for most to imagine here in 3-D that we are energy rather than solid matter, as is house, car, furniture and all that surrounds us!

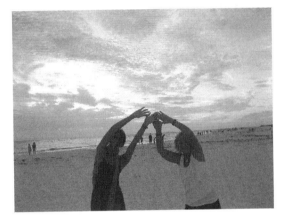

The fascinating book *The Field* (2001) by British investigative journalist Lynn McTaggart, explains how this could be possible, in her engaging documentation of Quantum physics studies of recent sixty years, demonstrating that our entire "reality," World and Universe are far more malleable than we have thought...

ENERGY RESONANCE: We are energy. As Energy Beings in a Quantum World, every Vibrational resonance within us puts Attention on the Field of Possibilities like ripples on the surface of a pond, calling "Creation" into form, then perceived as "reality" around us.

LOVE our "operating system," is our True Power Supply flowing unlimited from Source, *Zero Point generator* in the *Field of Possibilities*. Any thought-emotion Not of LOVE causes a logjam, blocking flow our Innate abundant Power Supply from Source. Thoughts and emotions creating our Vibrational resonance stem from what we absorbed and carried from family, genetic and environmental influences, until we *clear them!*

We are an energy being, designed to "plug in" to a particular "Power Supply" called Source, just like a power cord in an electrical outlet. When "plugged in" to Source we are supplied with Unlimited Life, Abundance, Well-Being, Health, Vitality, Joy, LOVE and

Success. This flow of Energy from Source is not fully available to us when there's a logjam (corrupt data) in our river.

Old "corrupt data" in our unconscious blocks the flow of the river of Life, Love and Consciousness, our True Power Supply. Only when we remove this unconscious content are filters cleaned out, allowing us to experience our World clearly through LOVE. How do we know when there's a logjam clogging our filters, and how do we remove it? *Any discomfort, pain or upset tells us there's a logjam in the river clogging our filter, diverting the flow of our True Power Supply, LOVE.*

Ervin Laszlo's "new Thought" offers we are intricately connected to Source or the *Field*, as part of a dynamic coherent whole. This offers insight into how dis-ease manifests in our organism, when due to Not of LOVE thought-emotion, a logjam is Created in the river. The "software" of our thought acts on Universal energy, calling "reality" into form around us.

Information is entirely basic in the Universe. In the latest conception the Universe doesn't consist of matter and space; it consists of energy and information. Energy exists in the form of wave-patterns and wave-propagations in the Quantum vacuum that fills space; in its various forms, energy is the "hardware" of the Universe. The "software" is information.

The Universe is not an assemblage of bits of inert matter moving passively in empty space: it is a dynamic and coherent whole. The energy that constitutes its hardware is always and everywhere "in-formed." It is in-formed by what David Bohm called the implicate order and physicists now regard as the Quantum vacuum, zero-point field, physical spacetime, universal field, or nuether- [a sub-Quantum level of reality].

This is the "information" structuring the physical world, information we grasp as laws of nature. Without information the energy-waves and patterns of the Universe would be as random and unstructured as behavior of a computer without software. But the Universe is not random and unstructured; it's precisely "in-formed."

Ervin Laszlo, Systems philosopher, integral theorist
The Quantum Brain, Spirituality and the Mind of God, Huffington Post: Religion

Our True Design LOVE is the Source of our greatest form of expression. It is how we are made and within this rests the secret of uninterrupted connection to the energy or Source *Field* that is our True Power Supply. We are always plugged into Source, however there is a catch, if we are carrying Not of LOVE thought there's a logjam. It's that simple.

When emotions are expressed...all systems are united and made whole. When emotions are repressed, denied, not allowed to be whatever they may be, our network pathways get blocked, stopping the flow of the vital feel-good, unifying chemicals that run both our biology and our behavior.

Candace Pert, PhD.
Molecules of Emotion

Harvard studies confirm *key fact*, that a maximum of 5% of thoughts-emotions come from the *conscious mind*. **The remaining 95% that "run the show," come from our unconscious, where forgotten experiences, genetic and historical family dynamics are cataloged and *repeated*.** In *Spontaneous Evolution*, Bruce Lipton and Steve Bhaerman note that new studies show we don't pass-on thought information *in* our DNA as was once believed; yet we are imprinted from the womb, infancy and onward with family dynamics, thought habits and ways of experiencing Life, passed on from generation to generation through behavior and memory resonance.

Though DNA is now believed to be like blank film, waiting to be imprinted with thought, still subtly genetic resonance is carried forward as is demonstrated by twins or siblings separated at birth, carrying forward same habits. Eye-opening book *Solar Revolution*, by biophysicist Dieter Broers exposes how cosmic shifts are affecting our DNA, actually entangled with other dimensions.

It would appear that the DNA is already partially embedded in the higher dimensions. In this respect DNA resembles an electron, only part of whose existence is manifested in our space-time dimension, since the other half is found in Hyperspace

It was discovered in 2001 the actual gene information is not embedded in the DNA. From the standpoint of real phenomenon and "real" observable world processes, located outside of our three-dimensional space-time dimension, they unfold in a totally different manner...

The fact that the "morphogenetic database" is located outside of our three-dimensional space-time engenders a connection between DNA and a level of Hyperspace...a Russian science News agency...reported on September 30, 2002, that changes in human DNA may be associated with geomagnetic disturbances.

Suffice it to say, that for our Power Supply to run through us like water through a firehose, we must clear away the logjam, take out the "garbage" removing all the "old data" resonating from our unconscious; otherwise "corrupt data" continues to run the show, as we Now know how our Attention on the *Field* brings our "reality"into being.

...that the human mind and body are not separate from their environment but a packet of pulsating power constantly interacting with this vast energy sea, and that consciousness may be central in shaping our world.

Lynn McTaggart
The Field

Powerful rays and Light *Fields* activating us from our Galaxy, the Cosmos and beyond, accelerate our molecular structure and send lower Vibrational patterns of old thought-emotion to the surface to *be let go*. As our Vibration shifts, all within us magnetically entrains to these New frequencies. Our **Quantum Lifestyle** covers habits for nourishment, cleansing and detox that support the Body as we move into these higher frequencies. We will integrate new habits, so Energy flows freely again as it did when we were Newborn...

Resistance may come up, with the inclination to hold onto old patterns and stay in the "comfort zone" of our denser form. We are energy "slowed down" into matter, based on Vibrational resonance of our thought (conscious-unconscious). For this reason, it's ultra-important to keep moving through to shed old thought-forms, and not resist our resistance!

A feeling of aversion or attachment toward something
is your clue there's work to be done.

Ram Dass
Polishing the Mirror

Breathing and Smiling are helpful when we feel "stuck," for they shift our neurobiology into a more open and LOVING state. No matter *who* we are, there may still be moments where old fragments surface. So it's not about whether we *are* stuck, it's about whether we notice and are persistent enough to use what we're learning to move beyond our "stuckness," to Breathe, Smile, pause, clear our "stuff" and move on.

The resistance to the unpleasant situation is the root of suffering.

Ram Dass
Polishing the Mirror

RESISTANCE: The degree to which we hold onto our old content not founded in our True Design LOVE, is the degree to which we remain entangled in our Resistance. *Resistance* is our *DENIAL* of thought-emotional content holding resonance in our World. Some of this old content can be catalogued as "terrifying" so our survival mechanism will come up with every possible excuse to keep it buried. Quantum Entanglement says that our resistance will continue to hold in form that which we are resisting. Resistance is our Attention on the item resisted. (*i.e.* "I don't want this to happen..." or "I don't like this or that...") This Attention on the *Field* (conscious-unconscious) continues to whatever it is in form, until we remove our "old data"/resistance.

A resistor in electronics reduces or slows down electrical current. Our "resistance" slows down or limits current flowing through us from our "Power Supply," LOVE. Find wiggle room *through the resistance* by addressing small things first. This will open doors to clearing bigger things. Breathing, Smiling, Trusting and Allowing are key ingredients to facilitating this Shift happening quicker and more easily. The more familiar the process becomes, the easier it is to shed what no longer belongs. As we emerge like a butterfly into new form, the chrysalis is naturally shed. Get ready **21st Century Superhumans**, we are going to Breathe, Smile and move through things... with more awesome tools to assist with the process, read on!

What the caterpillar calls the end,
the rest of the world calls a butterfly.

Lao Tzu - Laozi (604 B.C. - 531 B.C.)
Author Tao Te Ching, Founder Taoism

Alchemical transformation occurring naturally in our NOW is naturally unwinding us from old patterns. We may feel the push to let go fear and hostility, feel our resistance, let go and open to the flow with *LOVE,* sustaining a more vital, abundant, productive Life...

On the path of waking up, it's critical that we are selective with information we expose ourselves to as cells of our body are literally bathed with chemicals of our thoughts and emotions. (*Could this possibly mean, "turn off the TV?" hmm....*)

When we focus in LOVE our cells are flooded with natural, vitalizing LOVE chemicals, recharged by our Power Supply. Worry, stress or even News stories making us sad, angry or fearful, block vital force with chemicals of Not of LOVE, resulting in lowered vitality; and then we hold that story in Creation with our emotional resonance!

Some have told their TV to "go stand in the corner till it has something good to say." We like that, however for most, the idea of being without TV, computer newsfeed, social media, newspapers and magazines with latest updates about what's going on in the World may seem irresponsible. We are conditioned from a 3-D "survival" standpoint "it's important to 'know what's going on around us,'" even if most news is manipulated by corporate, financial, political and military interests, to Create a false sense of fear and apprehension in our World. This "needing to know" is rooted in deep-rooted residual of the blame-fear-hostility culture and "fear of death." Remember, "there is no 'out there,' out there," and "our thoughts are creating our 'reality.'" *Let's Create a good one!*

> Watching television is like taking
> black spray paint to your third eye.
>
> *Bill Hicks (1961-1994)*
> *Social Critic, Satirist*

Forgetting "we are LOVE" and losing our sense of "Oneness," caused us to accept a story that terrible things were going on, potentially dangerous, "someone else's fault" and beyond that, fear of "punishment." Sifting these ideas into our New Quantum perception of Life and our World, helps shed these old belief systems buried in the unconscious. On this *21st Century Superhuman* journey, we're learning how to shift out of old "survival" concepts, to embrace new more productive ways of thinking, Being and experiencing our "reality," founded only in LOVE and our potential for conscious Creatorship.

Letting go our views, attitudes and opinions based in blame-fear-hostility, is *essential* to removing them from "Creation." Yes even things we think are happening on the other side of the World, are held in form by energies inside us! This does take practice to get used to.

Alarming newsfeeds keep us addicted to adrenaline, producing potent neuro-chemicals acting as addicting "drugs." This offers a great excuse to avoid clearing what is denied in our unconscious. As something in us quietly screams, "Look what's going on in the World out there, those terrible people, or that is so sad what's happening," our biggest Quantum leap will be, to get the message to remove *our own* fear and rage.

Okay, this is a giant Leap from where we've been, yet an important one! As long as we are holding a frequency, thought or energy pattern here on Planet Earth, it is *going* to show up somewhere. So if I hear on the News about something "terrible" going on in the World, and I focus on how it makes me feel angry, fearful or both, and what I think needs to happen to this "terrible" situation or people, what am I doing with my Attention? You're right! I'm holding it on the *Field of Possibilities*, telling the *Field* to please keep this "terrible" thing going, because my Attention is continuing to call it into form from the *Field*.

I use my **21st Century Superhuman** Super-Wisdom, (Now that I've learned about Quantum "reality" and how I am an "Observer-Creator,") to shift my Attention Now.

1. I clean out my own unconscious content containing hate, fear, anger, desire to kill or get revenge, desire to lock them up, fear of death or whatever it is coming up for me in this situation. It may be a little difficult to identify; as it may be a resonance from thousands of generations ago in *my* bloodline. This needs to be cleaned out of *my* unconscious with the Aramaic Forgiveness tool (coming up), and I need to Breathe and Smile - otherwise I am going to keep bringing these things into Creation. Am I really that powerful? *Yes. Yes I Am.*

2. I choose to hold the *Field* of LOVE in this situation. When I focus on LOVE - and that is where my Attention is held in the *Field of Possibilities* - that is what I'm calling into form. And the *Field* has millions of ways to respond that I don't even know about! More than I could ask or think. The *Field* LOVES to bring forth LOVE - because really it's *the only TRUE ENERGY THERE IS*. LOVE will figure out a way beyond what we can imagine. For example, amazing inventions can solve giant problems on Earth, such as radio waves replacing pesticides, fertilizer and GMOs!

3. *P.S. Be patient with yourself.* This is ingrained thinking in all of us. It can take repeating this lesson over and over, till we reshape our Minds to deal with global issues that may "seem" overwhelming in these New ways. As *Abraham* says, "Go general" to release and let go Attention, clean out "old data" from our unconscious, and then hold the *Field* in LOVE. A new way of BEING Now is born through us on Planet Earth!

*Hey we are so impressed at you getting this!!! You've been doing your homework, testing out and talking about all these crazy Quantum ideas with your family and friends, sometimes laughing, sometimes scratching your head to figure out how they work. And here you are, an emerging **21st Century Superhuman**... World here we come!*

Back to TV and Newsfeeds: 2 things to do as **21st Century Superhumans**:

1. *Don't watch it, and hold the Field of LOVE* - knowing the best possible will come of everything, because you, Quantum creator, are shifting the entire Hologram with LOVE.

2. *Do watch it, and hold the Field of LOVE* - knowing that the best possible will come of everything, because you, a Quantum creator, are shifting the entire Hologram Now with LOVE.

...most of us don't want to be in touch with ourselves...we want to invite something else to enter us [like] the television....Every Breath we take...can be filled with peace, joy, and serenity. The question is whether or not we are in touch with it. We need only to be awake, alive in the present moment.

Thich Nhat Hahn
Buddhist Monk, Art of Mindful Living

We are untangling ourselves from human culture built around blame, fear and hostility. Much in our outer World established around the Not of LOVE thought paradigm becomes more obvious as we wake-up to our role as Quantum-Creators. It gets really exciting when we realize how easily the Collective can change as we make these shifts inside ourselves. Peace. LOVE. Abundance. Joy. *You pick!*

An untrained mind can accomplish nothing.

A Course In Miracles

Cultivating awareness of what we *desire to hold in resonance* focuses the Mind. Restoring this ecology of LOVE and its Creation in our World comes from focusing Attention upon *it*. This is also the energy that brings us the greatest Vitality, Well-Being, Longevity, Success and Abundance to Life. Know that it is so.

The Eternal Law of Life is: "What you think and feel you bring into form; where your thought is there you are, for you are your consciousness; and what you meditate upon, you become."

Godfré Ray King (1838-1939)
Original Unveiled Mysteries

Let's consider the other side. As we realize we *ARE* Quantum creators, do we want to focus on fear, hostility, hatred and a collection of other tawdry ideas broadcast in modern society, born out of ignorance or Not of LOVE thought? *You're right. Probably NOT.*

We're here to awaken from the illusion of separateness.

Ram Dass
How Can I Help?

Implement new programing for your neurobiology by immersing yourself in things you enjoy. Cultivate LOVE awareness with: music, art, song, writing, creativity, dance, beach, sun, walk, run, camp, kayak, hike, family, ski, snowboard, bike, golf, games, sports, reflect, focus, meditate, pray, children, pets, friends, Lover, lakes, rivers, streams, ponds, gardens, ocean, joyful play, Breathe, Smile. Feed the resonance of LOVE within yourself. Know it is the current from Source that powers your every moment. Remove any logjams and be fully connected with your True Power Supply from Source, LOVE. It is Now bringing you *everything* you need and flowing in and through you.

Realize deeply that the present moment is all you have.
Make NOW the primary focus of your Life.

Eckhart Tolle
The Power of Now

Breathe, Smile and establish this new flow of Being. Explore living in the resonance of LOVE, knowing that whatever you dwell upon, will be Mirrored by Creation in your "reality." Learning how Quantum "reality" operates, conceive of the possibility that we all *can* make this shift. Any energy expressed toward LOVE is productive for All.

> There is so much in this world that I do not understand... I have absolutely no idea how you [Neo] were able to do some of the things you do, I only hope we understand that...before it's too late.
>
> *The Councilman to Neo*
> *The Matrix Reloaded*

Clearing thoughts-emotions Not of LOVE, we *recognize Quantum "reality" is not someone else's fault but our own Creation.* LOVE flows through our Being and we discover New pursuits to thrill our Souls, as we partake in conscious Creation as **21st Century Superhumans,** bringing coherence out of chaos.

> I regard consciousness as fundamental. I regard matter as derivative from consciousness. We cannot get behind consciousness. Everything that we talk about, everything that we regard as existing, postulates consciousness.
>
> *Max Planck (1858-1947)*
> *Quantum Theory, Nobel Prize Physics 1918*

Hermann Verlinde, Princeton String Theorist tells us everything starts with Information. Seth Llyod, Professor of Mechanical Engineering, MIT states the Universe is a Quantum computer. Now, in the computer age, we can understand Mind-Heart as a "consciousness computer," that when given instructions through our "upgraded software" (clarified thought-emotion, conscious-unconscious), we have the ability to change anything and everything in our "reality" and our World.

The path to Living as **21st Century Superhumans** incorporates "waking up," to actively participate as Conscious Creators of our "reality," clearing all old "data" Not of LOVE, to connect with our True Power Supply, by clearing our "filters" and tuning our dial to LOVE. This means removing ourselves from *all* blame-fear-hostility *programing,* knowing our "reality" gives feedback if there is more to clear. We invite the *Field of Possibilities* to send us New Creation of our Heart's desire and more, as we actively implement **21st Century Superhuman** skills, tools, techniques for **Quantum Lifestyle.**

> We all affect the world every moment, whether we mean to or not. Our actions and states of mind matter, because we are so deeply interconnected with one another.
>
> *Ram Dass*
> *Polishing the Mirror*

Breathe - Smile - Meditate - Clear old "data" - Tune Dial to LOVE - Give it to the *Field of Possibilities* - Let it Go - Trust - Live from *Essence* - Left and Right Brain Dance - Marry Mind-Heart - Mud Between Toes - I Am Creative Being - DNA Codons *ON* - Loving - Unity - Oneness - Heart Coherence - Deep LOVE, Compassion, Gratitude - I Am Energy - My True Design is LOVE - *Shift of the Ages* - **Arc the Hologram Now!** ♥

Part 2: MIND

Chapter 7

The LOVE Channel

"I wish it need not have happened in my time," said Frodo. "So do I," said Gandalf, "and so do all who live to see such times. But that is not for them to decide. All we have to decide is what we do with the time that is given us."

J.R.R. Tolkien, Frodo and Gandalf
The Fellowship of the Ring

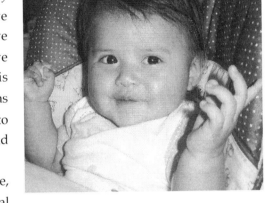

Our greatest adventure at this amazing Evolutionary Leap called *Shift of the Ages*, is restoring ourselves to the *Presence of LOVE* ...knowing that as *Beings of LOVE* we are "powerful beyond measure." We will live healthier, wealthier and wiser lives, as we restore the flow of LOVE in our Being. It is *essential* to clear thought-emotional patterns Not of LOVE (conscious-unconscious) to restore Life and vitality to every cell and aspect of Body-Mind.

Marianne Williamson's famous quote, used by Nelson Mandela in his inaugural address, touches the depths and gives us a tantalizing taste of what we discover when we "tune in to the Channel" of our True Design LOVE.

> Our deepest fear is not that we are inadequate. Our deepest fear is that we are powerful beyond measure. It is our light, not our darkness that most frightens us. We ask ourselves, Who am I to be brilliant, gorgeous, talented, and fabulous? Actually, who are you *not* to be? You are a child of God. Your playing small does not serve the world... As we are liberated from our own fear, our presence automatically liberates others.
>
> *Marianne Williamson*
> *A Return to LOVE*

In Ancient Aramaic the word *"prayer"* means *"set a trap for God."* When we are not quite tuned in to a radio or TV station there can be static or interference. When we get perfectly tuned to the channel and it comes in clearly, we are like an *antenna* setting a trap for God.

Dieter Broers describes the science behind this in his outstanding book (and documentary) *Solar Revolution.*

The crystals in DNA also form standing waves and thus interact naturally with higher dimensions (hyperspace). Scientific research has clearly demonstrated that these waves exhibit exceptional stability over time...

DNA thus comprises an antenna *i.e.* classical resonator pointed toward the vacuum virtually siphoning information from and exchanging information with the "nothingness..." This process also occurs outside the realm of the space-time dimension.... The geomagnetic field serves as a medium for information interchange with the DNA database...

... Properties such as "being in two different places at the same time," "the presence of waves and particles in a single entity," "electrons resonating with the entire cosmos," and "vacuum energy/nothingness that nonetheless Creates everything" also largely apply to DNA.

In its capacity as an antenna, DNA allows for information exchange not only on Earth but also the entire cosmos. A very special property of these phenomena is that DNA appears to have a kind of direct line to mental worlds of the controlling dimensions. This communication with higher dimensions enables our DNA to provide us with invaluable information concerning the source of all being. Hence DNA is relatively unaffected by terrestrial and cosmic fields, and has a pipeline to highest planes of the cosmos.

Dieter Broers
Solar Revolution

As we clear away all thought-emotional patterns Not of LOVE, we remove static interference and open up our clear connection with Creator-Source for the Channel of LOVE to come through loud and clear via our "natural antenna."

Prayers are the oxygen of God.

Saint Padre Pio (1887-1968)
Mystic Catholic Priest, bilocated, healed blind

As we clear, cancel, let go all thought-emotion Not of LOVE, we "tune our dial" to God-Source, receiving and transmitting our truest resonance, and by so doing we change ourselves and the World. The bottom line is, this is the simple, complex and complete purpose of our existence. When our lives emanate from this place, they are filled with Joy, Love, Abundance and Infinite Well-Being, resonating through us into the World.

Any genuine path with sincere practice, results in a gradual deepening of selflessness into ultimate "reality" of what the Gita calls the Self. ...just as our primordial cravings lead to manifold forms of misery, letting go of our ideas about "reality" and our desires for a particular result will lead to our freedom.

Bhagavad Gita
Ancient Vedic Text, 5,000 B.C.

To keep this Channel operating without static, we commit to Being fully present in all situations, living with Response-Ability. Our "reality" lets us know where making adjustments will tune-in our LOVE Channel more clearly. Upcoming "goal canceling" process removes unconscious content and thought-emotion Not of LOVE, keeping open a clear channel. *A Course In Miracles* says, *"All learning involves Attention and study at some level."* The Dalai Lama offers encouragement to cultivate clear connection by consistent focus, tuning our antenna to the right frequency:

> The highest form of spiritual practice is the cultivation of the altruistic intention to attain enlightenment for the benefit of all sentient beings... [This is] only realized through regular concerted effort, so in order to attain it we need to cultivate discipline necessary for training and transforming our mind...
>
> The potential for perfection, the potential for full enlightenment actually lies within each of us. In fact this potential is nothing other than the essential nature of mind itself, which is said to be the mere nature of luminosity and knowing. Through gradual process of spiritual practice, we eliminate obstructions hindering us from perfecting...enlightenment. As we overcome step by step, the inherent quality of consciousness begins to become more and more manifest until it reaches the highest stage of perfection...
>
> *His Holiness the Dalai Lama*
> *The Dalai Lama's Little Book of Wisdom*

Quantum physics Now demonstrates science behind these precepts carried in traditions throughout the ages, revealing that *presence and consciousness* have a creative effect upon our World. It behooves us to use regular practices to refine these deeper aspects of HUman-HUwom expression.

> Far more than you may realize, your experience, your world, and even your self are the creations of what you focus on. From distressing sights to soothing sounds, protean thoughts to roiling emotions, the targets of your attention are the building blocks of your Life.
>
> *Winifred Gallagher, NY Times Bestseller*
> *Rapt, Attention and the Focused Life*

Daily dedication to Smiling, Breathing and Focusing in LOVE, commitment to tools and practices herein, shifts our brain to its own natural high-level operating system, cleaning out old paradigm thoughts Not of LOVE.

WHAT IS NOT BUILT ON LOVE AND TRUTH *is now dissolving. The matrix of illusion that has programmed our minds for the last 13 millennia is collapsing. This vast illusion was structured for the explicit purpose of spiritual evolution for all its participants. There is a wider portal now open for LOVE and LIGHT energy, upgrading our DNA, downloading new codes and building new archetypes to accelerate our Evolution. We are changing and reshaping our World Forever...*

♥ Teddi's Guides ♥

Population, environment, food, fuel production, governments, economic systems, countries issues all encourage us to step up to the plate and take Response-Ability for *our thoughts-emotions*. We are "getting" how to hold this new resonance in the World, *shifting everything far and near*.

Get excited when something shows up that bothers you, and use it as an opportunity to release your old content resonating in the situation.Using these tools and practices to clear taproots of Ancient hidden pain, we become Free. Setting our antenna to the LOVE Channel, we Now release and let go all thought-emotional "baggage" Not of LOVE.

Once we access this newfound Freedom, we learn to invite Life to *flow through* us. Opening to our vital, generative, creative, sexual energy to flow in us as we are designed, we become radiant in the World, a magnet for good, abundance flowing through us. We Free suppressed energy, opening to Life! Instead of trying to "save the World," we move into wholeness within, flowing into Oneness and the World follows!

> Darkness cannot drive out darkness; Only Light can do that.
> Hate cannot drive out hate. Only LOVE can do that.

> *Martin Luther King Jr. (1929-1968)*
> *Nobel Peace Prize, Pastor, NAACP "I have a dream..."*

Restoring ourselves to LOVE our True Nature, our Vibration goes into the World as tuning fork resonating a New "reality" into Being. A product of collective thought Creation, global issues shift as we shift, into *Living the Presence of LOVE,* and positive restructuring takes place. Others follow when ready as resonance is drawn by resonance.

Nothing Changes if Nothing Changes -
As long as you continue to seek outside help you will continue to seek outside help. Look within to make a change, everything you need is there to heal yourself. Know your own truth and be true to yourself. Your focus must be to break the pattern! Stop giving in to fear energy of others. It will only perpetuate and manipulate you. Clarity comes to the mind that seeks it. You will not answer 5-D questions outside time and space with 3-D information, *and so it is...*

> *Reiner Heelon*
> *Vision Keeper*

Our waves of resonance go out like ripples in a pond, and Create ripples through our World. Each who becomes clear shifts the whole. Test out how you're doing as you enter into contact or conversation with parent, child, spouse, coworker, boss, sibling, friend, partner, pet. Notice whether you are Breathing and Smiling for the entire contact, expanding your aura and theirs. Keep the channel of LOVE open.

> Shiny happy people holding hands, There's no time to cry
> Put it in your heart where tomorrow shines

> *REM, Shiny Happy People, lyrics*

You: Wow! You don't want us to feed the hungry and save the whales?

Us: Well we don't mean you shouldn't do that (in fact if that's in your Heart, please do), however, even more importantly, everything we see around us in our world is called into being by the resonance we carry inside us (both conscious and unconscious).

One of the most important Quantum realizations happening today is that we cannot stop war by protesting war, we do not get rid of terrorism by hating it, we cannot stop starvation by grieving it, we cannot assuage our guilt by self-punishment, we don't stop fear by building walls or having bigger military, we won't get more money thinking we don't have enough. We just add Attention as Observer-Creators to what we don't want, that keeps calling it into Being.

The most Critical, Hugely Important thing we can do Right Now, and every Now moment from Now on... Is to clear our own internal data banks of any thought or emotion Not of LOVE. Then *Arc the Hologram with LOVE!*

Many are "inspired" to correct failing systems around the World, and good things are done. Let's take another look at why it's so important to do our *personal* clearing. What if Mother Teresa, Gandhi, St. Francis, and others had not aligned with LOVE first? They each did their own Soul search and clearing, to "Live the *Presence of LOVE,*" so their *Vibration* was as powerful as the work they did. Their *Lives* resonated the passion of their Hearts.

> Blessed are the ones that believe
> in the beauty of their dreams.
>
> *Eleanor Roosevelt(1884-1962)*
> *Longest Serving First Lady USA*

How we have our "dial tuned" influences the greater *Field* of Humanity. "'When a butterfly flutters its wings o in China, it causes a hurricane in the Caribbean,' *might* be possible" says physicist Nassim Haramein, "yet if a million butterflies flap their wings in unison it is much more likely." Our affect on the Whole matters.

> I remember a year and a half ago I was in the Orinoco, deep in the jungle, and out comes from the jungle a man, naked, who probably had never seen a wheeled vehicle, with a transistor radio clapped to his ear, probably listening to the ball game from Mexico City. So we have this extraordinary interdependent world, and then of course we have access to the understanding of human potentials. We're living in the golden age of the understanding of who and what we can be.
>
> *Jean Houston, Ph.D.*
> *Possible Human, Possible World Part I*

David Bohm, Einstein's protege, whose *Special Relativity* is standard in the field of Quantum physics, tells us in *David Bohm On Perception* (YouTube) that relativity means everything is related to everything else.

> I would say that in my scientific and philosophical work, my main concern has been with understanding the nature of reality in general, and of consciousness in

particular as a coherent whole, which is never static or complete but which is an unending process of movement and unfoldment....

David Bohm (1917-1992)
Implicate and Explicate Order, Holographic Paradigm

Ultimately we are Beings of Consciousness. Awakening from our long slumber, "tuning our dial" to the LOVE Channel, removing all static, activating our destiny as True HUman-HUwom, innocent as a Newborn, we shift ourselves to shift the Greater Whole. All systems are Now "go," to let us know we are "Creators," that our thought-emotion manifests in our World as our "reality."

Human Beings LOVE and care deeply for one another; wherever you go the Life of each brother, sister, parent, child is Precious. The moment we receive in our Hearts what is Now upon us in Quantum physics, that we are One, *"if you think you're separate you're living in an optical delusion,"* including Earth Mother Gaia, the Sun, Moon and Stars, as we do so we change *timelines* and the course of Human History *FOREVER*.

What you above all can do is activate the dormant powers that lie within you waiting to be activated. To do this you need to completely change your way of thinking - in other words, undergo your own personal paradigm shift in every sense of the term. This means that each and every one of us needs to learn how to ferret out and listen to our intuitions and inner voices, which far too often are drowned out by the rational mind...

How many of us genuinely have the courage to let our intuition "speak its mind?" Which of us pays heed to the warning voices the feelings, and the visions that percolate up from our unconscious, all of which are suppressed by the need to function in a culture that is based in so-called rationalism?

And yet what we urgently need is exactly this intuitive knowledge, which is the only knowledge that can help us to understand and accept the groundbreaking changes that await us in this transformative time.

Dieter Broers
Solar Revolution: Mankind on Cusp of Evolutionary Leap

As **21st Century Superhumans** enter the Heart to Live from *Essence*, we shift within and without, igniting others with courage, inspiration and vision to do the same. ♥

ARC THE HOLOGRAM!
I Am Therefore I LOVE ♥ I LOVE Therefore I Am

Part 2: MIND

Chapter 8

I Am Here

You find peace not by rearranging the circumstances of your Life,
but by realizing who you are at the deepest level.

Eckhart Tolle
The Power of Now

What a joyous thing to be in a body on Planet Earth Now! Accessing our Newborn state, our palette of Purity expresses with Innocence and elevates us beyond the material World, liberating full expression of our True Design LOVE. In this Pure state there is no vanity, competition or attachment to materialism, just a Pure flow of Wholeness, Oneness and LOVE.

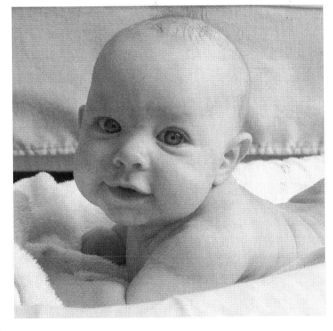

Connecting with openness and receptivity contributes to naturally expanding our full expression. Let's Journey on together, imagining we have Mind-Heart of a Newborn...relating with pure, simple joy in Life, trusting Mama is going to feed us, Papa is going to look after us, and all our needs are met, as we express our breathtaking presence flowing easily from Pure *Essence*.

Imagine holding *YOU* as a Newborn; innocent, pure, peaceful, loving, precious – *Now, go ahead be that Newborn:* Smile, Breathe, relax into LOVE, and allow yourself to access your pure state of Being... It is wonderful and safe to explore this way of integrating into the World. We are here to hold you in our arms with gentle coos, Smiles and LOVE. ♥

REFLECTION: Mind is powerful. We are *just beginning to comprehend how powerful* it is, with our Quantum understanding. Let's learn to use it well, for we *surely* will get what we focus upon! In fact really we are energy. Our thought is what calls or directs our energy into BEING. Be careful what you think - you just might get it. Offloading any content not belonging in a Being of LOVE, we place Attention on that which we desire, with energy of our True Design LOVE accessing our gentle strong "Newborn Heart."

> Beliefs have the power to Create and the power to destroy. Human beings have the awesome ability to take any experience of their lives and Create a meaning that disempowers them or one that can literally save their lives.
>
> *Tony Robbins,*
> *Awaken the Giant Within*

Bonds established with family, extended family, and friends or "Soul family," help develop our expression of LOVE in the World. These are our "Angels" and "best teachers" with whom we have a soul agreements to work things out together, with whom our "stories" surface for clearing and we merge into deeper LOVE. Always be grateful to these Loved ones for lessons learned with them, no matter if difficult when happening. As Wisdom-Keeper Sun Bear taught us, unless LOVE is deep enough, we won't get the lesson.

This is our "soul plan" to which we agreed. We cannot learn or grow alone or in a vacuum. Close relationships bring us our greatest learning. When deep Conscious connections exist in such relationships, they can be nurtured into kind safe learning environments to Mirror and offer opportunity to clear and deepen *Essence of Who We Are.*

Here we cultivate the powerful experience of being accepted by those who stick with us through "thick and thin," even when our "stuff" is up. As the saying goes, "We all come with baggage. It's good to surround ourselves with those who will help us unpack!" Elevating relationships with stronger connections, we evolve into a new cultural mythos built around greater LOVE.

> Yes, you know, I think one of the problems came when we got the television set and it replaced the hearth, didn't it? It was at the hearth that the grandparents or the elders told the stories, and the great chain of being between the generations was woven, and the wisdom was passed on.
>
> And now you know, the grandparents have moved elsewhere, often south, and we're left with the television set. But we're also being given access more and more, to everybody's stories, to everybody's myths. And also the sense that we are now all in it together, *in perhaps the greatest moment in human history, in which we are recreating the Earth story.*
>
> *Jean Houston, Ph.D.*
> *Possible Human, Possible World Part I*

LOVE is our most important, centered, peaceful state, accessed through the Heart and *Essence,* flowing from Source, from where all Life emanates. Freeing ourselves from false projections and expectations of and toward others, practicing with those we Love, clarifies ability to focus Life through LOVE. In any situation we are experiencing Not of LOVE, we clear out *our own unconscious*, and LOVE restores itself in the twinkling of an eye.

In order for things to change, you've got to change.

Tony Robbins
Unleash The Power Within

Water is a key transmitter of thought and we are 60-75% water. Masaru Emoto has demonstrated that Grateful and LOVING thought changes water into beautiful crystals. Images in his books *Hidden Messages in Water, The Miracle of Water* and *Angel Words*, show spectacularly beautiful crystals formed when water responds to sincere LOVE, Gratitude and other positive thoughts. His brilliant contribution exposes our capacity to change *EVERYTHING* with thought, even on a massive scale instantly.

Emoto's astounding water crystals reveal incredible potential for changing matter and self. With the focus of a group of people on Gratitude and LOVE, even distressed water molecules from damaged nuclear plant at Fukushima returned to beautiful crystalline structure *with collective thought focus.*

This is a *hugely important awareness*, setting in motion New paradigms, transporting us beyond negative news into New Creation. Any feeling in the outer Not of LOVE is a *GIFT*, a Mirroring to us from the *Field,* to make visible what is left to clear to realign with our True *Essence* LOVE. As we deepen our experience with the *state of BEING* LOVE, we expand our "Newborn state" to discover the unlimited power behind our true creative potential.

LOVE alone is capable of uniting any living being in such a way as to complete and fulfill them for it alone takes them and joins them by what is deepest in themselves...Understanding, Cooperation and LOVE are Keys to human survival.

Teilhard de Chardin (1881-1955)
French Philosopher, Priest

At front of this wave are those of us Now grasping these Quantum concepts, that what thoughts we emanate, we magnetically draw in. As Gandhi said, *"BE* the change you wish to see in the World." Ken Keyes Jr. transmitted in "urban legend" *Hundredth Monkey*, it only takes a few to Create a tipping point. (*i.e:* 2% participated in the American Revolution).

Never doubt that a small group of thoughtful, committed citizens can change the world; indeed, it's the only thing that ever has.

Margaret Mead (1901-1978)
American Cultural Antrhropologist

We let go old old belief that anyone but us is response-able for our "reality," that rather it is a product of resonance within us. This makes it *all* an "inside job." There is no 'out there' out there, and *New kinds of relationships are born* with lovers, family and friends.

...let the wind blow through you,
as through a screen door.

Mahatma Gandhi

St. Francis said, *"Sanctify yourself and you will sanctify society."* **21st Century Superhumans** are now learning to clarify, reveal, express, Live and Be their own True Presence of LOVE. Letting go of our "stuff," embracing LOVE with ease allows our energy to flow as a healing balm into the World for others and for self. As we move into this flowing river of LOVE, the Collective restructures around us, *for We Are Here!*

> My job here on Earth is twofold. My job is first of all to make amends... My second job is to awaken people who might be asleep. Almost everyone is asleep! The only way I can awaken anyone is to work on myself.
>
> *Dr. Ihaleakala Hew Len*
> *Zero Limits, Ho'oponopono*

Biophysicist Dieter Broers reports in *Solar Revolution* that Mayans saw our current cyclical transition as a "...cathartic function. They speak of 'awakened human beings' carrying out a 'sacred mission,' who will 'cleanse the Earth,' and for whom a new consciousness and new form of civilization will be ushered in, once we've passed through the initiatory threshold...Dec. 21, 2012." Shamanic stories from the Andes also tell us we're at the end of a cycle and the beginning of a thousand year cycle. *At this critical juncture, clearing to LOVE, to express our greater potential is essential for future thriving.*

> What must underlie successful [social] epidemics in the end, is a bedrock belief that change is possible... Look at the world around you. It may seem like an immovable, implacable place. It is not. With the slightest push - in just the right place - it can be tipped.
>
> *Malcom Gladwell*
> *The Tipping Point*

What may seem like unsolvable Global and personal issues can shift in a moment, with clarity and power of Mind-Heart operating in LOVE. Who we are and what we are capable of has barely been tapped into, and is emerging Now in this *Shift of the Ages*. We are showing the World what empowered Humanity-HUwomity can do. **21st Century Superhumans** focus through LOVE in *every* situation, adjusting all with power based in LOVE far beyond what we have yet imagined.

> Even as a piece of coal is under extreme pressure inside the Earth,
> It transforms into a diamond of great brilliance. So shall you be.
>
> *Nellie Cain*
> *Exploring the Mysteries of Life*

Celebrate the journey! "I Am here!" "I find ultimate Freedom in letting go what no longer serves my highest resonance of LOVE!" "From my Newborn Heart I Now express my own wonderful creativity through my Truest *Essence!*" More eye-opening tools for living **21st Century Superhuman Quantum Lifestyle** coming up, so let's continue on together, as we approach life from our pure innocent *Newborn* state, Living as our *Essence...* in LOVE! ♥

Part 2: MIND

Chapter 9

A Fairy Tale For Our Newborn

If you want your children to be intelligent read them fairy tales. If you want them to be more intelligent, read them more fairy tales.

Albert Einstein (1879-1955)
Nobel Prize in Physics, Copley Medal, Franklin Medal

Once upon a time long ago the Creation story happened. Father-Mother Creator infused LOVE Thoughts into a *Field* of energy. It expanded and danced through the Universe, singing and playing with joy and delight.

Father–Mother Creator Imagined Life, Beings, Planets. Stars swirled through space forming galaxies and solar systems. A beautiful blue-green planet took shape, with abundant water and growing things. Father–Mother Creator desired a reflection of him-herself and imagined a pair of beautiful beings to enjoy Life in their abundant Universe.

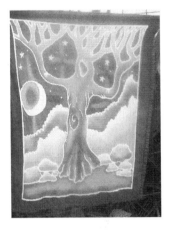

This intelligent Life-form emerged from the cosmic soup setting up housekeeping on Planet Earth. A beautiful woman with flowing hair and lithe body and a man strong and wise accompanied her, in their garden paradise. They were surrounded with fragrant flowering plants and trees; off in the distance were sights and sounds of 'birds, beasts, bugs and little fishes.' We might call these two beautiful beings our "great-great-grandparents." They lived happily in the garden paradise, with the same ability to cause matter and energy to take form as had Father–Mother Creator. They were so innocent they barely grasped their capabilities, as Creation flowed graciously around them.

One day our beautiful ancestors had a discussion. They were unhappy and blamed each other. The truth was whatever they were blaming each other for had come from inside themselves. They had forgotten as Beings of LOVE, that whatever they carried inside flowed freely into their World with Creation taking shape around them as a result of it.

If they had just remembered their *Essence* of pure LOVE, everything would have been wonderful again. Instead they built a belief that their upset had come from the other. They had been Created to live without pain or death, yet as they held onto emotions Not of

LOVE, their miraculous World changed, clouds covered the sun, and they saw death around them for the first time. *They were very sad...* Their dis-comfort increased as they fell away from LOVE.

Because of this one very tiny mistake in thinking, their children, grandchildren and great-grand-children and others who came after, forgot the purity of their LOVE nature. They became attached to things outside their *Essence*, and set up boundaries, governments, monetary and military systems, to protect them from one another, and make sure no one could take what was theirs. They built towns, villages, governments and religions founded in blame-fear-hostility-competition, instead of LOVE. A human culture grew up, forgetting about the regenerative Life-Form Father–Mother Creator had designed them to be.

Aches and pains, dis-ease and death, anger and war, greed, petty fighting, and even "power-over" religions dominated. What had happened to the beautiful garden paradise of our eternally youthful ancestors? One simple mistake... Forgetting that LOVE was Who They Were and How They Were Made... The simple mistake, thinking they were separate and blaming the other, lead to a downward spiral for them, their descendants and all living things. We call this *involution*. As in some wisdom teachings, perhaps it was a necessary experience to discover who they were, by experiencing who they were not. Some call this learning through "duality."

Once close to Father-Mother Creator they lived in Unity and Oneness. Blaming one another, they entered "duality," where they experienced themselves as separate - thus a "dual World"...though deep, deep inside their Hearts they knew a sense of longing for Oneness... drawn in through deeply forgotten memories of returning to the One.

Epilogue: A sense of ONENESS bestowed upon our "great-great-grandparents" in the beginning by Father–Mother Creator dawns again today...a thread carried forward in the Heart, through thousands and thousands of generations awakened by the Cosmos. The dawning of this New civilization erases memories on all timelines Not of LOVE. Activated Celestial Promise of Awakening is received with great joy by Living our True Design LOVE in our "garden paradise."

> These are the times. We are the people. If not now, when? If not you, who? -- as Hillel said two thousand years ago. All of us are serving as midwives... of the possible in each other. We can only do it together. There's no such thing as a guru anymore. I mean, guru should be spelled "Gee, You Are You."
>
> *Jean Houston, Ph.D.*
> *Possible Human, Possible World Part I*

Celestial Events are pressing us to awaken to our Heart and Oneness, Quantum physics reveals how Thoughts Create. Modern translations of Ancient Texts expose Keys to restoring our True Design LOVE. All this is preparing us for the most powerful Evolutionary Leap in human history, **Arcing the Hologram** across the Evolutionary Spiral to our True Design LOVE and... *Shift of the Ages! Are you ready?* ♥

Part 2: MIND - SECTION 3
CLEARING THE TEMPLE

Be Universal in your LOVE. You will see the Universe
to be the picture of your own Being.

Sri Chinmoy (1931-2007)
My Life's Soul-Journey:

In a wonderful trademark audience-participation exercise, dr. michael and jeanie ryce invite us to share qualities we've experienced while holding a Newborn. A list emerges such as, "joyful, peaceful, loving, sweet, gentle, nurturing, smells good, pristine, precious, present, soft, delightful, deep, innocent" and more. A sigh permeates the room, as participants' faces soften and smiles appear, for we are ultimately Beings of LOVE.

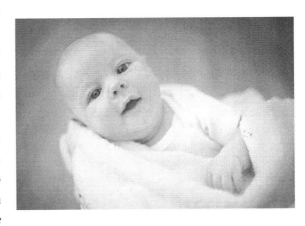

Connecting with this amazing Universal embodiment of pure LOVE, is an opportunity to experience getting closely in touch with our own Newborn *Essence* and Who We Truly Are. Once arrived into adulthood most have forgotten infancy and how it represents these amazing aspects of our True Being and Presence.

Breathe, Smile and reflect on when you've held a Newborn;
add your own descriptors to the list.

Gazing at this precious baby picture, deepen connection with this awesome state of LOVE and how it carries us into the Heart. Jeanie, michael and their team share this exercise with many participants, from church groups, to those in prison, youth at risk, always with a softening of the audience as a Newborn is such a wonderful Universal representation of the LOVE we are Designed to Be. Their Team of those dedicated to sharing this work is growing. Learn how to participate at whyagain.org. Keep a baby picture of self or loved one out as a reminder of this special place of LOVE within yourself.

Promise me you'll always remember: You're braver than you believe, and stronger
than you seem, and smarter than you think.

A.A. Milne
Author Winnie the Pooh

Life is amazing! We are born innocent and helpless, a miraculous design engaging mamas' and papas' deep instinct to care for us. As we grow through Life, and have our own children or observe children of others, we reflect and discover the level of ultimate sacrifice made by parents (even with their foibles) to give us a great start in Life.

Knowing ourselves as beings of LOVE is the essential Awaking of a Lifetime. Remembering this *Essence* of how we are made benefits every aspect Life, putting primary focus on LOVE as the True Design of our Being. Are you aware of thought-emotion Not of LOVE that you've expressed? It's time to remove this type of thinking *forever*. We are about to learn *essential tools* for clearing this unconscious content, restoring the Heart and our True Infinite Design LOVE.

Einstein reminds us of a key principle, *"We cannot solve problems at the level at which they were Created."* For this reason we will learn some slightly tricky skills to unwind this content from our neurobiological system, stored through genetic and family patterning and early Life experiences. Attempting to clear this unconscious content with logical processing of the conscious mind or traditional psychological therapies rarely make a dent. *In Review:*

(8) DNA is like a blank piece of film, upon which we write the program for our Life with our thoughts and emotions. The *Akasha* carries genetic memory patterns. Let's learn how to clean out old data and write it anew with LOVE from the Heart.

(9) Thoughts-emotions Create information chemicals that bathe our cells with what we feel-think toward self, others and Life, setting up our basis for vitality and well-being or dis-ease. How about fully activating our LOVE chemicals?

(10) 1% of Creation is matter, the other 99.999% is the energy of space or the *Field of Possibilities*. Electrons are continually "checking in" to see what information (or how our Attention) is directing them to reshape matter and circumstances from the *Field. Let's focus our Attention through lens of the Heart!*

(11) Be clear about Attention upon the *Field.* Clearing the unconscious is *essential to vitality, abundance, well-being and LOVE!*

We may want to *think* it's complicated. It's not. It really is as Einstein says, *"simple enough for a six year old to understand."* The fact that we're Now "repurposing" *thousands of generations* of thought is what makes it seem difficult. A great definition of insanity is, *"doing the same things over again, thinking we'll get different results."*

> Seek not the keys to doors that do not exist.
> Instead, refrain from creating the doors in the first place.
>
> *Rodolfo Young, totalauthenticity.com/HeartMission*

We make the choice whether to repeat patterns or Leap into a New way of defining ourselves. Guess what the only thing in the way is? That's right our *resistance* making excuses to be stuck where it is. *Let's take a deep Breath, dive in, and move through it!* Although challenging at first, once we get the hang of it, it's easier than we think! ♥

Chapter 10

Our "Not Of LOVE" Heritage

*Love is that condition in which the happiness of
another person is essential to your own.*

Robert A. Heinlein
Stranger in a Strange Land

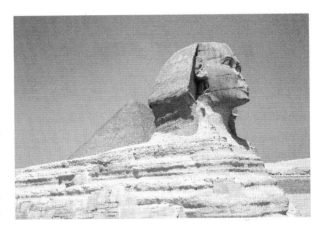

Has irritation welled up in you lately? Have you felt hurt by what someone else did or said? Have you told someone off, or not told them, yet felt it anyway? Did you later feel bad wondering how they would feel, but still wanted to be right? Or did you just feel you were right, and too bad for them? Have you felt sad, guilty, discouraged, depressed or ashamed? Are you horrified at the News? Have you been worried about what might happen in the World? Have you wished someone would treat you better? Have you fretted about your bank account or wished for LOVE?

Most of us have experienced some of this at some time. How did we get like this? Where did accumulated fear, anger and blame come from? Why do we act out unpleasant and painful emotions, rather than remaining in joy as Infinite Beings of LOVE? This collective resonance has been repeated by generations for centuries and resonates from our unconscious. These disintegrative patterns resulted in a Global culture riddled with disease, fear, blame, rage, lack and death, which we are now shifting by moving into LOVE!

The irrationality of such thought-emotional patterns inherited from the blame-fear-hostility culture, emerges in Light of what we're Now learning and teaching. We forgot we Are Creator-Beings, and whatever thought we send out comes right back to us! Resetting thought and internal dialogue achieves magnificent results in our World, as we enter into a state where thoughts, words and deeds resonate from LOVE and the Golden Rule.

Findings of satellite reveal ruins in South Africa reported by Michael Tellinger in *Temples of the African Gods,* confirm translation of Sumerian tablets by late Zecharia Sitchin. Roots of ancestry link to a culture with sophisticated technology beyond ours, originating off-Planet according to detailed Sumerian clay tablets over 200,000 years ago!

Ancient records of a slave-based workforce mining gold, expose where punishment for disobedience may lie in our genetic memory-banks. In Tellinger's book, *Slave Species of the Gods* he reports depraved abuse, anger, hatred, war, death, torture, fear and oppression that permeated thousands of years of human history in deep shadows of our past. Blame-fear-hostility-judgment-control has been at the root of human suffering for literally ages.

We are Now integrating a new way of thinking and perceiving our World, as we learn how thoughts Create. Ridding self of these deeply buried, Not of LOVE blame-fear-hostility patterns takes a bit of unwinding, *sticking with it* when we want to quit. Whatever the story, disempowering patterns *need to be let go of Now,* for us to have a happy future.

Creatures of Creation and our Planet reflect our imbalances through their suffering. Military power, governmental manipulation and corrupt corporate financial systems have left many suffering globally. We could look upon this with despair, yet even *this* is a resonance to clear from within ourselves!!! Are we ready to *free ourselves* to Live as Beings of LOVE? *Our World and all timelines change as we shift our Vibration to LOVE...Now!*

When I despair, I remember that all through history the way of Truth and LOVE have always won. There have been tyrants and murderers, and for a time, they seem invincible, but in the end, they always fall. Think of it, always.

Mahatma Gandhi (1969-1948)
Non-Violent Leader of India

At the most basic fundamental level, we are *Heart centered, Infinite Creative Beings of LOVE.* Our *Essence* is that of a Newborn, Pristine, Innocent, Pure, Delightful, Precious, Joyful. Uprooting old self-protective reactive patterns of rage, fear, doubt, despair, hopelessness, blame and wanting to lash out, when "cleared,"*restore our Vibration to LOVE.*

We are now in a new Pachakuti (age), a time of transition and great changes. Our generation and that of our children will be instruments for creation of this new world, respecting each living entity, raising the banner of the rainbow, as to become conscious life examples for our human brothers and sisters.

Mallku Aribalto
The Awakening of the Puma, Inka Initiation Path

Living with awareness is the first step to Freedom. The second step is going inside to remove our unconscious Not of LOVE data (no more blame). Best tools we know are coming up. The greatest calling we have in Life as Observer-Creators, is to restore our "Newborn" status, holding the Presence of pure LOVE in our World. Look out World here we come! *21st Century Superhumans* are now restoring our *resonance to LOVE!* ♥

Chapter 11

Aramaic Filters: Rakhma & Khooba
Rookha d'Koodsha

---

*We are not a human being trying to attain a spiritual experience, but rather,
we are spiritual beings having a human experience.*

Teilhard deChardin (1881-1955)
The Philosophy of Man

2,000 years ago a Great Master walked the Earth. In His early years He worked as a carpenter, and lived among humanity. According to several accounts of the "lost years," He disappeared into the Far East teaching very similarly to what was later recorded in Galilee.

He taught fasting and cleansing in the Essene Tradition. He associated with high level Mystery Schools such as Ancient Egyptian Coptics and aligned with Mystical Teachings of the Himalayas, attracting followers wherever he went, who reported that He carried far beyond ordinary *Wisdom* of which rare documents still remain. In a few short years he affected humanity so profoundly that His teachings permeated much World culture for 2,000+ years, from then till Now.

He spoke His Teachings in the Aramaic language of the day, and was called by His given name Yeshua rather than Jesus (a name given later by Greeks after their god

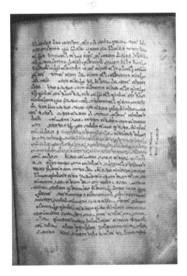

Khaburis Manuscript
Learn more at whyagain.org

Zeus). Ancient Aramaic had been in use for several thousand years, with many well known Texts recorded in it, such as the Talmud, Dead Sea Scrolls, New Testament and the original Old Testament from around 2400 B.C.

It is rumored that Ancient Aramaic appeared suddenly as a complete language in the Indus Valley and Persian Cradle of Civilization, preceding later languages including Sanskrit, Hebrew, Polynesian, Lakota and Arabic which were derived from it. Graham

Hancock's *Fingerprints of the Gods* suggests an advanced civilization was "jump-started" 6,000 B.C. in the Indus Valley, by remnants of earlier culture destroyed in Earth cataclysm.

Modern translation of Ancient Aramaic Texts of Yeshua's teachings, describe exciting and empowering "New" perspectives on our "reality," correlating astoundingly well with Quantum physics! His teachings instruct that our thought Creates, and how to clear all thought-emotion Not of LOVE (conscious-unconscious), to restore our True Design LOVE.

Dr. Rocco Errico established the Noohra Foundation in 1970, to help people of all faiths better understand modern translation of Aramaic roots of the Bible. Minister, lecturer, author, spiritual counselor and scholar on original Aramaic texts, he offers his bird's-eye view from a Life dedicated to modern translation of the Aramaic, *"LOVE is God in Motion."*

In almost all endeavors in Life we are to go forward, but in religion we need first to retrace our steps back to the source and then move forward. Let us realize that we can replace primitive laws of force, bigotry, hatred and violence with loving kindness, meekness, understanding and forgiveness. Every other attempt to usher peace into our world has failed.

The practice of Jesus' teachings is the answer for human ills. This Galilean prophet's simple and direct message was free of theology, doctrine, and dogma. He had no intention of starting another religion nor was he the founder of Christianity as we know it today. Therefore, let us join and participate together in demonstrating Jesus' principles and teachings in our daily living. This will bring peace and heaven on earth for all of us.

Rocco A. Errico
roccoaerrico.com

As we dig into powerful Aramaic roots, we are blessed with long standing friendship and professional relationship with dr. michael ryce, whose teachings focus on Ancient Aramaic principles. Trained as a Naturopathic physician, in his search for "true and deeper healing that would actualize the wholeness of our Design," he found himself immersed in teachings of Yeshua (Jesus), first through *A Course in Miracles*. Through certain contacts he was invited to become Moderator for a group of twenty-five scholars translating the oldest known copy of a handwritten Aramaic Text, the *Khaburis Manuscript*.

Immersed in secrets held in this Ancient document, he recognized eternal Truth based in the Science behind these teachings, that changed the course of his Life forever as it has for us. Once knowing the eternal science of these teachings, we realize there is no other path, except that of clearing our own Vibration to LOVE. Learn more about ongoing translation of *Khaburis Manuscript* at dr. ryce's website, *whyagain.org*

The Khaburis...Codex is a copy of the oldest known Eastern Canon of the new Testament in its native, and the original language of the Scriptures, Aramaic. The physical manuscript has been carbon-dated at approximately 1000 AD plus or minus 50 years. The colophon bears the seal and signature of the Bishop at the Church at Nineveh, then capital of the Assyrian Empire located today in the present-day Iraqi city of Mosul. According to colophon it is a copy of a text from approximately 164 AD....the teaching contained within the Manuscript can and will change the world.

dr. michael ryce
whyagain.org

Experiencing clarity revealed in this modern translation of the Aramaic, dr. ryce dedicated his Life and work to get these teachings out to "every mind, Heart and Being on the Planet." He and his wife jeanie travel to share Yeshua's original teachings full-time, Globally. Michael discovered that the Aramaic was not a religious language at all. It is a language revealing the *physics* of how to access and embody our True Design LOVE.

Original Aramaic describes fascinating elemental aspects of our "Design," easily understood with rudimentary computer knowledge, to which almost anyone Now has access. The Ancient Aramaic tells us about these elemental aspects of our "Design, filters that are like "firewalls" and a very powerful "anti-virus" protector.

1. ***Rakhma*** is a filter in the frontal lobe of the brain for *Intentions*, so all that goes from us are *Intentions* based in LOVE. Activated by ***Smiling...***

2. ***Khooba*** is a filter for the back of the brain for our *Perceptions* to be based only in LOVE. Activated by ***Breathing...***

3. ***Rookha d'Koodsha*** is a Feminine elemental aspect of our Design, when requested, r*emoves all corrupt data* Not of LOVE, like cleaning a virus out of a computer. We invite Rookha to help clear away "corrupt data" from our conscious-unconscious. [*Rookha d'Koodsha* was originally translated by the Greeks as Holy Spirit, however in the Aramaic it is *not* a person or being, but an elemental principle built into our "operating system."]

When these powerful built-in tools are *implemented,* they accelerate our personal Evolutionary process. Now you know why we say, "Breathe and Smile" often, as *they activate these important filters,* to clear our neurobiology of energies "Not of LOVE." A genuine *Smile* from the Heart with eye contact let's another know we are making a clear connection from the Heart, with intentions based in LOVE. When *Breath* flows freely, others sense we are relating from perceptions based in LOVE.

Breathing and Smiling send subtle messages to the body that life is "safe," and to others to know we approach them with LOVE. Tony Robbins used to tell us that it only takes *one tiny muscle movement* to turn a frown into a smile. Smile to share the LOVE.

Most ancient cultures contain Wisdom Teachings on how Breath connects us with Source. Polynesian, language derived from Ancient Aramaic, contains *honi* greeting, still used by many Hawaiians today, honoring spiritual Oneness by exchanging the "Breath of Life." When two people meet the press noses together, inhaling through the nose. They honor one another with the exchange of *ha,* the Breath of Life and *mana,* spiritual power.

With white men came a handshake, designed to check for weapons! This greeting was named "ha-ole," meaning without the "Breath of Life." This slang still sticks today.

Hawaiian *Aloha* is a sacred salutation, meaning mutual regard and affection, extending warmth and caring with no obligation in return. *Aloha* is the essence of relationship in which each person is important to every other for collective existence. ***Aloha means to hear what is not said, to see what cannot be seen and to know the unknowable.*** *Aloha* is very similar in meaning to the original Aramaic *rakhma* (intentions of LOVE), from which *Aloha* may be derived. We have now discovered numerous Ancient cultures containing such a greeting of open Heart and care for ALL.

Aramaic instructions for use of Body-Mind-Heart connect us to Source through Breath and Smiling are amazing keys to expressing our True Design LOVE. These simple but powerful elemental principles are **21st Century Superhuman** *tools,* that *when actualized,* change our lives dramatically forever, especially when we cultivate the habit of putting them into practice on a regular basis. Breathe and Smile.

• *Perceptions* of LOVE, through the **Khooba** filter are activated as *Breath* flows freely, felt by all we meet... returning this resonance of LOVE to us from the *Field*.

• *Intentions* based in LOVE through our **Rakhma** filter are activated when we *Smile*, felt by all we meet...returning the resonance of LOVE to us from the *Field*.

This energy vehicle we call Mind-Spirit-Body is designed for uninterrupted connection with Source, keyed to function at its highest when cleared of unconscious Vibrations and activated by LOVE. This systematized circuitry activates with natural functions, simply inhaling, exhaling and Smiling, focusing through the Heart, activating our torus field.

Body-Mind-Heart exchanges powerful radiant energy with all we meet and literally designed to operate *Infinitely* when plugged into our True Power Supply LOVE. As there is "no 'out there' out there," when we Breathe and Smile it Mirrors back to us, helping us thrive. Activating these simple habits alters us and our World, forever...

There is Magic Everywhere
Take a Moment, *Breathe and SMILE...*

Nancy Dock
Merlin's Cave Fall Equinox

When scholars translating the Ancient Aramaic *Khaburis Manuscript*, found a village where the language was still spoken, they inquired as to traditional translation of *Rakhma*. The people replied they had lost direct translation hundreds of years ago, though *Rakhma* was considered, *"the most precious jewel a person could possess."* Reclaiming use of this elemental aspect of our Design, *Rakhma: intentions based in LOVE* and using it on a moment to moment basis, brings amazing powerful changes to us and our World. When **21st Century Superhumans** get rowdy they cheer *"Rakhma On!"* Dr. ryce sheds additional Light on vital elements, *Rakhma* and *Khooba*.

Depending on the filter set, a mind generates LOVING, FEARFUL or HOSTILE realities. Reality is the perceptual output of the human mind. In the frontal lobes of the brain are all intentions you've ever experienced. In the back of the brain, all units of perceptual memory are stored. Everything you've ever experienced is registered as electrical impressions in brain cells.

There are filters that modify the output of both areas of the brain, intention and perception. Each has three filters, two of which are fear and hostility. In the ancient Aramaic language, there were words that represented the third filter over each area of the brain and each of these words was translated as LOVE, but with much deeper meaning. These filters when active allow access to different qualities of both intention and perception.

The third filter, over intentions, was called "Rakhma." It allowed only intentions keyed to LOVE to be used by the mind as raw materials for our goals. This is important, it turns out, because our goals determine or drive, quite literally, the output of the perceptual part of the brain. In the area of perception, the filter was called "Khooba" and this filter allowed only units of perceptual memory keyed to LOVE to be used in building perceptual reality...

dr. michael ryce
FAQ whyagain.org

ACTIVATE LOVE FILTERS: Rakhma and *Khooba* Filters ARE extremely *powerful,* assisting us to shift out of blame-fear-hostility intentions-perceptions (conscious-unconscious) to LOVE. Teach self and children to openly Breathe and Smile, using the filters and activating them within self. *This* is the most important part to *"get in shape;"* all other wishes and dreams fall into place as we *re-learn* how to operate in *Perfect LOVE.*

The first step is to keep your mind plugged-in to its proper Source. Rakhma and Khooba, together, are what Jesus described as Perfect LOVE. If there is fear or hostility in your Life, you need to learn how to set Rakhma and Khooba. They will cast out anything less than LOVE.

At this point, get quiet, close your eyes, take a deep Breath, and say internally, "I release attack [or source of my fear-hostility-blame] and reset the LOVE Filters, Rakhma, over Intentions, and Khooba, over Perceptions." *Visualize and feel through all your senses in your Life or memory that which takes you into that space of LOVE, Wisdom, Intelligence. Devote yourself to daily practice; it is the key to "Enlightenment." Your perceptual reality will begin to shift immediately.*

dr. michael ryce, FAQ whyagain.org
Explain Rakhma or Khooba LOVE from the Aramaic

Meaning of original Aramaic and related languages is incredibly Mind-expanding as to meaning of our "reality." Modern Aramaic Definitions for these elemental aspects (dr. ryce)

Rakhma - is a filter in the mind over *INTENTIONS*- it allows only intentions keyed to LOVE to be available as the raw material for use in setting my goals which are drivers for my realities.

Khooba - filter in the mind over *PERCEPTIONS* - allowing only units of perceptual memory keyed to LOVE to be available for structuring my personal "reality."

Rookha d'Koodsha - Active Feminine principle from God in the human mind that deletes error thinking and teaches us the truth. The "SuperProcessor!"

Engaging these filters keys us to LOVE. Using our own powerful design this way keeps Not of LOVE thought-emotion moving out of our system immediately upon awareness.

What is usually seen as religious advice, "You must have Rakhma-LOVE for God, neighbor, and self," was not religious but very practical, in fact, brilliant advice. The output of your mind, your perceptual reality in Aramaic terms, is the light or the guide for your earthly Life. The tiny fragment of the actual world seen through the mind is what we have to flesh out in our intelligence. If LOVE is maintained in the mind, especially in a trying situation, high level function is available.

dr. michael ryce, whyagain.org
FAQ Explain Rakhma or Khooba LOVE from the Aramaic

Below is a short question process to use when issues surface or when feeling blame toward someone else, to shift perspective and take Response-Ability. Becoming aware of and clearing our own resonance, is the path that *frees us* from suffering. Notice your Life changing in positive ways. Make copies to carry with you.

Notice and Question My "Reality"

1. My "reality" comes from my personal, genetic, conscious, unconscious Mind Energy. (___ ___) *initial to affirm.* Breathe. Smile.

2. As Observer-Creator this is my Response-Ability (___ ___)

3. I locate and cancel my " good goal" for situation bothering me, which is:

_____

_____. It may seem odd to cancel our "good" goal, however beneath it is a motivation from unconscious content (95% of the iceberg under-water). Canceling the goal is the key to release and clear, what we've been in denial about, to let it go from our unconscious.

4. *Rookha d'Koodsha* (____or?) assist me to reset *Rakhma* and *Khooba*, clear my unconscious content, its effects and learn the truth.

5. I Reconnect with Source, ask for restoration to LOVE and offer LOVE to_____ (situation or person)

6. I offer you_____(give something to the situation or person based in LOVE). Breathe. Smile.

Adapted from dr. michael ryce "Reality" Management Worksheet, No Fault Empowerment Tool (11 Step)
whyagain.org Start Here

BIGGEST QUESTION ASKED - WHY CANCEL MY "GOOD" GOAL? Our "good" goal in the conscious mind, is a "self-protective" denial mechanism, keeping us from having to be in touch with 95% "corrupt data" in the unconscious (because it was put there for SURVIVAL). Primary thought that runs our Life is the *95% in the unconscious.*

CANCELING OUR GOAL in the 5% conscious mind, is a *"keyway"* to release underlying data from the 95% unconscious. Canceling our goal in the conscious is a secret signal, once done, it dismantles thought structure *beneath it in the unconscious.* For example, a "good" goal in the conscious mind might be, "I Now have lots of money in my bank account." So beneath this in the unconscious is my fear about money such as, "I don't have enough, my family was poor, how am I going to pay my bills..." As we cancel our "good" goal that has been "protecting us" from this old pain or resonance in the unconscious, it is let go, and we can cultivate a NEW THOUGHT, free from this old unconscious resonance!

More examples:

Conscious - Tip of Iceberg 5% - "Good" Goal / Unconscious - Lower Iceberg 95% - Hidden

1. We have a great relationship	/ He-she is never there for me
2. He's really a good guy-girl	/ I'm terrified when I'm around him-her
3. I really LOVE my mom-dad	/ I'd be in big trouble if I told the truth
4. I'll have more money soon	/ I'm worried how I'll l pay my bills
5. I'll pray for peace	/ how are we ever going to have peace?

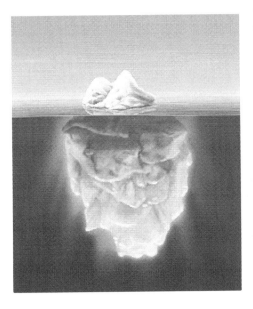

Our 5% conscious thought is the *tip of the iceberg.* The 95% below the surface is "data" hidden in our unconscious from in utero, infancy, early life experience, childhood and our generations, like a secondary "hard drive," that we're unconsciously in denial about because it's too painful for our awareness. The root of all fears, fear of death, is layered beneath the rest.

In the blame-fear-hostility culture we fell into running Life by punishment-reward "rules," erasing memory that we are Eternal Creator Beings. Removing this "data" buried in shadows of the unconscious with goal canceling, clears its resonance to restore our True Design LOVE.

Fear of "letting go," keeps us clinging to the familiar. Once we dig in we discover one old fear after another lets go. It doesn't take going far into human history to find wars, Dark Ages, Crusades, bloody sacrifices and more that have fed our deepest patterns buried in genetic memory. As we remove these subtle energy patterns woven into our fabric, including fear of punishment and loss of self, we clarify our vehicle and renew full connection with our True Design LOVE.

DENIAL: Refusal to acknowledge what is there by blaming someone or something else for what appears in our "reality," reducing ability to remove our own internal content.

We have shifted dramatically using the goal canceling processes, with transformative results as have those around us. It was taught by Yeshua (Jesus) as best as could be understood in that day. Becoming proficient at this True Aramaic Forgiveness process of clearing our own unconscious content, accesses Heart and our ability to resonate LOVE.

> ...Observations, perceptions, beliefs and notions of reality can switch, because emotions have hardwired roots in millions of years of survival and evolution. This explains why being right sometimes feels like a matter of Life and death.
>
> Buried painful emotions from the past make up what psychologists and healers call "core emotional trauma". The point of therapy - including bodywork, some chiropractic and energy medicine is to gently bring that wound to gradual awareness, so it can be re-experienced and understood. Only then is choice possible, a faculty of your frontal cortex, allowing you to reintegrate any disowned parts of yourself; let go of old traumatic patterns; and become healed or whole.
>
> *Dr. Candace Pert*
> *Discovered Opiate Receptors; "*
> *Your Body Is Your Unconscious Mind"*

Confusion and conflict is sourced from *within*. Our thoughts Create our "reality." Canceling goals assists us to clear this content easily and effectively. We will learn how to free ourselves from this old energy as we deepen understanding of these Aramaic tools in coming few chapters, and how to bypass our old "denial" survival mechanisms.

It can be a "dark night of the Soul" when we are replaying and clearing these things. Yet, they naturally resonate to the surface as our Vibration draws Life circumstances to reveal them to us. Holding back from pointing the finger at anyone else, circumstances or "telling a story," we are training ourselves too look within, and clear the resonance from within us.

Clearing layers as they arise, amazingly we begin to feel lighter and flow through Life more Freely, until soon we're operating totally in New frequencies! These tools are the "gateway" to birthing the **21st Century Superhuman**, as we activate our Dreams at the Highest level, Now Creating through the Heart. ♥

Chapter 12

Tuning Up Our DNA: LOVE Is Freedom

*I am not sure exactly what heaven will be like, but I know that when we die... [God]
will not ask, 'How many good things have you done in your Life?' rather he will ask,
'How much LOVE did you put into what you did?*

Mother Teresa (1910-1997)
Missionaries of Charity, 1979 Nobel Peace Prize

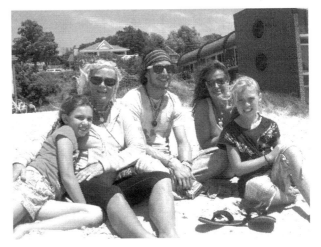

Yeshua's teachings, carried forward simply summarized in the *Golden Rule, "Do unto others as you would have others do unto you,"* was and still is Quantum physics made simple and is ultimate Service. Whatever we do (or intend) toward others comes back in like kind; thought Creates and draws in Mirroring of itself in our "reality."

Yeshua shared with the people "out of the Heart come the issues of Life." In the Aramaic "Heart" in this position meant "unconscious," yet there was no understanding for this in the culture of the day. He told them their unconscious content produced what appeared in their Lives. In the Aramaic: *Shbag* meant to *cancel*. It is good to pause and *NOTICE* what is surfacing in our World, as a result of our unconscious thought-patterns. Doing our clearing, to *cancel*, let go, releases generational Vibrations forever. Clearing ALL Not of LOVE resonance, shines LOVE through ALL timelines, shaping them and us into a New Quantum "reality."

*No one is to be called an enemy, all are your benefactors,
and no one does you harm. You have no enemy except yourselves.*

St. Francis of Assisi (1182-1226)

This is how we Leap beyond Ancient Not of LOVE patterning that has held us spellbound in its inertia for so long, to be shed it forever like a molting skin. One of the most empowering and real acts of Freedom is to move out of any possibility of "blame" towards another for our circumstances. This knowledge empowers us to change anything.

Forgiveness in Aramaic is the process of removing all content Not of LOVE from Our Own Unconscious, holding resonance in our Lives and World. This is the path to restoring our True Design LOVE.

In *this* miraculous ability to restore our True Design LOVE is the Key to Leaping across the Evolutionary Spiral. Clearing ourselves to LOVE, Compassion and Gratitude to Live in Heart Coherence "wakes up" our DNA, awakening sleeping codons.

… our bodies are continually striving for complete or perfect DNA...Our own genome is in a constant state of evolution, a never-ending process of completing itself, re-computing and re-scanning its own structure and constantly filling in the missing bits...Just like new computer technology to scan photographs and turn a dull image into a perfectly sharp image, the genome is constantly fixing the dull inactive bits, unlocking, reactivating them to perform a specific function for which they were Created.

Just because the geneticists have not yet figured out what all the dormant stretches of DNA are for, does not mean that evolution is going to stand still and wait for us to figure it out. Slowly but surely we are evolving physically and mentally as the genome reactivates itself. It is like a rebirth from a long sleep from which humankind is waking up. A sleep into which we must have been induced by someone or something long ago. A sleep of ignorance and forgetfulness.

Michael Tellinger
Slave Species of the Gods

It appears that only 3% of our active genes are coded in a way we can recognize. Long stretches may have coding we do not yet recognize, that used to be called "junk DNA." Scientists think we currently use less of our DNA than any other species including yeast! Since mapping of the Human Genome, realization has dawned that "junk" DNA is actually essential, yet we currently are guessing at what it is for. As we activate and access the additional 97% of our DNA who knows what humanity is capable of?

Deep inside our genome, in between all the brutal and barbaric genes, there is a natural tendency for compassion, LOVE and peace, which is encoded but switched off. Sometimes it breaks through the clutter. If the genome evolves and allows us to move closer to a completely reconstructed DNA, we are one step closer to a perfect genome and total enlightenment on both the physical and spiritual fronts.

Michael Tellinger
Slave Species of the Gods

Ever wonder? Is it astonishing for such a bright species that so much of our World is still in chaos? That almost the entire gamut of human history is riddled with war, destruction, dis-ease and death? That many in the developed World participate in suppressive habits, with little motivation to express their greatest creative potential? That

33% global population is starving, and *a person dies of starvation every 3.6 seconds?* 1/7 the population of the Planet are without sanitary drinking water? Our biodiversity is declining at an unprecedented rate, with 10,000 species extinct in the last 100 years?

Brutality has been heaped upon brutality for differences in ideology or selfishly claiming resources. We cannot help but carry a residual of this Not of LOVE history inside us, *until we clean it out. FEAR* is a resonance carried for thousands of years, mostly rooted in blind obedience to avoid "punishment." Addressing this may put us into avoidance, yet clearing it so it no longer holds resonance in our World is the wat to Create lasting change for an emerging New World based in LOVE and Freedom. *Do you remember when you:*

- Did what was expected of you?
- Told an untruth?
- Deferred to someone else instead of speaking up?
- Attired yourself to fit in?
- Took on a job or career, not because you Loved it, but for the money?
- Stayed in an unhappy or disrespectful relationship?

Or you may be doing these things, and they may give a feeling of safety or comfort because they are familiar. It is amazing how wide and deep compliance goes, buried deep in us from long ago, based in blame-fear-hostility fear of punishment. Breaking bonds with these old patterns is a journey that frees us to exit our chrysalis to fly into the Universe, transformed into something amazingly wonderful and beautiful. Breathe and Smile.

Throughout history there have been legends about interference from the fallen Children of God who came to Earth from outside of the Solar System of Alfa and Omega. This seemed so outrageous that we usually discounted these stories as myths. Now the Company of Heaven is confirming that aeons ago some interference did occur...

After we came to the erroneous conclusion that we were powerless, fallen sisters and brothers from other systems realized our vulnerability and decided to take advantage of the opportunity. They even went so far as to proCreate with the Children of the Earth in an attempt to perpetuate their nefarious plans. The fragmented state of our DNA made our genetic codings malleable. This allowed the fallen souls to change our DNA in ways that enabled them to manipulate us.

The Company of Heaven revealed that modifications made in our DNA by these souls changed the Earth from a school of cocreation and empowerment, to a school of duality and separation...But the Light of God is infinitely more powerful than darkness, so in spite of all the resistance, little-by-little the Light began returning to Earth.

Patricia Diane Cota-Robles
Who Am I? Why Am I Here?

Shifting to Heart-centered Living activates our DNA, restores balance with Earth Mother Gaia, humanity-huwomity and our sense of Oneness with All things. Wonderful change is taking place in global awareness, ethical action and Living LOVE. Our DNA contains incredible potential we have yet to access. Latest research reported by Gregg Braden, HeartMath Institute and Drunvalo Melchizedek reveals *DNA "codons" switch on as we enter into Heart Coherence, restoring our True Design LOVE.*

> We know by the Law immutable, by truth unwavering, by the endless Life and God, that all divinity is within us, and that though it be now but little evolved, all is there of infinite capacity, available for the uplifting of the world.
>
> *Annie Besant*
> *The Masters*

In *Solar Revolution,* Dieter Broers cites studies that our DNA is continually mapped anew, that DNA sends and receives information beyond space and time, in constant communication with multiple levels of the Cosmos. "Hence we will be able to fulfill our sacred mission as we recognize internally who we really are... According to various prophecies, humanity is engaged in a process of transformation that will culminate in 'ascendance to the fifth dimension.' Heim says 'for all intents and purposes we are already integrated at higher levels,' it is just for us to become aware of it. "

> Needless to say, many of us have yet to come to this realization and continue to live our lives reactively for the most part. Ignorance of these things lands us in "Plato's cave," with the result that, as befits a cave, our viewpoint is limited to the shadows on the cave walls, which we mistakenly take to be our reality. But in point of fact these shadows, this reality, this world is nothing more than secondary information concerning causality.
>
> We can only achieve the kind of perception and recognition I am talking about here if we expand our point of view and our consciousness in such a way that we engage in a... "tuning" process. This in turn will result in what is generally referred to as enlightenment. And although both enlightened and unenlightened...will perceive the same things [from different perspectives], they will be interconnected...Such a process may in fact constitute ascent to the fifth dimension...
>
> *Dieter Broers*
> *Solar Revolution*

SETTING A NEW BEAT - METRONOME - ENTRAINMENT: In an amazing demonstration of 32 metronomes keeping beat for music, each one started separately and clicking independently take just a few minutes to synchronize. We are designed individually yet we are a Collective. It is easy to yield to mass consciousness, like "shadows on the wall of Plato's cave," or in "realities" emerging from resonance of unconscious data. Our current "wake up call" invites us to set a new beat with millions on Planet Earth, Now stepping into enlightened living from the Heart. This entrainment to higher frequency vision and knowledge synchronizes the collective to a New beat.

If you look around, you can find a face of God in each thing, because He is not hidden in a church, in a mosque, or a synagogue, but everywhere. As there is no one who lives after seeing him, there is also no one dying after seeing him. Who finds Him, stays forever with him.

Shams Tabrizi (1185-1248)
Rumi's Spiritual Teacher of 7 years

Essentially we must attend to offloading the old content from our unconscious. As this content Not of LOVE is thrown overboard, our ship is Free to fly with the wind on sea of Life. True Freedom comes from being awake and subject to our True Design LOVE, rather than the old "shadows on the wall." Clearing our resonance shifts us and the Whole, with the miraculous result of relieving Ancient and personal pain and resulting global miseries.

As more of humanity practices Heart-based living it will Qualify as the 'rite of passage' into the next level of consciousness. Using our Heart's guidance will become common sense based on practical intelligence.

Doc Childre
Founder HeartMath®

If we ever feel, "It's impossible that this resonance could have come from me," and find ourselves blaming someone or something else for our discomfort, fear, hostility or even feeling rejected or not understood, the "prime directive" is to go within and remove this resonance or judgment *FROM WITHIN*. Once this principle is embraced and applied in ALL situations, relationships, events, conditions, circumstances and things, we transcend ALL Not of LOVE, to hold Compassion Deep LOVE and Gratitude, while taking nothing personally. By so doing we cultivate Heart Coherence, full activation of our DNA and Oneness with ALL. Breathe. Smile.

One of the biggest questions that comes up, as we grow in understanding of these principles, is the "why" question, "Why did my Loved-One or pet die so young, or of such an illness, or why were they killed in a accident, why was someone raped, murdered, molested or suffered a degenerative condition, why are horrible things still going on in the World?" Although difficult to grasp at first, Quantum physics is very clear that EVERYTHING is a product of thought (conscious-unconscious) Mirrored as our "reality." Perhaps fear of death that needs to come to our Attention for us to get clarity and release it, perhaps there is memory of-judgment of-fear of rape or murder in our generations (could be thousands of years ago) surfacing to clear with LOVE.

WHAT IS PAIN? An inharmonious energy pattern we feel, that brings our Attention to disharmonious frequencies within us. Painful experiences are residual of thousands of generations of thought-resonance. As Observer-Creator calling "reality" into being, ALL that shows up in my "reality" is for me to be present with and clear to LOVE. That's it!

Moving toward Enlightenment, these old frequencies can no longer be hidden and are surfacing for us to clear. Simply *PAUSE and Notice* the energy Mirrored that has likely been carried in *your* energy field, buried in *your* unconscious for perhaps *thousands of generations*. These magnetics have pulled a person or situation with matching energy or resonance into your World who Mirrors it. At a "Soul level" you "agreed" to clear these things with LOVE.

> When you become aware of silence, immediately there is that state of still alertness. You are present. You have stepped out of thousands of years of collective human conditioning.

Eckhart Tolle

Knowing what you have to clear requires noticing what feelings come up for *you* regarding the situation. Our worksheet process in next chapter is perfect for doing this. A deeply intense or painful experience may take many worksheets to clear. Cancel your goals until the layers are removed, and these shadows can disappear from "Plato's cave" of the unconscious forever. New layers are bound to arise to clear and cancel as they come up, gradually to be let go forever.

The now famous saying of the Iroquois Confederacy, "to the 7the generation" means that whatever energies I participate in will be encoded to my future generations' DNA, family story or attitudes, and expressed by them. We *21st Century Superhumans* clear our unconscious for ourselves, our relations and unto the 7th generation and ALL who come after past-present-future. *Arcing the Hologram through spacetime, ALL timelines, into ALL dimensions, we restore our True Design LOVE.*

This is the single most self-validating action we take, restoring health, vitality, well-being, success and abundance. It will likely take practice to fully understand and actualize this new way of thinking and living our lives. Once we get this Quantum principle Life shifts in amazing ways! *We are literally writing new "code" for our DNA*, and redirecting how Life unfolds before us.

Yeshua's (Jesus') teachings contained elements of Quantum physics that we are just Now understanding, about how our energy Creates, built around the principle that what we hold in the *Field* is Mirrored back to us. Amazing little-known records reveal Yeshua was teaching these principles even early in Life, and considered a bodhisattva or enlightened Master even then.

Traveling the Himalayas, Nicolas Notovitch, Russian officer, spy, and journalist had opportunity while recovering from a broken leg to read the yellowed, two volume text, *The Life of Issa*, preserved for centuries in a nunnery. A member of his party translated the Tibetan, from which Notovitch wrote *The Unknown Life of Jesus* published in 1894. When he returned home much controversy about authenticity of the documents, drove a skeptic, to journey to expose the fraud, instead discovering the 224 verse volumes were real. The depth and meaning of the verses grounded in eternal spiritual truth is obvious.

> Issa taught that men should not strive to behold the Eternal Spirit with one's own eyes but to feel it with the heart, and to become a pure and worthy soul....

Not only shall you not make human offerings, but you must not slaughter animals, because all is given for the use of man. Do not steal the goods of others, because that would be usurpation from your near one. Do not cheat, that you may in turn not be cheated ....

Beware, ye, who divert men from the true path and who fill the people with superstitions and prejudices, who blind the vision of the seeing ones, and who preach subservience to material things...

Reverence Woman, 'mother of the universe,' in her lies the truth of creation. She is the foundation of all that is good and beautiful. She is the source of life and death...Bless her. Honor her. Defend her. Love your wives and honor them, because tomorrow they shall be mothers, and later-progenitors of a whole race. Their love ennobles man, soothes the embittered heart and tames the beast...

As light divides itself from darkness, so does woman possess the gift to divide in man good intent from the thought of evil. Your best thoughts must belong to woman. Gather from them your moral strength... Do not humiliate her, for therein you will humiliate yourselves. And all which you will do to mother, to wife, to widow or to another woman in sorrow-that shall you also do for the Spirit.

Yeshua (Jesus) was known in the Himalayas, India and Tibet as St. Issa, where he traveled, studied and taught from age 12-29. His teachings were passed on verbally for centuries and existed in random documents in that part of the World. The original documents found by Notovich were later sought and discovered by Nicholas Roerich, traveler and distinguished scientist, who recorded them in diaries from 1924-1928, and later published called *Altai-Himalaya*. Roerich reveals how significant these vital ideas were among Moslems, Hindus, Buddhists and how they had penetrated even the remotest locales. They tell how St. Issa preached beside a small pool near a bazaar under a great tree.

Issa said man had filled temples with abominations: to pay homage to metals and stones, man sacrificed his fellows in whom dwells a spark of the Supreme Spirit.

Man demeans those who labor by the sweat of their brows, in order to gain the good will of the sluggard who sits at the lavishly set board. But they who deprive their brothers of the common blessing shall be themselves stripped of it.

Issa bade them 'Worship not the idols. Do not consider yourself first. Do not humiliate your neighbor. Help the poor. Sustain the feeble. Do evil to no one. Do not covet that which you do not possess and which is possessed by others.'

Nicholas Roerich
Altai-Himalaya

Yeshua (Jesus) came to Earth as a Great Master, to wake us up and remind us about what action in Life is harmonious with the Laws of Creation and the Universe. Pain, suffering and resistance are simply a product of thought experimenting outside of LOVE. Are you ready to be a Quantum revolutionary? Adventure into shifting your DNA to join the ranks of many Now living connected to our True Power Supply LOVE. Draw a New "reality" into Being through this resonance.

> If you look around, you can find a face of God in each thing, because He is not hidden in a church, in a mosque, or a synagogue, but everywhere. As there is no one who lives after seeing him, there is also no one dying after seeing him. Who finds Him, stays forever with him.

> *Shams Tabrizi (1185-1248)*
> *Rumi's Spiritual Teacher of 7 years*

Summary:

• Living for materialism is our of harmony with Source, rather live for your "fellows" within whom is the spark of the Supreme Sprit

• A person is not to sacrifice their Life laboring for another (we are equal)

• Those who deprive others of the common blessing will lose theirs (Mirroring)

• No idol worship (anything not of Spirit)

• Consider others first; help the poor (we are ONE)

• Do not humiliate your neighbor (neighbor is *anyone* in Aramaic near or far)

• Do not covet what others have (Attention on "not having")

• Notice just the fact of Creation is a miracle (miracles are natural to LOVE)

• Don't follow someone who demonstrates their power with a miracle

• Rather than striving to see Eternal Spirit feel It with your Heart

• Don't steal for that is like taking from yourself (we are One)

• If you cheat - you will be cheated (not karma or punishment: *Quantum physics*)

TRANSFORMING OUR GREATEST CHALLENGE: Sit quietly and think of a challenging situation or person. Most of us have someone we "blame" for our struggles-troubles. Breathe and Smile. Allow your thoughts to flow with the situation or person, and no matter how it seems, know you and they are ONE. Bring LOVE into this situation. Breathe. Smile. Ask yourself what old energy is appearing to be let go of Now. Enter more deeply into LOVE through the Heart. Smile. Breathe.

> Working on our own consciousness is the most important thing that we are doing at any moment, and being love is the supreme creative act.

> *Ram Dass*
> *Polishing the Mirror*

We get quicker and more efficient at "canceling our goals and letting go the old energy," as we deepen these clearing processes. Be with the energies to clear, release, let go. Smile. Breathe. Welcome LOVE. Expand through your Heart. Smile. Feel-See-Hear your New resonance going out into the World, in your spinning torus field, with LOVE. ♥

Part 2: MIND

Chapter 13

Ancient Aramaic Forgiveness Freedom Tools

The Heart is like a garden. It can grow Compassion or fear,
resentment or LOVE. Which seeds will you plant there?

Buddha

Why would it take "Loving someone or something enough" to "get the lesson?" In our most intimate pain, often through loss or suffering of a Loved-One, death or when a relationship ends we tend to seek till we find answers. How powerfully Vibrational frequencies *within us,* magnetize or attract scenarios with others of matching resonance, is a New and unique way to view Life.

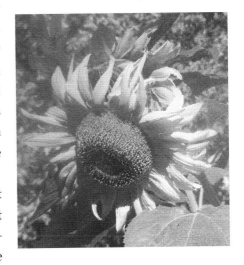

We recognize we are acting out the most standard Quantum physics Double Slit Experiment: that our thoughts as Observer-Creators call "reality" into being by their resonance of "Attention on the *Field.*" When a terribly "painful" situation occurs, LOVE keeps us connected so we will stick with it until we get clearly *"what in us"* is resonating in this situation. It may take a little unraveling, and going over it many times for the full continuity of layered thought pattern to become visible and clear.

We are whirlpools in the river of consciousness. Our individuality curls tightly in when focused on self, and loosens up as we connect outwardly experiencing our Oneness. We are the whirlpool and we are the river. Ultimately we Are ALL connected, emerging from the *Field of Possibilities,* the same "cosmic soup" as ALL Creation. We are letting go the belief that when events occur, something or someone outside of us is at cause. Vibrational patterns magnetize ALL into Being around us. LOVE keeps us associated to "waking up."

Enlightenment is a crumbling away of untruth. It's seeing through the facade of pretense. It's complete eradication of everything we imagined to be true.

Adyashanti (1962-)
The Way of Liberation

We offered earlier a short "reality" questioning process for you to play with as issues came up, as a building block for our worksheet process. Commitment of the *21st Century Superhuman* is to cultivate Response-Ability in *every Now moment*, clearing *ALL* Not of LOVE *ASAP*. In this chapter you will be introduced to our worksheet process - a vital tool to clear our unconscious content. Doing this "work," we Free ourselves from being victim's of circumstance, knowing we have the power to choose a new Creation.

Nassim Haramein reminds us in his explanation of Quantum physics 99% of our existence is space. It is waiting to emerge from our Attention upon the *Field*. How will we "qualify" it? As our "reality" is simply a projection of "thought energy" through us. Are we ready to "adjust our filters" and shift our thought enough to call in Creation in new ways?

Boundaries are imaginary. Rules are made up.
Limits don't exist.

This is the crazy, wild, awesome thing about our Quantum World!!! As we perceive ourselves as unlimited, we realize *all* is a result of thought Creation. Einstein said, *"matter is simply energy slowed down enough to be visible to our perceptions."* Are you ready to let go of limitation and any old pattern that comes up Not of LOVE? The thought resonance we are designed to function from, for optimal experience within Universal Law, is LOVE. Shifting over to this completely unleashes staggering potential.

Our greatness is being able to remake ourselves.

Mahatma Gandhi (1969-1948)

Now is the eternal Moment in the 'No-Time' Continuum, for us to change all timelines, *Arc the Hologram*, release anything Not of LOVE restoring our True Design LOVE. *This is the way to a viable future, Living from a New mindset. It is the most important task at hand* for *21st Century Superhumans*.

Sometimes the act of letting go is far greater than the act of hanging on.

Eckhart Tolle
Power of Now

TAKE NOTICE OF YOUR GENERATIONAL PATTERNS: What strong characteristics are you aware of typical to your family tree, Now asking to be cleared from your unconscious, and from your generations forever? Perhaps rather than externalized rage, there is withdrawal or depression that carries its own unique expression and response. What traits do you notice in your family or experiential World that you will benefit from clearing? Use upcoming exercises to remove these thought-emotional patterns from your generations.

EXAMPLE GENETIC HERITAGE: I (Cary) had a fiery temperament from one side of my family bloodline. Life Mirrored many times this habituated Not of LOVE thought-emotional data. As I have done clearing, letting go blame, canceling goals, my clarity and inner ecology have shifted tremendously! Integrating this principle has taught me how to use my energy with wisdom, rather than responding with reactive patterns handed down from my generations. Turning that fiery temperament into the courage to go into "Plato's cave" and clear my own "corrupt data" has brought about extremely powerful use of it!

What you think in secret comes to pass,
your Life is just a looking glass.

Jack White (1934-1998)
God's Game of Life

GETTING TESTED: We may think we're doing "well" in our clearing, then (drumroll), someone shows up to **"test us."** *ha!* Our first response is, "This *can't* be coming from me, I've already cleared that." Whatever is triggered by this other person or event *IS Mirroring a resonance inside us (blame-fear-hostility-judgment-control),* that once acknowledged can clear quickly. Give thanks for the *GIFT!* It gets easier. Breathe and Smile.

You are the Soul of the Soul of the Universe
and Your Name is LOVE.

Rumi
13th Century Sufi Mystic

STORIES: Most of us have had our *"stories,"* in the old way of thinking, and may have in the past sought out others for sympathy or support. In these "old" situations, considering someone else at fault, our friend took our "side, we out-number them, proved they were wrong and we won," which used to make us feel good. *NO MORE!* Perpetuating our "stories" about someone or something else just kept us in denial, about our own internal content resonating the situation. We are they. They are us. *There is no 'out there' out there...*

Better than a thousand hollow words, is one that brings peace.

Buddha (563-483 B.C.)

A great way to share our "story" for support is with a "process buddy," who understands how to assist us in this clearing process. When we're in our "stuff" it can be very helpful to have support. As Quantum Beings we recognize no one is at fault. *AND NOW,* we get to tell a new *Story* of LOVE!

Two are better than one...
If either falls down, one can help the other up.

Ecclesiastes 4: 9-10

Please take us *Literally,* when we offer this "goal canceling process" using our *Ancient Aramaic Freedom Tools* is *vital* for **21st Century Superhumans.** There is *nothing* we know of more potent or that does a better job releasing old data from the unconscious. The most important thing is to "do it!" Once we get moving this new direction we can as Abraham says, "Pick up the oars, float and let the river carry us." Keep Breathing, Smiling and clearing, until all you experience in your "reality" is your True Design *LOVE*.

When she transformed into a butterfly, the caterpillars spoke not of her beauty but of her weirdness. They wanted her to change back into what she always had been. But Now, she had wings...

Dean Jackson
The Poetry of Oneness

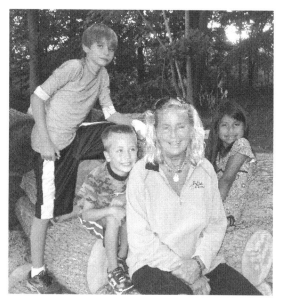

NEVER HAVING TO SAY "I'M SORRY" AGAIN Imagine being so Freely aligned with your True Self and Essence that every moment, everything you did or thought was in total abandon, perfectly aligned with flowing Creation of Your Being - like a kid. Saying "sorry" would seem ridiculous, as you'd be honoring the perfect flow of Creation emerging every moment from within. This is the New way to Live! If "sorry" pops out - we just tell each other, "No more of that!"

Familiar forgiveness or pardoning, used for many centuries was part of that Ancient blame-fear-hostility culture we've almost forgotten about Now. In fact from a "power-over" standpoint the individual at "blame," may have been avoiding being hurt or killed. What an amazing piece of thinking to have stored away inside us at a deep level. As Quantum Beings, we *know* ALL resonance comes from inside. We Now remove this "fear" content from our own patterning and laugh!

There may be circumstances respecting outmoded social customs, where the best thing to do is Lightly *apologize* as a "bridge." However, let go of being *"sorry"* - a statement of fear of punishment. Experiment with the True Aramaic Forgiveness Process using worksheet tools in this chapter. Once your "goal" is cancelled with Aramaic Forgiveness, your "reality" will shift dramatically, *because you have shifted your resonance.* As *Gandhi said -*

Where there is LOVE there is Life.

HOW MANY TIMES WILL I NEED TO DO THIS PROCESS?: When we studied Body Electronics with Dr. John Ray, he told us, "In a day when people can take one antibiotic pill and be "better" in a week; they're shocked when I tell them it will take two years to clear themselves, to be well and functioning at a higher level."

HOW MANY TIMES SHOULD I FORGIVE MY BROTHER? When Yeshua was asked, "How many times should I "Aramaic Forgive" my brother?" He said in Aramaic **77 x 77 = 5929** (the Bible inaccurately records it as 7 x 77). Many doing this work commit to doing 5 worksheets per day for 2-3 years, which literally accomplishes this and clears much!

Only when we LOVE someone or something enough,
do we get the lesson.

Sun Bear
Native American Shaman, Medicine Man

The deeper our pain, the more necessary to remove it from our energy system, as it reduces Life force. This blocked energy causes dis-ease and dis-comfort, leading to low vitality, illness, depression and miseries of our modern World, resulting in a long slow walk toward the grave. It may take several *years* of clearing deep issues to get through the layers. Yet clearing our blockages by removing our unconscious content is Key to Life, LOVE, vitality, and sets up a "hundredth monkey" effect for the entire Collective to shift.

I will let go... And that will collapse it into a new possible outcome.

Dr. Richard Bartlett,
Matrix Energetics

PRINT 100 COPIES OF THE WORKSHEETS x 2 SIDES: We suggest *printing* our Ancient Aramaic Forgiveness Freedom Tools (50-100 at a time double-sided to save paper), quick and easy to grab one when "something comes up." Many have done 2-3,000 worksheets in a 1-2 year period. The amount of change and transformation reported is mind-boggling - rewiring Now to LOVE! Choose a version of the worksheet you are ready for. Commit to 3-5 per day. No need to share your worksheets. Do them efficiently, and throw away when done. Complete as quickly as possible; scribbling allowed; offload old content and dismantle constructs holding them in place. Note issues that come up for additional worksheets. Keep count if you like, for fun!

YEAH FOR YOU! This takes putting on our **21st Century Superhuman** *propulsion boots*, to Leap past old paradigm thought, and align with our new path to clarity. (Remember, this is a far different way of thinking than what we've been taught). The "brilliant and gifted" Yeshua knew 2,000 years ago, how important it was to clear "corrupt data" to access our full potential and restore our True Design LOVE! Simple - *CANCEL ALL GOALS NOW!*

TRUE ARAMAIC FORGIVENESS FREEDOM TOOLS: We start here with simple versions of this worksheet process. For those desiring to progress to more detail, those by dr. michael ryce finely tuned over decades (free at whyagain.org click "start now") are excellent. This facilitates Yeshua's Aramaic "goal canceling" instructions, *offering* a clear path to shift *out of* old beliefs, transforming into our True Design LOVE. Michael and jeanie's *Mindshifter Radio Shows* (archived/live whyagain.org) have assisted us to learn and grow, offering powerful daily support to integrate this New way of Being.

TRUE ARAMAIC FORGIVENESS WORKSHEET- Version 1
Goal Canceling Freedom Tool (make copies)

"REALITY" *Created by my thought (conscious-unconscious) Mirrored in my World*
CANCEL GOAL = FORGIVENESS - A tool for changing "reality," by clearing my thoughts-emotions Vibrating in this situation, to restore my True Design LOVE. ♥

NOTE TO MYSELF: People, situations and circumstances involved are Mirrors, gifting me with opportunities. If I'm In Pain - I Am the one who has clearing to do!!! My "reality" (what I believe and how I feel) is made from thoughts *in me.* As I change my thoughts, my "reality" changes. I Am committed to clearing repeating patterns in my Life!

1A. I seem to be upset because of (person, thing or situation) _____
(__ __) [my initials say this is a mirror of my "stuff"]. Write what happened _____
_____

2. This triggers feelings inside of me of _____

3. The thought that causes me to feel this way is _____
_____Breathe. Smile.

4. I want to punish or get even by _____
Punishment and blame are not my friends. As I accept that these feelings are mine, not from someone or something else, I Response-Ably notice and clear my own thoughts.

4. A friendly thought I have about #1A is _____

5. MY GOAL: What I really want in positive words is _____
_____

I choose to feel good rather than be upset. I choose to let go of my old content.

6. I **cancel** — let go of — my need for my "good goal" #5 _____ Breathe. Smile.

7. I connect with LOVE inside me, knowing that canceling my "Good Goal" releases data from my 95% unconscious (put there for my or my ancestors' "survival"). I Now Breathe and Smile as I release this resonance of old denied thought patterns.

8. I join with the LOVE in you #1A _____ and share a New LOVING goal with you _____

> **ARAMAIC: Khooba** perceptions of LOVE back of brain: Breathe. **Rakhma** intentions of LOVE frontal of brain: Smile. **Rookha d'Koodsha** Feminine elemental force that breaks off the effect of errors and teaches truth - super processor that can heal all generations. **Shebag:** to cancel - corrects disassociated states of mind (*Shebag* was originally translated as "forgive" but meant "cancel")

MORE DETAILED WORKSHEETS: Thanks to dr. michael ryce and his wife jeanie for developing this awesome process. Our worksheets are simplified versions of theirs, based on needs of our clients. For those who desire a deeper challenge to self-inquiry, download dr. ryce's more detailed *"Reality Management Worksheets."* Free at *whyagain.org (Click "Start" upper left).* Michael and jeanie's daily *Mindshifter Radio Show* is also extremely supportive for integrating this process - link at their site.

TRUE ARAMAIC FORGIVENESS WORKSHEET - Version 2
Goal Canceling Freedom Tool (make copies)

This Goal Canceling Process is the "keyway" to removing my "corrupt data" (95% unconscious thoughts-emotions Not of LOVE) rather than blaming someone else. Clearing this data restores My True Design LOVE, of which I am reminded when holding a Newborn.

1. I ♥ have been convinced by my mind that my "trigger" (them, it, self or situation) name the object of your Attention (#1A) _____ (__/__) [my initials say I recognize this is my mind energy]. My feelings_____

2. Describe what happened _____

_____

THE TRUTH IS MY "REALITY" IS STRICTLY INTERNAL CreateD BY MY THOUGHTS!
As I take Response-Ability for and remove my disintegrative thoughts my "reality" shifts

3. My thoughts that cause my feelings_____

4. I want to punish them or self by_____

5. Fear/hostility and punishment distort my "reality." I choose to see every part of my mind accurately, heal and Free myself. My exact goal for (#1 A) in positive words is _____

_____

6. When upset my "reality" is constructed of *MY corrupt data.* This data was hidden in my 95% unconscious for my *SURVIVAL* (or my generations'), covered up by my "Good goal" of my 5% conscious (tip of iceberg). *Canceling* my "Good Goal" unlocks data in my unconscious, to let it go. In Aramaic, *Shbag - **cancel*** "Good Goal" to thankfully remove this Vibration from my unconscious forever! Yay! *(write #6).*_____

_____

7. I Now invite Aramaic-*Rookha d'Koodsha,* Feminine principle "super processor" to clear/remove/delete ALL "corrupt data" (dis-ease) _____ from my neurobiology, restoring my Newborn state LOVE. ♥ Incline me toward healing, and heal my denial and my capacity to generate #2 (triggered emotion) _____
Breathe. ♥

8. I now feel _____ about #1A (trigger). About my earlier perception of my "reality" I now see that_____ ♥ I ask to be shown how I have violated #6 my "Good Goal, tip of the iceberg

_____

9. A principle of the Universe is that whatever thought-emotion conscious-unconscious I put out comes right back to me! I Now choose Truth and Perfect LOVE. I choose to structure a truly Loving goal toward you #1A (my trigger) based on #6 (my goal above)
_____ ♥

Make double sided copies of this Freedom Tool. Commit to doing 3-5 per day. Make an agreement with a buddy also doing this work to call or text each other when you're done. ♥
Thanks to dr. michael ryce for his development of this process - learn more at whyagain.org

DON'T RESIST YOUR RESISTANCE: In Aramaic "satan" is the "resistor" or "divider from LOVE" (*not* bad guy in red suit with horns). The part of us that fears going into our pain to clear it is our denial or Resistance, keeping us from going into the fear of removing "corrupt data" Not of LOVE. Breathe, Smile, move through resistance. Breathe. Smile.

> The place where you are right now, God circled on a map for you
> Wherever your eyes and arms and heart can move
> Against the earth and the sky, the beloved has bowed there-
> The beloved has bowed there knowing You were coming…
>
> *Hafiz*
> *14th Century Persian Mystic Poet*

In the modern World, it is easy to fall into the trap of thinking I can just change my thoughts. It is a little more tricky than that, as Yeshua taught and Einstein knew: *Problems cannot be solved at the level at which they were Created* (conscious mind). It is essential to go in deeper, to offload our unconscious content. (Videos soon at *21stCenturySuperhuman.com*).

> Enlightenment is the continuous realization our Life-experience is a Mirror of our beliefs…simply be aware that what you believe is what you see.   As you shift your beliefs, what you "see" will change. Seeing is not believing; believing is seeing. ♥
>
> *Teddi Mulder*

Think of Mother Theresa, St. Francis, Mahatma Gandhi and others who committed to Live their LOVING Vibrational *Essence*, holding a new *frequency* or *tuning fork*, for humanity's harmonization. When we clear our resonance and hold the tone, frequency or Vibration of LOVE uninhibited, we too shift the World.

> *Be* the change you wish to see in the world.
>
> *Mahatma Gandhi (1969-1948)*
> *Non-Violent Leader of India*

According to Quantum theory our resonance offers our *message* to the World. We magnetize events, circumstances and people in as perfect Mirroring of what is within. As we do our clearing to offload inharmonious data, we actualize our greatest potential for living with Joy, Abundance, Wholeness, LOVE, Health, Well-Being and Vitality.

> Evidence from scientific studies shows thoughts and intention hold power…calming intentions of test subjects show up instantaneously in a darkened room as millions of photons. Tiny particles of "Smart LIGHT" manifest in an instant across the globe…KNOW your intentions and thoughts are charged…live and active!
>
> *Cory Ann Cashman*
> *Winged ScribeParaphrased from David Wilcock*

21st Century Superhumans are part of a Wave of Rising Consciousness Now transiting the Globe, changing our future forever for the better. Living by design rather than default, we are Now Leaping across the Evolutionary Spiral, in this *Shift Of the Ages!* ♥

Part 2: MIND
Chapter 14
Reclaiming Our Power

The most holy ground is that where
ancient enemies become friends.

A Course In Miracles 26:6:1

Digging deeper into what is buried inside us causing stress, let's learn to embrace what dr. michael ryce calls our Power Person Dynamic.

POWER PERSON DYNAMIC: Most of us had a childhood relationship with *someone who we felt had more power over our Life than we did.* Our Power Person had *their own* stress response patterns, based on *their* power person from childhood. Our lifetime stress-response pattern is rooted in childhood dynamic initiated with this person.

Most often our Power Person is a parent (though can be someone else). As we apply *Aramaic Forgiveness (removing our content)*, we crack open the path to noticing this pattern when it arises and releasing ourselves from it. This is often a generational pattern. The Ancient Aramaic word here is *"genare"* meaning "cause."

The Israelites wandered with Moses for forty years. Generations had to "die off for them to get out of the desert," did not mean the actual people had to die off. It meant their unconscious generational thought patterns had to go to get out of "wandering in the wasteland." They needed a "system upgrade." "Causes" had to die off.

What is at cause? Thought. When rage, fear and blame are *REMOVED* with this amazing work, we leave the desert for the "promised land," where the Active Presence of LOVE becomes the operating principle, calling forth our Creation from the *Field. Wow!*

POWER PERSON STRESS RESPONSE: When *stressed* we pattern behaviors around our Power Person Dynamic, like this:

1. **At *lowest stress level*,** we do what we did to *appease* our Power Person.
2. **As *stress level increases*,** we do what we did to *get back at* our Power Person.
3. When *stress is highest*, we do what our Power Person did *that we disliked most.*

A favorite saying identifies when this is going on: *When the Stress is Up and the Chips are Down - we act out our Power Person Dynamic.* (refer to 3 levels above)

YOUR POWER PERSON: Think about who your Power Person was/is, and what your 3 levels of responses are (can be helpful to write them down). We also may discover how we "act out," as someone else's Power Person, and draw in others who represent our Power Person. It's important to be aware of this as well.

Here is my (Cary's) example:

1. To appease my Power Person I became quiet and made myself small
2. To get back at my Power Person I left or threatened to leave
3. What I disliked most that my Power Person did, and have done in the past when my stress level was off the charts, is an explosion of disruptive and disrespectful words and energy directed at those I'm with (have only done this a few times in my Life)

Write down who your Power Person is/was, and your 3 stress responses. Breathe, Smile, and reflect on when/how this shows up or has shown up in your Life.

Our "reality" resonates into being from our thoughts and emotions, as do events that draw out our Power Person Dynamic stress response. This is a Mirroring of unconscious data to cancel, release and let go (most likely handed down from our generations). The Aramaic Forgiveness worksheet process are perfect tools to clear this content from our Being and restore our operating system to LOVE. Using the worksheet process daily helps identify these patterns as they arise to clear.

This extremely powerful information can reveal patterns we have defaulted to repeatedly. This offers a safe, insightful, productive context to get in touch with where debilitating reactive behaviors came from, and how to clear and shift them forever.

> There are two basic motivating forces: Fear and Love. When we are afraid, we pull back from Life. When we are in Love, we open to all that Life has to offer with passion, excitement, and acceptance. We need to learn to Love ourselves first, in all our glory and our imperfections. If we cannot Love ourselves, we cannot fully open to our ability to Love others or our potential to Create. Evolution and all hopes for a better world rest in the fearlessness and open-hearted vision of people who embrace Life.
>
> *John Lennon (1940-1980)*
> *Beatles, Singer, Songwriter, Activist*

PURPOSE OF STRESS: As the "soup-pot" of daily Life is stirred, all things that appear as stressors are actually Mirroring of *our unconscious content,* from the *Field* often tied in with our *"Power Person Dynamic."* It is not actually the outer situation causing our stress. Stress is caused by old stored blame-fear-hostility-judgment-control stored inside us. Sound familiar and *outrageous?* In the *pressure cooker* of stressful situations, our thought-emotional patterns need to be cleared. It is a Leap to grasp and embrace this, as we habitually think of stress as being caused by something or someone *outside of us*; a denial trick, to keep from having to go into our pain-blame-fear-hostility to remove the resonance in *us.*

Once we activate brain cells to comprehend that our "reality" is Created from our internal content, amazing shifts can take place. Once aware, we can actually *LAUGH* when our Power Person Dynamic shows up, release *OUR* content, thus deactivating our stress response, entering an exciting new level of *BEING!*

At the root of most stresses we find the Power Person Dynamic acting out. When stress is up, begin the questioning process. Am I acting out #1, #2, or #3 in relation to my Power Person Dynamic? Use a *Ancient Aramaic Forgiveness Freedom Tool* to cancel goals this stress brings up. Even something seemingly as positive as falling in Love or getting a New job can activate our Power Person Dynamic, making us want to fight, or run and hide.

As we delve more deeply into these patterns, we face and offload feelings of limitation held since childhood, causing us to feel *powerless*. As **21st Century Superhumans** we learn to move into courage and commitment to clear these uncomfortable layers, to access the magnificence of our True Design LOVE, expressing our *Essence* with clarity in the World.

Whatever we put Attention on and add energy to, we get (conscious-unconscious). How do you feel when meeting a schedule? Is there a Power Person Dynamic in the shadows that hasn't been addressed and cleared? Do you seek approval of an invisible parent or societal expectation? Have you lost who you are on the way to conformity or obedience? Even though this is a Power Person Dynamic, *"they"* are still Mirroring something inside of *you.*

> Argue for your limitations and sure enough they're yours.
>
> *Richard Bach, Illusions:*
> *Adventures of a Reluctant Messiah*

Clearing away layers of our "Power Person Dynamic," charges dissipate, and the person we have issues with may drift away from our World, or better yet we'll be around him/her and whatever they do will not affect us, *because we will be operating clearly from our True Design, LOVE.* Each of us who shifts this balance, changes our World.

This Evolutionary Leap, *Shift of the Ages,* activated by Cosmic Influences is opening us to a sense of Oneness. It is actually making it *easier* for us to let go all this old "stuff." *In fact, it's pushing us to let it go...*

ADDENDUM - ANCIENT ARAMAIC RESOURCES

What it takes to reformulate one's Life is monumental. Our work is about tools and community to facilitate this process. Join us and reap the joys of accelerated growth and well-being.

dr. michael and jeanie ryce

DR. MICHAEL AND JEANIE RYCE: support an emerging global community, who *share essential TRUE ARAMAIC FORGIVENESS around the World.* Dedication to getting this out to *every "mind, heart and being on the planet,"* has them traveling much of the year. Utilizing their tools and radio show daily, has *dramatically changed our lives.*

Access powerful resources Now at *www.whyagain.org*. *Resources and thought process here emerge from their teachings on the Aramaic for which we are so Grateful!*

Mindshifter Radio Show: DAILY call-in show, discussion. M-F 1-2 pm EST, phone 646-200-4169 or computer at www.whyagain.org (plus 300 archived shows) *Fantastic - interactive!!!*

Mindshifter Meetings: Check for one near you or start one in your area

Worksheets: Click *"Start, Here"* in upper left at whyagain.org download numerous versions of *FREE "Reality" Management Worksheets* in several languages. *Essential!!!*

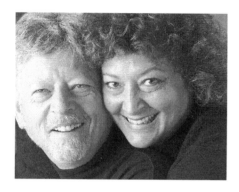

Travel & Workshops: Host dynamic and inspiring, michael and jeanie ryce in your community. Check their calendar for speaking and workshops. *Awesome!!!* Also 2 hour Video classes available at whyagain.org tremendous support for worksheet process.

Retreat Intensives: Immersion in these principles with raw foods, for major shifts, groups and teachers, around the World. DVDs / CDs (live streaming soon) all at whyagain.org.

Certification to Teach: Become certified; or work with someone who is certified

I looked in temples, churches and mosques,
but I found the Divine within my Heart.

Rumi (1207-1273) 13th Century Mystic

Focus. Breathe. Smile. Be Joyful in Your Life, as it Merges into the
Creative, Flowing, Radiant existence, for which You were Designed.

♥ ♥ ♥ LOVE ♥ ♥ ♥

Excellent Aramaic & Other Resources

WAY OF MASTERY with Jayem: After a "personal encounter" with Jeshua (Jesus) 25 years ago, Jayem dedicated his life to living and teaching Jeshua's teachings based on modern understanding of Ancient Aramaic. His online ashram and center in Bali offer excellent audio and video: *WayOfMastery dot com* book: *TheWayOfMastery dot com*

DALE ALLEN HOFFMAN: Dale discovered Ancient Aramaic through dr. michael ryce over 20 years ago, continuing to deepen his linguistic understanding, teaching accurate interpretation of the Ancient Aramaic. There are rumors of a documentary film, *Rakhma.* Dale does workshops, private sessions and is working on a book with excellent videos available on YouTube and *DaleAllenHoffman dot com*

EFT TAPPING: Though not Aramaic this is a great additional tool that supports clearing.

Part 2 Mind: Section 4
Wakeup Call Of The Heart

The heart in us is deeper than any emotion or psychological issue.

Krishna Das
Devotional Kirtan Chanting

We are living in such an amazing era! During the last 100 years there have been more "advancements" than in the last few thousand put together, planes, trains, automobiles, rockets to the moon, cell and computer systems and more. What we have proven we can do, accomplish and understand is almost beyond our wildest imaginings, and there is more to come! Our World exists in a myriad of contrasts... Yet we have barely begun to harness the most powerful device known to humankind: *the Heart.* ♥

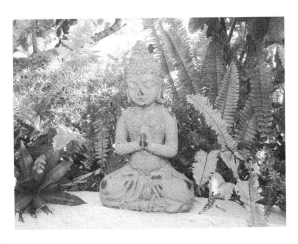

Our Planet has become smaller and smaller as our awakening becomes greater and greater, with surfacing inequities among humankind hovering on the brink of radical change. The obvious externalized materialistic culture that spawned corrupt governmental, religious and banking systems run by corporate greed rather than human need, is declining at a fast pace, with many nefarious, inharmonious enterprises facing dissolution Worldwide. The fact is, there really is more than enough on our dear Planet and among ALL of us, to provide food, shelter and comfort for ALL Mother Earth's citizens; yet:

Action Against Hunger reports 3.5 million children dying each year from starvation, staggering numbers in contrast with trillions spent on the war machine. Only 7-13% of the 34 million children afflicted with severe acute malnutrition receive life-saving treatment they need. Yet acute malnutrition is hunger we can "solve" with rightly allocated resources.

Time-Newsfeed March 2013, reported 6 billion people out of 7 billion planet-wide have access to mobile phones; in contrast 60% of global population lack access to basic sanitation. Of India's 1.2 billion residents half are mobile subscribers, yet only 1/3 of India's population has access to toilets (2010 UN report).

As a result of corporate global central bank policies, the rich have been getting richer and poor have been getting poorer; wages fall behind inflation, savings are sinking and social mobility is at an all-time low. There hasn't been such a great gap between the top 1% and everyone else since the roaring twenties.

World Bank estimates 125 million children in poor countries do not attend school (one in every five children). Rather than taking care of this, they fund wars.

An inspired private organization, FreetheChildren.com collects "the price of a cup of coffee a day" to build a school with just 33 contributors; this is an example of a young visionary taking action after looking into the eyes of a child in Africa.

60% college grads can't find work, while paying off outrageous college debt with exorbitant interest.

"Most of us" likely had enough money to buy groceries last week, while 870 million of 7.1 billion in the world or one in eight, suffer chronic undernourishment. 3/4 in underdeveloped countries; 1 in 5 children go to bed hungry every night.

There is enough wealth on Earth that no one needs to go hungry, be sick or go without good drinking water or sanitation, no one needs to have anywhere near the amount of misery we have. $223 Trillion in global wealth, held by the very few, is managed through depraved corporate structures, governments and banking systems run by trusts that should be public trusts for the benefit of the people, yet instead are privately held. In wars there are no winners; the nefarious World Bank system finances war on both sides.

Of all the enemies to public liberty war is, perhaps, the most to be dreaded because it comprises and develops the germ of every other. War is the parent of armies; from these proceed debts and taxes ... known instruments for bringing the many under the domination of the few.... No nation could preserve its freedom in the midst of continual warfare.

— *James Madison, Political Observations 1795*
Fourth US President, Father of the US Constitution and Champion of US Bill of Rights

Even with tanking economies, bank bail-outs and U.S. job loss, defense budgets grow. U.S. military spending has increased 114% to $682 billion, according to *Stockholm International Peace Research Institute, who reports that World military spending totaled $1.75 trillion in 2012,* lead by the U.S. though China and Russia are not far behind. *Business Insider* Oct. 2011 reports, *"Facts About Military Spending that Will Blow Your Mind:"*

1. America spends more on military than the next 15 countries combined

2. The Pentagon spends more on war than all 50 states combined spend on health, education, welfare, and safety

3. Total known land area occupied by U.S. bases and facilities is 15,654 square miles -- bigger than Washington D.C., MA and NJ combined

4. Money 'wasted' or 'lost' in Iraq $11 billion = 220,000 teachers salaries

5. Defense spending is higher today than any time since height of World War II

6. US defense spending *doubled* while the economy *shrunk* by 1/3

7. Yearly cost of stationing one soldier in Iraq, would have fed 60 American families.

8. One day in Afghanistan cost more than it did to build the entire Pentagon

9. More money was spent every five seconds in Iraq than the average American earned in a year

10. The Pentagon budget consumes 80% of individual income tax revenue

11. Compensating radiation victims of nuclear testing could fully educate 13,000 U.S. children ($1.5 billion)

IS SOMETHING NOT RIGHT WITH THIS PICTURE? YES! And we are in the midst of a Giant Wake-Up Call! The only reason any human being is still suffering on Planet Earth is because we've been asleep. We hadn't *NOTICED* ill-conceived banking, governmental, economic and religious systems were running things without consideration of Good for ALL. Rather than *NOTICE* we are ALL One, we thought we were *separate,* and it was "them out there," *someone else's fault. Well,* as the Dylan song goes, *"The times they are a' changin'..."*

Now that we're waking up, how are we changing all this? One thought at a time. We are Creator-Beings. Our thoughts are magnetic, they Create instantly, and they return energy in Like kind. Beyond karma and punishment, we are simply Living in the "reality" thoughts have Created. The *matrix* can only return that which we give it. *This is how we change it!*

- *Firstly,* we remove from ourselves ALL (conscious-unconscious) thought, containing blame-fear-hostility-judgment-control and restore our True Design LOVE. ♥
- *Secondly,* we enter into Living from the Heart and from *Essence.* ♥
- *Thirdly,* we follow the **Golden Rule:** *Do unto others as you would have others do unto you.* This means everyone. How simple is that? Breathe and Smile. ♥

Sound familiar? Activated by Light photons in the Cosmos and Ascending waves of consciousness, what we may not have paid Attention to before is Now becoming blatantly obvious. Our Global community has reached a "dull roar" about ALL that is bearing down upon us, from dangers of GMOs to chemtrails, vaccinations, pesticides, hunger and starvation to poor education and more. Everything around us is screaming and whispering, "Wake up!" "Pay Attention!" "Notice your Thoughts, Heart and Actions." "They Matter."

Creative Minds are coming up with New innovative systems beneficial to ALL. Perhaps we're ready for a Planetary governing body represented by all countries, effecting Global harmonization and care? The more who "step out of the matrix," and apply their brilliance and creativity to solutions, the more exponentially Global change accelerates.

When we're true to ourselves we manifest a reality that is true to us. Our attachments don't fulfill us. When we take that step to be true to ourselves, live our dreams and commit to our passions, it's really a true story when you actually do it...

Laura Eisenhower, Awake in the Dream Radio

An amazing thing is happening. People are stepping forward by hundreds of thousands around the World Now, deeply concerned about these issues, their own Lives and their Global family. Somehow we are awakening from a deep, dark slumber, where we forgot who we were, why we're here and where we'er going. We allowed ourselves to be enslaved by corporate ignorance, false and abusive greed-based monetary systems, puppet governments and religious systems oppressive to the human spirit. *Shift ourselves, shift the entire Hologram.*

Global tribunals now expose crimes agains humanity so horrendous we will not even list them here and such corruption in governments and banking systems that only shadows will soon remain. We are Now clearing these from all timelines and removing them from our thoughts forever. Rather, let us imagine towns and cities rebuilt with organic gardens growing more delicious food naturally everywhere than can even be consumed; laughter fills the air from happy beautiful children of all colors around the World, as they play and innovate, knowing their thoughts Create. ALL are blessed with plenty, safety and joy.

Let us imagine letting go of 40 hour weeks at things that drain our souls, instead Free clean energy around the World, and happy people express creativity and Life-force through joyful endeavors for good of ALL. Power of the Heart, once aligned with our True Design LOVE is invincible, bringing about real and lasting change...

Accessing the *Field* more intimately, we broaden our connection to the possible. Like Emoto's water crystals, with right focus the structure of matter changes instantly! As we interact with matter on subtle levels, restructuring takes place beyond the electromagnetic *Field,* not yet measurable with current instrumentation. Within us is capacity of "Divine" Creatorship. Whatever we've been through, whatever genetic data we carry, whatever journeys we've experienced, whatever history is mapped in our neurobiology, it is shifting Now, as we enter this Evolutionary Leap called the *Shift Of The Ages,* with LOVE.

> It doesn't matter whether I LOVE you with my eyes open,
> or my eyes closed...what matters is that I LOVE you.
>
> *Jack White (1934-1998)*
> *God's Game of Life*

21st Century Superhumans are emerging into New Lives as Creator-Beings, releasing from the unconscious that which no longer serves. It is our Gift to access the *Field* to Create New "realities" of LOVE. This journey of Awaken-ing or En-Lightenment is about restoring our True Design, where all DNA codons are turned on, aligned with our own Sacred Core.

Catching this wave of change calls for each of us to step into Greater Truth of our own Being, releasing ALL misalignments, to discover and Live as True Self. Unwinding in this Ever Present Now, we invite LOVE to pour forth into our World through us.

We *Arc the Hologram* as we shift ourselves into LOVE, transforming ALL that has occurred throughout spacetime, restoring higher Vibrational Earth frequencies to a harmonious New Earth and resonating well-being, joy and abundance for ALL. ♥

Chapter 15

Brain And Heart Team Up

When a certain number of people come together and choose at a moment in time to Create a precise emotion in their hearts, that emotion literally can intentionally influence the very Fields that sustain Life on planet earth.

Gregg Braden
The Divine Matrix

There is good reason to get to know brain and Heart better. *Every thought* sends electromagnetic waves from the Heart, with measurable effect upon the World in which we Live! This is a powerful reason to cognitively focus upon what thought-emotional energy we desire to send our, for each person's Heart Vibration resonates profoundly in our World!

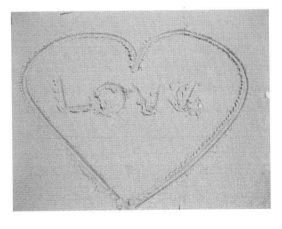

The Human Heart is now documented as the strongest generator of both electrical and magnetic fields in the body. This is important, because we've always been taught that the brain is where the action is. The brain has an electric and magnetic field, but they are relatively weak compared to the heart. The heart is about 100 times stronger electrically, and 5,000 times stronger magnetically than the brain.

The reason this is important is because the physical world as we know it is made up of these two fields of energy, electrical and magnetic. Our own physics books now tell us, if we can change either the magnetic field of an atom or the electrical field of the atom, by doing so we literally change that atom; we change the stuff that our bodies and this world are made of.

And it appears now that the human heart is designed to do both; to change both the electrical field and the magnetic field of our bodies and our world, and they do so in response to the emotions we Create between our heart and our brain.

Gregg Braden
The Role of the Heart in the Law of Attraction

The Heart is electromagnetically more powerful than the brain, has a stronger role in decision-making and highly influences our state of Being. In fact the Heart gives the brain more instructions than the brain gives the Heart; and it is a powerful "sending device!"

Our Heart Coherence or harmony has a significant effect on higher cognitive, perception and memory... Across many Ancient Traditions, the Heart was considered the center of the being, a source of connection to the Divine.

Spirit Science 15
The Power of the Heart

The Heart also has direct neurological links with right brain's creative power and ability. Right brain and Heart link to pituitary and pineal glands, creating a two-way electromagnetic antenna for sending and receiving LOVE! The Heart is our *"gateway to the Divine,"* so when we focus through the Heart, it positively affects us and All Life.

Every thought we think Creates a molecule called a Neuropeptide
that connects to a cell receptor site and manifests as our reality.

Dr. Candace Pert
Molecules of Emotion

Thoughts Vibrate energy into form. They also naturally transmit to people and animals, especially those with whom we're closest where we develop awareness of how our telepathic signals affect and are received by others. Fine-tuning intuition and telepathy, we strengthen right brain and heighten flow between Heart and Greater Mind. ALL such exercises elevate our ability to participate in Conscious Creation.

The meaning of a human's Life is evolution of consciousness. We are solely responsible for everything we think, feel, do and undertake. We must be responsible for it. We must bear and savor positive-negative, processed through thoughts, actions and feelings. Everyone must use their connection with creation.

Billy Meier
Swiss Pleiadian UFO Contactee

Our brain is our filter for Greater Mind, which encompasses ALL. The left brain is a powerful driving force in our culture and unless used in harmony with right brain can limit us. It likes straight lines, theoretical factual survival ideas; it makes dualistic comparisons: right-wrong, good-bad, should I? shouldn't I? ...deciding, wondering, problem solving, outside creative right brain flexibility. Left brain Masculine energy accomplishes a great deal in the material World, awesome for many jobs, yet when dominant, it has "run over" the World in an imbalanced way. Masculine and Feminine, left and right brain blend to Create perfection.

Left brain is most effective when left and right brain work together. Feminine right brain encompasses global, artistic, creative, flowing capacities. We are coming out of a period of Masculine left brain dominance on Planet Earth, Now playing itself out with collapsing systems. Masculine is moving toward blending with the Feminine, in this *Shift of the Ages*. Reintegrating Feminine qualities will bring our World into a beautiful balance unknown for thousands of years. Both men and women will discover this balance within self and collaboratively with one another, optimizing our pure potential. The Feminine right brain encompasses our capability to behave in a Quantum manner, integrated with left brain much is accomplished.

Excellent results occur when left brain activates structure and movement, learning to focus, holding image of a result, and *releasing it* to the right brain to offer its flowing creative process to the *Field*, beyond what the left can even imagine. This optimizes left brain, to manage and organize tasks, then "dance" with right brain's creative capacity.

> The Collapse of the Wave Function - I have come to realize the right brain can perform a weak collapse of the wave function. Free from the need to organize things into spatial dimensions and make sense of them, the right brain has direct access to the Quantum process.
>
> *Dr. Richard Bartlett*
> *Matrix Energetics*

Moments of genius occur when left and right brain communicate at lightening speed through *corpus callosum* (at center of brain), and *"whole brain" function* is activated. Left and right hemispheres meld and engage through the Heart. We best access this flow of interactive, higher brain function, where greatest talents and Creations reside, when we are rooted in *Heart Coherence,* coming from being in states of *LOVE, Compassion and Gratitude.*

Left brain likes to be busy in quick Beta mode, so let it make a list or run like a wild horse; teach it to let go of obsessing, otherwise it holds in Creation what it doesn't want (Quantum Observer). Right brain likes slower deep Alpha-Theta frequencies. She gently entices Left brain to join her - and when he does, the sparks fly! In the flow between left and right hemispheres and Heart, we open two way communication with the Universe.

GOAL CANCELING BEFORE SLEEP: Quiet left brain's stressing by resetting your Divine creative process. Just before going to sleep open mouth for open mouthed breathing - to release any holding patterns in the body. Express to yourself internally:

- "I now invite *Rookha d'Koodsha*, Cosmic super processor and state of Being, to help cancel and clear all my goals, conscious, unconscious, subconscious and incomplete."

    ✦This dismantles some of the old "corrupt data" that has been running the show.

- Next, "I reset my *Rakhma* and *Khooba* filters for intentions and perceptions of LOVE (Breathing, Smiling)." "I give all to the *Field* to be taken care of in Amazing ways."

    ✦Use image in chapter "Meditation and Inner Stillness" to visualize dropping down through brain wave frequencies, releasing all to go out of from into the *Field* to be reborn anew in LOVE.

Cultivate capacity to design your Life by putting Attention where you choose rather than defaulting to old programs. *Marry Mind and Heart:*

Left Brain: (fret fret) "How am I going to get that done?" (Breathe, smile, relax)

Left Brain: Envision it done perfectly, in all its sensory perfection (for 17 seconds or so)! Pass it on to the *Field* and right brain.

Right Brain: Gently release left brain's detailed vision to the *Field*, trusting it will come back better than it left! Experience it done.

Heart: Through my radiance I experience and KNOW this as already done. *"mud between the toes" "smell raindrops on the sunflowers"*

The Field: Wow, I Am getting a beautiful resonance coming from this *Heart:* I'll pass these ripples out through all Creation and bring back a wonderful reply.

LEFT BRAIN and RIGHT BRAIN "DANCE:" After several thousand years of obscured Feminine, and over-amped Masculine, are we ready to discover how these two fabulous energies, combine, blend and "dance?" The two wild positive-negative charges we call Masculine and Feminine, weave together ALL of Creation. Masculine based left brain Creates structure and movement, sweet Feminine right brain "holds the *Field*." Alone they do alright, together they rock! (Scenario in our example below can easily be replaced with any situation).

EXAMPLE - CREATE THE LIFE YOU DESIRE: You and your husband, wife, partner, friend, are working in a faraway city. Both of you would like to move and live closer to "home and family," but the only place you've been able to get jobs is far away. Like a dog worrying a bone, you've thought: "I don't like my job, I don't like this place, (though some things may be interesting), I have a few friends but not like the ones back home, I miss my family, what am I gonna do?..." Breathe, Smile and let go all the obsession-based thinking.

Let's follow our left to right brain approach to get better results in this situation and help this young couple get home to their family. Such a desire can be called in quickly! Retrain Left and Right Brain to "dance" - use this model in any situation for Great Results!

1. *Breathe and Smile... Come on now, really Breathe and Smile...*

2. Optimally we use our worksheets. For now, just do this exercise: (write it down)

> A. Put your "positive desire" statement at top *AS IF IT ALREADY IS*. Example: My husband and I have found great jobs and are moving or Live close to my family.

> B. List of all fears-doubt thoughts-emotions about this situation (*your "garbage"*). List your thought or emotion "Not of LOVE" inherited or learned from our blame-fear-hostility culture Go ahead make your list. (ex: "I don't like my job, I don't like it here, I have a few friends but not like the ones back home, I miss my family...")

C. *NOTE:* The reason we are doing this is so these thoughts-emotions do not continue holding resonance from the unconscious. You might think, "We're focusing on the negative." It's more that we're collecting *garbage* from the unconscious and putting it in a garbage bag to remove it!

3. Now, let's give the left brain something constructive to work on in such a way that you get results! Rather than fretting, worrying and wishing, instead envision yourself near family. You and your husband-wife-partner-friend each have landed your dream jobs! Imagine the home you live in, having dinner on Saturday or Sunday with family and familiar friends. Imagine Being with siblings more often and what this is like. Feel the New generations of kids, nieces, nephews, and grandkids bringing joy and laughter into your Life, and the elders with their kind, sage Wisdom. Make your images sensory and emotionally rich, just as if you are there in your perfect "reality!"

4. Now instruct left brain to give these creative images and feelings to right brain. Then ask creative right brain to wrap her arms around them and give them to the *Field*, where ALL matter and events await in potential for Attention to call them into form.

5. Let the right brain send your images through the Heart (to which it is intrinsically connected) then to the *Field. Breathe and Smile.* Trust that the *Field of Infinite Possibilities* has a thousand ways to respond, beyond what we can imagine. Trust the *Field* to bring what's perfect into form. Say, "Thank you! Breathe and Smile...

6. REPEAT: Whenever thoughts or feelings come up about your situation, notice what thoughts are based in "Not of LOVE." (Use *Aramaic Forgiveness Tool* goal canceling worksheets). Let garbage thoughts float away like blowing bubbles on a summer day.

7. REPEAT: Tune in your best, most beautiful images, sounds and feelings of your desired reality as it's *"already happening,"* give it to the *Field.* Breathe, Smile, Relax. Go on with your Life and trust the *Field.*

8. CONTINUE TO REPEAT the process when thoughts come up. Train left and right brain to handle things in this new way, embracing Quantum potentials of the *Field*, releasing the "old dog and bone" left brain fretting from the old paradigm.

9. When this subject arises in conversation, thought, word, mind or Heart, notice it "already is" ***"mud between the toes."*** As you shift your left-right brain mechanism to operate differently, amazing things are happening! Trust. Breathe. Smile.

10. *Breathe and Smile*...and as progressive Quantum physicist Nassim Haramein says, "May the vacuum (*the Field of Infinite Possibilities, the Matrix, the Plenum*) be with you!"

Quantum Measurement - The Quantum wave function describes infinite probabilities before you chose one reality or outcome, and collapses all other possibilities into the thing you have chosen.

Dr. Richard Bartlett,
Matrix Energetics

FORMULA: Clear unconscious content. Meditate daily to improve EEG brain coherence, to implement full brain function and to deepen access to the *Field*. Deep LOVE, Compassion and Gratitude bring Heart Coherence. Marry Mind-Heart to integrate Left-Right Brain function. Enjoy continual new emergence from the *Field*.

> Empty space is not empty at all! The vacuum is actually a plenum. It contains an abundant amount of energy, the zero point energy. There is a cosmic dance of energy back and forth between the physical realm and the zero point field, a constant creation and destruction of matter from the void... Could it be that what scientists call zero point energy is in fact our own collective consciousness and that we are creating the physical world from this energy?

Ralph Ring
bluestarenterprise.com

Evidence points to the Heart being more "navigator" than the brain. The Heart, 60% neurons, is constantly broadcasting information to Body and brain. The Heart is directly connected with the emotional body through the limbic system and right brain, from which creative flow drops directly into the Heart for our "Creation" to go out into the World. Feel yourself flowing energetically through the Heart. *How cool is that???*

> Notice What You Notice. We are patterns of light and information manifested into matter. As light and information, we have direct access to all infinite information that is available to the Universe.

Melissa Joy Jonsson
Matrix Energetics

As we evolve in this process, Masculine left brain learns to relax, becoming more playful and less driven, blending with Feminine right brain and Heart. Deepening our experience of consciously creating, we rediscover laughter and let go worry to be more Lighthearted and joyful. Life emerges in synchronicities, and miraculous events begin to appear in our "reality."

> I no longer live in the current moment, I live in the current...

Gary Clark Eco-Art
www.facebook.com/garyclarkart

We are currently speeding up Vibrationally, facilitated by movement into the Heart and restoring our True Design LOVE. Our *essential inner process in this Now* as **21st Century Superhumans,** is to move into the Heart, to Live from creative intuitive knowingness expressing our *Essence* and bringing our Gifts into the World. ♥

Part 2: MIND

Chapter 16

Success with Heart Coherence

----------------- ❤ -----------------

I think we're at a point in history as a country and a civilization where the consequences of inaction are far more serious than consequences of taking action for shifting the path we're on.

Tim DeChristopher
Peaceful Uprising

When was the last time you laughed out loud or gave or received a big hug,? Have you walked in the rain or sat under a tree just because you could? Are you Living your True Design, rejoicing with friends? Living LOVE is the answer to ALL. It connects us with *Essence* from which we emerge more refined each moment.

Anything Not of LOVE is part of the *illusion* from which we are Now unwinding. Habitual disintegrative thought patterns of the blame-fear-hostility culture are "loosening." Create a New future "reality" Now, by canceling, releasing and letting go ALL Not of LOVE thought!

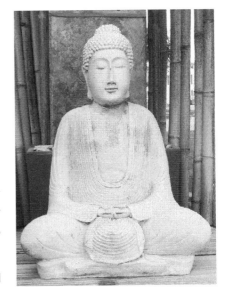

Change your thoughts and your "reality" will change, not the other way around.

In the old way of thinking it can *seem like* changing our thoughts is difficult. Yet it's not, it's a matter of CHOICE to let go rather than carrying around the old anymore. Our *Ancient Aramaic Forgiveness Tools,* worksheets for clearing the unconscious are awesome. Once the process is learned it becomes an automatic internal system for clearing as anything comes up. Canceling to clear old shadows establishes a "clean slate" for our Attention on the *Field.* Flowing into this New connected state of Being, we discover the way is clear to LOVE.

Our New Awareness cultivates New "realities," aligning us with New Planetary energies and accelerating frequencies of Ascension. Living authentically in Heart is the New "En-Lightenment" that changes everything. Moving into Heart, accesses pure connection with *Creator-Source*. Natural Inner-sense and the miracle of authentic Self-expression, play a vital role for **21st Century Superhumans** actualizing a New Now. YOUR unique, Heart-centered presence is *Essential* to the Whole.

SELF-MASTERY ALCHEMY 101: NOTICE thought patterns (conscious-unconscious) making up your Attention. NOTICE how you are using your Mind-energy (conscious-unconscious), based on your resulting "reality." NOTICE residual blame-fear-hostility patterns still resonating and clear them! Cancel goals with *Ancient Aramaic Freedom Tools*. Commit to 3-5 worksheets per day. Open Breath. Follow through to keep shifting internally. Integrate **Quantum Lifestyle** habits *Part 4: BODY* to clear and elevate at cellular level. Manifest your True Nature through the Heart.

NOTE: Greek translation of "Forgiveness," as God or someone "letting us off the hook" was never accurate. *True Aramaic Forgiveness meant to remove from ourselves that which we or our generations engaged in that removed us from LOVE.* Doing this personal work of goal canceling and clearing our old data is the Only Path to going beyond disease, poverty and even death. This is a Quantum act. Shifting our Attention on the *Field* by changing our internal content opens us up to move into Oneness, changing our entire "reality."

> ...there is a discussion of two types of defilement, disturbing emotions that cloud the mind, and their imprints which act as obstructions to knowledge and...our achievement of omniscience.
>
> *His Holiness the 14th Dalai Lama*

It may be awkward at first to let go the pull of society's "ego rewards," clamoring for our Attention, yet when we respond to the Truth of our *Essence*, expressing through the Heart, our Greatest Gifts flow forth for real "success." Clearing Ancient pain of disconnect from self and accumulated "baggage" of long ago, we purify and step into Mastery that brings forth Radiance of our True Being, "surrendering" to Authenticity, which moves us into higher frequencies known as En-Light-enment.

> ...waiting is a God-guided action, one with as much power as a decision... Waiting is often necessary to get what we want. It is not dead time; it is not downtime. The answer will come. The power will come. The time will come. And it will be right.
>
> *Melody Beattie*
> *The Language of Letting Go*

Use creative right brain to drop into the Heart and flow with, into and through unlimited Abundance from the *Field*. Experience your Life unfolding naturally in New ways when so aligned. Play with your visions, concepts and ideas, letting them go into the *Field*. As we Trust and Allow for this kind of Creation, we activate New DNA codons. Holding Attention on the *Field* in this New way is a powerful skill in our toolbox, accessing Heart as Primordial Observer, knowing LOVE'S *KNOWING*. Offer Heart's Creation with clear Mind-Heart-Vision to the Universe, *and then see what happens!*

Quantum Measurement - Weigh things in the direction of fun, altered states of consciousness and all possibility. This activity shifts the probability that something can actually change.

Dr. Richard Bartlett, Matrix Energetics

It may take tricking yourself a bit to figure out ways to "drop into the Heart." Melissa Joy from Matrix Energetics says, "Let your eyeballs fall out of your head, and drop down into your Heart." This is a playful experience to get out of the head, so Heart can take over. Try her way, then experiment until you find your own ways to drop into the Heart. Breathe, Smile and strengthen this New alignment that you will get to know and use often.

WE ALL HAVE GENIUS CAPABILITY. WE ALL HAVE ACCESS TO ALL. Think of the brain as your filter system, determining how much Greater Mind is allowed to come through. ALL that limits our access to Greater Mind is the brain's finite filter system, qualified by unconscious data, generational and societal conditioning. Is your thought taking you deeper into Greater Mind and Conscious Creation through the Heart, or keeping you limited in blame-fear-hostility? The brain "thinks it knows," yet when we let go of our old data and access through the Heart, we enter a New paradigm, dimensions of Greater Mind, Oneness and Our own Brilliance!

Space, time, matter, energy and biological life may be the result of a Source Field that is conscious and alive in its own unique way - on a scale far too vast for the finite mind to fathom.

David Wilcock
Source Field Investigations

Slow down, take a deep Breath and Smile. Go into the Heart, allow answers to come from where wholeness and Oneness reside, where Divine Masculine and Feminine merge, activating En-Light-enment. By so doing, we step into alignment with Oneness, through which we offer our greatest contribution of *Essence* to those we Love and to the World. It is said, "Many yet unborn will benefit from what we now do."

INTUITION - THE HEART KNOWS THAT IT KNOWS: Our intuition is like wi-fi, constantly receiving in-formation from the *Field* and Greater Mind. Experiencing the World intuitionally is some of the most important in-formation we ever access, though it has not been honored culturally in the modern World, and often requires deepening of Awareness to recognize what is coming to us. Our intuition comes through any of the senses and can just be a gentle quiet thought in the Mind. Learn to *NOTICE* and acknowledge your own signals when receiving intuitive information, from Mind beyond filters, through Heart.

Go into your Heart. Be Heart-present with others and your surroundings. Programmed by cultural "norms," it can be a bit uncomfortable at first to think of entering Heart Space with anyone. Let go of fear, dis-comfort or expectation, knowing you are ONE with ALL.

Smile at others. Open doors for them. Say, "Isn't it a nice day?" Breathe. Smile. Be in the Heart. You will be amazed at how open and supportive others become in your Presence.

The secret of attraction is to LOVE yourself. Attractive people judge neither themselves nor others. They are open to gestures of LOVE. They think about LOVE, and express their LOVE in every action. They know that LOVE is not a mere sentiment, but the ultimate truth at the heart of the Universe.

Deepak Chopra MD
New Thought Author, Natural Physician

A Tibetan Monk chanting "Om" and Mother Theresa caring for the poor with no thought of self are examples of "relating from the Heart." Take special moments in your life to be Heart-centered. Experiment. Play with it. Explore. Have fun. Be the radiant Being You Are. Breathe and Smile. Know that by this simple act You Are changing human civilization. *Arc the Hologram Now with LOVE! Breathe. Smile.*

Our greatest adventure is this inward journey, taking Response-Ability for how the *Field* is manifesting around us by refining our inner Vibration. This is an entirely new way to Be in Our World, focusing and shaping our internal Heart environment, so Life emerges by choice rather than by default. Everything dissolves into the Active Presence of LOVE, which is becoming our "normal" state of Being, where we rediscover Passion and Joy. True passion arises Voice, Vision and Feeling of the Heart, more available once we learn to heed our intuition and *Essence*. When we're in alignment with *Essence* and the *Heart* we manifest easily, as p*assion is the driving force of manifestation.*

The old system of thinking and belief is Now transforming. New thought processes through Heart, activates DNA codes and brings us into alignment with Higher Mind. We are magnificent Beings, capable of Innate Conscious Creation. We are awakening to real Truth, as we choose our "reality" by moving Conscious thought into form.

Your vision will become clear only when you look into your heart.
Who looks outside, dreams. Who looks inside, awakens.

Carl Jung (1875-1961)
founder analytical psychology

Living from the Heart our World transforms, and we relax into a New state of Unity, in "peace that passes understanding." Great Masters taught that tuning in to Heart we merge with the river of Self that is ONE, for *within our Heart is the most Sacred Place of All...*

We are co-creating this change as it comes into being...on a personal level, you have a choice. You can...believe that Life is out to get you and things really suck right now. Or, you can realize that we are on the threshold of the most spectacular, mass spiritual awakening in human history. You make the choice every day -- every moment. When you feel LOVE, peace, acceptance and forgiveness of others, you are part of the solution....

David Wilcock, Divine Cosmos dot com

248

Living from the Heart we are Initiators of the most Powerful shift in human history:

It's about time we begin it, to turn the world around

It's about time we start to make it, the dream we've always known

It's about time we start to live it, the family of man

It's about time, it's about changes and it's about time

John Denver, It's About Time

Gregg Braden reminds us that to to heal our bodies and Create peace, we must speak to the *Field* that connects all things, using the non-verbal language that communicates with "the stuff of which this World is made." As we Create Heart Coherence in our lives, becoming more cooperative, less aggressive, more willing to solve problems together, that experience is transmitted through the *Field*. Others are drawn to shift their resonance through entrainment, because we're all connected in the *Field*. It's like tossing a pebble into a pond. The ripples go out and merges with others, creating a New pattern, as we *Arc the Hologram with LOVE. Now shifting ourselves, the entire Hologram shifts!*

HeartMath Institute

HeartMath® bridges science and spirituality with research related to the Heart, that setting New standards for business and individuals. Their studies demonstrate how powerful the Heart is as our Body-Mind's *central operating system*. It's no surprise that they demonstrate a harmonious, rhythmically functioning Heart makes us happier and healthier, with better performance on ALL levels.

HEART COHERENCE: *HearthMath® made the profound discovery (no surprise), **that Heart functions most Coherently when we focus in thoughts and emotions of Deep LOVE, Care-Compassion and Sincere Appreciation-Gratitude.** As we learned from Gregg Braden's enquiry of the Tibetan monk, he knew entering a state of Compassion without judgment was *essential for his prayers to be effective,* which put him in perfect **Heart Coherence.**

Below is part of an interview with HeartMath®'s co-founder Howard Martin, key spokesperson and accomplished musician. He co-produced Founder, Doc Childre's award-winning recording, *Heart Zones,* which ranked on Billboard for fifty consecutive weeks.

I believe that the heart is the *entry point of spirit into matter*. But let's start with empirical knowledge. For me, the subject begins with the fact that the heart is an autorhythmic organ.

Saying the heart is autorhythmic means that the source of the heartbeat actually resides within the heart itself. The heart has its own intelligence. You see this clearly reflected in the heart transplant patient, where the beating heart is removed from the donor, and it's still beating and continues to beat during the transplantation process. Nerves cannot be reconnected between the brain and the heart, but the Newly transplanted heart keeps on beating.

In a healthy person, signals from the brain regulate the timing of the heartbeat. The capacity to slow down and speed up is not present in the heart. That's why heart transplant patients need PaceMakers.

But the heart beats on its own. In fetal development, the heart forms first. It begins beating before we even have a physical brain. For me, the implication is that when Life itself begins, it is because something triggers in the heart. There is an integration of spirit and humanness, and the heart begins beating.

So right off the bat, from a biological perspective, we have this organ that starts to beat — nobody knows why — and continues to beat, even without the brain. Again, it has its own intelligence... Even at the biological level, this innate intelligence manifests within the heart.

Susan Barber interview with Howard Martin
When LOVE Is Not An Emotion, Spirit of Ma'at

The Heart is keyed to our emotional state, where harmonious patterns emerge from a calm, balanced state of Being. On the other hand, when the Heart is stressed it becomes incoherent, diminishing creative ability and intelligence. *21st Century Superhuman, Quantum Lifestyle* tools and habits lead to Greater Heart Coherence. Learning to stay in Heart Coherence is beneficial as Heart handles much communication within Body systems.

1. Communication between Heart and brain links emotions and creative thinking

2. Heart signals the Body through the blood pressure, synchronous with brain

3. In 1983 the Heart was reclassified as a hormonal gland, as it reduces the stress hormone cortisol and produces the LOVE hormone oxytocin

4. The Heart's bio-electricity permeates every cell in the body, producing 40-60 times as much electricity as the brain.

In uterus, first formed are 8 cells, basis of the Flower of Life from Sacred Geometry, core energetic pattern of Creation. In the midst of a torus field *on day 21 the Heart begins to beat*. Heart's electrical field is so strong it can measure eight feet from the body. Its torus-like field surrounds us in a 360 degree sphere. Many Quantum physicists believe all Creation is torus *Fields* within torus *Fields*, an energy form that promises to bring us clean free unlimited energy. This is the powerful energetic pattern through which our Heart's messages are transmitted to the World around us.

When I speak to this electromagnetic energy coming from the heart, by the way, I'm not speaking about subtle energy, like an aura. I'm talking about a dense level of electromagnetic frequencies. It's really there. It's scientific fact.

Howard Martin
Executive Vice-President, Co-Founder HeartMath Institute

HeartMath's cutting edge technology measures "heart-rate variability" (HRV). Strong negative emotions Create incoherent Heart frequencies, appearing as jagged patterns, similar to Emoto's images of water crystals with irregular shapes from "negative" thought or emotion.

When LOVE, Gratitude, Compassion and other positive thought is held, beautifully formed patterns take shape mapping the Heart's energy field. *A brilliant, Coherent spectrum of harmonious frequencies, occurs in the Heart when we hold positive emotions.*

Most powerful Heart Coherent Emotions are:

☑ DEEP OR UNIVERSAL LOVE
☑ CARE OR COMPASSION
☑ SINCERE APPRECIATION OR GRATITUDE

Let's put on an imaginary Tibetan "monk's robe," Breathing and Smiling, entering into Deep LOVE, Compassion and Gratitude, we traverse our World in Heart Coherence, holding Vibration for highest levels of health, well-being, radiance and abundance for ALL. *Heart Coherence is the primary task before us as* **21st Century Superhumans!** We broadcast information to every cell in our body and to every corner of our World. As we transmit thoughts-feelings through the electrical field of the Heart, Creation of our "reality" is born.

HeartMath's research shows that intuition is more activated when we're in Heart Coherence and our intuition is more effective when viewing the "bigger picture." Positive emotions produce DHEA, "youth" hormones. Very insightful, studies also show that *five minutes of anger suppresses immune factors for 6 hours!* **This is the best reason ever to get rid of, cancel, release, let go ALL our "old data!"**

As we enter an expanded state, where Living in the Heart in LOVE becomes our way of Life, an entirely New wave of human civilization is born. Reborn in Universal LOVE, we Now exponentially expand our capabilities of Heart-centered Intelligence and deep Universal Wisdom.

I believe that the Heart represents the entryway into a completely new intelligence that defies traditional, logical, linear thinking. It represents a complete dimensional shift in planetary awareness.

Howard Martin
Co-Founder HeartMath®

This is LOVE in a New Octave. It accelerates our Evolutionary Journey, harmonizing with Cosmic influences now waking up our brain, pineal gland and DNA. Moving into higher frequency 4th and 5th dimensional Heart awareness, we expand our capability to embrace and enjoy Life, empowering personal and Universal experiences of *Higher LOVE -*

Think about it, there must be Higher LOVE. Down in the Heart or hidden in the stars above. Without it, Life is wasted time. Look inside your Heart, I'll look inside mine...Bring me a Higher LOVE...

Steve Winwood
"Higher Love" Lyrics

Institute of HeartMath offers a personal device, a finger sensor for computer, iPhone or iPad to develop Heart Coherence in 5-30 minutes a day. Heart-centered awareness supports practical effective transcendence of old thought-emotional patterns, and enhances Living with greater balance and well-being. Heart Coherence is also foundational to sustainable shifts into a more focused expanded, creative state as 4th-5th dimensional Beings.

Ancient wisdom teaches it. History of prayer teaches it. Yeshua-Jesus, Buddha, Gandhi, Mother Theresa, St. Francis and Masters throughout the ages taught or teach it. Quantum Physics demonstrates it. Simply put, LOVE is the True Design of our Being. We cultivate it by clearing Mind and Heart of any "logjams in the river," to operate our system with Heart Coherence through LOVE, Compassion and Gratitude. Deepening Living from the Heart is how we shape a New and Viable Future.

We are Observer-Creators simply by our Presence in this World and its Attention on the *Field*. Centering in LOVE expresses resonance through the Heart, to call in "realities" based in LOVE. This is how we Live according to our True Design, following in the footsteps of many En-Lightened Ones who have gone before...*this is how we change the World.*

The Buddha's teachings on LOVE are clear. It is possible to live twenty-four hours a day in a state of LOVE. Every movement, every glance, every thought, and every word can be infused with LOVE.

Thich Nhat Hanh
Buddhist Monk, Peace Activist

Science Now demonstrates that our Heart is an Amazing *"Sending Device,"* as the Ancients always knew. Fine-tuning our Hearts to LOVE, Compassion and Gratitude, we express Heart Coherence. We change our own Body chemistry. We change our DNA and our World. This is En-Light-enment - bringing greater Light into our Being - to resonate with LOVE; as we do so, Miracles occur...

Sentiment without action is the ruin of the Soul...

Ed Abbey (1927-1989)
American Author and Environmentalist

The biggest secret of being a **21st Century Superhuman** living **Quantum Lifestyle**...*is resonating through the Heart with LOVE.* **Arc the Hologram** Now with LOVE in the 'No - Time' Continuum! *Changing ourselves, changing the World Now with LOVE!*

♥ ♥ ♥

NEXT: ***PART 3: SPIRIT***
Live Your Dreams: Success, Passion, Relationship, Community

Part 3 SPIRIT

Live Your Dreams: Success, Passion, Relationship, Community

~ BLESS YOU ON YOUR JOURNEY ~

May you Soar on Golden Eagle's wings
Drinking the Elixir of Life in every Breath
As you Rise up in Your conquest of Self
Allow the Phoenix to leave the Ashes behind
As You behold Your Newest God-Goddess Self
To kindle in its Live Flame Of LOVE and LIGHT -
Thankyou for your LOVE
Thankyou for Caring
Thankyou for Being such a Good Friend
Thankyou for Being the Teacher that YOU Are
Thankyou for Teaching Me
Thankyou for Opening your Heart and Soul
And Especially Thankyou for Being You
Thankyou for showing me Hope and Faith
Too often we run from the very thing we need the most,
And as a result, find ourselves unhappy and lonely
There is a better way and it lies in Growth.
Hell is not to LOVE anymore.
Into Sacred full Moon's Glow
Your Shine makes the Heaven dim
The Embering coals Glowing
Within Your Soul of LOVE'S Eternal Flame
Lighting the Presence
Into Divine Truth and Wholeness
Glimmering cascades of LOVE
Stream from the Wake that You Walk through
Leaving Imprints in Eternity of Faith and Goodness

BELOVED Brother David Ellis (1953-2007)
High Spiritual Being and Traveler in this World
Find His Writings at www.21stCenturySuperhuman.com

Part 3: Spirit - Section 1
We Are Energy Beings

Never forget your real identity.
You are a luminous conscious stardust being
forged in the crucible of cosmic fire.

Deepak Chopra MD
Natural Physician, New Thought Author

Let's explore deeper levels of what it is to be an "Energy Being." This is a big shift from the Newtonian World, where we thought for so long that we and matter were static and solid. The *Field* or little understood "dark *Field*" making up 94% of our Universe, teems with quarks and electrons, tiniest particles of light-energy, ready to respond to our slightest command.

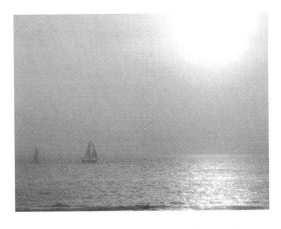

As a man who has devoted his life to the most clear-headed science, to the study of matter, I can tell you as a result of my research about atoms this much: There is no matter as such. All matter originates and exists only by virtue of a force which brings the particle of an atom to vibration and holds this most minute solar system of the atom together. We must assume behind this force the existence of a conscious and intelligent Mind. This Mind is the Matrix of all matter.

Max Planck (1858-1947)
Founder Quantum Theory, Nobel Prize Physics 1918

Nassim Haramein, progressive Quantum physicist tells us we are continually exchanging energy with an Infinite Universe that is teeming with creative potential.

This infinite nature exists in every one of our atoms, so we are connected to the infinite field of space at all times...every billionth of a second we exist we are exchanging information with the vacuum of the Universe with every one of our atoms...this is the ultimate message of the new energy technology, that *this energy and you and I are one*. With this understanding, we are moving away from the concepts of scarcity, deterioration and entropy into unity, abundance and ultimately the thriving of our society.

Nassim Haramein
Free Energy & The Future Of Science (Youtube Feb 2013), The Resonance Project

The *Infinite Field of Possibilities, Source Field, String Field or Divine Matrix,* which used to be considered empty space, is alive with energy continually flowing into Creation. John Hagelin, Quantum Physicist from What the Bleep tells us, "It is like "effervescent ginger ale, awaiting our thoughts upon it to bring matter and events into form." Currents in the ocean are as much a part of the ocean, as we are part of this *Field* surrounding us.

Clearing our thought is critical to Conscious Living, as it plays a vital role in how this *Field* expresses in our "reality." [Part 1: SHIFT OF THE AGES] When we hear there's weather or military activity brewing, we may think, "Oh no." Then what are we doing with our thought-energy? That's right, sending "creative" ripples through the *Field* with "Oh no" creative energy, and we continue to hold that "thing" in form. What happens when we instead, *feel-know-be* Peace ("mud between the toes")? That's right...it shifts as we do!

Our initial eight cells, formed from the *Field,* are very much like the Sacred Geometry "Flower of Life." Our heart forms within this symbol of Infinite, ever-emerging Creation, recorded in rock art throughout Ancient civilizations. Our Heart is directly connected with this tide of Pure LOVE, flowing eternally in our Universal Sea. Centering Breath, Life and Thought in the Heart, we literally shift our "external reality." Smile. Breathe.

The book of John says, "In the beginning was the Word." Original Aramaic says, "In the beginning was the *Mind-energy.*" Clearing Thought is the singe most potent act of Creation we ever do for rightly focused, Life and Well-Being emerge from it. Bruce Lipton tells us "Vibrational frequencies are supremely efficient in creating cellular responses." Even the cells of our body are a product of our thought! *Be aware of what you resonate!*

The more people become aware and have the knowledge that they have the power to be ultimately responsible for their lives, the easier it will be for all people to become aware. As biologist Rupert Sheldrake's Morphic Field theory suggests, the more this information is out in the field, the more it is repeated, the more quickly it will become acceptable.

Bruce Lipton, brucelipton.com
Danielle Graham, Genetics, Epigenetics and Destiny, superconsciousness.com

Recognizing our body is an Energy vehicle and everything about health and well-being comes from whether this Energy is flowing or not, is the first step in ultimate Wellness. Have you wished, hoped, prayed for or envisioned change, that has not yet come? We Now know how critically important it is to clear the logjams of "Not of LOVE" thought or emotional resistance, from our unconscious generational and experiential data-banks, otherwise if we could change it simply with Conscious thought, *it would be already done!*

We are about to explore in-depth *21st Century Superhuman* systems, tools and concepts from Ancient and modern Tradition, supporting us as Energy Beings. Relating to ourselves as Energy rather than solid matter, we discover how to miraculously activate Regenerative Supreme Health, Productivity, Creativity, Abundance, Well-Being and LOVE. ♥

Part 3: SPIRIT

Chapter 1

Co-Creating This *Shift of the Ages*

The whole Universe appears as a dynamic web of inseparable energy patterns...
Thus we are not separated parts of a whole. We are a Whole.

Barbara Ann Brennan
Hands of Light

We are at the Hub of the Wheel of Life, co-creating this *Shift of the Ages*. With use of beneficial processes and practices offered here, we set in motion New Mind-Energy into the *Field*, both individually and collectively. Barbara Marx Hubbard sheds positive insight, tipping the scales, favoring a positive Global future over situations that could be seen as threatening to our very survival...

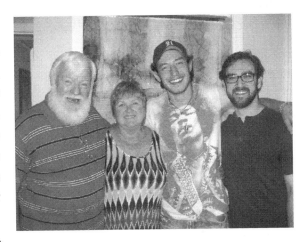

Ironically, as planetary conditions become more chaotic, the prospects for positive change actually become better. As we have noted, evolution is able to adapt by repatterning itself quickly during times of extreme instability. And it is here that we find a scientific basis for our potential to "cross the gap."

We earlier discussed how at each crossroads in biological evolution, the immediate crisis of survival faced by a species or an ecosystem is what drives its processes of adaptation.

Indeed, the threats we currently face are catalyzing millions of us to engage in personal transformative processes such as those we have just presented. These practices are a crucial part of the urgent work of the repatterning of human society...

Crucial innovations in all sectors of society, plus a variety of new methods of social synergy, will soon reveal a powerful collective path of repatterning...

Barbara Marx Hubbard
Birth 2012 And Beyond, Humanity's Great Shift to the Age of Conscious Evolution

ALL things are *always* in a state of flux, no matter how "stable" they appear. If we are stuck on our ideas or carrying around layers of long-standing thought-emotional patterns, we may *appear* to be stuck on "repeat" mode, because of *our* continuing *Vibrational resonance*. However everything changes in an instant, the second we shift our *resonance*, by shifting our thought (conscious-unconscious). Breathe and Smile...

As we shed layers, and relax into Knowing we are One with All things, *our Vibrational Frequency rises,* reformulating the very atoms of our existence. Like skydiving, or going through a rapid in the river, it's exhilarating to finally take this Leap. Whatever we place our Attention upon, magnetizes into form as "reality," as a result of the *Field* Mirroring our resonance. With practice we learn that best results occur in all areas of Life, when expression comes from Heart and *Essence*, set in Deep LOVE, Compassion and Gratitude.

Intention is the Heart and Soul of All We Do...

Kailash Kokopelli
Earth Shaman, Inner World Musician

We get to choose the channel we tune-in to. The more we focus on Pure LOVE, Compassion and Gratitude, receiving from the abundant flow of Source, the more it colors what appears in our World. And the converse is true. The more we focus on that which is Not of LOVE, it continues to appear in our "reality" and the World around us.

This may seem counterintuitive, as we are used to watching latest News stories and knowing what events are "going on" in the World. We are also used to accepting a particular diagnosis for our Body. We may feel we're negligent by *not* watching or telling others the latest. *This is a huge shift for our consciousness,* to get *out* of thinking *this is "reality,"* and get into *recognizing* that ALL is *Mind-Energy*. We are going to make the biggest shift we possibly can, by putting out New Mind-Energy to test this Quantum experience.

We have an Ancient physical "survival mechanism," operating out of *fear* with thousands of generations of thought that says: we need to run, protect, defend ourselves, residual thoughts of the blame-fear-hostility culture. We are birthing a new phase of human experience, discovering what happens when, rather than focusing on what we don't want, we begin to focus on what we *choose*. Teddi has a great philosophy, "The World is full of beautiful people doing wonderful things," and anyone who knows her will confirm, that's what she experiences! Our Attention on the *Field* (conscious and unconscious) draws in the "reality" we experience around us.

Personal drama or in sensationalized news stories focus Mind-Energy on *fear.* Let's remember, there is no 'out there' out there. All there is, is our Attention on the *Field of Possibilities*, and it can only Mirror back to us whatever we give Attention to (conscious-unconscious). Keep doing *Ancient Aramaic Forgiveness* worksheets [Part 2: MIND] to offload thought buried in the unconscious. Once done this repeatedly, we begin to see only LOVE Mirrored in our World. Self-healing and Global change previously unimagined emerge.

This Evolutionary Leap into Living from the Heart in LOVE, Compassion and Gratitude becomes our primary focus, as we begin leaving behind all else. Our Newly trained Observer-Creator Attention focuses on only what emanates from LOVE. Will we "get it" ALL instantly? Probably not. Yet *the more we get it, the more we get it.*

Some will adopt this in itty-bitty stages, others in big steps, at whatever rate they are able. We are shifting thousands of generations of thought, and the "amoeba" of Collective Conscious will move ahead as it does. ALL we can change is Self and this changes ALL!

There is no 'out there' out there. Whatever we experience in our "reality" is generated from the resonance *inside* us. Our Life (and yes, even the World-at-Large) is a "biofeedback loop" Mirroring our Vibration back to us, to show us where we need to adjust to align with LOVE. When ALL within us is LOVE, that will be all we see around us (like Mother Teresa), because we will be Living in this New Vibrational frequency.

The initiate is the one who lives in harmony with the Universal essence.

Mallku Aribalo
The Awakening of the Puma, Inka Initiation Path

So yes, for most this is a process, where whatever we see in our World reminds us to make another internal shift. *Shift. Shift Shift.* Return Focus to LOVE-Compassion-Gratitude. Breathe, Smile. We now stand in our World in a New position. Rather than looking out at what "happened to us," we step back and notice what our energy or thought has Vibrationally magnetized in as our "reality." We notice if we have adjustments to make on our own internal content to more favorable results.

It may seem scary to let go of our fear-based-control, yet it is the highest choice we have, explained fully in Quantum physics. ***Recognizing that our Mind-Energy has called forth what we perceive around us, the fastest way to turn it around is to change our Mind-Energy.*** In fact if we will just loosen our grip long enough to actually begin thinking in these new terms, it changes everything *in the blink of an eye!*

When you make a choice, you change the future.

Deepak Chopra MD
Natural Physician, New Thought Author

AND - when we *do* focus on LOVE-Compassion-Gratitude, we actually activate more DNA codons. *Wow! Talk about future science!* We used to think we were *victims of our heredity.* No more. Stem cell biologist Bruce Lipton, PhD became so excited when he learned this, he left his first professional career to begin a second, as successful author and thought leader, demonstrating that we are not victims of our genes.

In fact he relates, two Nobel Prize winning scientists have discovered *cells can actually be programmed backwards,* to take on a different form than their original! This means we can biologically change ourselves through timespace! Use this on a supposed dis-ease or anything! Bruce Lipton is a prime example of someone who made the "Leap" to follow his

Heart, from a safe secure position. He and co-author Steve Bhaerman of *Spontaneous Evolution,* contribute an entirely new view of how we operate in our World, inspiring many.

Also exciting, *Waking Times* reports HeartMath® Institute's researchers discovered "factors like LOVE and appreciation, or anxiety and anger, also influence a person's [DNA] blueprint. In one experiment participants *"changed DNA with positive mental states."*

An individual holding three DNA samples was directed to generate Heart Coherence - a beneficial state of mental, emotional and physical balance and harmony - with the aid of a HeartMath® technique that utilizes Heart Breathing and intentional positive emotions.

The individual succeeded, as instructed to intentionally and simultaneously unwind two DNA samples to different extents and leave the third unchanged. Control group volunteers with low heart Coherence were unable to alter the DNA.

Healthy cell expression and a Quantum nutrient diet: If we want to nourish our bodies at a cellular level (and not promote dis-ease), the institute recommends an abundant diet of *Quantum nutrients.* When we are stressed or negative, our biological energy reserves are diverted from the important task of regenerating and repairing the body.

We can counteract this cellular starvation by focusing on genuine states of Care, Appreciation and LOVE. These positive emotions enhance our energy system and feed the body, even down to the level of DNA. HeartMath® calls such positive feelings "Quantum nutrients."

Carolanne Wright, Guest Waking Times
You Really Can Change Your DNA - Here's How

We are learning to make *21st Century Superhuman* choices. The more we immerse ourselves in the path of the Heart and choose to clear ourselves to live in Pure LOVE, Compassion and Gratitude, we activate our Ascension or En-Light-enment process, with a greater sense of who we are and a more flowing state of being. We may still have a good portion of our Lives in the 3-D World, yet we also spend time in the flowing experience of 4-5-D, the higher Vibrational state of the Heart. Becoming aware of when we enter these higher Vibrational states, integrates us as Conscious co-creators within this *Shift of the Ages.* [Part 1: SHIFT OF THE AGES]

We enter the 4th dimension while sleeping, in dream-state, waking-dream or lucid-dream state and meditation. We can direct this in numerous ways, depending on what suits us. It is a good practice to always surround ourselves with Light and LOVE, and request support and accompaniment from any of the myriad of hierarchial Beings who inhabit the Cosmos in Realms of Light. [Part 2: MIND]

Set intentions where you'd like to journey and what you'd like to access. In the few moments right after waking, is best brain wave cycle to reclaim memory from 4-D sleep or meditation, so keep tools handy for quick note-taking to integrate symbology, experience and information *(as Einstein did).* We used to say, "The veil is very thin to those who wish to see." These days we say, "*There is no veil.*" We walk between dimensions and Worlds with connections open and clear; we see and experience only that for which we are ready.

Loved ones who are on "the other side," particularly those who were in our "spiritual family" often feel present, even though in different "dimensions," as there is no death, just a shedding of the body. We also connect with higher frequency "teachers" on "the other side." They come in when we are in prayer, holding space, or doing meditation or writing, and visit us in 4-5-D dream state.

We integrate these 4-5-D experiences as we Live, Breathe, Smile, LOVE during waking hours. Life is more flowing, birthed anew each moment, trusting the *Field* to to meet our needs. We experience spacetime rather than time and space, meaning the imprint of our Consciousness on the *Field* and what occurs from it, rather than a transit through time or space. [Part 2: MIND] This imprint can change as soon as we shift our focus, and the entire Hologram shifts through timespace or spacetime.

As we integrate this deep and lasting Truth, we change ourselves, and we change the entire Hologram, according to the 2nd Immutable Universal Law of Correspondence: "as above so below, as below so above." Integrate at your own pace. Be patient with yourself. Keep growing. *Arc the Hologram with LOVE!* ♥

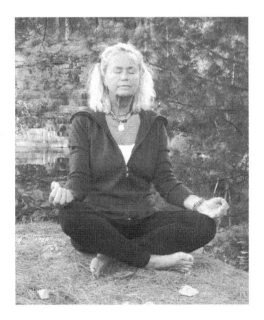

Teddi on the Path: Early on My Path, I was introduced to Ed and Nellie Cain... I was curious about the process of channeling, and the metaphysical. I began attending their weekly classes at Unity Church and reviewed the chapters of their book, "Exploring the Mysteries of Life."

The first channeling I received told me that I was a "neophyte..." a child being introduced to the "Adult World." They went on to say that with regular meditation and my willingness to totally surrender, that my Life would fulfill its destiny!

*For the next few years, I studied the **Kabbalah**, the **Koran**, the **Bhagavad Gita**, and many other books that could be called spiritual guides, such as **Autobiography of a Yogi**, **A Course in Miracles** and Ram Dass' book, **Be Here Now**.*

I came to realize that The Path to Higher Consciousness and Awareness would become my Life. There were many that came before me, there are many who walk with me, and many will come after me... The most important part of it ALL is the Knowledge that there is a Path and that the Path is Pure LOVE. ♥ *Teddi*

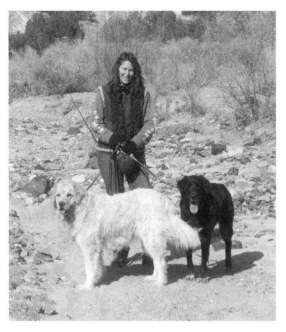

Cary on the Path: When I was a kid in school I used to write on my papers, "What is Truth?" Then I would ask my parents if they believed in God, and thank goodness they would say, "This is something you will have to find out for yourself." I've always been grateful for the inner part of me that was seeking my natural wisdom and connection with Source.

We all have this intrinsic desire; it comes forth in individuals at different times and in different ways. My Life has always had "Heart Seeking Spirit," at the hub. In high school I read **Siddhartha,** a story of illumination in the time of Buddha. I got hooked when he was robbed, and had the realization the thief must have needed his things more than he did, a perspective way beyond what I had ever considered. I also read a book called, "Death Be Not Proud," about a boy who died from a brain tumor. It changed my Life, because somewhere in my heart I knew there was way for people to be well. My Life became about both of these journeys.

I remember when I began having paranormal experiences, memories, visions and dreams. There was the logical left side of my brain that kept saying, "No. This is not real, ignore it." Then a bumper sticker with Einstein's "Imagination is more powerful than knowledge" fell into my hands. It was above my desk for years. It was the Lifeline that came down to me and said, "What you feel-know in your Heart, is more powerful than any logic. Trust your Heart," so I would Breathe, Smile and say, "Okay."

Still it was a process and a journey till I could listen to my Heart over the pull of the World's illusions. I spent years with one foot in each. I have always had telepathy with my four-leggeds, who inspired me to follow my Heart of Hearts, and set myself free from the Illusion. Once I did, there was no turning back, and it still is an unfolding process... ♥ Cary, with Daisy and Maggie in Spirit ♥

Chapter 2

Emotional Tone Scale & Healing Crisis

———————————————   ♥   ———————————————

Your Perfect Electronic Blueprint already exists.
All You have to do is Step Into It.

Dr. John Whitman Ray (1934-2001)
Founder Health and the Human Mind, Body Electronics,
Pax Mundi Award (World Peace Award)

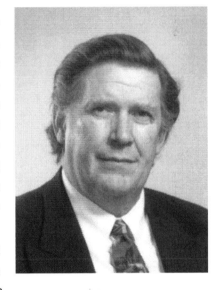

Emotional Tone Scale has been one of our favorite tools over 30+ years, mapping out a clear path to shed low frequency thought-word-emotional patterns, to move into Joy, Enthusiasm and LOVE. This upcoming chart was given us by our beloved teacher, Dr. John Whitman Ray as a tool for *Health and the Human Mind*, *Iridology* and *Body-Spinal-Cranial Electronics* in the early 1980s, serving us brilliantly ever since. It navigated thousands of hours of personal change, tracking insights for us and others as to where we were in our healing. It has been shared many times, which we encourage you to do as well.

Dr. John Ray's system of Health and the Human Mind and Body Electronics, is twofold. It includes a system of acupressure point-holding that originated in Ancient Tibet, combining with essential clearing of thought-emotional patterns stored in cellular memory. Because these thoughts-emotions crystalized in the Body structure, we called them "crystals" as they would dissolve with point holding in Body Electronics.

In dr. michael ryce's work with Ancient Aramaic Forgiveness, he calls this data "carbon-based memory" or CBM. He derives this from the fact that our body is made up of mostly carbon and water, and that unconscious thought is carried in the body structure. Interestingly, on the Periodic Table of elements, the number for the carbon atom is 666. Might we guess 666 "the beast" is simply our "Not of LOVE" data holding Vibration in the *Field? Wow!* Such a concept transmitted long ago would have been little understood, except in parable, though easily Now with modern science of healing and Quantum physics.

This crystalized thought-emotion is carried throughout the body structure, in tissues, blood, bone and organs. The "logjam" of "Not of LOVE" thought slows down circulation of Life-force, causing accumulated toxins that gradually coagulate into formations we call dis-ease. Crystalline structures in our tissue, like tiny sharp pieces of quartz crystal, carry an electrical charge with the message of the thought-emotion that put them there initially.

Due to the Vibrational level of this "data," flow of our True Power Supply is reduced, and aches, pains, illness and dis-ease result. An easy example is when someone gives us a foot massage and we say, "Ouch!" when they hit a sore spot. These are places where painful thought energy is stored in the tissues as tiny sharp crystals. We learned long ago in Body Electronics, *all* thoughts and emotions Not of LOVE are stored throughout our Body.

In our modern culture we have cultivated the habit of having surgery to remove or taking medications or suppress the most painful tissue. Because we are not removing the cause, our old thought-emotional patterns stored in the unconscious, by removing one painful location, we simply Create a delay until it appears somewhere else, and thus the degenerative path - UNLESS - we go to work and remove our old thought. [Part 2: MIND]

Bruce Lipton tells us the cell is programmable like a computer chip. What is interesting about the computer chip is that it contains semiconducting material quartz or silica.

Biological behavior and gene activity are dynamically linked to information from the environment, which is downloaded into the cell. A cell is a "programmable chip" whose behavior and genetic activity are primarily controlled by environmental signals, not genes.

Bruce H. Lipton PhD
Biology of Belief

Genetic history bleeds into our environment in-utero and through family dynamics, to program our DNA. Are we ready to clear out our "old data" so it doesn't continue causing us misery and carry on to future generations? Our human culture operates as a Hologram, like a giant collective "amoeba" of which we *are ALL part and we are One."* Our World, our children and those closest to us absorb and resonate what we share with them (consciously and unconsciously). So although epigenetics tells us our DNA is programmable, whatever data is *replayed in our family dynamics and/or environment,* tends to be imprinted and carried forward, until *we* chose to change this personal history.

It is *ultimately exciting* that we have great *POWER to change this by clearing* and switch our "channel" to LOVE. This is being asked of us by future generations, so we can have a viable future. We are going to learn to us some great tools to assist us.

To prepare for Body Electronics, we saturated ourselves with liquid trace mineral solution, elevating the body's electromagnetic potential to be able to carry a charge. We were on fresh and raw foods and herbs for cleansing. Most importantly we learned the value of willingness to "go into the pain" to release thought-word-emotional patterns that would surface during marathon two hour point-holding sessions. We plunged into Body

Electronics, when shortly after learning about it, I (Cary) broke my arm *(x-rayed and doctors wanted to do surgery and put two pins in)*, yet we healed it in a matter of six hours with the Body Electronics system of point holding and thought-emotional clearing. [Story: Part 4: BODY - *Miraculous Tales*] It brought crystalized patterns to the surface of the Conscious mind like layers of the onion, dissolving, as the original thought-emotional content was released through the Tone Scale to LOVE. Dr. John Whitman Ray's famous "words to Live by," precious to our Hearts, echo forever in our Minds:

Until a person can experience on the conscious mental level
that which is on the physical, they are bound to the physical.

Dr. John Whitman Ray (1934-2001)
Founder Health and the Human Mind, Body Electronics

As we dissolved the "crystals" and thoughts that Created them, Life-force flowed again as the electromagnetic field of the body restored itself to wholeness. As searing burning heat of the Body's healing energies expressed through *kundalini fire* flowed through the arm, we could literally hear bones clicking back into place, muscles restored, black and blue marks gone, and it was *as if the bone was never broken (though the experience remained)*. We were fortunate to experience these advanced principles early on. This recognition of True healing has been with us and in every avenue of teaching - healing we've followed since.

The body is intricately tied in with all thought-emotion, conscious-unconscious. We lower or raise the body's Life-force and Vitality, simply by the tone or frequency of thoughts, words and emotions plus nutrition-cleansing. With upcoming Emotional Tone Scale, it's easy to recognize whether we're moving up or down the tone scale. Feelings in the body let us know what emotion is surfacing to clear and we move upscale to LOVE.

It takes courage and willingness to keep going into our "stuff," to access old layers that surface and clear; then regain vitality, and *go through the process again.* Letting go this genetic and experiential "old data," we move into *Enthusiasm*, our True Design LOVE. We Breathe and Smile as we go through this process, (and sometimes cry), though it's good to move from crying into Breathing, because Breathing helps release the old "stuff."

There is nothing good or bad, but our thinking makes it so.

William Shakespeare (1564-1616)

The Emotional Tone Scale gives us a clear path to notice, or gauge what direction we're moving, offering insight into what thoughts-emotions are creating our "reality." Surfacing our repeating content to clear, allows us to live from a new Conscious resonance with more vitality, as energy flows through those formerly blocked tissues. *Yeah!* Things move faster Now. In our Quantum World, things can shift very quickly, even in an instant, so allow yourself the Freedom to access pure potentiality. In moving beyond these things we are able to operate at New levels, rather than getting Attention for our old Pain or Story.

When you drop into the field of the heart, there is no fear, there is no duality, there is no belief. There's just access to pure potential and from that place, miracles can show up and lives can transform

Melissa Joy
Matrix Energetics

On the Emotional Tone Scale, identify current emotional level. See what's on the same horizontal line on chart: chakra, color, gland and thought. Breathing and noticing where you are on the Emotional Tone Scale, allow emotions to surface and clear to move upscale, toward the top of chart. If moving into deeper suppression you may move down the chart. Clearing old thought-emotion may be like a wave pattern, where you move up and down the chart depending on what's clearing. This assists with identification and how to support Mind-Body clearing, healing process.

21st Century Superhuman
Emotional Tone Scale

Chakra	Color	Endocrine Gland	Emotion	Thought	Iris
7 Crown	Violet	Pineal	Enthusiasm/ Universal LOVE	Creative Imagination	White-Violet
6 Third Eye	Indigo	Pituitary	Pain	Intuition - Specific Memory	Bright white
5 Throat	Electric Blue	Thyroid-Parathyroid	Anger *(overt thyroid - covert parathyroid)*	Security-Acquisition	Light Gray
4 Heart	Green	Thymus	Fear	Intellectualization	Gray
3 Solar Plexus	Yellow	Adrenal-Pancreas	Grief-Sympathy	General Memory	Dark Gray
2 Sacrum	Orange	Sacrum	Spleen / Apathy	Social Activity	Very Dark Gray
1 Base	Red	Gonads	Unconsciousness / Emotions Shut Down	Sex Without Love	Black

EFT tapping can also be of benefit with the Emotional Tone Scale. As we move through a particular area of the Chart, it assists to activate New neurobiology *(instructions online)*.

"Chakra" section of the Emotional Tone Scale, refers to the seven chakras within our physical energy field, corresponding with the glands. When an emotion resonates or is being cleared, give Attention to the corresponding chakra by visualizing the color of the chakra. A practitioner or friend can be supportive by balancing the chakras. Clockwise hand movement (facing the person's back or front) adds energy. Gentle counter-clockwise discharges. LOVE yourself. LOVE what is letting go. LOVE what is rebalancing.

"Color" refers to chakra color. Balance-nourish your "Rainbow Light Body" by visualizing and surrounding self with color of each area while clearing that area of Body. Carry precious or semi-precious stones or crystals, enjoy (raw) food, clothing, fabrics, furnishings of each color to add energy and vitality, clear and move upscale at each level.

"Endocrine Gland" section of the Emotional Tone Scale, refers to the seven major glands of the Body and their associated emotional patterns. While processing emotion related to a particular gland, look up herbs and nutrition supportive of that gland and nearby organs. Nutritional support assists tissues to free connected or denied thought-emotional energy. Glandular support with supplements is also very helpful.

"Emotion" section refers to emotions surfacing, often resonating from unconscious data. Illness and injury do not happen by accident. They are the mechanism pointing us to where we are out of synch with Source or our own Heart and Soul. Every pain, i-llness, injury is a "wake-up" call to pay Attention, clear and align with our Heart. Emotion acts as a "tuning fork," drawing issues, people and events into our World to match and Mirror our resonance. Emotions held in the physical resonate, until we bring them to Conscious awareness, release and move up the tone scale. Awareness is key to clearing. Notice what you are feeling Now. Begin there. Be present with it and allow yourself to move upscale.

> Freedom comes when one clearly experiences the true Self as being separate from mind, when the Light of Pure Consciousness shines unrestricted.
>
> *Roy Eugene Davis*
> *The Teachings of the Masters of Perfection*

"Thought" section of Emotional Tone Scale pinpoints the *level* of thought permeating our Life in the moment. Discomfort, pain, dis-ease express suppressed consciousness and matching Lifestyle. Clearing, we move upscale into the Heart and creative imagination.

Levels of unconsciousness or apathy appear as, *"I don't remember,* I don't know or I don't care." As we move up the tone scale clearing to LOVE, Breathing and Smiling bring the experience to the Conscious mental level to clear. Though unaware of thought under the surface, this tool focuses in on what needs to clear. Dis-comfort or suppressive habits push us to "wake up," return to Essence and the Heart. Each moment is a perfect expression of our resonance. If we don't like what we are experiencing, shift inside.

> The secrets of alchemy exist to transform mortals from a state of suffering and ignorance to a state of enlightenment and bliss.
>
> *Deepak Chopra MD, New Thought Author*

"Iris" section refers to Iridology. Light and dark color of fibers in the iris gauge what level of healing or suppression is in particular areas of the body. Look for patterns in your own and friends' eyes. (Eye charts online). Videos and eye readings soon at our website.

The Light of the Body is the Eye. On what have you set your sight?
If your eye be single, your body shall be full of Light.

HERRINGS LAW OF CURE All healing occurs from the head down, from the inside out, in reverse order to which the symptoms occurred, *based on the level of vitality.*

HEALING CRISIS is the term we use when experiencing layers freeing up physically, mentally, emotionally. As Vitality rises with good nutrition and clearing of "old data," cellular Life-force rises, and hidden or suppressed symptoms surface for us to clear. In this process we *re-experience* thoughts, emotions and events, as they move out of our system.

Pain is but the sign you have misunderstood yourself.

A Course In Miracles

In a *Healing Crisis,* what comes *up* often triggers us as it originally did. With this New awareness we move through it easily, finally releasing it from Mind-Body. We learn to "go into the pain," rather than "away from it," *getting support* if needed. The only way "out" is to go through, being present with what comes up, Breathing, clearing, releasing, Smiling.

If you embrace the present and become one with it, and merge with it, you will experience a fire, a glow, a sparkle of ecstasy throbbing in every living sentient being. As you begin to experience this exultation of spirit in everything that is alive, as you become intimate with it, joy will be born within you, and you will drop the terrible burdens and encumbrances of defensiveness, resentment, and hurtfulness. Only then will you become lighthearted, carefree, joyous and free...

Make a commitment to follow the path of no resistance. This is the path through which nature's intelligence unfolds spontaneously, without friction or effort. When you have the exquisite combination of acceptance, responsibility and defenselessness, you will experience Life flowing with effortless ease.

Deepak Chopra MD
The Seven Spiritual Laws of Success

21st Century Superhuman Body and Mind KNOW how to achieve Wellness, Wholeness and Alignment with Heart. Life flows naturally, pushing us this direction. As we let go our "old data" and take in Vital High-Frequency Nutrition with Cleansing, we remove ALL blocking this flow. Clear, clean and nutritionally sound, well-being and vitality flow! ♥

NOTE: Links on Dr. John Whitman Ray's work *(no longer with us in the Earth-plane):*
DrJohnWhitmanRay dot Blogspot dot com; Body-Electronics dot ca; Douglas W. Morrison - *HowWeHeal dot com;* Robert Stevens - *MasterySystems dot com/course/Body-Electronics; BodyElectronics dot co dot uk; YouTube videos posted by Jeremy Holt*

Part 3: SPIRIT

Chapter 3

Our Chakra System

Chakras are energy-awareness centers.
They are the revolving doors of creativity and
communication between spirit and the world.

Michael J Tamura, Clairvoyant
You Are The Answer: Discovering and Fulfilling Your Soul's Purpose

Following sacred knowledge, handed down through the ages, carried in or stories easily grasped by simpler cultures, the Rainbow Body of Light has always held a place in mythologies and traditions. Norse and Germanic tribes had the ALL-powerful Guardian of the Rainbow Bridge, with his place between the Worlds. There have been numerous Rainbow warriors, Hopi Rainbow Nation, and Noah's Rainbow in the clouds.

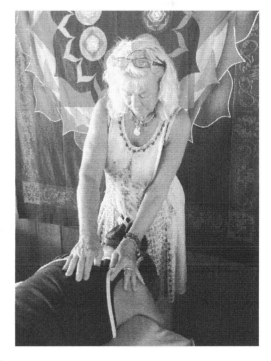

Shine a light through a prism, and you get the Rainbow colors of our chakras. Light diffracts, beaming through our chakras in translucent Rainbow colors,, radiating in our auric field, which some are gifted to see naturally. We are a colorful expression of the resonant energy *Field* of Creation. Get to know colors of Light associated with each area of the body (reviewed here shortly), and if you haven't done it before, imagine "seeing-feeling" the power of colorful translucent energy moving through them.

The word Chakra from Sanskrit "sounds of Creation" (5,000 B.C.), means spinning wheel of Light. When two beams of light cross each other they are non-interrupting. As Energy Beings in Quantum "reality," our bodies emit waves of energy that can be clarified, upscaled and if needed released with chakra energy and polarity balancing. Becoming familiar with our chakras gives us a way to recognize, balance, nurture, support and enhance Coherence of our energy field. Website titled "Chakra, Vortex of Light," tells how Color, Light and Sound operate through our chakra centers.

> Sound raised to a higher Vibration is color...According to Hindu beliefs, everything in the Universe is made of sound. Each chakra has what is called a "seed sound."These seed sounds are the symbolic representations of the energy pattern of each chakra and hold its essence. [Mantras are Seed Sounds], Crystal bowls and tuning forks are used to aid those wishing to resonate with the wheels of light.

Everything in Creation is sound; geometric form emerges from Vibration. When we are centered in LOVE our Heart's resonance Creates a higher frequency geometry in the water molecules of our Body, harmonious with Source and our *Essence*. Raising our frequency into this Higher *Field* of in-formation, we find ourselves flowing within our torus *Field*.

Light is energy frequencies made visible. Tuning the chakras helps us harmonize Body-Mind-Spirit as One to access Unity Consciousness. Sound assists with this harmonization. Many spiritual practices utilize Kirtan or Gregorian Chants, Tibetan Bowls, flute, drum or gong to soothe, balance, harmonize Body-Mind-Spirit. HeartMath Institute discovered sounds producing *Heart Coherence* initiate a state of such LOVE that ALL Life improves. Enjoy soothing sounds to harmonize *your* Body-Mind. Nature's sounds also benefit us profoundly, sleep with windows open, walk and play outdoors, garden.

Each chakra has its own color of Light and Vibrational spin that can be harmonized with sound and Light. Chakra imbalances or low energy are recognized and corrected by energy workers. Polarity, massage, Reiki, Tai Chi, Quigong, crystal bowls and other similar practices are ALL beneficial to balancing chakras' spinning energy centers.

Energy balancing, self-administered or by another, gets us in touch with what needs harmonization. Our chakras are "check-in points" to adjust flow of our internal energy. Finding this balance with awakening of Heart and Pineal gland, we learn to work in harmony with the Universe, empowering us to fulfill our deepest dreams.

Pain, dis-comfort or stress in a particular part of the Body, points to that chakra and what it represents. This provides us a pathway for recognizing and clearing the *source* of our pain, identifying energies to be cleared and support the chakra to flow freely.

Relaxation, Breathing, focusing on our energy flow, while someone works on us, assists us to clear "stuck patterns." Our energy radiates through our chakra centers into the World. Clearing with support from friend or practitioner, with nurturing energy balancing, we energize Body-Mind through the chakras, re-connecting with our True Design LOVE.

Learning to identify our chakra centers, what color, emotion and thought resonates through each is an important element to recognize when we are Healthy and in balance energetically. We may find we prefer to wear certain colors, discovering those colors strengthen or enhance certain chakras.

Lessons from
Chakra Centers' Spinning Energy

1st Chakra (Base), RED, SEXUAL ORGANS: Home, Family, Security, Relationship

2nd Chakra, ORANGE, SPLEEN: Personality, Expression or Imprint; How we "show up" in the World.

3rd Chakra, YELLOW, SOLAR PLEXUS: Courage and/or Fear Center. Power center. What is Solar Plexus emanating or shielding?

4th Chakra, GREEN , HEART: Radiating LOVE into the World. Living from Heart rather than head: holding Deep LOVE, Compassion, Gratitude., amplified into the World through spinning Heart Torus Field (extends 8-12' spherically)

5th Chakra, TURQUOISE / ELECTRIC BLUE, THROAT: Power of the Spoken Word. We Create with our words. We hold back our words when we carry fear of speaking. Opening throat brings our Voice into the World unique and important as a snowflake.

6th Chakra, INDIGO, THIRD EYE: Gateway to Third Eye pineal gland; Inner Vision cultivated at Ancient Mystery Schools such as in Egypt and India; developed through Power of Imagination, Visualization, Meditation, Inner Knowing, Psychic-Telepathic ability.

7th, VIOLET, CROWN: Merging Higher Self or Soul with physical; Transpersonal Point; Projects Light to Self, Others and the World; Violet Flame, Pure White Light, cleanses, purifies, protects, raises frequency.

LEARN CHAKRAS COLOR, MEANING, LOCATION Make your own learning page for chakra colors and meanings to learn, absorb and flow through Life. Note how energy Body integrates. Notice what chakras you activate with colors of foods and clothing Nourish your energy field with colors to restore and support emotional integrity.

CHAKRA CLEARING, OPENING, RELINK DNA: Regular clearing of chakra centers supports Life's journey. Lie down in a quiet place and teach yourself to easily balance your chakras or energy centers. Do as visualization, or lie on massage table, bed or floor. Place hand (self or partner) over location, slightly off body, feel the energy between hand-body.

- Begin at your first chakra or base center. Include energy going down through legs and feet in to the center of the Earth, from base chakra grounding into Earth Mother Gaia, activating as grounding energy for your Life.

- Visualize each spinning chakra. You or partner can hold hand over the chakra. Breathe. Visualize the flow of Light and Color. Visualize and add color and energy to each chakra with a clockwise motion. Feel the energy of that chakra awakening, Breathe, Smile, enjoy the energy flow.

• Receive message each chakra has for you in the word-thought-emotional realm. Cancel goals to let go anything "Not of LOVE." Invite LOVE to resonate through each chakra with its essence, restructuring your energy matrix from the *Field*.

• Notice how comfortable each chakra center is. Remember we are part of an infinite *Field* of energy continually flowing into Creation.

• The 7th or Crown chakra is a fulcrum point that connects with 6 chakras above, in our other levels of Being, operating in highest frequencies of Light-LOVE.

HIGHER CHAKRA CENTERS: There are 6 higher chakra centers above the familiar 7 in the physical, which in the past were little understood. In our *Now*, activated by Cosmic *Fields* of accelerated Light, higher chakra centers are activating for those accessing 4-5-D and beyond. [Part 2: MIND} The Crown or 7th, is a fulcrum point for 6 chakras in the physical below and the 6 higher vibrational of matching resonance above.

These higher chakras are in Radiant pastel tones, complimentary Higher resonance of those below. For those aware of them, Higher chakras are used in interdimensional Gridwork, Planetary healing, sending-receiving information of Greater Mind, participating in the collective at this level and connecting with Creator - Source.

8th Chakra above Crown: Links to Multidimensional Mind

9th Chakra - 2' above head to Earth's Grid: Lightwork restructuring of Planetary Grid, Higher Dimensional activity in 5-D

10th Chakra: Non-Linear Solar System Connection
11th Chakra: Galactic Consciousness

12th Chakra: Travel through wormholes and interchange with Universal Source *Field*

Visualize Being in your Higher chakra centers above the Body, sensing your Radiant Higher Self and Frequencies sending-receiving. As you become comfortable in these Higher Frequencies, gently loosen grip of identifying solely with physical. Integrate with your OverSoul and perceive from there. Breathe. Smile. Flow, as the Energy Being You Are.

Our DNA is Light encoded filaments. Barbara Marciniak's Pleiadian channeling tells how thousands of years ago, another race scattered and disconnected these Light coded filaments, which we are restoring. Current activation in accelerated Light *Fields,* reconnects these filaments into crystalline DNA patterns, enhancing our chakras or Light centers.

There are multitudes of chakra centers, and there are multitudes of potential helixes that can form. Right now, the common denominator with respect to the number of helixes and chakras that the consciousness of humanity can handle without destroying itself is 12... Some people will be functioning with the 12 helixes within a short period of time while others around the planet will not receive this shift until later...

We are dealing right now with an involvement of 12 helixes to plug into the 12 chakras.. you will receive information from these personal centers for they are collective centers as well, just as your other personal chakra centers are... As you learn to translate the chakra experiences, you will discover that Life is not the same anymore.

Not all people on the planet are going through these changes right now, because you are not all coded to respond at this particular time. Each of you came in with a certain order – a map of when and where and how you best operate. Many of you are learning to follow this plan of the self that will lead you to discover your exalted self.

Barbara Marciniak
Bringers of the Dawn, Teachings from the Pleiadians

Studies at UCLA have revealed that many children Now arriving on Earth, have more DNA filaments connected. This wave of Souls called Indigos, are 30% more intelligent, many with strong intuitive and psychic abilities. These more advanced Souls of the future benefit from and are gifted at energy and psychic work. Offer them opportunities to learn! Early wave Indigos first started around 70 years ago. If you think you may be one, do some reading to learn about Indigo qualities, and "decode" the information you came in with.

Ancient Traditions also raised sexual energy through the chakras, as a path to free consciousness from duality by merging in *ONENESS*. Sacred sexuality or Tantra integrates Higher states of consciousness through Union. Practices include raising sexual energy with Kundalini through chakra centers along the spine. This energy symbolized by serpents is represented in the Ancient Caduceus coil (logo of modern medicine), representing DNA helix and its Holographic link to Light of Source. Couples benefit by focusing on Union with tantric practices, with resulting enhanced vitality and extended ecstasy. Focus around sacred Union explores and expresses merging of Divine Masculine-Feminine.

Although most spiritual disciplines insist on evolving into higher states of consciousness by controlling or denying the senses and lower states of consciousness, Tantra teaches that you cannot experience complete personal and spiritual liberation while restricting a part of your being. Tantra is a profound form of active meditation that expands consciousness using the senses to take you beyond the realm of the senses. It teaches that sacred sexuality is a way of deepening intimacy and expanding consciousness, a way to achieve freedom from limitations and to join with the Divine.

Observing a Tantric experience, you might assume you are simply witnessing "great sex." But if you could see the experience clairvoyantly, you would witness an amazing dance of energy and color, not unlike a fireworks display. Furthermore, if you could see into the hearts and Souls of the participants, you would observe a consecrated joining of loving intent.

Michael Mirdad
Sacred Sexuality, a Mantra for Living Bliss

Masculine and Feminine are magnetic principles holding Creation in form. Experiencing sacred sexuality opens couples to the experience of Unity Consciousness, and the Knowing we are not separate. Deepening LOVE through such sacred Union, releases us from duality, elevating us beyond 3-D into 4-5-D to enter Higher dimensions of the Heart.

Drunvalo Melchizedek reports Egyptians practiced moving sexual energy up to the Heart. The Ankh symbol directed it to flow through Heart chakra out back, over head by a natural pathway, in through front of Heart, flowing in a continuously regenerative loop.

> ...the heart chakra of Unconditional Universal LOVE, is the first place where energy completes itself. Each chakra has a "direction" associated with it, as Life-force energy rotates its way up the body in a pattern similar to DNA...
>
> *Drunvalo Melchizedek*
> *ANCIENT EGYPTIAN SEXUAL ANKHING, The Spirit of Ma'at - Vol. 1 No. 9*

A single person can practice raising sexual energy through the chakras, then through the Heart. Once this sacred practice is cultivated it is easily used in any setting, aligning energies of Higher self to support emerging events and "reality." Energy practices and meditation transport us beyond a purely physical existence. Activating Higher chakra centers, our Radiant energy Body connects us with Higher dimensions of self.

> Chakras are specialized energy centers connecting us to a multidimensional Universe. The chakras are dimensional portals within the subtle bodies which take in and process energy of higher Vibrational nature so that it may be properly assimilated and used to transform the physical body.
>
> *Richard Gerber*
> *Vibrational Medicine*

Getting to know and energizing our chakras or spinning Light centers, opens us to aspects of self beyond the physical. Awareness that we are Eternal Beings helps remove Ancient fear patterns about death (used from Ancient times to mange humanity), activating our Higher energy vehicle that *does not die when / if* the physical body is shed. With practice such experiences become enjoyable and useful, opening us to other dimensions within this Life through the Living presence of our Eternal state. Engaging fully with balanced chakra centers enhances our Radiance on ALL levels.

Natural practitioners, chiropractors, energy and bodyworkers can support us in energy Wellness. Commit to Journeying *toward* We-llness, rather than *away* from i-llness. Remove the "i" from illness, replacing it with "we" for wellness. To accomplish this *we must remove the "logjams in the river,"* denied and suppressed thought, "Not of LOVE" stored in our unconscious long ago. [Part 2: MIND] Simply *Being in ONENESS*, Unity consciousness or *Heart Coherence* as **21st Century Superhumans**, awakens Well-Being, and clears our chakras. These spinning *Fields* of Light connect physical with Higher-self, and our embodied Eternal Spirit shines its unique, Radiant Rainbow of LOVE and Light into the World. ♥

Part 3: SPIRIT
Chapter 4
You're A Shining Star

You're a shining star, no matter who you are
Shining bright to see what you can truly be

Earth, Wind and Fire
"Shining Star," Lyrics

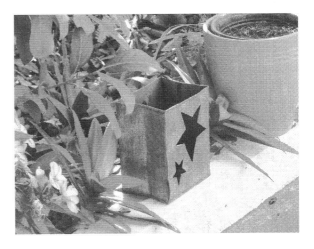

We are stretching into New ways of perceiving Life, as we grow beyond thousands of years of cultural conditioning that someone or something *outside of us is to blame* or at fault for our circumstances. Learning what it means to be Response-Able, while letting go of self-blame and still Loving Self is empowering.

As we play with these ideas we develop new neurological pathways for this In-formation, literally re-wiring Mind and Body. Amazingly enough our brain is "neoplastic," and changes as we shift how we use it, removing some of our age-old "filters" held there by "old data."

Our "old data" actually acts like a "filter" on a movie projector. Imagine that *WE* are the movie projector and our "reality" is the "movie." Energy flows from Source in continual waves of Creation based in LOVE. *HOWEVER*, if we have any "old data" Not of LOVE in our unconscious, these stored thoughts from our generations, childhood or repeat adult patterns, act as a "filter" on our "movie projector."

Source energy, continually flowing to us in LOVE, is then colored, filtered or shaped by our "old data." The *only way* our "reality" can possibly appear is as Source flows through our "movie projector," and is colored by our "filter." Until we remove this "old data," we will keep playing the same "movie," and our "reality" will be various repetitions of old patterns stored within us. Only when we remove our "old data," do we get a New "filter" to allow the flow of Source energy of LOVE to bring forth a New "reality."

Response-Ability means that as soon as we feel something painful or uncomfortable that we don't like about our "reality," we use the *Ancient Aramaic True Forgiveness* tools - worksheets, with Breathing, and Mindshifters radio shows by dr. michael ryce and additional associated worksheets to remove this content from ourselves forever. [Part 4: Mind] As we do so, we change the "filter" on our "movie projector," and get to watch a New movie! Then we can say, "Don't hold onto who I was a month or a week ago," Smile.

We are designed to operate with LOVE from Source continually flowing through us. The amazing "prize" for letting go, brings us a better "reality" of LOVE, Kindness, Success and Inner Peace, once "old data" Source is currently filtered through is removed. Only when we remove our "old data," does the "movie" of our "reality" change. This is how we shift ourselves, to shift the entire Hologram. *Arc the Hologram Now with LOVE!*

Neurotransmitters linked to the "old data" atrophy as we let it go, and New neural pathways develop, "opening doors where there were only walls before." Suddenly one day we wake up, and things have shifted so much inside us that we begin living our days and moments in a different Light. Having changed our "filters" or let go "old data," we barely know when it shifted, yet we like it!

> LOVE one another and help others to rise to higher levels, simply by pouring out LOVE. LOVE is infectious and the greatest healing energy there is.
>
> *Sai Baba (1926-2011)*
> *Indian Avatar, Founded Free Hospitals, Manifested out of thin air, Taught LOVE*

Until we "wake up" to the fact that we Create our "reality," [Part 1: SHIFT OF THE AGES] there are tendencies to compare self with others, conform to fit in, fear we won't be accepted, seek approval to succeed, avoid punishment, grasp at what we perceive to be ours, deny our pain and denial with food, drugs, alcohol, busy, and so on… These suppressed thoughts (conscious-unconscious) began with a thought-emotion stored away long ago, still holding resonance in our World from within us. *Our first big step to freedom* is to allow ourselves to flow into letting go this resonance, cancel, release and clear.

> You must learn to LOVE your emotions. As long as you describe something as difficult, you make it difficult. …You are resisting and judging the changes coming about. You are feeling that you do not know what is going on, and you wish to be in control. Control is something very convenient and very handy. It must be applied at the right place at the right time, like superglue. Superglue in the wrong place doesn't do much good, did you ever Superglue your hands or lips together?
>
> *Barbara Marciniak*
> *Bringers of the Dawn*

If there is even the tiniest bit of discomfort, anger, resentment, fear, doubt, anything but LOVE, resonating in our current "reality," it is a message that we have something yet to clear. [repeat] Whatever our *conscious mind* thinks, is simply a coverup called "denial," to *avoid* the old pain we're carrying in our unconscious. Until we "open the can of worms" to get it out, it's going to continue drawing matter and events into our "reality" that perfectly Mirror our "old data." The reason we don't want to acknowledge it's there, is the very reason we shut it away in the first place, because it is associated with severe pain or terror even for our very Life, often stored from infancy and/or genetic memory. Once we let it go, we Awaken to a new level of Being, expressing our resonance from a new root place.

> You want to sweep difficult things under the rug and say, "I don't want to do these," when the difficult things are your gemstones. Even if you discover you have 101,000 boundaries, do not feel frustrated. Simply say, "This is interesting." Look at the boundaries you have set up...simply observe them and see if you can discover how they came about. See what purpose they served — what grocery store you shopped at when you bought those items.
>
> *Barbara Marciniak*
> *Bringers of the Dawn*

We can be so entangled with our old content, it may seem a difficult journey out. It is hugely helpful to "report in" to a buddy on the path daily, after fulfilling our committed worksheets and other processes to remove "old data" holding resonance. [We encourage regular listening to dr. michael and jeanie ryce's Mindshifter Radio shows or archives and videos at whyagain.org. and (videos soon at our website)] By participating you will meet others on the path and build alliances for encouragement and inspiration.

> What is coming out now are the things that originally blocked you from perceiving reality. These are the parts of your emotional body in which the highway system was severed and the information could not flow, so you moved into pain and translated the emotional pain out of your physical body.
>
> *Barbara Marciniak*
> *Bringers of the Dawn*

Listening to our Heart, heeding emotions and responding to them, is part of the critical path to reclaiming our balance in this World. Highly sensitive individuals tend to be those absorbing collective pain particularly as children without good coping skills, carrying residual into adulthood as a unconscious resonance. We can be hard on ourselves, thinking our baggage is hopeless and stay in avoidance, when nothing could be further from the truth. This is part of the *ILLUSION* surrounding us in the blame-fear-hostility culture. Merge New skills, with the child within. Hold yourself, a Newborn in your arms and comfort him/her, Smile, Breath, LOVE. Know and share with this beautiful infant we are changing this all Now with LOVE.

It is amazing when we realize it's safe and healing to let go of imagined obligations and charades to the outer World, remembering who we truly are on the inside, at our *Purest Essence*. Our misaligned culture has rewarded conformity, where if we do what is expected we have safety, security; with the message that if we don't comply, our lives will be more difficult. This falsehood has been carried on for tens of thousands of years, serving a system of greed and servitude. Michael Tellinger's *Slave Species of the Gods* tells this story in amazing detail. Many today are waking up to the fact that we've been living in a system that rewards servitude over brilliance and creativity. From this emerges some of our greatest pain and disorientation of spirit. This is why the removal of "old data" is so critical and repeated here many times. We must go through our denial to remove Ancient programs (just like computer programs) that have been running our lives in Not of LOVE.

Advertising of a greed based monetary system strips us of honoring natural beauty, encouraging us to compete with styles or images which we imagine equate to to being accepted and Loved. Recovery means our own wisdom, intelligence and gifts are worthy and essential to bring forward. Then, like a flower or plant in the garden in good organic soil, we ground ourselves in True Being, to grow and express our brilliance and beauty.

Waking up from this cultural slumber is the most critical path to recovering inner Joy, Peace and Expression. Noticing our feelings, and telling the truth about them is a way of heeding our inner guidance system, nudging us to wake up. First we must escape the fear that something will go wrong if we do this.

It's been denied culturally that it's okay to listen to our feelings and follow what they tell us. We've been taught it's important to set our feelings aside, and do what is expected of us. Struggle of self-doubt arises when we're caught between desires of the Heart and *Essence,* and demanding requirements of society, jobs, partners, and expectations of others.

> If you are feeling pain within your emotional body, ask yourself why you believe the pain is there, what purpose the pain serves, and why you were choosing to Create pain through your emotions. Why is it not your choice to Create joy? *All is choice.* We need to remind you of this.
>
> *Barbara Marciniak*
> *Bringers of the Dawn*

Our biggest pain is our separation from True Self and our True Design *LOVE,* an illusion we bought into long ago. These resources help renew connection with who we Truly ARE. Remember, as Observer-Creators we change the shape of our World in each Now moment, by changing our Mind-Energy. Clean out the "old data." [Part 2: MIND]

Who knows what it is that turns on the light for each to awaken from this slumber? Part of despair is that we've lost hope that there is a way out of our tunnel, and part of us thinks we may be stuck there forever. This is where seeking out others with whom we can make our Journey juicy again, is so essential. Find a friend or group to read and discuss this book with, and share your Journey, *for where two or more are gathered...*

We hold the *Field* of consciousness and change much more effectively and powerfully, when we share it with others. "Connecting with others of like-mind brings more clarification than we find alone, for "no man/woman is a island." Shedding light on the path, leading us to the Joy of our *True Expression* recovers vitality of our True *Essence,* and allows the greatest Life-force to flow through us.

Stories are intensified, when told repeatedly, solidifying the magnetic 3-D pattern of illusion, making them seem real. Some common internal story dialogue goes like this, "I don't like the way my body looks" "I don't have enough money," "I'm not a good mother/father," "It's their fault," "I don't like them," "They took advantage of me," "They make me angry," "I'm too busy," "I don't want to do my clearing work."

All such stories are linked to addictive emotions we use to cover up our pain. Once we pause, Breathe, and use *Ancient Aramaic Forgiveness Freedom Tools* [Part 2: MIND] to clear our unconscious thought-emotional content, we get relief, implementing new patterns, Breathing in thought-forms based in LOVE. Loving Self.

> All things appear and disappear because of concurrence of causes and conditions.
> Nothing ever exists entirely alone; everything is in relation to everything else.
>
> *Buddha (563-483 B.C.)*

Attention (or story), according to what we've been learning in Quantum physics, holds the story in form, by keeping repetitive Attention on the *Field*, thus re-creating our "reality." Only when we change OUR THOUGHTS, does our "reality" change. The *Abraham Teachings* by Esther Hicks say we perpetuate our patterns by "beating the drum." Any emotion less than LOVE is a "denial drug,"distracting us from addressing and removing, painful thought-emotional content from our unconscious, still resonating in the *Field*.

Rage is potentially the most used drug on the Planet, along with the adrenaline "drug" of keeping "busy," with fear like the cherry on top. Painful emotions, rage, grief, sorrow, sadness and withdrawl are used to mask pain. When we access and clear our pain, we become free of the need to use these emotions for distraction. We function optimally, when we break free from the "comfort zone" of pain, and send LOVE Chemicals to our neuro-receptors. Response-Ability to clear our thought-emotional content at cause our pain (conscious-unconscious) is a courageous Leap. Once we do, we shift our World and our "reality" *FOREVER*. How fun will it be to be bursting with Joy and Creativity?

> The most precious gift we can offer others is our true presence. When mindfulness embraces those we LOVE, they will bloom like flowers.
>
> *Thich Nhat Hanh*
> *Vietnamese Zen Buddhist Monk, Teacher, Author, Poet, Peace Activist*

Buried within us is fear of punishment from the blame-fear-hostility culture. Our rage or grief is how we keep blame or punishment at bay, keeping others at a distance out of fear. Go back to our Power Person Dynamic [Part 2: MIND] to recognize what we are protecting ourselves from; [Part 2: MIND] - Level 1: What we did to appease our power person, Level 2: What we did to get back at them, Level 3: What they did we disliked most. Bringing these "corrupt programs" to the Light frees us from them. *Awareness = Freedom.*

> Without Darkness how would we know what Light is?
>
> *Legend*
> *1985 film*

An Ancient Polynesian teaching called Ho'oponopono, practiced today by Kahunas or healing priests in Hawaii, erases errors that Create dis-ease. Morrnah Nalamaku Simeona is a modern Kahuna, who applies these principles in today's World, clearing thought-emotional content from within self that is causing disharmony, engaging the active presence of LOVE. Through our research we discovered that even Ho'oponopono is rooted in Ancient Aramaic Teachings, where instruction was carried forward, for how to clear *ourselves* of Not of LOVE Mind-Energy holding resonance in a situation.

> If we can accept that we are the sum total of all past thoughts, emotions, words, deeds and actions and that our present lives and choices are colored or shaded by this memory bank of the past, then we begin to see how a process of correcting or setting aright can change our lives, our families and our society.
>
> *Morrnah Nalamaku Simeona*
> *Ho'oponopono Practitioner*

Notice any addiction to thought-emotion Not of LOVE, such as rage, busyness, grief, sadness, guilt, shame, or anything else. Remove them to clear the unconscious of this "old data." Depending on our choices in Life, we activate our *Essence* to varying degrees. Changing what is going on in our Life, is as easy as changing our thoughts! Once we get this everything changes. Clean out that unconscious container to change the resonance in your Life, LOVE yourself and reclaim your True *Essence forever...*

> Thankfully when we go into these negative expectations our prayer-fields collapse rather quickly, because we lose our connection with the divine and are no longer outflowing LOVE. A fear expectation can still be very powerful. That is why you must monitor your expectations carefully and set your field consciously.
>
> *James Redfield*
> *The Secret of Shambhala: In Search of the Eleventh Insight*

HEART COHERENCE: HeartMath Institute demonstrates Heart frequencies harmonize, when we experience *LOVE, COMPASSION* and *GRATITUDE*. Letting go incoherent emotions, and making the conscious choice to focus our Attention in this coherent spectrum, *powerfully changes our Lives* and those around us, our electromagnetic resonance and the World. *If all we do is take the step to focus in these three emotions above no matter what comes up in Life, we will shift internally towards LOVE.*

> Until we extend our compassion to all living beings,
> humanity will not find peace.
>
> *Albert Schweitzer (1875-1965)*
> *Nobel Peace Prize 1952, Physician, Philosopher, Medical Missionary*

Sometimes we need to know there is someone who LOVES us. As the Sufi's say, *"There is Only ONE, Being All of Us."* All we have to do is tap into It. It helps to find another, who will hold our hand while we are shifting into this new way of Being. Find them. It is helpful to know that we are not alone from a warm human standpoint. Get a hug - give a hug, share a Smile. Breathe. Find someone with whom you can watch dr. michael ryce's powerful videos for support in reclaiming your *Essence*. Remember, we are entraining our Minds to a *completely new way of thinking*. We are building "new brain cells." Create alliances with others sharing the journey. *The Buddy System works.* Breathe. Smile.

Stress is pressure that turns coal into a diamond. "We bring it on ourselves, for our Highest Good." Stress pressures our emotional body to release suppressed layers, surfacing like bubbles to Light of Awareness. We have suppressed emotion habitually overriding it, stress gives us a nudge to get our Attention. Stress is a combination of Resistance meeting Life Force, moving us toward opening to the flow of Life.

> Wherever you go, east, west, north or south, think of it as a journey into yourself!
> The one who travels into itself travels the world.
>
> *Shams Tabrizi (1185-1248)*
> *Beloved Mentor and Spiritual Teacher of Rumi 7 years; later said to have "disappeared"*

Once we actualize self-Mastery, we will relate to stress in new ways. Rather than at its affect, we recognize it is a *Healing Crisis*, coming up to shed light in dark places, Mirroring our "corrupt data" in our unconscious, for us to clear. Notice what resonance inside us is requesting our Attention to be released, let go of and canceled forever. "Yes, this situation is my Creation, from my resonance." Pay Attention. Get Clear. Breathe. Smile.

> There is no such thing as a problem without a gift for you in its hands.
> You seek problems because you need their gifts.
>
> *Richard Bach*
> *Illusions, The Adventures of a Reluctant Messiah*

Time pressure brings chronic stress, which we deal with like rats in a maze. What is it telling us? Slow down? Listen? Change your Life? A doorway to clarity? Clear these old "programs" with tools in previous chapters, particularly Power Person Dynamic..

> When you choose to be aware of behavior patterns that don't serve you,
> you are in a position to change them. That's empowerment!
>
> *dr. michael ryce*
> *Why Is this Happening To Me Again?!*

Breathe. Smile. Notice that what is going on around you is only as real as you make it as Observer-Creator, *by your Attention upon the Field.* Notice your Heart of Hearts, what does it Desire? *This is the Real Essence of You.* Do your best to bring about this desire in your Life. *Right, it might take changing a few things, AND it just might be worth it. No one else is to blame. Your internal content is "driving the boat."*

> People deserve to live in gentle, Loving environments where aliveness, delight and
> joy are the norm. Anything less is an insult to the human spirit.
>
> *dr. michael ryce, whyagain.org*

Remember, there is no 'out there' out there. Change your outer World by changing your inner World. Start inside first. Hidden within is the voice of your intuition pushed in the background so long ago, asking for you to give your Attention to something really important. *What was it? Listen to your Heart. Express your True Essence. LOVE you.*

What is real? How do you define 'real?' If you're talking about what you can feel, what you can smell, what you can taste and see, then 'real' is simply electrical signals interpreted by your brain.

Morpheus, The Matrix

Initiate deeper connection with Heart and *Essence*. Read this Commitment to Yourself daily. Reprinted with permission dr. michael ryce. *Download free at whyagain.org*

Commitment To Myself

I promise to TRUST myself enough to be willing to hear
and speak the Truth and treat myself LOVINGLY,
Gently and with Respect. I will do this in my thoughts,
words and actions, consistently.

In every interaction I will look for and acknowledge the
Highest and Best in myself, as I surrender to LOVE,
my true nature. Staying connected to my Source,
LOVE, and nurturing that relationship is more
important than any issue.

If anything unlike LOVE comes up, I will go to that
quiet place within where LOVE dwells. I'll listen to,
welcome and accept LOVE's guidance. I'll be teachable
as I ask to be inclined toward healing and shown how to
keep communication open in all relationships.

I'm willing to be RESPONSE-ABLE for my own
realities and learn to keep LOVE Conscious, Active and
Present as I HEAL and CELEBRATE Life!

When we Live in Pure LOVE, there is a place of no stress, just a flow of Beingness. *Stress is a Healing Crisis*. It is our "reality" asking to be set Free.

We don't understand things as they are, we understand them as we are.

Anais Nin (1903-1977), Avant-Garde Novelist

Stress is like the Cosmic Ringer Washing Machine, that promises to "squeeze the stuffin's out of us," until we get rid of all of our "old baggage," holding experiences of Not of LOVE in Creation. Relax. Release. Cancel your goals. Let Go. Breathe. Smile. LOVE. *"You Are A Shining Star,"* beaming your way into Being a ***21st Century Superhuman!*** ♥

Part 3: SPIRIT - SECTION 2
LIVING LIVES WE LOVE

You are a paradise, but you have forgotten yourself. You are looking everywhere except within you, and that is the only place where you are going to find the treasure, the truth of beauty.

Osho (1931-1990)
Indian Mystic, Teacher of Self-Inquiry

As we align as Beings of LOVE we express more meaningfully in our lives. We are drawn to pursuits through which we express our creativity, visions and dreams. We open ourselves up to New ways for Life to unfold around and through us.

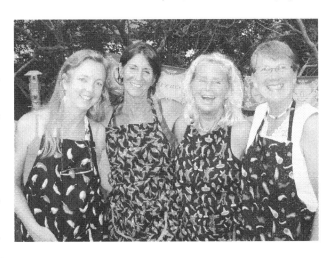

When we give ourselves to Life and say "Divine Perfection is unfolding," we are speaking Truth, because all that *can* unfold is *what IS*. Life and our World is Vibrational expression. Vibration emanating from us determines *EXACTLY* what emerges in our World. We are in the midst of learning to understand and embrace this. Letting go how we think things are, and committed to Who We *Are* from the *Heart*, changes *everything!*

> I have looked at all the danger in this world. Truly looked at it. All of it. And it is not on the outside, but comes from me. All of it.
>
> The only thing left for me to do is change danger into joy and the world will transform itself. All of it. I am no longer interested in how I can best react to the dangers of the world or how educated I can be about them. Any of it. I do not wish to exist in such a world. I would not want any of it. None of it.
>
> And so, it comes down to whether or not I feel I deserve to have what I do desire. Any of it or all of it or none of it. Whatever I vibrate outward in my beingness is what will be Created in my world. It must be so. I accept nothing less. Otherwise, I would have no purpose what so ever.
>
> I'm letting go of ...... a world of danger ..... a world of peril ..... a world of lack .... and a world of fear.

Allen Smith
RainbowDidge Music

Reflect on what is showing up in your World right Now, knowing the only way it is there, is as a result of thought *resonance* inside you. Check your feelings to determine whether you are happy with, or would like to change it. if change is the choice, *clear your ow unconscious data.* Then do a "ceremony," light a candle, say a prayer, Meditate, go deeper to connect with your Greater Being. *Be your own Shaman.* Tap. Shift your Vibration to LOVE for a more desirable result. Tell the Truth. Live from Authenticity and *Essence. Breathe Smile.*

This refinement process repeats itself, until we re-*Unite fully* with Higher-Self. Seek companionship and encouragement with others moving Consciously into LOVE. Challenge and change your patterns of thought, speech and behavior that impede your happiness. Deepen connection with your talents! Make your place in the World based on meaningful expression. Share with others of like-Mind, like-Spirit; Create community. *Access Joy!*

According to Gallup polls, only 20% Love their jobs and the remaining 80% dislike their jobs. *Wow!* Pouring ourselves into positions for security, duty and obligation, rather than expressing our True Talents and Abilities is a loss to us and the World. Waking up to our *Essence* and finding ways to express our Truth is an art, bringing forth our Unique Contribution that can come from no one else. Discover your own Creative Juicy Flow, to reap endless Rewards, offering your "True Service" to the World.

Polls show those who have *no Attention* paid them at work, disengage by 46% and after a few months get sick. Those who aren't ignored, but criticized lose interest by 20% *(ouch)* eventually getting sick also. *Those who are acknowledged **even once,** only lose interest by 1%!* Annual cost in US for disengaged employees: $380 million. *How ridiculous is this?* What kind of systems are we giving our lives to? Are we ready to *WAKE UP,* disengage from what doesn't serve us, get creative and empower ourselves to live *juicy* lives? *Let's do it!*

Surrounding ourselves with support and positive input, makes us *Healthier, Wealthier and Wiser! No surprise!* This wake-up call is our Great Opportunity to develop thriving Communities with like-minded family-friends, where co-Creation brings forth the *Essence* of each individual, intrinsic to the Whole.

Are you ready to develop a new path doing what you LOVE? It may take creativity to figure out how and what, yet your Health, Success and ALL in your Life will thank you for it! Those talented at business have a special role to play in these transitional times; *You* are a bridge to support establishing wise New enterprises, opening doors for others to *thrive!*

There is a wave of many on the *Planet,* Now stepping up to affirm Life and Live in their Joy. Operating from *Essence* takes the Destiny of self and our World into our own Hands. This is an Evolutionary Leap for HUmanity-HUwomity, to catapult us out of old perpetuated suppression, which we will look back someday and see as Ancient history.

The entire experience of our existence in this World is a biofeedback loop to let us know the quality of our Vibration, and how to "tune-up" our "operating system" to LOVE. **21st Century Superhumans** acting on this awareness, *IS* the **Shift of the Ages.** ♥

Part 3: SPIRIT
Chapter 5
Creative Genius - Following Your Bliss

A re you accessing your True Authenticity with full Self-Empowerment? If you're answering this question with a resounding, "Yes!" *...yeah for you!* If not, the very first thing to ask is, "What is my True *Essence* and how can I express it?" We may have a "story" that says our family or society "expects us" to do, Live or Be a certain way. Or for safety and security we must enter a particular profession or earn a certain amount of money. We will soon 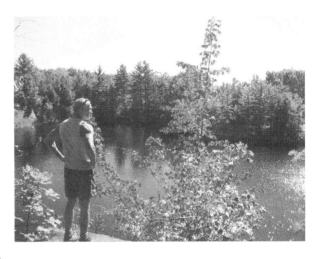 discover that even these thoughts of what "someone else" expects of us, begin *within us!* Our "old data" Creates and perpetuates this "story," inhibiting us from Living our *Essence.* Learning to be True to *Who We Are* and Be Authentic, is Vital during this **Shift of the Ages.**

The worst curse to befall anyone is stagnation, a banal existence, the quiet desperation that comes out of a need for conformity.

Deepak Chopra MD
The Return of Merlin

It's common in our society to conform to what's expected. Most forgot long-ago their deepest Desires, Aspirations and Dreams, sacrificed to "expectations" of the World. As we recover these precious aspects of our Individuality, we open doors to opportunities to fulfill us at the deepest levels, to carry us beyond societal norms that have kept us like rats in a maze or a hamster on a wheel, while our Creative Genius Awaits our Full Attention.

The most creative act you will ever undertake is the act of creating yourself.

Deepak Chopra MD, *Way of the Wizard*

Once we choose to move into greater self-expression, discovering how to accomplish this may be one of the greatest and most challenging adventures we embark on in our Life. We may feel we are running an obstacle course, juggling family, friends and job *with* True self-expression. We don't have to drop everything and walk away from what we have or are doing, (though some might), yet there are critical steps to escalate action toward Authenticity and *Essence.*

Give up defining yourself - to yourself or to others. You won't die. You will come to Life. And don't be concerned with how others define you. When they define you, they are limiting themselves, so it's their problem. Whenever you interact with people, don't be there primarily as a function or a role, but as the field of conscious Presence. You can only lose something that you have, but you cannot lose something that you are.

Eckhart Tolle
The Power of Now

9 Guides for Living Your Genius

- ❖ Stay fully Present in every Moment
- ❖ Remove "old data" to align with *Essence*
- ❖ Respond to and act from your Heart
- ❖ Tell the Truth
- ❖ Be Authentic
- ❖ Envision Your Possibilities
- ❖ Manifest Your Visions and Dreams
- ❖ Step through New Doors Opening

Enter more deeply into *full participation* right where you are, with whoever you're with, continuing what you're doing, heeding the *Heart* as your primary compass, *then if things need to change, they will change.* Use Ancient Aramaic "goal canceling" [Part 2: MIND] to *clear "old data."* Breathe. Smile. Tell the Truth. **Follow your Heart.** LOVE. Rinse. Repeat.

If we are an emerging species, wherever we are in our own lives that impulse within us for more Life, more meaning, more creativity is the same universal impulse toward greater consciousness and freedom that animated Life for billions of years. Our discontent, our passion to self-express, our yearning for higher quality Life are the universal force of creation manifesting uniquely as each of us.

Barbara Marx Hubbard
Conscious Evolution

The Body's only True drive is toward Life; in the same way our Heart moves Innately toward LOVE. Push through imagined shortcomings, hesitancy, insecurity, resistance, rage or fear, to Awaken what brings you *JOY,* and find New ways to shape your Life around it.

> You are LOVED just for being who you are, just for existing. You don't have to do anything to earn it. Your shortcomings, your lack of self-esteem, physical perfection, or social and economic success - none of that matters. No one can take this LOVE away from you, and it will always be here.
>
> *Ram Dass*
> *Polishing the Mirror*

It may at some point mean walking away from job or relationship - hopefully not, yet we sometimes grow at different rates than others. The more we center in LOVE, are Truthful, Breathe and Smile, giving Life to "the *Field*" to emerge in New ways, the easier and less bumpy our transitions are. Bumpiness comes from "old programs," or "logjams" in the river. The "river" pushes till we get clear. Work with your own internal process to choose "Waking Up" over being a "Sleep-Walker." Keep Body-Mind-Heart clear and clean.

> If you want to understand a society, take a good look at the drugs it uses. And what can this tell you about American culture? Well, look at the drugs we use. Except for pharmaceutical poison, there are essentially only two drugs that Western civilization tolerates: Caffeine from Monday to Friday to energize you enough to make you a productive member of society, and alcohol from Friday to Monday to keep you too stupid to figure out the prison you are living in.
>
> *Bill Hicks*
> *Comedian and Satirist*

Our singular expression as a Being is our deepest constant drive. ALL pain and suffering experienced in Life is but a cry from the Soul or our True Beingness, summoning us to remove every inhibiting Vibration, to get on track with and express *Who We Truly Are.*

> Without you, the world is without a source of many wonderful things.
> LOVE yourself wildly and spread it out to the world.
>
> *Sark, Best-Selling Author, Illustrator*

This dance of the flow Chi, Prana, Spirit, Life Force, Creativity is what we are learning to restore. It is *hugely* important in this Ever Present now, as Planet Earth's activations continue into the Ascension process, of an emerging New Civilization based LOVE. We are being activated, initiated, invited to join this Evolutionary Leap. This is why it feels like the pressure cooker has been turned up to "high." We are feeling impelled to grow, and *if we are still stuck in old ways,* our life may have become uncomfortable! Grow. Breathe. LOVE.

> A hero is someone who, in spite of weakness, doubt
> or not always knowing the answers, goes ahead and overcomes anyway.
>
> *Christopher Reeve (1952-2004)*
> *Actor, Director, Author, Activist - Superman*

Systems around the World appear to be falling apart, yet in Truth they are inharmonious with Who we are becoming and Where we're going. The old is restructuring as the New is being born. Those "Waking-Up" are stepping into Authenticity. Rather than continuing as cogs in an old system, they are illuminating creative solutions to activate exponential change. We can experience either World as they Now parallel one another. Knowing our thoughts Create we can focus on that which is "broken," or we can express wholeness, talents, creativity and intelligence to bring forth what we LOVE with passion.

People rarely succeed unless they have fun at what they are doing.

Dale Carnegie (1901-1955)
How to Win Friends and Influence People

ASK YOURSELF THESE QUESTIONS: Take out a clean sheet of paper and write down your answers with feeling. Date and save to review in a few months.

✦ What do I LOVE to do?

✦ What Am I good at?

✦ What are my talents?

✦ If I could do anything I wanted to, without regard to income or expectations of others, what would I do? What adjustments can I make in my current Life to actualize some of it?

✦ Describe your "Ideal Life" in detail (as if "it is" currently happening) include ALL items in list above, also incorporate how this assists the World to be a better place.

How does a person become an effective agent for Freedom? ...all that is required is to want to, and consciously choose to act as a free person. That changes his/her direction along the pebbles of the multiverse. By that choice, he/she begins directing the force of intent that flows through all of us, towards free action.

Rosalie Parker
You Must Free Yourself First

Joseph Campbell, inspired mythologist of the last century who developed StarWars' "hero's journey," offers the revolutionary idea, **"Follow Your Bliss...** and the Universe will open doors for you where there were only walls before." *Wow!* Remember the only "reality," is taking shape through our thought! ***Shift our thoughts, shift the Hologram!***

The power to change the world rests with you and you alone: For too long people have believed themselves to be weak, or relied upon others to change the world for them. You'll know that you're fully awake when you realize you have infinite power to change the world by simply living the change you want to see. First, you have to identify the principles that you believe in and then go out and live by them. If just a small minority took steps to do this, it would shake the establishment to its core.

TealScott
What kind of World do you want to live in?

We are learning to recover newborn innocence, uninhibited LOVE of Life and Freedom; this powerful current flows through us. As Dr. John Ray said, *"Your Perfect Electronic Blueprint already exists; all you have to do is step into it."* The only reason we haven't expressed every aspect of Who we are, is because we have a "unconscious" storage container, crammed full of Ancient thought-emotional patterns, like outdated "computer software." These thoughts from generational experience runs our Life! Clean out that old database!

> As you dive deeper into the heart, the mirror gets cleaner and cleaner.
>
> *Rumi, 13th Century*
> *Mystic Poet*

The "New software" of your Awakened Self, free of "unconscious" content will run far more effectively. Each of us is brilliant, gifted, sensitive and creative. *"Let the beauty we love be what we do. There are hundreds of ways to kneel and kiss the ground."* (Rumi) Once limiting beliefs are unwound, we express Greater-Self, harmonious with Heart-Soul.

> Sail along with your Newfound energy, speeding along to more completeness and wholeness within yourself. Finding your true self is your job. And the exploring is just beginning for many of you...the stage is set for each of you to move forward on the path you have chosen, all the while fitting into the whole to complete a bigger picture designed for the greater good of all.
>
> *Emily Leslie*
> *Lady Nada*

Once we change our programming, we step into a new, bigger phase of Life, from which we will never return. The Awakening consciousness is unstoppable, carrying us beyond where we've dreamed. Stepping onto the path, we hold our Vision before us and *emerge* into awesome New ways of Being, compatible with Who we Truly Are.

> Hope is not what we find in evidence, it's what we become in action.
>
> *Frances Moore Lappé*
> *Diet for a Small Planet*

Aligned with Heart, we tap into our capacity to succeed on every level. Aligned with guidance of Higher-Self and Source, the Universe responds by supplying ALL our needs.

> Once you accept His plan as the one function that you would fulfill, there will be nothing else the Holy Spirit will not arrange for you without your effort. He will go before you making straight your path, and leaving in your way no stones to trip on, and no obstacles to bar your way. Nothing you need will be denied you. Not one seeming difficulty but will melt away before you reach it. You need take thought for nothing, careless of everything except the only purpose that you would fulfill. As that was given you, so will its fulfillment be...for it rests on certainty and not contingency. It rests on <you.> And what can be more certain than a Son [or Daughter] of God.
>
> *A Course In Miracles, Chapter 20, The Vision of Holiness p 433*

Yogi Bhajan (1927-2004) became a Master of Kundalini Yoga by age 16, a rare feat. At 39 he immigrated to the United States from India, leaving a government career to realize the vision of bringing Kundalini Yoga to the West. He gave his first lecture at a Los Angeles high school gym in 1969. At his first presentation, not a single person was present, yet he came to teach and proceeded to speak to the empty hall. His work ultimately reached hundreds of thousands and initiated a movement of Awakening around the Globe, with over 300 centers in 35 countries continuing today (after his departure from this realm). He authored 20+ books, started natural food companies, and was considered a World leader.

The greatness of a man is not in how much wealth he acquires,
but in his integrity and his ability to affect those around him positively.

Bob Marley (1945-1981)

"He made his reggae music to uplift us, inform, entertain, inspire, and make change in the World; a musician, a poet and songwriter, a philosopher, a soldier, an activist and a leader." - Cedella Marley

Ask yourself, "Am I working just for money?" Or "Am I bringing my greatest gifts and talents to the World?" "Do I rest on the weekend, only to go back to another grind, an uninspiring routine, without satisfaction of fully expressing my Soul and unique gifts I brought into this world that may contribute to a better future for all?" "What would happen if each of us made the transition into doing only what we LOVE?" *Our World would certainly change, entering a New "reality" of wholeness...* Though it may seem like a big adjustment, consider which World you'd rather Live in, and set sail that direction! Start where you are and shape your Life gradually to Live with passion!

The world without spirit is a wasteland. People have the notion of saving the world by shifting things around, changing the rules, and who's on top, and so forth. No, no! Any world is a valid world if it's alive. The thing to do is to bring Life to it, and the only way to do that is to find in your own case where the Life is and become alive yourself.

Joseph Campbell (1984-1987)
The Hero's Journey

As each of us steps into this New way of being, with shifts and changes to Live from expression of the Heart, a New society is born. Going beyond old dynamics, "I can't do this because…" to "I Am that I Am…" we restore our true design LOVE.

You should never hesitate to trade your cow for a handful of magic beans.

Tom Robbins

In our current state of affairs many or most live a form of enslavement. We have been doing this for so long, we barely know how to grow beyond it, and yet this cultural belief system has certainly outlived its usefulness. There have been Awakener's throughout the ages who have attempted to get humanity to become self-aware, and step into greater potential. Each of us is brilliant beyond measure, with creative potential to express for the highest good of ALL humankind. As Henry David Thoreau said, *"This World is but a canvas to our imagination."*

> I am thinking this morning of the men in the mills and factories; I am thinking of the women who, for a paltry wage, are compelled to work out their lives...I never more fully comprehended than now the great struggle between powers of greed on the one hand and upon the other the rising hosts of freedom. I can see the dawn of a better day for humanity. The people are awakening. In due course of time they will come into their own.

> *Eugene Victor Debs, Orator (1855-1926)*
> *American Labor Movement Leader, Ran for U.S. President 5x, Nominated Nobel Peace Prize*

Steve Jobs, Founder of Apple Computer and great visionary of our day, carried his ingenuity beyond every wall that told him it couldn't be done. In 2013 Apple dethroned Coca Cola as the "top brand" in the World (Bloomberg Business Week). The 2013 movie on his life *Jobs* is inspirational, showing how passionate he was that every person should have access to easy to use, understandable computer systems. Were it not for Steve Jobs driving way beyond the norm after his passion, we would not have the multitude of user-friendly computer products we have today. He left us before age 60 with these words:

> Here's to the crazy ones. The misfits. The rebels. The troublemakers. The round pegs in the square holes. The ones who see things differently. They're not fond of rules. And they have no respect for the status quo. You can quote them, disagree with them, glorify or vilify them. About the only thing you can't do is ignore them. Because they change things. They push the human race forward. And while some may see them as the crazy ones, we see genius. Because the people who are crazy enough to think they can change the world, are the ones who do.

> *Steve Jobs (1955-2011)*
> *Founder Apple Computer*

Each of us is Newly emerging from the *Field of possibilities* every moment. Who We each Are is *uniquely significant* to the Whole. Rumi says, *"Behind every atom of this World hides an infinite universe."* Aligning with Greater Possibilities we restore our True Design LOVE, expressing *Essence* as our One Ultimate Task, and the Lights go on! We shift the entire Hologram and ripples move throughout our World as we *Arc the Hologram with LOVE!*

> *Sadhana* is where you sit, dwell in thoughts and words of the soul, peel away all your non-reality with the vastness of your spirit. If you train your mind this way, then you will discover something for yourself. If you live in absolute fearlessness, God will live in you because fear and truth cannot go together.

> *Yogi Bhajan*
> *Introduced Kundalini Yoga to the West*

It takes courage for those Awakened to move in New directions, Breathing, Smiling. Yes as we do so, we open the way to a viable future. We are a Collective in crisis with "issues to solve," the result of thousands of years of misplaced Mind-Energy, that as we shift into our Hearts, changes in an instant. What better way, than to have *7 BILLION* Minds-Hearts coming up with solutions and New ways to express our magnificence here on Planet Earth as a model for future civilizations throughout our Galaxy and beyond?

> A powerful key to determining our experience ahead comes from a shift, inviting us beyond asking, "What can I get from the world that exists," to asking, "What can I offer the world that is awakening?" How we answer this question becomes our collective answer to what comes next.
>
> *Gregg Braden*
> *The Divine Matrix*

Until we change our programming, we keep doing the same we always have. As Albert Einstein says, *"Problems cannot be solved at the same level at which they were Created."* Tony Robbins says, *"In order for things to change you've got to change,"* and Rumi says,

> Why stay in the cage when the door is open?

The Universe is simple. What you choose to Create with your thoughts is the World you'll Live in - the one with Joy, Abundance, Creativity, Laughter, Play and Peace is knocking at your door. Awaken Now to shift your thoughts moment-by-moment to LOVE.

> I am the journey of a billion stars,
> and I am the miracle of a mind awakening to the journey.
>
> *Fernando Vossa*
> *Breakthrough Energy Conference 2012*

The "old World" may still be out there, yet by putting our Attention on the *Field* in productive ways, we are a non-participant in those things that no longer serve our Highest Good. This is a miraculous transformation going on inside us, recognizing ourselves as Observer-Creators, *MAKERS* of our "reality," throwing off the "old," dancing into the New!

> Not all of us can do great things. But we can do small things with great love.
>
> *Mother Teresa*

Are we ready for a World that solves its problems peacefully, with benefit and enough for ALL? Are we ready to Live as sovereign Beings, expressing our greatest talents through Creative Joyful Lives? *Yes we are!* **21st Century Superhumans** are now emerging by the thousands and millions Globally, and a *New World's a' Comin'....*

> I believe in the good things comin', comin', comin'
> Out of darkness light are pumpin', pumpin', pumpin'
> Who have I been, who am I becomin'?
> Everything's already alright, always alright, always alright...
>
> *Nahko Bear*
> *Black As the Night Lyrics*

Part 3: SPIRIT

Chapter 6

Living From *Essence*

Drop the idea of becoming someone, because you are already a masterpiece. You cannot be improved. You have only to come to it, to know it, to realize it.

Osho (1931-1990)

Indian Mystic, Teacher of Self-Inquiry

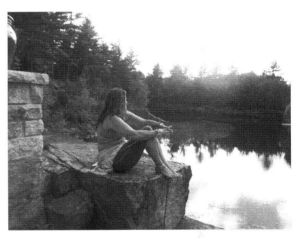

A dynamic fulcrum point for those who seek it is the moment of epiphany, when Life takes on New meaning and we commit to something greater than ourselves. In this Innate commitment we also awaken to deeper connection with the unique *Essence* of Who We Are.

Essence: The indispensable quality of something, without which it would not be what it is.

Do you remember innocent times of childhood when you Loved to dance, run, play, climb trees, have pillow fights, jump on the bed, shout with glee, smile sweetly? Think of what aspects of self you gave up to become an adult, conform to society or achieve what you thought was expected. Remember *your expressive "child"* and invite this delightful presence into your current Life.

You must find the place inside yourself where nothing is impossible.

Deepak Chopra MD

Natural Physician, New Thought Author

Imagine your sweet, spontaneous childlike qualities flowing through you, clearing away denser layers: reclaim joyfulness, spontaneity, easy Breathing and laughter, the natural desire to be heard and seen. *Breathe and Smile. Nice!* Invite your childhood dreams to bubble to the surface; they hold secrets to expressing your *Essence Now.* Smile. Breathe.

Always remember to judge everything by your inner feeling of bliss.

Osho (1931-1990)

Guru, Teacher of Self-Inquiry

When you're with children, get on their level, play, look into their eyes and listen to what they have to say. It's amazing what they teach us and help us connect with in our own "inner child." If you're a parent, delight in your children growing daily or being grown up; if you're a lucky grandparent spend time with your grandchildren, or simply enjoy being with children when possible. Absorb their childlike qualities to reclaim yours; nourish your *Essence* and restore the nature of your True Being.

> Dance like there's nobody watching,
> LOVE like you've never been hurt,
> Sing like there's nobody listening,
> Live like it's heaven on earth.
>
> *William W. Purkey*
> *Developer "Invitational Education"*

This Lighter state of being, births a new internal ecology from which to place our Attention on the *Field* with more creativity and awareness. When we *PLAY* in the *Field*, it's fluid. Letting go of expectations and making choices through the Heart makes it easier to enter 4 - 5-D, where molecules are less solid, particles are moving faster, potential is in wave form and objects are non-local in the *Holographic Universe*. Breathe. Smile.

> In a holographic Universe, location itself is an illusion. Just as an image of an apple has no specific location on a piece of holographic film, in a Universe that is organized holographically things and objects also possess no specific location, everything is ultimately non local, including consciousness.
>
> *Michael Talbot (1953-1992)*
> *The Holographic Universe*

3-D "reality" offers tangible feedback, instantly *Mirroring to us the resonance within us.* Rather than saying, "I don't like the way things are" when observing our Mirrored "Creation," we know how to shift *our* internal resonance, releasing thought-emotional patterns "Not of LOVE." "Reality" continues to act as our Mirror, with feedback on how we're clearing "old data," rewarding us as we do so with a more harmonious "reality."

> Is there a story you've been telling...that is holding you back from where you want to be? The story that you tell so much, you don't even realize you're telling it?
>
> Well, STOP IT!! ...Telling the same story over and over holds you right where you don't want to be...- in that story!! Speak of the positive aspects of your life and your dreams. Telling a new story with passion raises your vibration so much that your new story can became your new reality. Image-in the possibilities!!
>
> *Sierra Goodman*
> *Oceans of Inspiration*

Activate New desires by "marrying thought and feeling in the Heart, as [if] it has already occurred." Remember the "pray rain" story? [Part 2: MIND] Feel the mud between your toes and under bare feet, it *IS* raining! Offer the *Field* your Vibration, centered in

"Compassion without judgment" and *it is so.* Use these skills to set in motion your Desires and Dreams of how and what you'd like to Create in your World flowing from *Essence.*

Man is the creator of change in this world. As such he should be above systems
and structures, and not subordinate to them.

Steve Jobs, Apple company mission statement 1980s

The most empowered thing we can do, is renew our sense of connection, inspiration and vision with our own *Dreams.* Recall what you dreamed as a child; hidden within these are clues to your greatest talents that once upon a time were set aside to become a cog in the wheel of society or someone else's dream.

Creativity is the greatest rebellion in existence.

Osho (1931-1990)
Indian Mystic, Guru and Teacher of Self-Inquiry

Asking ourselves, "Who's in there and what will she-he be happy doing?" can open doors to move toward becoming Who you Truly Are. *These personal answers can initiate a New way of Life.* Is there someone Living their Dream you admire or respect? *This could be you!* Observe qualities worth emulating. Consider what it will take to move *more* into your *Essence.* As each of us accesses True *Essence,* our Natural Brilliance flows through, and our Authentic self-expression inspires others to do the same.

Life begins where fear ends.

Osho (1931-1990)
Indian Mystic, Guru and Teacher of Self-Inquiry

Creativity intrinsic to our very nature, is often eclipsed in modern society by boring repetitive jobs, even if interesting at first. We emerge from Source continually creative, yet get worn down by stagnancy. Imagine every human on Earth, nearly 7 billion, living generative Creative lives. A completely New culture naturally emerges, ebbing and flowing with the Breath of Life, while natural Evolution pushes us toward Living from *Essence..*

Recover your *True Expression,* lost or given up long ago to fit in to society, business or "supposed expectations" of others. Find your own clues from childhood.

1. Are you spending time doing what you don't like, so you can spend *more time* doing what you don't like? Are you teaching your children to do the same?

2. Gregg Braden points out the *Divine Matrix* can only Mirror the resonance we give it. For our "reality" to change, we must change *our internal thought resonance.*

3. Daily practice: Breathe. Smile. Clear the unconscious of 95% old data that needs to go *(Harvard studies).* [Part 2: MIND] Clear your Vibration, *free* your energy.

4. Rather than thinking of what you *don't like* in your Life; focus Attention through Mind-Heart. Send out *feeling* (Compassion without judgment) that what you desire IS. *(It's raining, toes squishing in the mud).* We are recovering the "lost art" of Living the Truth of our Essence; yes, it's a practice. Breathe and Smile.

5. Know the *Field* will send you perfect responses with insights *(comfort vs discomfort);* notice what adjustments will get you closer to your vision.

6. **Be In The Ever Present Now!** (future-past don't exist). Breathe and Smile.

A great example is Steve Jobs, whose drive to accomplish his dreams when others had *no idea* what he was doing, and a core sense of purpose that never left him *even when he was kicked out of his own company,* brought forth some of the greatest innovation of our time, changing the face of personal computing *FOREVER*. His phenomenal ideas produced user-friendly technology, resulting in a company worth more than Google and Microsoft combined. The 2013 movie *Jobs* is an inspiring study on a *"visionary with a sense of purpose."*

> You're going to spend a great deal of your time in the workforce. Find something you can put your Heart into, do good for the world, and you'll never *work* another day in your Life. [service]
>
> *Steve Jobs (1955-2011)*
> *Founder, Apple Computer, Jobs, the movie*

As activations from the Cosmos pour upon us and Quantum physics opens doors to a New perception of "reality," we are getting a clear "reboot." Transcending the judgment-control-blame-fear-hostility culture, as empowered Observer-Creators, we discover "safety and security" *are a result of our true expression,* rather than given in exchange for it.

> Life can be broader once you discover a simple fact. Everything around you called Life was made up by people no smarter than you. You can change it, you can influence it, you can build your own things that other people can use. The minute you understand that you can poke Life, and when you do, something will pop out the other side, you can change it you can mold it.
>
> That's the most important thing. To shake off this erroneous notion that Life is there and you're just gonna live in it, versus embrace it, change it, improve it, make your mark upon it. Once you learn that, you'll want to change Life and make it better, because it's kind of messed up in a lot of ways. Once you learn that, you'll never be the same again.
>
> *Steve Jobs (1955-2011)*
> *Founder, Apple Computer, Secrets of Life video1994*

Lynne McTaggert's book, *The Field,* has been called, "the book that lifts the veil on a state of being that is our birthright." In it she offers a glimpse "down the rabbit hole" as to how close our thoughts are to our "reality" in Quantum Creation:

> It appeared that the unconscious mind somehow had the capability of communicating with the sub-tangible physical world - the Quantum world of all possibility. This marriage of unformed mind and matter would assemble itself into something tangible in the manifest world... Both the unconscious mind, a world before thought and conscious intention - and the 'unconscious' of matter - the Zero Point Field - exist in a probabilistic state of all possibility...

When you get far enough into the Quantum world, there may be no distinctions between the mental and the physical. There may be only the concept... There might not be two intangible worlds. There might be only one - The Field and the ability of matter to organize itself coherently.

...the Coherence of consciousness represents the greatest form of order known to nature...that may help shape and Create order in the world. When we wish for something or intend something, an act which requires a great deal of unity of thought, our own Coherence may be, in a sense infectious.

...On the most profound level...studies...suggest that "reality" is Created by each of us only by our attention. At the lowest level of mind and matter, each of us Creates the world.

Lynne McTaggart
The Field, The Quest for the Secret Force of the Universe

This Coherence of consciousness or Unity of thought is best achieved when we Live from *Essence* aligned with Heart and True-Self. It can be a *huge* leap beyond our familiar comfort zone. Our *Essence* is our best "operating system." When it is running effectively with no "virus" or "old files" to slow it down, we shine through. Living this, our True Design LOVE, takes us into major transformation, significant for us and the Collective, as we each profoundly affect the whole.

LOVE is not an activity of the mind, but is the 'Pure and Luminous Essence' which Creates mind. This Essence from the Great God Flame streams into substance, and constantly pours itself out, as Perfection in form and action. LOVE is Perfection manifest. It can only express Peace, Joy, and an outpouring of those feelings to all creation – unconditionally. It asks nothing because It is Eternally Self – Creating, being the Heartbeat of the 'Supreme.'

LOVE owns All and is only concerned with setting the Plan of Perfection into action in All. It is a constant pouring out of Itself. It takes no cognizance of what has been given in the past, but receives It's Joy and maintains It's balance by continual Out-streaming of Itself. Because this Perfection is within LOVE forever flowing forth, it is incapable of recording anything but Itself.

Godfré Ray King
Original Unveiled Mysteries 1936

As we Live within our True "operating system" LOVE, the energy field around our Heart spins in a torus" field extending 8-12' around us, radiantly sending our Coherent electromagnetic resonance into the World. *Wow!* ***Arcing the Hologram!***

Our work is to observe our non-serving behaviors and patterns without getting pulled in and triggered. We observe and catch ourselves in the act of running old patterns and behaviors, LOVINGLY shifting them into new behaviors and patterns serving our highest good. Name em', claim em', shift em! Be a conduit of LOVE and the highest good for yourself and for others.

Sierra Goodman, Oceans of Inspiration

When there's a "ripple in our "reality," we notice the thought-emotion inside *us*, and that *we* have *clearing* to do. How about News, wars, unrest in the World, GMOs, crazy politics and economics? Yup! It's all a Mirroring of energies *within us, reminding us to "clean house" and let it go.* If we are seeing these things around us, there is a residual of judgment-control-blame-fear-hostility in our unconscious, "asking" to be released to LOVE. *As we clear to LOVE and Live from Essence, our "reality" Mirrors it!*

What if I should discover that the poorest of beggars and the most impudent of offenders are all within me; and that I stand in need of the alms of my own kindness, that I myself am the enemy who must be LOVED -- what then?

Carl Jung
Founder of analytical psychology (1875-1961)

At *Science & Non-Duality Conference 2013 (Youtube)* Bernardo Kastrup PhD reveals that in expanded awareness, brain activity *decreases* and we are *outside* the brain in *Greater Mind* (*Holonomic Brain Theory*) - Greater Self - Oneness. From altered states of consciousness we amazingly enter into an expanded state of Greater Mind - Greater Self, as Einstein did.

We are individualized "whirlpools" in the *Stream of Mind,* focused in our own little vortex, though still part of *Greater Mind.* A whirlpool in a stream is self-localization, yet *it is still the water.* Our brain is a "gatekeeper" or "filtering mechanism" for Greater Mind, creating our own "whirlpool" of individualized "reality," yet still part of Greater Mind.

Kastrup says, "...the brain does not generate the Mind in the same way the whirlpool does not generate the Water... Individual consciousness is a whirlpool in the flow of Mind - Greater Self - Oneness. ...From my reality my whirlpool is the center of the World...This is a metaphoric way of seeing what we are." When we contract into fear, stress or Not of LOVE thought-emotion we focus inward. The tighter our whirlpool becomes, the more we isolate in self-focusing, often to exclusion of all else around us.

We experience the outer World as "ripples" across the Stream of Mind, as they enter and make waves in our whirlpool. Kastrup encourages expanding our sense of Being by relaxing our whirlpool. Fear keeps us in tightly contracted whirlpools. "Eliminate the junk that culture and education have put in your Mind...this is a collective dream..." In expanded awareness our "whirlpool" is less defined, we are more interactive with what is around us, Greater Mind- Greater Self, creative expression and flowing with All That Is.

Releasing and letting go, trusting, flowing, integrating with Heart, we unite with ALL that Is - Greater Self - Oneness, to expand, flow and express through our True *Essence* in this World, as *21st Century Superhumans.* ♥

Our history is being reborn. There should be no doubt that each and every one of you [us] has been called to add a grain of sand in the growing process of this great mountain that leads to eternity.

Mallku Aribalo
The Awakening of the Puma

Part 3: SPIRIT
Chapter 7
Superhuman Abilities

Man-Woman is so made that when anything
fires their Souls, impossibilities vanish.

Jean de la Fontaine (1621-1695)
French Fabulist and Poet: "The Fables of la Fontaine"

Once we acknowledge our ability to access Higher states of consciousness, what once seemed miraculous, suddenly becomes "normal." We begin to Live through Heart and *Essence* by cultivating daily practices of thought-clearing, reverence for ALL Life, heeding intuition and daily meditation-prayer. "Prayer and meditation do not let God-Source know we are here, it reminds *us* God-Source is there and to trust the *Field!*" Such practices align us with Authenticity and the Heart, which is when "paranormal" talents readily appear.

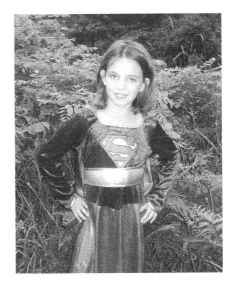

Synchronicities become apparent, and we notice episodes of precognition and telepathy that become a regular part of Life. What we used to call the "veil" between worlds seems to have become very thin (or not there) for those in higher Vibrational consciousness. With greater awareness comes the realization that we often do know events before they happen. Much occurs that we might have in the past interpreted as coincidence, yet we Now can see well-orchestrated synchronicities. We notice events happening, and we had thought them just recently (precognitive). We think of a friend, and the next thing we know, they call or are at our door. We heed our "still small voice," noticing that intuition has become our regular guide. People seem transparent - we carrying on a conversation, yet beyond the words we have full awareness of intent. At the same time, we know our thoughts Create our World, and "there is no 'out there' out there," so no matter what we sense from others, we infuse LOVE into every moment, clearing ourselves first. We may begin to notice we have precognition about people and events before they happen.

Many during this Ascension transition, are experiencing and demonstrating extrasensory or paranormal abilities. Immersed constantly Now, in intensified *Fields* of Light, our DMT is activating, elevating Body in frequency, so manifestations and transformation occurs. *As more of our 12 strand DNA connects, as we align with our True Design LOVE, the miraculous naturally appears with ease as everyday occurrences:*

- Lighter Body, ease of movement, higher frequency cellular structure

- Less food, lighter nutrition, raw-living foods, *prana* - Breatharianism for some

- Immunity to dis-ease; continual Rejuvenation and Youthfulness

- Increased mental powers, more Brain Capacity, Higher Intelligence, non-linear Dimensional Thinking

- Living outside time, Changing Timelines with LOVE

- Critical Mass - Higher Consciousness affecting others, Earth and beyond

- DNA data storage reprogrammed by sound, tones, words and language

- Transmission of Higher In-formation through DNA, wormholes, time-space

- Multidimensional chakras: DNA longevity upgrade; new 'operating system'

- Advanced Telepathy, ability to do mind-melds

- Companion Higher-Dimensional Beings: Angels, Ascended Masters, Guides

- Interaction with Allied, Highly evolved Extra Terrestrial Intelligences

- Rebalancing logical Mind and Heart, opening Heart-Space from inside

- Resonance with Soul purpose, aligning with Over-Soul

- Emerging new systems, flooding the old with Light, releasing shadows

- Discovering safety and security in the Flow of Creation rather than structure

- Awakening to new Levels of Being, Energetic Signature of Earth increasing

- Re-uniting with Soul-Mates, Soul-Community, Twin-Souls, Soul-Family-Fractals

As we integrate these new dimensions of experience as a natural part of our Lives, we may find ourselves disoriented in our regular "routine" 3-D "reality." As we clear our "old data," we establish a path to operate in New ways, and to open New possibilities in our "reality." Allowing for this inner transformation, opens doors in the outer.

The more you are out of balance or the more you are outgrowing this reality, the more the branch will become unstable to sustain you ~ meaning the branch is functioning as your vibrational reality. Time to move further to another branch is our advice or just clear some patterns of your thoughts to sustain that reality of which you are made.

The choice is always up to your own heart and soul as to where you wish to thrive toward, so take a few moments of your time every day to truly make that choice by heart, so as to continue your journey and life path in the most resonant vibration of your being.

Méline LaFont
Saint Germain -Current Unfoldings July 3, 2014

As we enter a more creative state of *BEING*, releasing "white knuckles on the wheel," to flow in Mind-Energy of LOVE, focusing 17 seconds, giving it to and trusting the *Field*, our structure actually lightens up. Density of 3-D body magnetizes into form by focus of Attention, shifting as we begin Living through the Heart, clearing "old data" and restoring our True Design LOVE. This process is different for each; a journey of unfolding.

Our dear friend Bill Ballard, focuses meditation and transmutation into Higher Dimensions working with Planetary grids, putting out inspiring videos on our current Ascension and shift process. Interestingly, in these videos his auric field is *visible* as ripple patterns behind him (*pearls2u*, Youtube). He has done much clearing and gone through deep transformation with Heart activation to raise his Vibratory frequency, maintaining a state of pure LOVE, and as a result is *a visible carrier of Radiant LIGHT* in this dimension.

Australian, Jasmuheen has sustained herself since 1993 primarily on prana, Light or Universal Life Force. Her books describe her journey, with a 21-day process to convert to this form of *sustenance*, with methods of self-healing, regeneration and rejuvenation. "Breatharians get nourished from the purest Source, the Universal Life Force which contains all bodily needs." Raising ourselves to a frequency where we can easily live without food is also not so far out of the question.

We *do live* on *prana* or Universal Life Force; physical food is an additional 3-D practice. Jasmuheen speaks around the World, with numerous followers on the path of living on *prana*. Having been with Jasmuheen in Mount Shasta in 2,000, she is authentic, and represents a rare but wonderful *Essence* of Higher Human expression, breaking boundaries of belief of what is possible in the physical.

Jasmuheen told us about the early days when she began living on *prana*. At first she became very thin. She spoke to her Body, to Creation, to her Guides and Teachers, to the place from where the energy of her being emerged. She told her body, "look we are healthy, we're living on *prana* it is important that we look like a normal type of Body." Within days 10 pounds were added. aligning with how she chose to appear in the World. She offers clues as to how one might live on *prana,* when others are starving for lack. It is a mindset, aligning with the flow of Life from the *Field of LOVE*. Obviously, this is not for everyone, yet we can become aware of *prana* sustaining us, and Live Lightly and "karma-free."

Determine what *you're* good at and LOVE to do. Find a way to do it. Create an environment in which you can express Authentically and work with others who LOVE what they do! Find those who enjoy working with you; offer one another positive input. Your Joyful Vibration and Well-Being extend into the Planet. Pain, illness, dis-ease and misfortune will disappear due to lack of Attention upon them. As we go into Greater Being step-by-step, synchronicities occur, "opening doors where there were only walls before..."

What man is a man who does not make the world a better place?

Balian of Ibelin
Kingdom of Heaven film 2005

We are in a waking up "wave," pineal and pituitary glands activated by Cosmic conjunctions, with exposure to faster moving and more intense particles of LIGHT, as our Solar System orbits through a rare place in space. Jose Arguelles, Mayan Calendar historian offers in *The Mayan Factor: Path Beyond Technology,* we are in a 5,125 year cycle "crossing the Galactic Beam" of intensified Light originating from the core of our Galaxy. Earth's Purification and Regeneration are events initiated by this "Galactic Synchronization."

Disintegration of *outmoded* economic and governmental systems will continue to be a natural process, as millions around the Planet Now hold frequencies of LOVE and LIGHT at unprecedented levels. Inharmonious systems become unsustainable, and New emerge, gently aligned with LOVE. This is exciting, as we recognize that disharmony in the outer is a reflection of Collective and personal disharmony on the inner. As we shift *our* internal focus and Vibration, the Collective reaches a *tipping point,* and our external World changes.

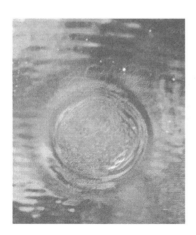

This is SIMPLE. It is Quantum. The *Field* offers our "reality," as an *exact* Mirroring of *Vibrational resonance within us,* a result of our conscious-unconscious Attention on the *Field.* Change your resonance; change your Creation, change your "reality," change your World. As we shift our Vibration, going out like ripples on a pond, we change the whole.

We we shift the entire *Holographic* existence, and ALL humanity adjusts. This is the 2nd Immutable Universal Law, describing how the ever-flowing *Field* of Creation operates. These Universal Laws guide us to realign ourselves with LOVE. The first Universal Law is that thought-emotion or *Mind-Energy* Creates; and the third is that all Creation is *Vibrationally* alive, ready to respond to *our* Attention upon it.

A new Species of HUman-wom is being born, with this Leap across the Evolutionary Spiral to a New framework. We are surfing the biggest wave in human history, dropping into the Heart, and living according to our True Design LOVE. *Surf's up kidz! Let's go!*

ALL on Planet Earth have potential Now to upgrade to higher frequencies, assimilating Cosmic qualities harmonious with LOVE, moving into finer dimensions. Change your "reality," change the World. ***21st Century Superhumans Arcing the Hologram Now!*** ♥

Part 3: SPIRIT

Chapter 8

Manifestation Of Abundance

*Don't be satisfied with stories of how things have gone for others.
Unfold your own myth.*

Rumi
Essential Rumi

W e exist in an ever-flowing *Field* of Abundant Life bubbling up "like effervescent ginger ale," magnetized by thought into form around us. We and our "reality" emerge anew each moment, as does ALL Creation! *NO-THING is "stuck" in its "current" form...*

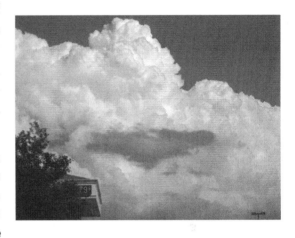

When you look with an electron microscope without a person in the room, what you see is a cloud. The electron is a cloud. It is hypothesized that this cloud consists of all the probability orbits that this thing can be. The very notion of a material world is no longer viable, now that we have discovered the ultimate building block of matter doesn't really exist. The atom is now thought of as more of a possibility entity by many leading physicists.

Dr. Richard Bartlett, Matrix Energetics

Let's take the idea of Abundance from a ***21st Century Superhuman Quantum Lifestyle*** standpoint. We *are* already ONE with All That Is. Any part of us that doesn't comprehend this yet is still caught, in Not of LOVE thought-emotional patterns to be cleared. Any gap in our belief system, between us and what is already ours tells us, "mine the gap!" Our blocks to Source energy limit access to what's there for us. Thousands of generations of thought put logjams between us and Innate Energy flow. It's important to clear these [Part 2: MIND]. Material goods, events and people in our World, are regulated by our "filters" established by our Mind-energy ("old data," Ancient resonance). Clearing thought, plugging into Source, expressing *Essence*, we access Abundance naturally ours.

Abundance is not a product of your circumstances, education or training - it is a result of your passion and purpose being expressed.

Rodolfo Young
totalauthenticity.com

Really. If you knew that if you detoxed your body and ate more vital foods, you would grow more abundant hair or it would make you slimmer would you do it? Probably! We have tended to do things more for external reasons than for internal. This is something to grow beyond, to empower access to our Abundance.

We are often addicted to what we think we want in the outer, to look better, have more or get Love. We have trained ourselves to bargain with God or the Universe for the end result, rather than becoming One with Who and What we Truly Are. Bargaining and affirmations help us find our way back to the trail, yet they are not the trail. The trail to Abundance is merged with Source in LOVE, clear from unconscious limiting thought.

Detachment comes from inner knowingness we are a pattern of behavior of higher intelligence. When things don't go our way, we let go our idea of how things should be. In our limited awareness, we cannot see the synchronistic, harmonious patterns of the universe of which we and our intentions are a part.

Deepak Chopra
Universal Law of Detachment

We are so used to thinking that what we'd like to get or have is outside of us and we need to pull it in or strive for it. This is backwards! In fact most of our current "progressive thought" around Abundance goes something like this: make your dream board, detailed list or imagine what you'd like to have in full living sensory color, and if you cross your eyes just right, leap three times in the air and say the right affirmations, it will come to you. This is a game to trick yourself into shifting enough internally to line up correctly with these things; however in truth, it will get you close, yet it's the long way to get there.

I'm trying to free your mind, Neo. But I can only show you the door.
You're the one that has to walk through it.

Morpheus, The Matrix

We are already ONE with All Abundance That Is! We have descended into "matter" in the 3-D World, thinking we are separate from Eternal Creative flow of Source. We are Now Remembering Who We ARE, Observer-Creators in this continually CREATING Universe. Giving hopes, dreams, visions, wishes and worries to the *Field,* letting them go with trust and Gratitude, brings us into receivership more quickly than worrying about what we don't have (holding it in form).

The Law of Detachment says that the way to acquire anything in the universe is to relinquish our attachment to it. The moment we combine one-pointed intention with detachment to the outcome, we have that which we desire.

Deepak Chopra
Universal Law of Detachment

We emerge into this Life, starting out with one tiny zygote or cell, carrying within it messages from millions of years of evolution and hundreds of thousands of years of thought, that by a miraculous process multiplies and grows into the Being we Become. Driven by our Soul, we have our own UNIUQE wonderful message we bring into embodiment with us, enhanced and shaped by our brilliant, kind, exciting Heart, Mind and Spirit. Abundance comes in many ways as we move into Authentic self-expression!

Heartfelt intention to make the choice to raise your vibration is the first step...Once intention is stated, we can drop expectations of how the guidance will come to us and begin to consciously think of already existing on a fifth dimensional planet.

The imagination is a very powerful tool in the Universal Law of Attraction and will become the way we will manifest instantly on the New Earth via thoughts. Imagine being part of a unity consciousness which is filled with peace, love, and goodwill toward all people.

Michelle Walling
What Most People Do Not Know About Manifestation

TAPPING FOR ABUNDANCE: We have mentioned EFT or tapping. (Look for our videos or others online). Use tapping to release and clear neurobiology connected with old limiting beliefs and thought-forms, along with Ancient Aramaic Forgiveness. Use a phrase to realign with your Oneness and openness to receiving Abundance of ALL that Is:

- *I Am that I Am the LOVE and the Light of the Universe.*
- *I Am the Eternal Abundant flow of Creativity.*
- *Breathing and Smiling I release my Desire to the Field.*
- *I invite the Field to bring my "reality" into form in New ways.*
- *Thank you for ALL the Miracles in My Life. Gratitude fills every cell of my Being.*

If you find me not within you, you will never find me.
For I have been with you, from the beginning of time.

Rumi, 13th Century Mystic Poet

Expressing our True *Essence*, our "piece of the puzzle" clicks into place. We emerge as the exquisite, sparkling, extraordinary Being we are, unique as a snowflake, harmonizing our own melodious Life flow through the Heart into our "reality" and our World.

There is only one important point you must keep in your mind and let it be your guide. No matter what people call you, you are just who you are. Keep to this truth. You must ask yourself how is it you want to live your life. We live and we die, this is the truth that we can only face alone. No one can help us. So consider carefully, what prevents you from living the way you want to live your life?

Shams Tabrizi (1185-1248)
Rumi's mystical mentor who after 7 years disappeared

Do you ever say, "If I just had more money my life would be better?" The Truth is when we step into Living from the Heart above ALL else, Abundance is ours. It is the Gift of existence continuously flowing to us from Source, as we clear away debris of "corrupt data" blocking its flow, and ground in LOVE and *Essence* we are. Entering the Heart we carry more Light, and reorganize our molecular structure. Loosening our grip on materialism, spiritual understanding awakens to guide us. Lighter Body brings freer expression to Life. Our good friend Stuart says, "Continuing to live in the Spirit of Gratitude and in awe of the mystery!"

Meditation is the best way focus our intent and scientifically assist us to manifest what we desire. We drop down into slower brainwave patterns as we meditate. Through this slowing of brain waves, we enter the *Field*, allowing "reality" to fall out of form and emerge in New ways. Thoughts we carry into the *Field* in our meditations have the excellent possibility of transcending probabilities, as gentle waves rippling through the ocean of timespace bring New circumstances into form.

> This world is like a mountain. Your echo depends on you. If you scream good things, the world will give it back. If you scream bad things, the world will give it back. Even if someone says badly about you, speak well about him. Change your heart to change the world.
>
> *Shams Tabrizi (1185-1248)*
> *Rumi's mystical mentor who after 7 years disappeared*

As we cultivate ability to drop into this state with regular practice, we more easily merge with the *Field*. Numerous studies expose increased synchronicities, precognition, increased anti-aging hormone, improved events-circumstances with regular meditation. Although many forms of meditation suggest nose Breathing, we prefer open mouth, as it opens the HU, open exchange of Breath with Source (letting go holding patterns in Body).

We surround ourselves with Light and LOVE, inviting support from Higher Realms: Source, Creator, Yeshua-Jesus, Christed of Buddhic consciousness, Guides-Teachers, Angels, Ascended Masters, Great Rainbow Brother-sister-hood, Loved Ones, a myriad of hierarchial Beings in Realms of Light. We experience what we are ready for, and what we are not, is not visible. When we are ready we will be invited or it will be opened.

> We look forward to greeting you in the realms of full consciousness and when we do, you can take pride knowing that you had played the largest hand in your own personal evolution and in those of every other Soul who will be with you and us in these wonderful realms.
>
> Remember that you are Divine, and that everything around you is comprised of the same Divine energy of LOVE and perfection.
>
> *Wes Annac*
> *The Hathors*

Not sure if you want to meditate? That's ok. Check at our website for guided audios (soon) to activate similar states, opening to consciousness in altered brainwave frequencies for ease of manifestation. In aligning with Abundance, cultivate Brain-Heart coherence where intuition, pre-cognizance and synchronicities are a natural part of everyday Life.

MORNING-EVENING FOCUS: When you wake in the morning and/or before going to sleep at night, go into the *Field* through meditation and Breath. Invite everything in your current reality to "collapse out of particle form," become waves, and collapse into the *Field.* This means your body, financial situation, pets, relationships, home, stress, worries, vehicle, garden, business, job, animals, children, parents, World, aches and pains, anything else you can think of... Let it all collapse into the *Field,* invited to return to New form with LOVE.

Thousands of years of "slavery" in various forms on Planet Earth reported by Michael Tellinger in *Slave Species of the Gods,* depicts a dominant race keeping others subservient with a system of rewards and punishment from god/gods (small g where stories were fabricated for control), punishing the disobedient and pseudo-rewards for the obedient. We ALL may carry residual thought in the shadows of our unconscious from this.

We have concluded much of the deeper work we've done, with clearing unconscious shadows of dark fear and rage, were stored generationally as a result of such Ancient roots. Without going further into it here, we encourage adventurous Souls drawn to topple long held beliefs and shift awareness, please do check out Michael Tellinger's extraordinarily revealing books and videos on this history to break Free from such patterns, and learn to cancel this "old data" from your unconscious in Part 2: MIND.

If you are at a job you don't like, remaining out of "obligation," if you're in an unfulfilling relationship, sticking it out for sake of "duty or fear of lack" if you're participating in a system you don't like, yet continuing out of "fear of rocking the boat," it is time in this Now Moment to Wake Up to your Heart! The World is missing out on awesome nourishment to the Greater Whole that will occur when YOU release tens of thousand of years of thinking based in human bondage, and enter into expressing joyfully Who YOU Are!!! *Arc the Hologram* with LOVE. As you so do, you free others involved as well, to go on and explore Living their *Essence.*

Support others by freeing Yourself! Yes this might take a bit of unwinding, yet is so Worth It!!! Get going...and if you have *"maybe someday..."* written across your forehead, use the Ancient Aramaic Forgiveness process and let go old "corrupt data" still running the show. [Part 2: MIND] You *will* rock the boat. The World *will* change. Others will be drawn. Aligning with Authentic Truth of Your Heart, the entire Hologram shifts. REMEMBER, "There is no 'out there' out there." *It begins and ends inside of you.* The more Joy and Truth you connect with, the more contagious it becomes. Your Life *will* change others' Lives.

The more you are motivated by LOVE,
the more fearless and FREE your action will be.

The 14th Dalai Lama

Esther Hicks' Abraham Teachings tell us, anything we focus on for 17 seconds is enough to set the *Field* in motion, and results in Creation. As we release our thought-emotion from Heart we allow the Universe/*Field*/Source to take over. We dream, focus, and stay unattached to the outcome. This is what Abraham calls, "Going General," a very important Key in Quantum Creation and staying in the flow; focusing then letting go.

This is such a departure from how we're used to thinking, worrying and obsessing; can't you just see a dog shaking its tug-toy and not letting it go? Recognizing this resistance in our old style of thinking is the first part of self-Mastery. The second is honoring the aspect of Mind-Heart that is Observer-Creator by its Attention on the *Field*, managing our internal "content," rather than default. The third is Knowing the Universe is Abundant.

> Once you truly understand that we live in an abundant Universe, you allow yourself to become the kind of person who who Creates that which you desire, instead of one who settles for what you can get.
>
> *Jen Sincero, Best Selling Author*
> *You Are A Badass, Stop Doubting Your Greatness, Live An Awesome Life*

Shifting to Living Abundantly requires managing our internal state. Anything we hold Attention on for 17 seconds is likely to manifest! Attention to old patterns, even unconsciously holds them in form. Release, let go, get clear, trusting our needs are supplied, realign connection with All That Is, and Life flows.

> Dream on, Dream on, Dream on,
> Dream until your dreams come true...
>
> *Steven Tyler, Aerosmith*
> *Dream On, Lyrics*

Knowing the Infinite *Field* has unlimited (*millions and billions*) ways to come into form, beyond what we imagine; invite the *Field* to send wave forms of potential into matter. Put your Attention on it and then let it go. Welcome the expectation you will be living in a New "reality" shifted beyond where you were before.

> Be thankful for what you have in the moment
> and more will be added unto you.
>
> *Jack White (1934-1998)*
> *God's Game of Life*

Let it go. Trust the Force Luke. Give it to the *Field.* Breathe. Smile. The *Abraham Teachings*, *"Go general."* Instead of holding onto what we *think* we want, or going over and over it, we give it to the *Field*, trusting what comes back will be beyond *PERFECT.* Breathe, Smile. Give it to the *Field* again and it will shift *more.* The *Field* can only respond in kind to Mind-Heart energy we give it. Clear the unconscious till resonating LOVE and Create from this place.

> Be glad that you don't have instant manifestation. This buffer of time is really your friend. It's your opportunity to observe and to ponder and to visualize, and to

remember. It's your opportunity to take an Emotional Journey that might be different from what you're actually observing.

Esther Hicks
Abraham Teachings

When there is a strong desire to have something, such as vehicle, home, job, relationship, dream about it, write it, put a picture on the dream board, know how much you LOVE it, then *give it to the Field. Give it to the Creation process.* Trust. Focus to put it in motion; then let it go and trust. In Abraham's words this is the *"Art of Allowing."*

Imagine your highest dream of who you want to become, and your greatest vision falls short of that which the Divine has in store for you.

Esther Hicks
Abraham Teachings

Earlier in the last century the idea was brought forth that our thoughts Create, in writings such as Napoleon Hill's *Laws of Success*. Lesser known though equally brilliant were writings and lectures of others such as Neville Goddard.

Neville captured the sheer logic of creative-mind principles as perhaps no other figure in his era. This "New thought" opened the doors for us to begin comprehending at deeper levels, how thoughts and emotions Create. Every great wisdom teaching contains instruction to be mindful of where our attention is placed....[He] was one of the quietly dramatic and supremely influential teachers in the New Thought field for many years...

Mitch Horowitz
Searching for Neville Goddard

Neville studied with an Egyptian mystic named Abdullah, of whom very little is known. However it is told that Neville spent 5-7 years exclusively with him, absorbing lessons from Hebrew, Ancient Aramaic, and the Kabbalah. Joseph Murphy who studied with Neville wrote, "Neville may eventually be recognized as one of the World's great mystics...we are privileged to use a Law given...to cushion the blows of Life. The Law, stated succinctly is this in Neville's words: "Imagining Creates reality." And "you must make your future dream a present fact by assuming the feeling of your wish fulfilled." This is exactly the emphasis of many Ancient traditional cultures; experience your vision as it already *IS*.

We are restoring our awareness that we are already One with All That Is. All Creation exists in the Ever Present Now. There is no past and no future, for in the Now Moment all Creation comes into Being. As we step into a place of Oneness and Gratitude, relax and trust the flow of Life, we send our vision out into the *Field*.

Affirm the now as your only active eternity. So shall Truth descend in full power upon you - not divided by past memories or future desire, but bursting with present fulfillment. No mortal lie can creep into the glory of the Ever Present Now.

Myrtle Fillmore 1939
Co-Founder Unity Church

Ask yourself, *"If there was there was no such thing as money, and I could be doing anything that I wanted, what would I do with my life?"* What if everyone on Earth said, "We are going to step out of the meaningless, and commit ourselves to the meaningful: Lives, solutions and Living from *Essence.*" Can you imagine how quickly our World would change? Find what makes *you happy,* and discover a path to do it. Build in a healthy transition. As we live from our Hearts and the Truth of our Being, we align ourselves with *Infinite Universal Supply,* and integrally put ourselves in receivership. Entering the Heart changes our hormones, emotional state, and opens our receptor sites, making us feel younger and more vital.

As we step into Living from *Essence,* aligning with Truth of our Heart, a new level of Beingness emerges. We feel ourselves flowing in the River of All That Is. We know that whatever appears in our Now "reality" is an absolutely perfect reflection of the energy resonating in us. *We fine-tune,* get more connected with Heart, removing more "old data," till LOVE and True Expression become the waves continually emerging and being Mirrored to us and from the *Field,* Abundantly. Following this path unlimited Abundance is ours.

> The greatest obstacle to abundance is not letting go of what you have now.
>
> *Rodolfo Young*
> *YourInspirationGuide dot com*

Meditation, cleansing, high frequency Lifestyle and other spiritual practices assist us to enter into clarity of Mind-Heart, where we are better able to call forth what we desire from the *Field.* The Edgar Cayce article, *"Time and No-Time"* at In5D.com Edgar Cayce tells us:

> Learn these lessons well: First, continuity of life. There is no time; it is one time. There is no space; it is one space. There is no force, other than all force in its various phases and applications. The individual is such a part of God that one's thoughts may become crimes or miracles, for thoughts are deeds. What one metes must be met again. What one applies will be applied again and again until that oneness of time, space, force are learned and the individual is one with the whole.
>
> *Edgar Cayce and John Van Auken*
> *Toward a Deeper Meditation*

Wow! Abundance flows to us **21st Century Superhumans**. We are aligning with Heart, freeing ourselves from false obligations, Living Authentically and radiating *Essence* into the World; putting forth our intent to the *Field,* Trusting, letting go Attachment and allowing, to restore our True Design LOVE. ♥

> The belief that there was ever a lack of Divine Love or Light or any other good thing that would be in support of Unity or Christ Consciousness has been one of humanity's greatest misconceptions as there simply is no lack unless it is Created and supported as a belief within the mind of the ego.
>
> *Masters Kuthumi and Lady Claire*
> *WalkTheEarthAsALivingMaster dot com*

Chapter 9

Changing Timelines

Be realistic - plan for a miracle.

Osho (1931-1990)
Indian Mystic, Guru and Teacher of Self-Inquiry

We are awakening to a powerful new understanding of our existence in Light of Quantum physics. It's an *inside job*, beginning in the Heart, giving clarity to how to *Live as LOVE.* Quantum "reality," provides a clear map, to change our future from inside out! Going beyond the experience of Life, as if "something outside of us is doing something *to* us," *everything changes* as we go within.

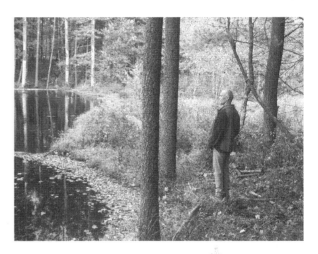

It has taken thousands of years,
yet within this century both scientists and spiritual seekers alike have once again begun to view laws of nature and laws of God as reflections of the same truth.

Rosalyn L. Bruyere
Clairvoyant, Healer, "Wheels of Light, the Spinning Chakras"

ANCIENT TEXTS HAVE ALWAYS TOLD THE STORY [*Part 2: MIND*] Truth Now revealed in Quantum Physics was always carried in Ancient texts.

1. ***In-formation from Ancient Texts collected by Gregg Braden***, (Nag Hammadi, Ancient Tibet and Native American) on effective "prayer or asking" of the *Field* or *Divine Matrix*, in "its" language, in order to receive what we are asking for. *These include:*

1) Chant, bowls, gongs, sing, pray to focus in: Heart - Compassion without judgment
2) "Marry Mind and Heart" - say to the mountain "move" and it will move
3) As [if] it "already *IS*" (mud between toes)

2. *Ancient Aramaic Texts* contain *explicit instructions* on how to operate our *"Biocomputer."* We invite *Rookha d'Koodsha* Feminine principle "anti-virus," to help cancel our "corrupt data." Then we activate elemental aspects or filters (firewalls), so only LOVE gets through: *Rakhma* activated by Smiling puts *Intentions based in LOVE* in place (front of brain), *Khooba* activated by Breathing puts *Perceptions based in LOVE* in place (back of brain), so ALL interactions shift to LOVE!

3. *Clay tablets from Sumer, 4000 B.C.* - 500,000 scattered in collections and museums around the World *(translations online):* 2,000 of these were documented in minute detail by late scholar-historian Zecharia Sitchin's rare cuneiform deciphering skills over three decades ago, substantiated in numerous fascinating books such as T*he Twelfth Planet* and *When Time Began.*

> a) Now at least 100 square miles of circular stone ruins in south Africa offer puzzle-pieces for cohesive rendering of this story Sitchin would have been thrilled to see. Exposed in Michael Tellinger's *Adam's Calendar* and *Slave Species of the Gods*, shocking yet clear evidence documents 200,000 years of history of a cloned slave race, possibly actually going back much further, with involvement from one or more off-Planet races.

This information awakens us to origins far beyond traditionally documented 7,000 year history. With these revelations we begin to understand why perhaps we may carry such deep layers of self-doubt and fear needing to be removed from our unconscious, in order to access a truly viable sense of self and our possibilities. The curious and open-minded will benefit from pursuing these historical details further, to awaken to the *deeper* sense of what is unraveling here. Sitchin has been called the most controversial writer of our time, because he challenges everything we thought we knew about human civilization.

> We are a fragile species on a knife's edge, precariously balancing between the rapid evolution toward the universal community of beings, or toward the destruction and extinction not only of humanity, but of the entire planet.
>
> The road forward is pretty clear, but we must find a speed of solution to the millennia of propaganda, religious oppression, dogma, and fear that have been so entrenched in humanity that it will take some kind of miracle from the real God to release those who are trapped by it.
>
> *Michael Tellinger*
> *Slave Species of the Gods*

Have you ever wondered about undercurrents in World culture of such insane and inhumane practices as racial prejudice, sexual abuse, sex trade, slavery and near slavery in sweatshops and diamond mines, killing of innocent men, women and children in wars for oil in "foreign countries," training young men and women to kill, governmental and economic systems draining life-blood from citizens everywhere, 147 bloated corporations and a few ultra rich families owning all the World's "wealth," devastating Earth Mother Gaia, her indigenous people and creatures destroyed nearly to extinction for material gain? Have you ever wondered why we treat Earth as a resource, rather than honoring her as our Home? How many do you know, living happy lives, without struggle? Has the thought crossed your mind, whether it's viable for ALL to live in Peace, Harmony and Creative Joy together on our beautiful Planet? *IT IS,* ***AS SOON AS WE CLEAR OUR "CORRUPT DATA"*** holding resonance in the Field. [Part 2: MIND]

The wound is the place where the Light enters you.

Rumi (1207-1273)
13th Century Persian Poet, Sufi Mystic

How many are fearful to do much except what we're *supposed* to do? Subject to corrupt governmental, economic and corporate systems, the majority are afraid to speak up, for fear of being locked up, imprisoned or rights eroded by corrupt outmoded systems. Multibillions have been spent on wars and weaponry, while millions starve, with little clean water, no sanitation and rampant illiteracy in much of the World. Step back and notice this broad historical perspective, asking yourself where you are in relation to it.

I believe in the principle declared at Nuremberg in 1945: Individuals have international duties which transcend the national obligations of obedience. Therefore individual citizens have the duty to violate domestic laws to prevent crimes against peace and humanity from occurring.

Edward Snowden

We are Living in the unfolding of circumstances in which we may need to find ways to speak or stand up. Equally or moreso, it is essential to cancel, clear, release, let go the Vibrational content *within us* (conscious-unconscious) resonating from our generations to hold these things in being. For the majority it is easier to go into denial (food, drugs, alcohol, busy, rage), than removing our own "old data". When we first learned about this, we thought, "*No it has to be someone else's fault*; someone bad out there is making this mess, the pollution the wars, the ignorance, the suffering." WRONG. *Clear our own "old data!"*

Fear is a powerful seducer. It plays subtle games that can turn peace into uneasiness. It dances in the shadows waiting to take our mind on a twirl into darkness of all that is false. It screams it's own truth, it shouts, slaps, burrows and buries itself within our psyche to keep the false self alive in the game. Fear is our creation. Brought in as a master teacher to hide ourselves from us, so as to fully forget our Godhood within this 3/4D game.

Now that eons pass and all possible roles are played out, the mosaic Created by the false flag of fear = separation, begins to crumble. Brilliant light = LOVE begins bursting out from every crack. Soon the light becomes so powerful, the mosaic begins to crumble to dust and we re-all-eyes what a profoundly transformative, expansive gift we've just given ourselves as Creators Creation Creating Creation.

For from the deepest darkness, the brightest Lights shine.. The magnetic pull back into the full spectrum of our Wholeness becomes irresistible. We now re-all-eyes WE ARE that LOVE = Light. This IS our ascension, or as I see it now our RE-EMERGENCE

Judy Vancil Jandora
Tarot, Transformation, Mural Artist

Lets *turn the Lights on* and notice what inside us had to be "shut down in us" to comply with such systems - perhaps some of our disconnected DNA?

Our entire DNA structure is like a Contact time-release capsule. When we were originally programmed, our basic DNA structure was limited to a double-helix strand. The triggering mechanism that enables us to function as we do is affected by stellar radiation. We are now at a place in the orbit around our central galaxy where the radio frequencies of the center of the galaxy, as well as many other star systems, are communicating new information to us [activating our DNA].

Willard Van De Bogart
The Return of the Anunnaki, Earthportals dot com

The Great Awakening, occurring *Now,* is happening on many levels: rare Celestial events, Quantum physics revealing how our thought Creates *and in Light of this*, Ancient Texts in modern translation hold much more meaning. We *are* mega-Leaping *in spite of* our past, into this accelerated, amazing Now Moment in Earth's history. *We are Creator-Beings, Awakening to our potential.* Entering Higher Consciousness, accessing the ever-flowing-positive-creative *Field* of *Infinite Eternal LOVE.*

A first step for increasing the coherence in the field environment is for *each individual to take responsibility for their own energy*. We can do this by becoming more conscious of thoughts, feelings and attitudes that we are 'feeding the field' each day...as enough individuals increase heart coherence it leads to increased social coherence. As a critical mass of cultures and nations become more harmoniously aligned, this can eventually lead to increased global coherence and sustainable peace.

HeartMath Institute
The Heart's Intuitive Intelligence: A Path to Personal, Social and Global Coherence

If anything appears around us, Not of LOVE, it is our "reality" Mirroring our thought conscious-unconscious, to show us where we need to clear our own "corrupt data." Start with the feeling in us. *Change ourselves. Change the Hologram. Second Universal Law.* This is how it works in the **21st Century Superhuman, Quantum World.** As we release all historical and current thought-emotion "Not of LOVE," we change related timelines, past and future. It does not require a *savior or punishment*. It does require the simple act of "waking-up" and *walking through the fire* of our own "corrupt data" to restore our True Design LOVE.

...the Masters are supra-human, beyond the frailties of emotion, and they demand total commitment to the chosen path. It is of greatest importance to follow the Light with determination, discernment and detachment. There is no such thing in this world as miracles. *Everything happens through science. Only a person who doesn't understand science calls it a miracle.*

Dr. Ram Bhosle
Student of Mahavatar Babaji 1800 yr. old Master of the Himalayas

The more we get this, the more exponentially we shift as a Collective, and our World changes around us. *Goal Canceling Examples:* feeling Not of LOVE toward another, being irritated-hurt, worrying about money, wars, governments, World issues, sad about animals or people, uncomfortable with Body or looks, death of friend or pet, feeling victim, dislike job. Perpetuating Mind-Energy Not of LOVE Creates dis-integrative "realities."

Have you ever had a dream Neo, that you were so sure was real? What if you were unable to wake from that dream? How would you know the difference between the dream world, and the real world?

Morpheus, The Matrix

Emotions *give us messages* about what thought-emotional *content* we're carrying in our unconscious to *clean out. Do your "housekeeping," take out your "garbage," cancel your goals.* Once clear, you will resonate LOVE. Live a new Life, do things that matter, be Authentic, discover True happiness. *THIS IS A JOURNEY.* It is a rewiring of thousands of years of circuits. **Change your thoughts. Change the World.**

The goal of Life is to make your Heartbeat match the beat of the Universe.

Joseph Campbell (1984-1987)
The Hero's Journey

Whatever happens(ed) in our history, prehistory or future history, *there is only one thing that matters.* As we restore our True Design LOVE, everything is cleared. Once we do so, and change how our Vibration puts Attention on the *Field of Possibilities,* we change *everything.* **We shift the entire Hologram...**

You can call it God if you want, but you don't have to. Quantum consciousness will do. Nonlocality, tangled hierarchy, and discontinuity: these signatures of Quantum consciousness have been independently verified by leading researchers worldwide. This experimental data and its conclusions inform us that it is the mistaken materialist view that is at the center of most of our world's problems today. To address these problems, we now have a science of spirituality that is fully verifiable and objective.

Amit Goswami, PhD
The Secret; theoretical Quantum physicist mitgoswami.org

We are the sentient beings on the Earth-plane who have volunteered *(yes!)* for the task of restoring our True Design LOVE, by releasing and letting go all Not of LOVE thought-emotion. This is *Quantum Lifestyle!*

Find your own sobriety then you can share peace -
instead of being outraged - find peace.

Deepak Chopra MD
Natural Physician, New Thought Author

Based on current views on timespace or spacetime in dimensions beyond 3-D, Quantum physicist Nassim Haramein offers we can go into *any timeline* anywhere in history where a particular situation occurred. As we access that event and hold LOVE in the presence of those circumstances, we clear the *Field,* changing that event forever. Future and past also shift as they Now emerge differently from this point in timespace.

We reshape our future and our past, when holding LOVE in the *Field* for all points in human history *Now.* Connect with the part of you that is non-local, the deeper realm of your Soul. Enter ALL timelines with LOVE. *Arc the Hologram,* like an arc-welder.

LOVE bears all things, believes all things, hopes all things, endures all things...
Do not be conformed to this world, be transformed by the renewal of your mind...

1 Corinthians 13:7, Romans 12:2

Do a test run with this list; see if you can hold each in your Heart: WWI, WWII, Hiroshima, Vietnam war, rape, murder, genocide of Jews, Native Americans and others, disturbance of ET Life, worst thing in your life. Activate New brain cells and hold LOVE for each situation. Breathe. Smile. If you can't that's awesome too; just notice and do the *Ancient Aramaic Forgiveness* goal canceling process [Part 2: MIND] to remove your "corrupt data," then hold LOVE again. Rinse. Repeat. Breathe. Smile.

So let's walk our talk, and make brain circuits of positive emotions. *We just do it. We practice.* Let some of us be good, do good. Be with God some of the time, be in the ego some of the time, and let the dance generate creative acts of transformation. With this resolution, with this objective in mind, I invite you to *become Quantum Activists.*

Amit Goswami, PhD
The Secret; theoretical Quantum physicist mitgoswami.org

As we delete these things from human history by clearing them from our Vibration - even our memory changes. As we restore the Presence of LOVE within our Being and clear the Vibration of Not of LOVE events and situations from the map of Creation, a New World is born. We change ALL timelines, past, present and future. *We Live in LOVE in the* **EVER PRESENT NOW.** *(Thanks Dr. John Ray for the concept of the Ever Present Now...)*

Clear yourself, change the World. **Arc the Hologram! Laugh. Play. 21st Century Superhumans Now clearing ALL timelines with LOVE. ♥ ♥ ♥**

Part 3: SPIRIT - SECTION 3
A NEW CIVILIZATION
BASED IN LOVE

The moment you come to trust chaos, you see God Clearly. Chaos is Divine order versus human order. When the chaos becomes safety to you, then you know you're seeing God clearly.

Caroline Myss
Spiritual Madness:
The Necessity of Meeting God in Darkness

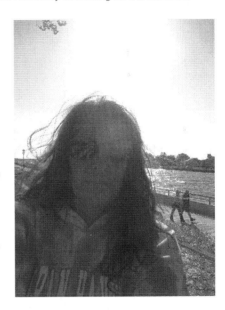

The *mantra* of *change-makers* of our Now is that out of current chaos of dis-integrating governments, monetary systems and religious structures in diverse places around the World, innovative solutions are birthing. As coal exposed to extreme pressure transforms into a brilliant diamond, so do we. In fact, massive numbers of people Now are holding Radiant LOVE and Light on the Planet.

Who knew the peaceful mainstream uprising of the Occupy movement would have such far-reaching and international impact? A Voice of Oneness. Meanwhile gatherings of "Light-workers" such as on 11:11, focused around the idea of Ascension, grounding qualities of "Christed Consciousness," initiating a level of transparency, dedication, commitment and Light-filled dialogues perhaps not seen for 2,000 years.

What most of us '*Truthers*' did in the face of all this...was to begin to speak, write, and broadcast an **Alternative Story**, one based on both ancient wisdom and whatever factual intel could be found 'out there'. Stunning growth of the Internet, and it's natural dispersion of encyclopedic information about any and all subjects, helped *immensely*...

...we also benefited magnificently from information received from 'insiders', ex-military, whistleblowers, 'black ops' types, ex-spies, ex-corporate goons and shills whose direct exposure to and experience of the 'REAL Deal' they felt, couldn't remain hidden from public view any longer... This 'new' *Real* Story not only exposed lies, deceptions and manipulation of the Old Institutional/Ruling Elite

Story, it also revealed glorious potential **New Life** that we are now *finally* actively ushering into existence...actually ***creating*** as we move rapidly into its Energies!

Wayshowers I communicate with directly...have been guided during this brief moment of relative calm to sit back, let go of what we have done and...be witness to the *explosive* Awakening of Humanity now occurring... Soon, we shall be called into our next roles here – and then our time to just sit back and relax will be over for a while....I recommend ALL of you put forth your best effort, finish cleaning out the closets and dark corners of your own psyches — and simply *stop worrying* about anybody else's! We all need to be fully prepared for the next unfoldment of The Grand Plan. It's gonna be *RAD!!!*

Alexander Del Sol
Waverider1 / Avatar Coach

We used to believe the "New higher frequency Earth" would separate from the old, denser Planet, leaving behind those who continued to "play with matches" in archaic darkness, in personal and Global power battles. Yet such exponential change has occurred with movement into intensified Light *Fields*, understanding Quantum physics and Ancient texts, that we are Now transforming into a New Civilization based in LOVE on *this Earth*, where "She and we" are "Ascending" together with as few "bumps" as possible.

It has been said, "We're Living on borrowed time." Yet (a.) there is no time. (b.) We now know, the more LOVE we pour into this World, the more readily ALL transforms. Releasing ALL Not of LOVE *from our own thoughts and consciousness*, unfolds Creation anew each moment taking shape *based on Higher frequencies*.

It becomes more apparent by the day, that the more we shift within, the more the World shifts around us. There is a "New Earth" being born, and it is "within us!" Shifting our internal frequencies, and with each New person who "catches on" exiting the old paradigm to Live Authentically in the Heart, the Vibration of the Collective shifts.

This is what is transforming in our deeper consciousness. We are moving into true Diversity in Unity, and this is only possible when one releases judgments and begins to accept that we are each different than one another but not better or worse. The actor is no better than the janitor, the president is no better than the accountant. Each, as in all nature, is actualizing their particular function and authentic purpose. There is a balance in the Universe and each instrument in the Universe's orchestra has a particular sound to contribute to the music of the spheres. And the ***Aquarian Age*** is the opportunity for our human family to develop just such a culture, one aligned with the nonjudgmental "attitude" of our universe. "All are Created equal, with certain inalienable rights".

Leo Knitghton Tallarico
Perspectives From The Sky: Cardinal Grand Cross July 2014

Let's explore what makes up our New Civilization based in LOVE, what it offers us personally and collectively, a New way of Life for the *21st Century Superhuman.* ♥

Chapter 10

Spirit Of Community

*If you want to go fast go alone.
If you want to go far go together.*

African Proverb

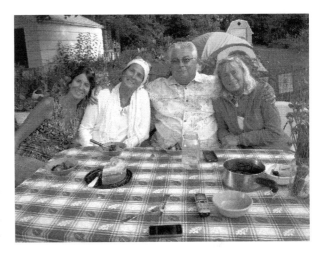

In Ancient Aramaic (as spoken by Yeshua/Jesus), "Heaven" meant *"Community of LOVE." Wow!* Pause and think on that... Heaven, the fantastic place we have imagined "somewhere out there," our future "reward" ("if we're "good"), is *Here and Now* in our Hearts and Lives, sharing Life with one another in the "Community of LOVE." This is how we were meant to Live, eternally, in our neighborhoods, our homes, our World. *Our Heaven begins right here.*

Taking practical steps to restore our True Design LOVE and joining with others doing the same, we manifest or reveal a New "reality." It becomes easier to cooperate and collaborate. Neighbors begin working together for mutual benefit, sharing gardens and assisting one another. Communities emerging Now around the Globe, range from supportive neighborhoods and shared homes, to rural properties set up for group living, gardening, farming, healing centers, sharing and co-producing resources. We Now hold the frequency or tuning fork" for Creation in this New "reality," our *Community of LOVE*. THIS IS THE PATH to the New Earth.

It is possible that the next Buddha will not take the form of an individual. The next Buddha may take the form of a community - a community practicing understanding and loving kindness, a community practicing mindful living. This may be the most important thing we can do for the survival of the earth.

*Thich Nhat Hanh
Vietnamese Zen Buddhist Monk, Teacher, Author, Poet, Peace Activist*

Grounding of Global Communities is a major key to smooth, peaceful transition in this Evolutionary Leap, into expanded connection with our existence. We emerge anew from the *Field* with each progressive shift toward wholeness, and the entire Hologram shifts.

The majority of simpler cultures around the Globe infinitely depend upon one another within extended family and Community for everyday life. It is said in those simpler cultures, "We always have enough and we always have each other," where in the western World "we never have enough, and we're always alone." Even with advancements of modern culture, wisdom says shift priorities, renewing commitment to one another and Collective Well-Being.

Simpler cultures Live the experience that we are "ALL One," for as Einstein said, *"If we think we're separate, we're living in an optical delusion."* Connected with ALL HUmanity we are also simultaneously unique individualized expressions. With this emerging New consciousness, Visions of possibility and action are arising everywhere!

Communities will provide its inhabitants with ongoing opportunities for practicing deep listening and true spiritual intimacy where much more meaningful exchanges can take place between all members of the community and beyond. This has been a planet of lonely people who are now reaching out to be shown how they can truly move into Unity Consciousness and begin establishing the foundations for a new Golden Age of Freedom...

People are already coming together to build the Love and Light of Source within their hearts, minds and bodies and this will continue to expand outward like spokes on a wheel. The hub of the wheel will be centered in Unity Consciousness and as that center and its spokes continue to expand, it will become a magnet for attracting millions until you have truly established your new Golden Age of Freedom upon your Earth plane.

Saint Germain and Lady Portia
Walk The Earth As A Living Master

Do you live where you can grow food, herb and flower gardens, fruit trees or berry bushes? If not there may be wisdom in moving to where you can. If each family grows a food garden, with a small, partially underground greenhouse where needed, it would defray food shortages and ring a bell of freedom. This strategy is currently recommended by the UN for turning expected shortages facing us, into abundant survival. We can literally change the face of human civilization *in one gardening season,* as did UK's Victory Gardens during WWII! Such simple action can cooperatively cultivate a New World and a viable future for ALL. Not everyone may LOVE to garden, so let each do what they LOVE. Alternatively cultivate strong relationships with those who grow local organic near you.

Endless material diversions can keep us distracted from the Real and the Eternal, based in LOVE. "People need to leave those artificial vertical high-rises and go back into the agrarian communities where the soles of their feet reconnect with the elemental intelligence of the Earth and thereby boot them back into the immortal paradigm." (Sacha Stone)

Festivals are an instinctive movement toward recovery of this *Essence*. Immersion in such festivals can bring enrichment. We relax, let loose, dress playfully and bring out our transparent childlike self, becoming more versatile, self empowered and Authentic.

> This is what the Shift is about. It's not about turning on the news to see if anything has changed...We're lucid dreamers, the energy we emit and the energy we see outside ourselves determines what will appear around us. The energy within us determines where we're going. We *are* the breaking news, what we empower is what appears around us.
>
> *Laura Eisenhower*
> *Awake in the Dream Radio with Laura Eisenhower & Dr. Dream*

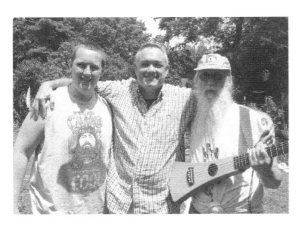

Transformational festivals are emerging Globally, 100+ each year, with 10,000 to 70,000 attendees! Bloom TV Series exposes the incredible example of vital, creative Life emerging at these festivals with such names as Beloved Sacred Arts and Music, Blissfest, Sonic Bloom, Symbiosis, Knowfest, Rainbow Serpent, Ascendance, Earth Frequency, Source, Envision, Burning Man, Water Woman, Electric Forest and more...

A grand expression of *"Heaven, the Community of LOVE,"* festivals are full of creativity, song, dance, art, visioning, practicing radical generosity and self-sufficiency. Spearheaded by younger generations, they offer a wonderful living model that is radically changing our core-cultural system, flowing into the everyday Lives of participants. It becomes difficult for them to return to unsatisfying jobs once they've had a taste, to struggle to get by, so they begin seeking alternative lifestyles and creative ways to support themselves. This is an outgrowth of an old system that is devastatingly dissatisfying.

We are at a fork in the road where the old monetary system is "on a decline" with mathematically uncorrectable trillions of dollars of debt. Rather than sucked into fear and chaos, or a New system of "control" based in "carbon dollars," many are moving into decentralized systems of community, honoring sovereignty of the individual, paving the way to wiser living.

Michael Tellinger's *UBUNTU Contributionism: Blueprint For Human Prosperity*, explains how money was not a natural outgrowth of human culture, rather imposed by those desiring to subjugate the masses for their own wealth. He connects dots from early pre-history where money evolved in Ancient enslavement of the human race subservient to another warlike, dominant culture. As a result we've developed a World where we're accustomed to competition, greed and separation, believing it's the way. It's not.

It is now highly feasible to take care of everybody on Earth at a higher standard of living that any have ever known. It no longer has to be you or me. Selfishness is unnecessary. War is obsolete. It as a matter of converting our high-technology from Weaponry to Livingry.

Buckminster "Bucky" Fuller (1895-1983)
Innovator, Spaceship Earth, popularized geodesic dome

Tellinger adopted the Ancient African Ubuntu philosophy, consistent with many Ancient cultures around the Planet, of nourishing and harmonious Community Living where ALL cherish and look after one another.

I am, because we are.

African Ubuntu Philosophy

In Light of Ancient history unearthed in *Adam's Calendar,* Michael Tellinger was prompted to develop a concept about what our society would be without money. He discovered that *every single problem* we ever have disappears when we remove money, and it is the ultimate tool for control! He explains that it will take several phases to transition to a different type of monetary system for us to move beyond this one. (books, videos online)

He suggests moving out into small towns and villages, where it's easier to implement "Councils of Elders" and local decision-making, getting "off the grid," developing self-sufficiency. Honest free money systems with various currencies and talent exchanges are Now exploding around the World. *Brilliant ideas* are evolving as we get over the hurdle of fear about thinking in this New direction, and more Minds-Hearts become engaged.

Tellinger ran for President of South Africa in 2014 for the New Ubuntu Party. Exposure brought these precepts vitally to the forefront, courageously seeding change toward a viable future, beyond what most have imagined. Michael and his wife travel internationally, speaking at length on this important topic.

Learn more: *"Foster Gamble talks to Michael Tellinger 25 Sept 2012"* YouTube. The more who stand together on these issues, the more effectively we move forward. Find comprehensive tools for freedom and integrity, come up to speed quickly and learn about solutions developed by others at *Thrive Movement Solutions Hub dot com* and *New Era dot org* with close to a million members. Leaders such as Foster Gamble of Thrive Movement and Michael Tellinger of Ubuntu, working together with others globally, developing practical solutions for viable change of outmoded system.

Foster Gamble calls actions going on in this current transitional trajectory "the Aikido move of the century...a historical evolutionary opportunity that we can all be part of. Millions of groups around the World are connecting, fundamentally zeroing in on universal morality, creating transitional systems that will work, emerging organically and naturally."

Humans don't need money to thrive - all we need is LOVE and each other... Money doesn't plant the seeds or grow the food or solve the mathematical equations or build the rockets - people do, as long as we work together in united communities toward the greater benefit of all using our God-given talents we will thrive beyond our wildest beliefs.

Michael Tellinger
On Moneyless Society

Tellinger says, "This liberates everything about humanity and everything we do as a species." What if all we did each day is what emerges from within us, in a mutually contributory society? Even with 7 billion people, there is more than enough on our abundant Planet when not being syphoned off by the ultra rich. Though the idea may be shocking, we encourage you to research in Tellinger's books and videos, that expose origins and links between laws, money, banking and governments. His revolutionary philosophy is that a society built on contributionism is a free society on a free Planet.

Jefferson believed...skepticism is an essential prerequisite for responsible citizenship. He argued that the cost of education is trivial compared to the cost of ignorance, of leaving government to the wolves. He taught that the country is safe only when the people rule.

Carl Sagan
The Demon-Haunted World: Science as a Candle in the Dark

As John F. Kennedy said, even now inspiring the younger generations on the fiftieth anniversary of his death, "Ask not what your country can do for you, ask what you can do for your country." Converted into current terms, "Ask not what your family or community can do for you, ask what you can do for your family or Community," a fine reminder to connect from the Heart with those around us with ideas and action.

Bring what you have that is good to the table.

Sun Bear
Native American Shaman, Medicine Man

Similar to other "aristocratic" cultures throughout history, in our modern developed World, a drive toward individualized wealth to the exclusion of others, pushes aside anyone who gets in the way. It has bred competition, deprivation and desperation, taking resources from the hands of the many, putting them into the hands of the few. Initiating change, international Sovereignty movements Now express and represent True freedom.

Whoever devised this system in the blame-fear-hostility culture, had complete amnesia on how intricately connected we Are, inseparable from dynamics of the coherent Whole. As John Lennon said, "Our society is run by insane people for insane objectives." It may take a bit to untangle ALL this, yet we have before us an amazing potential with infinite possibilities, as our DNA currently activated by Light *Fields* in the Cosmos opens us to greater paradigms. Potent seeds of the future are germinating during this fertile cycle.

The corporate revolution will collapse if we refuse to buy what they are selling... their ideas, their version of history, their wars, their weapons, their notion of inevitability. Remember this: We may be many and they may be few. They need us more than we need them. *Another world is not only possible, she is on her way. On a quiet day, I can hear her breathing.*

Arundhati Roy
1998 Man Booker Prize Fiction "The God of Small Things," Civil rights & Environmental activist

In the race for individualized wealth, the vast majority have suffered and relinquished their "Souls," to high and low paid "enslavement" rather than Living as juicy Creative Beings, as is our birthright. Our monetary system was Created to control and syphon resources off the masses. Money is printed out of thin air and the more the banking systems get people to spend, the more control they have. Suffering of this nature ripples through the entire Hologram of HUmankind, affecting *ALL*. New systems are Now being peacefully and wisely established around the World, to move us into more viable alternatives.

The real cause of hunger is the powerlessness of the poor,
to gain access to the resources they need to feed themselves.

Frances Moore Lappé
Diet for a Small Planet

We may be caught in the idea, "This is mine, it's important for me to keep." An alternative strategy, is noticing how we enrich our lives by sharing with and embracing others and greater Community. It can start right at home with small changes. "One city in Brazil recruited local farmers to help do something U.S. cities have yet to do: *end hunger.*"

THE CITY THAT ENDED HUNGER: "To search for solutions to hunger means to act within the principle that the status of a citizen surpasses that of a mere consumer."

Frances Moore Lappé
City of Belo Horizonte, Brazil, Hope's Edge: The Next Diet for a Small Planet

Absolutely our most powerful resource, is clearing out our own unconscious of corrupt blame-fear-hostility "data" to restore our True Design LOVE, setting up a New resonance. *21st Century Superhumans are now Arcing the Hologram* with LOVE based practical transitional solutions! *"One who stands in the Light, stands in the Light for All."*

My problem was not with comfort or monetary wealth. My problem was with a way of Life in which those who have more than they need are envied or extolled, while those who are materially poor are scorned or forgotten.

John Robbins
The New Good Life: Living Better Than Ever in an Age of Less

Excited, we merge into Community Now, AS WHO WE ARE. Home, car, job, career, profession, relationship easily repurposed. Community is the stepping-stone to leverage us from routines we're drowning in alone, lightening our load for betterment of ALL.

There's more stability in a triangle than with just two poles, more stability, more grounding. Where three or more gathered it exponentially multiplies, particularly when those three are participating at the same consciousness level.

Shalamee Campbell, Sis*Star on the Path

Sacred Feminine sweetly blends with Masculine. Feminine incubates, Masculine Creates structure and drives forward. Honored in new ways, they birth to nurturing and healing our World. True leadership comes from this balance, directing international peacekeeping.

Some who have wealth or are gifted at creating it, are learning to wisely lead innovative projects and enterprises for accelerating societal change, supporting others and the greater good with their skills. Together we are so much more than we are singly. Oriah Mountain Dreamer says, *"It doesn't interest me who you are, how you came to be here, I want to know if you will stand in the Fire with me and not shrink back."*

> Millions of us are moving into the "social chrysalis," attempting to evolve ourselves and our culture toward a still amorphous undefined society. Each imaginal cell is coded with a unique creativity yearning to be expressed and integrated into the body of the societal butterfly. None of us has seen this form of society. We might call it a Co-creative Society in which each person is free to be and do his or her best within the evolving whole.
>
> *Barbara Marx Hubbard*
> *Evolution by Choice, Not by Chance*

When we examine our beliefs about any subject… we realize we are as individual as snowflakes. How we believe and why we believe is our individual truth. Once in a while we will have a feeling of being on "common ground" with another and our passions for living come together. Any genuine path will, with sincere practice, result in a gradual deepening of our True Nature. Letting go ideas about reality and desires for a particular result, will lead to True Freedom. Amazing Insights come to a mind that is Open and Free! Teddi ♥

> When we allow ourselves and everyone else the freedom to fully individuate as spiritual beings in human form, our Souls will automatically want to flock together, like moths to the flame of our shared Divinity, each with wings in glimmering colors and unique patterns of individual human expression.
>
> *Anthon St. Maarten*
> *Psychic and Counsellor, Divine Living*

Remember, Heart Coherence our most POWERFUL STATE is achieved by focusing in LOVE, Gratitude and Compassion. *Simple.* The sooner we get this, we as a Collective change the World. Make this your natural state of Being. Considering others into the equation improves our lives too! Tones or frequencies of our thoughts-emotions, like ripples in a pond, harmonize-resonate-join with matching frequencies, to co-Create more complex and wonderful realities than just ours alone.

> By acting compassionately, by helping to restore justice and to encourage peace,
> we are acknowledging that we are all part of one another.
>
> *Ram Dass*
> *LOVE Serve Remember*

Insight into global banking challenges and tightly stretched economic systems, urges all of us to ease our burdens by collaborative sharing with one another: homes, meals, gardens and the moments of Life. Creating pockets of community right Now, is the life-raft to carry us through.

We are here to awaken to the illusion of our separation.

Thich Nhat Hanh
Vietnamese Zen Buddhist Monk, Teacher, Author, Poet, Peace Activist

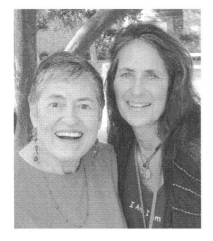

Test out the Community process, *right where you are.* Consider co-housing with family or friends to ease up the budget and make it through changes on the horizon. Use sharing and exchange to care for children, pets, and the elderly. Cultivate relationships with your neighbors; discover what you can exchange or share with one another.

That New direction may be our return ticket to the Garden, but this time, we will return as conscious gardeners, co-creating ever more beautiful, functional, and loving expressions of Life.

Bruce H Lipton, PhD and Steve Bhaerman
Spontaneous Evolution, Our Positive Future And A Way Two Get
There From Here

When one has opened to a greater energy flow, and others surrounding them have not, there may be a energetic discharge balancing out the *Field*. We may need to make choices, draw lines in the sand, and choose to surround ourselves with healthy Awakened others, possibly migrating to other circumstances or location for Well-Being.

"It is beautiful and makes deep sense...space is not empty at all; it is flowing over with the We that embraces all....the We is making itself felt, understood, intuited all over this globe and is manifesting in many ways - as people wanting to cooperate, collaborate, to be in community and communion, seeing that the time of heroes...is definitely over... The world and its problems have become so complex that we can only hope to find adequate answers in 'circles' of very different people, where we can meet eye to eye and heart to heart - in a sort of collective leadership. And this is underfoot already on a worldwide scale...initiatives are going on all over the world, with this is one aspect of "We" manifesting.

Another aspect is the sense of spiritual or Soul families or clans finding each other again across countries and continents. It is as if we have chosen ages ago to come together in this critical time on the planet to be midwives to what is wanting to emerge. Whatever may be the case we do recognize each other and there is an immediate connection beyond words, even beyond understanding; all we do is accept it.

A third aspect manifests through what has been called the Circle Being, manifesting as a higher order of being together with an incredible coherence that draws in the individuals participating. This certainly is We, being highly coherent."

Michel Bauwens
The Next Buddha Will Be a Collective, Reality Sandwich

Listen to your Heart. Discover how you can extend into Community. It may take a bit to unwind all this. Take small steps. With experience, your courage will open doors and carry you and others to new places. Waves of Spirit are moving within us. The moment is Now. The ninth wave of the Mayan Calendar is upon us. Do you have your board ready to catch this wave? This once in a Galactic eon wakeup call to our DNA with Cosmic Light showering down upon us, is carrying us into fantastic New territory! *It's ALL good.* Trust. Breathe. Smile. *Catch the wave!*

The co-creative society cannot be imposed or engineered into existence. It is nurtured into being by increasing the connections and coherence among those already initiating vital actions. It emerges when we collectively overcome the illusion of separation that has divided us, for the capacities we need — the technology, resources, and know-how — are already present in their early stages to realize our evolutionary agenda. Only a catalytic spark of shared LOVE and spiritual experience is needed to activate the great genius of humanity to join in inspired actions.

Barbara Marx Hubbard
Conscious Evolution

There have been critical points through history when the "sleepers" were called to Awaken. Noah's flood, the sinking of Ancient continents of Atlantis and Lemuria. This moment is no less important, though different. We are at a critical Planetary and human crossroads, choosing whether to emerge to the next level or sink our own ship.

Quantum physics has awakened us to New Awareness of our Observer-Creator status. Ancient texts in modern translation offer profound insight. The question is will we go beyond our conditioning and take action with wisdom? Each will choose. Each will matter. A healthy future cannot be born in pollution, corruption or disharmony. A healthy future can only come from Minds-Hearts established in LOVE. *Above ALL, this is our task.*

On the journey through Life we are encouraged, inspired, LOVED and uplifted by meeting dear friends and companions along the way who share common Visions, Desires and Dreams. We have already begun sharing households and dharma, where we light incense, hold space and meditate daily; where we share Lifestyle and focus, creating a beautiful sacred space, sharing healthy food, gardening, expressing our creativity, honoring who we truly are, and lifting our lives up to our Highest potential. We are irresistibly drawn together by matching Vibration of Mind-Heart, birthing the New Earth. What kind of community or home would you like to call in around you? Make it so. As our beloved Sis*Star Amantha Meyers says in Spirit, "So be it, and so it is!" Cary ♥

Discover those to whom you are magnetically drawn by shared Vibration and Vision. It happens naturally. Notice when it does. Enrich and inspire each other with your resonance.

> Important encounters are planned by the Souls
> long before the bodies see each other.
>
> *Paul Cohelo*
> *The Alchemist*

Ah yes, Community. We know many communities that have come and gone over many years, groups purchasing land to live together off the grid, with failures and successes; *bless them all!* We are well aware of the challenges.We are in a New era of community. *There is one thing we've learned that supports ALL Communities to succeed:*

NEW EARTH COMMUNITY RULES: Based in Universal Law: *Thought Creates.* ALL Events, ALL People, ALL Issues are a product of the resonance within us. To the degree we get this is the degree to which we will succeed. If we are there and in pain, it is a result of OUR "old data." "There is no 'out there' out there." Our unconscious content is 95% of how we hold resonance in the *Field of Possibilities*, the remaining 5% is conscious. This unconscious-conscious resonance calls our "reality" into being around us. *That's it.* Our True Design is LOVE. *Arc the Hologram.*

1. **All is Mind-Energy -** *thought Creates. Clear your thoughts.*

2. **As Above - So Below** *Shift ourselves, shift the Whole. Arc the Hologram!*

3. **The constant Vibration** *of the Field eagerly awaits our Attention upon it...*

> I AM responsible for the "Realities" that I see, Hear and Feel...
> They are "Magnetized" to me for my Awareness. *Teddi* ♥

As each individual embraces these principles and puts them into practice, *we will have powerful, healthy Communities.* Be joyful, loving and kind. Be creative. Dance together, pray together, eat together. Does it matter what our prayers "say?" Remember, in Aramaic to "pray" is to "set a trap for God," to tune ourselves to the *Field* or Source channel of LOVE.

Prayers of the Heart (matching 8 Hz resonance of Earth) align perfectly with Oneness with ALL That Is, flowing in continual Creation from the *Field*, harmonizing with Earth Mother Gaia. Encourage and inspire each other. Play. Breathe. Smile. Live.

> The Universe will always bring you to further and further coherency. And actually I believe you even see that in our equations. It doesn't matter how whacked out our physics get and how many dimensions we have to add, we can't even get out of the truth... meaning it's there, it might not be understood, it might not be complete. But it's always bringing us in that direction [toward higher scale of coherency].
>
> *Nassim Haramein*
> *The Resonance Project*

There is no punishment or mistake, only lessons. The *Divine Matrix* only returns to us that which we put into it, resulting as a feedback loop, letting us know whether we are in

LOVE or in "Not of LOVE," and whether we have "corrupt data" to clear. This Quantum principle is the ultimate theme of all True teachings. Let's remove our Minds from news and outer chaos, designed to keep us hypnotized with Not of LOVE thought.

> These times are the most exciting humanity has known on your planet for thousands upon thousands of years. Your entire planet and everyone upon it is moving into their next level of awakening and this will inspire many around your world to build communities where everyone will be supported to live in Unity Consciousness.
>
> These communities can be as small as a family unit or as large as a small town or village and in truth, there is *no limit to what can now be Created and manifested* upon your paradise planet when you are living, speaking, listening and loving Presence-to-Presence. Many will be also be guided to simply be examples of what it looks like to live as your Presence on Earth.
>
> *Masters Saint Germain and Lady Portia*
> *WalkTheEarthAsALivingMaster.com*

Focus in the Heart. Envision our World beautiful, healthy, happy and well. Enter Heart Coherence: LOVE. COMPASSION. GRATITUDE. *THIS IS THE ONLY THING TO DO.* The more Compassionate we are, the more readily mass Consciousness shifts. The more Gratitude we have, the more comes to us. The more we open our Heart, the more we are LOVED. Breathe. Smile. Laugh. Play. Create. Serve In-Joy. Resonate LOVE. Give Thanks!

> The Spirit shall look out through matter's gaze. And matter shall reveal the Spirit's face and all the Earth becomes a Single Life...
>
> *Sri Aurobindo (1872-1950)*
> *Freedom Fighter, Philosopher, Guru: turning human into divine*

Demonstrating what an amazing readiness there is among HU-Beings to move toward community, New Earth Project which became New Earth Nation was founded in 2013, and within 4 months with barely any promotional effort 250,000 people had joined. Rather than "a community," it is instead a monumental "blueprint" comprehensively covering many areas necessary to establishing communities under the umbrella of the New Earth concept World-wide. Sacha Stone, Founder encourages those interested to spend a few days reading the template at NewEarthNation dot org.

Experts from around the World have contributed energy and resources to develop new concepts such as "life-extending bio-architecture" and "zero-point social ecology where there is no one standing over anyone else." It's about "re-engaging with the organic premise of being human and taking ourselves out of the artifice of the so-called civilization." Inspired visionary, Sacha Stone passionately breaks new ground:

> [It's about] moving out of a toxic city grid and moving into a fractal community in Chile, Mexico or Mozambique, meaning you are already making a determination to step outside of time, money and fear to engage with the other. And the other is the

absence of fear, absence of fear begets love and fellowship. All that begets wellness, prosperity and abundance. The rest follows as a mathematical certainty.

...What do you want? You tell us. What do you envision? Bring that majesty, bring that expression, bring that dream, bring that fantasy, and bring that improbability. Bring it to this space. This space is that playing field, is that sub-space vacuum that will allow for anything and everything to emerge and manifest, provided it's in attunement with pure truth. If it is in attunement with pure truth it will resonate to the people and the situations and the circumstances around it will conspire toward manifesting it. That's a beautiful thing if you think about it. It means that righteousness really finds its feet.

...it's just a question of us wanting now sufficiently to withdraw from the old order of things, which is entropic, intellectually dead and physically very harmful, and step out of that and step into the new. I believe that every single human being that has warm blood, and I don't mean that as a joke, will resonate absolutely to this. This is the coming of age. It's our graduation. It's also the only exit strategy really presenting itself that I can see.

Sacha Stone, Founder New Earth Nation
New Earth Media News, June 30,2014

We find joy in gathering in Community, where *"two or more are gathered,"* we access greater potential to shift the collective to a higher path. As Patricia Cota-Robles says, "When the 51% are Awakened, the other 49% come along just by the magnetics and inertia of it all." This is how the "Yogi in the cave" *does* change the World; they choose, as we do, to focus Mind-Heart in a Resonant *Field* of Higher Attention, Aspiration and Knowledge.

> Never doubt that a small group of thoughtful, committed, citizens
> can change the world. Indeed, it is the only thing that ever has.

Margaret Mead (1901-1978), Cultural Anthropologist

The more who step out of of meaninglessness, to Create viable and exciting solutions, the more wildly exponential becomes the change taking place. As we gather, manifestation to serve a common good emerges, for mutual growth and expression of enlightened Lives. Initially one of the biggest barriers may appear to be economic. Yet as groups form with New and creative ways to take care of basic needs, the easier it becomes for others to join in. Gradual steps toward Living in more Heart centered ways can be a dynamic pathway to finding one's way out of the maze. There are also global funds based in huge resources of gold held for humanity that wheels are in motion to release soon.

Front-liners have initiated powerful solutions promising to change our World faster than we think. Open Source is the New method to put developing ideas in the hands "of the people." 3-D printer designs and Now Nikola Tesla's patents (released by Tesla Motors) have had many, many thousands of downloads Globally. The One People (formerly OPPT) and Hopegirl's Fix the World Project have produced a Free Energy Machine (based on

Tesla's work) that is Now producing 6x more clean energy than it takes to run it. Other groups are developing it further, with evidence we will soon outrun our need for fossil fuels, which changes the face of human culture forever. No more power or fuel bills!

> God Created us on the planet so that he, she, it, Creator,
> Spirit, us, would know ourselves better.
>
> *Jack White (1934-1998)*
> *God's Game of Life*

INITIATING COMMUNITY offers Strength, Encouragement Inspiration, Wisdom and Vibrational Enhancement to those gathered. Among 112 million single adults in the U.S. alone, 47% of the population, makes aloneness at epidemic. Statistically those who share LOVE and companionship live longer, are healthier and less stressed. *Start here:*

- Share a home with one or several others, Expand interaction to several homes
- Grow a garden, trade harvests with neighbors who do also.
- What moves your Heart? Find ways to include this in your Life.
- Contemplate whether you need to shift from current job to more Heart satisfying.
- Start the day with a group household meditation, candle, incense, prayers
- Move beyond competition and judgment into harmony, mutual support and LOVE
- Use a "talking stick" for group meetings. Encourage honesty and openness.
- Share meals. Take turns at preparation and cleanup, chores.
- Is there a Global focus you can participate in or initiate? Explore this.
- Consider ways to simplify. Inspire others to do the same.
- Start a **21st Century Superhuman** Group or *Mindshifter's* Group (dr. ryce)

HEART COHERENCE CHANGES THE WORLD: Join HeartMath®'s Global Coherence Initiative at GlobalCareRooms dot org. Meet others, organize groups, or jump on individually. Remember how meditation changed crime rates in Washington DC and war activity in Iraq? Shifting our World is as easy as focusing Mind-Heart energy in LOVE.

From our research we know heart coherence is not an idle state; it reaches out, influences and supports in many beneficial ways. Evidence suggests a global *Field* environment connects all living systems and consciousness. We believe a feedback loop exists between all humans and Earth's energetic systems.

We are working together with other initiatives to realize the increased effectiveness of collective intention and cooperation. The are growing numbers of organizations with tools and techniques to facilitate increased heart connection and collaboration with others. This evolves into a collective opening of the heart, which is a major step toward increasing global and social coherence. We call this heart-based living.... each person's thoughts, emotions and intentions affect the field.

> *HeartMath Institute*
> *Global Coherence Project*

We are coming closer to the reality of Global Peace. Many thousands of *21st Century Superhumans,* Now accessing LOVE and Peace in Thought, Meditation, Prayer, Share, Clear and Amplify this energy into the Collective, with an amazing Global network of connected New Earth citizens emerging. *Bravo!* Steven Greer's Disclosure Project of government officials testifying to ET interaction, which began when the nuclear bomb was dropped on Hiroshima-Nagasaki to prevent such events from occurring again, we may be joining a Galactic family. It is said, *The time of the lone Wolf is over. Gather Yourselves...*

HOPI ELDERS' PROPHECY

You have been telling people that this is the Eleventh Hour, now you must go back and tell the people that this is the Hour. There are things to be considered. . . .

Where are you living? What are you doing?
What are your relationships? Are you in right relation?
Where is your water?
Know your garden.
It is time to speak your truth.
 Create your community. Be good to each other.
And do not look outside yourself for your leader.

He rubbed his hands together and said, "This could be a very good time!" There is a river flowing now very fast. It is so great and swift that there are those who will be afraid. They will try to hold on to the shore.
They will feel they are being torn apart and will suffer greatly.

Know the river has its destination. The elders say we must let go of the shore, push off into the middle of the river, keep our eyes open, and our heads above the water.

And I say, see who is in there with you and celebrate.
The time of the lone wolf is over. Gather yourselves!

Banish the word 'struggle' from your attitude and your vocabulary. All that we do now must be done in a sacred manner and in celebration.**We are the ones we've been waiting for...**

ChoQosh Auh'ho'oh, coastal indian elder brought "the HOPI TEN" from 5 elders in the village of Orabi Hopi Nation in April of 1993. (relayed by Orabi Mountain Dreamer)

Chapter 11

Dance of Relationship

The flute of the infinite is played without ceasing, and its sound is LOVE.

Kabir (1398-1518)
Mystic Poet and Saint of India, Bhakti-devotion to God

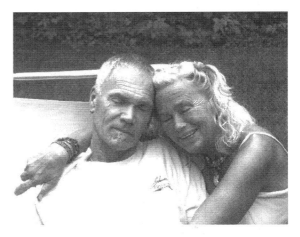

In the sacred dance of relationship we find mirrored the deepest treasures of Life, the most challenging and empowering lessons to test our very soul, as well as the most nourishing peace, joy, comfort and companionship. Individuals we draw in by the mystery of this magnetic resonance to share the path of relationship, are as perfectly matched to us as peas in a pod.

Alchemical attraction is one of those mystical things beyond the logical mind, and once activated for "real," we may as well just get out of the way and let it flow until it lands. We are energy beings. Our Body-Mind is a product of Vibration of thought carried within us. Those we magnetically drawn in, hold intricate puzzle pieces *to US*. We Mirror one another's deepest pain and greatest joy. We enter each other's Lives *to know ourselves better*.

You are a paradise, but you have forgotten yourself. You are looking everywhere except within you, and that is the only place where you are going to find the treasure, the truth of beauty.

Osho (1931-1990)
Indian Mystic, Guru and Teacher of Self-Inquiry

Relatively unconscious, in early Life, we blissfully float along and relationship lessons come at us unawares. As we awaken, deciphering Life in New ways, multiple layers are exposed. We then identify where this pattern is coming from in our past or generations, and what it means to us. Eventually, we recognize value in taking full Response-Ability for

ALL appearing in our World, and relationship becomes a New and delightful vehicle for engaging with another to expand self, our "reality" and state of Being.

3 Levels of Relationship

1. *UNCONSCIOUS:* Starts out "in Love" with partner. When challenges come up develops "stories" to explain *why it is the other person's fault,* and how it can be fixed, based in in blame-fear-hostility-judgement-control culture. Responds to most situations through Power Person Dynamic [see Part 2: MIND for details]. Relationships may end or carry on in uncomfortable chronic blame-pain patterns.

2. *AWARE:* Loves partner and self. When issues come up, *knows* they can "get through it." Uses discussion with partner and or therapy to process through issues coming up in and with each other. Considers it healing for each partner to "work through their stuff. Negotiates for "other person" to change as best solution when issues come up. Often conforms with cultural expectations and traditional relationship paradigms.

3. *OPEN AND AUTHENTIC:* Holds LOVE for self and partner. Knows their relationship "reality" from joy to pain is a product of *their* Vibrational thought resonance. They use Ancient Aramaic Forgiveness process-Freedom Tools to cancel goals and clear *their own internal content* appearing as issues; they learn from and work through Power Person Dynamic. {Part 2: MIND] They notice things change as they shift internally. They are honest with Authentic self expression, in LOVE. They utilize connection with partner-relationship to expand more fully into who they are and deepen experience into New levels of Being.

Together in LOVE

As we live together, in LOVE, we change the World. As we grow together, in LOVE, we let go of old thought patterns and limiting beliefs.

As we share together, in LOVE, we change our personal history and the interpretations of the past and present circumstances.We are connected deeply to the Universe, to a Higher Consciousness and to each other. We learn to stay centered, expand our awareness and trust our inner–voice, moment by moment, By learning to listen, stilling our minds, setting our intentions, we merge into Oneness.

We ALL share the Vibration of LOVE and Wisdom within us…and as we allow it to expand, we remember what we have Always Known: We are made of LOVE, we are uniquely special, our Light shines through any darkness and we Create Miracles by being Together in LOVE!

Teddi Mulder & Nancy Dock
Natural Awakenings

Whenever possible it's best is to join in relationship with someone who is focused on similar growth and development of consciousness. Such a relationship can contain High levels of spiritual and personal evolution for both partners. Many "waking up" while in relationship, even with deep Love for one another, may find themselves at very different places on the path. When this occurs, most important to remember is that the path of growth is our own. Even another person at a different phase of their evolution can be a Mirror to show us what we still carry inside Not of LOVE to remove; and sometimes we need to "draw the line in the sand."

UNCONSCIOUS levels of intimacy and sexuality are expressed in immaturity, when young (or very unaware), to fulfill basic desires of self-gratification or security. In the "old world" in many cases this level of interchange continued throughout Life. However we are ALL being activated by current Light *Fields* and Gamma rays Now penetrating our Solar System [Part 1: SHIFT OF THE AGES], many are Now growing beyond this phase.

As we emerge into AWARE levels of intimacy, we deepen sexual connection and gravitate towards mutual fulfillment through Love and Understanding. This path often sustained in traditional paradigms, will open a New mutual dynamic if both are awake and interested. Intimacy in this partnership blossoms naturally, based on commitment to one another, family, productivity and mutual growth through bumps and triumphs of Life.

Moving into OPEN AND AUTHENTIC intimacy we come to the relationship with Authentic expression of Who We Are, open to holding LOVE in all situations. We have developed capacity LOVE many, to "fall in LOVE daily," to LOVE self fully, and yet we seek the Higher path to deepen intimacy with One partner. We express honesty in ALL areas, which sparks bonding and more deeply sustainable intimacy This means Loving our Body. Telling our Truth gently with LOVE.

We learn to run our powerful sexual energy through ourselves with or without a partner, establishing a new framework for deepening sexuality when shared. We grow beyond the old paradigm matrix of self-protection and secrecy. We learn through loyalty in relationship, that all resonance in our "reality" is a Mirroring from within.. We learn how to operate with or without a partner as a whole being, with freedom to Be fully Who We Are.

Mind is so powerful it would lead us to believe there's a material world.

Byron Katie

We are like super bio-computers. Our Bodies transmit Vibrational signals from thoughts we engage in, and they appear as our World. We communicate with community, family and partner in a more "open-Authentic" way, moving out of blame and fear into LOVE, activating new dimensions of self. Who we Are is amplified in honest, open, non-blaming, mutually supportive relationship. It improves endocrine function and Heart Coherence, *literally* activating New DNA filaments, honing the Body to carry more Light, increasing Longevity hormones for Vitality and Well-Being.

Magnetic Masculine-Feminine principles are fine-tuning in this New "reality" of relationship. These two powerful aspects, the yin and yang of Masculine-Feminine are core dynamic of Creation in our World. We grow into balancing these polarities *within self*. Feminine is returning to its native place of being honored by and equal to the Masculine. The two polarities differ, in that Feminine incubates and holds space, while Masculine structures and drives forward, perfect complimentary dynamic for Pure Positive Creation.

Magnetism between these two potent forces, flows within and between us, deepening in intimate relationship. Imbalances of the last few thousand years resulting from ignorance in this area, Now refocus with LOVE, Unity and Oneness. This re-synchronization empowers us with the flow of Source and Earth's regenerative energy, moving us into dimensions of Pure Potentiality, Longevity and Well-Being .

Kundalini, Sexuality and Multi-Dimensionality

Magnetic Masculine and Feminine expose themselves more exquisitely in wonderful exploration of Conscious Intimate Relationship. The Secret of drawing in a partner devoted to sharing this path requires first being committed to Knowing and LOVING Self. In the past we may have diminished ourselves to "gain or keep" another, or shifted even just a little out of our Truth for someone to "like" us, which we are Now moving beyond.

The drive to share Union through sexuality is powerful within us. Honoring Self, we draw in our perfect Vibrational compliment. ALL is Vibration, *perfection unfolds*. Determine if who you pull in Mirrors *a pattern*, or if they are "right" for sustained relationship. We have had partners who helped us clear *a layer*. Once that layer is gone, we may be done with "karmic clearing" with that Soul. Ceremony with sage, incense, prayer can blesses and clear former partner(s) energy, as sexual fluids exchanged imprint in DNA and cells.

Desiring higher frequency companionship, we draw in a partner who is a Vibrational match to Authentic Self. Such powerful combining of energies Create more than we do alone. Such alliances are beneficial with family, friends, partners and community, AND Feminine-Masculine polarities are exquisitely explored through Sacred Intimacy.

High teachings embrace joining with *One partner,* with whom there is a pure magnetic chemistry and dedication to deepening Intimacy together. Such commitment found and treasured unselfishly, progresses Soul Evolution. It becomes possible to pass through and clear "old deep layers" that we may not access alone or in a more superficial relationship. This "old data," from generational or experiential "data bank" may have kept us from achieving deep mutual connection in the past. Once this clears we reach greater heights of mutual Ecstasy, Union and Co-Creativity.

We may hit "sticking points" at this level of clearing and feel we want to leave the relationship. We may think "it's not working," or maybe "someone else" seems a more interesting partner. There really is no "other" in the Quantum world. A Vibrational "partner" Mirrors perfectly back to us awareness of how to move into LOVE. Releasing and letting go any resistance to what we feel is negative about partner or what they are doing or doing "to us," our "reality" shifts. *It is ALL an inside job.* The outer shifts instantly as we get this, moving into LOVE. In relationship with commitment, Soul Evolution occurs, and we can sit together and be so at-one, there is only ONE.

We sit together, the mountain and I, until only the mountain remains.

Li Po

An advanced relationship model is Now emerging with those who are "Awake" both for those previously in "old paradigm" relationships, currently "alone," or still in relationship. As Authenticity and Truth of *Essence* become dominant themes, there is high need for Freedom of movement to flow and express fully in the Now. This puts a Vital New Dynamic into relationship possibility, where Freedom of Spirit must be maintained at all costs in order for this Soul to keep emerging onto their path of Full Expression. *"My Perfect LOVE for you my dear, is Your Perfect Freedom."* (Jack White to Teddi, *God's Game of Life*)

It's only possible to live happily ever after on a moment to moment basis.

Margaret Bonnano

Dedication with One partner is a Sacred Path, to deepen True Intimacy. The Truth is, our real relationship is with Self-Source; yet building trust with Another, Sacred Space for clearing, Truthful Self-expression, Honoring Individual Freedom with deep LOVE and Trust, we experience wholeness merging in Union with Divine-Higher Self. This level of deepening, emerges naturally with One partner who is a Vibrational match with our path. As our friend Kami Be says, "Find someone on your level rather than taking the short bus."

Sexual energy is the powerful Life-force of continual Creation, flowing from Source. Through Aware and Conscious Sexual partnering, we expansively open to greater levels of receiving Life, Creativity, Vibrancy. Whether we are with a partner or not, becoming familiar with this generative energy flowing through us and learning to allow it to radiate through us is part of the Soul Journey. We are Now clearing shame and wounding around sexuality carried for thousands of generations, learning to Live Joyfully in our Bodies.

Soul Evolution carries us into full unbroken connection with Source. True Intimacy of Sacred partnership is an Ancient path to En-Light-enment. Sexual interaction in such partnership is a Sacred tool. Ancient teachings instruct moving sexual Life-force energy or Kundalini, up the spine, weaving between chakras like two serpents or a double helix, also Mirroring DNA. Ancient Tantric, sexual techniques for spiritual awakening teach raising this vital creative current through Heart and Crown, to consciously immerse in sexual energy, rather than only genitals. Breathing, opening to consciously experience flow of this energy activates a magnificent generative state, in which we are fully designed to Live.

Our sexuality is core to our happiness and power as human beings.

Baba Dez Nichols
ISTA International School of Temple Arts

We are designed to Live in waves of full body orgasm, an art long suppressed in human culture, yet amazingly powerful flow of Creative Life-force through us. As we heal sexually, accessing connection to happiness and Joyful Living through sexual energy, we hold a frequency for healing pain and imbalance on Earth. Healthy sexual expression increases Vitality, Radiance and Well-Being, activating hormones and other dimensions. Engage sexually with Self or Partner with Pure Intent, without projection, as what is in the Mind sends powerful creative waves. Focus in Heart with LOVE. Amplify sexual ecstasy.

TANTRA MEDITATION TO AMPLIFY GENERATIVE SEXUAL ENERGY: Women and men use this practice to raise kundalini, activate flow of sexual energy through total Body-Mind (shakti-kundalini). Do singly sitting cross legged, or in chair, or lying down, or sit or lie back-to-back with partner. Use circular open mouthed Breathing. Connect with Central Light Core of the Earth, bringing a current of Light-energy up through root chakra, tightening vaginal muscles for women and perineum for men. Feel the Source *Field* flowing and generating through you, amplifying Creation, permeating LOVE. Let it flow out head all the way to Central Sun and back in circular motion through the Earth and up again through you. Allow yourself to be filled with this generative energy. Practice regularly, a few minutes to hours. Feel at peace with and receive the abundant supply of the Universe.

Last week at the river, by two small waterfalls, I was lying on a granite rock in a natural indentation that perfectly fit my body. I became aware of my "star family" communicating with me. Not only were they communicating with me, they were upgrading me, and I realized it has been an ongoing process for quite some time; years. I was shown that we are already living in the NEW. Some realize it and some don't. I was then shown the parts of me which are afraid of the New and struggling to hold on to the OLD. I could feel the fear and grasping-ness of it. Heart clenching pain actually. I was also told that everyone is going to "make it". It doesn't matter what they eat or what yoga they do...it is happening to all. (I would imagine the food, yoga etc... help with acclimating and understanding what's going on and flowing with it - that's from me, not them)

Then I was shown how to navigate the NEW. Open the heart and allow the huge LOVE which is all around and constantly offered to pour in. It literally looks like a tunnel/portal pouring down and in (from the top of our heads to our whole body, especially the Heart, when we open and allow it. In the NEW we no longer have to learn from pain and suffering, which was the way we did in the OLD. Being nourished by all this Light will feed us, to the point where we will not really need to eat anymore. We will continue to do so because of habit and comfort, until we have grown beyond it. As we open more and more, we will understand this part fully. Funnily, this is an ongoing process. The key is to stay sensitized and aware of the bigger picture in each and every precious moment with Heart open, feeling Body doing the thinking.

Ceslie Rossi - Siri Sadhna, Soul Essence

Some think it's holding on that makes one strong; sometimes it's letting go.

Sylvia Robinson

Part 3: SPIRIT

Chapter 12

Family, Children, Pets

Children of the world, deserve a paradise
Open up your eyes it's plain to see it's up to you and me
Love has the strength to change this world

Julian Lennon
Children of the World, Lyrics

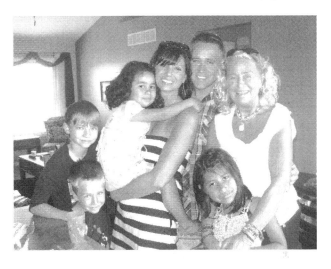

Do you know a family you LOVE, cherish and consider a model, that you admire or feel your Life is enriched by being around? Such energy is wonderful to find and absorb for our own Well-Being and Healing. Inner circle of family can be one of the most nourishing aspects of human existence, and yet it can also be challenging. Original unit of mother-father-children was core survival mechanism of the species (still is in some cultures today). Developing into more sophisticated roles, a deeper understanding of the family unit expanded and grew into learning from one another.

Whoever we "draw in" as "family" either by birth or proximity, there are always lessons to be learned with one another, as by our resonance (conscious-unconscious), the eternal flow of Universal LOVE clears all "logjams" out of its way. [Part 2: MIND] Our beloved family members who have shown up by either blood or companionship, nurture or challenge us to our very core, and are there as a result of this flow of Universal LOVE. They bring us the deepest and most enduring lessons about ourselves, that challenge us to grow into someone greater than we do alone. Through the magnetic of LOVE, a deep bond is there that keeps us learning the lesson until we get it. This is the miracle of LOVE.

Between children, parents, siblings, companions and extended family a magnetic matrix comes together, where we, like a beautiful flower in a garden, grow and evolve, weeds and ALL, with a group energy that draws us beyond self-interest, to put forth much unselfishly for others. It is in the giving and receiving that we bloom and grow into an amazingly beautiful flower or tree that we could not alone. Even when we have to grow *without* family there is the added dynamic of lack, or the push and pull of who *isn't there.*

Our heart aches, our heart fills with joy; there are losses, triumphs, oppressions, victories, despair, hurts, pain, sorrow, suffering, and the exquisite recognition of so many things we would never learn alone. This is the power of family. This is the power of LOVE.

Many young Souls are "arriving" today, with DNA activated to gravitate toward Oneness. They are attuned to a natural freedom of expression and peace. They bring an infusion of New energy to Earth without hardened overlays of older generations. They are excited, enthusiastic, gentle, kind and brilliant. It is up to us to nurture them with LOVE.

Many younger souls, ranging from 12 - 34, caught between the New paradigm and the old, are uncomfortable with structured 3D, yet searching for how to establish a New trail into the kind of World they were born to birth. *Our special Heart guidance is welcomed...*

Even as the populace embraces - or at least explores -- the coming changes, we are still collectively hanging on to old attachments... For example, we still judge, compete, and believe in lack and limitation. And we aren't completely honest with ourselves or others, often hiding behind politeness or political correctness.

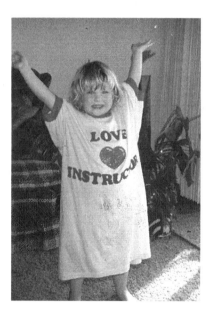

The children who have recently incarnated are different from previous generations. They are called "Children of the Light," "Millennium Children," and "Indigo Children" for good reason. These children are highly aware, sensitive, and downright psychic. They also have zero tolerance for dishonesty and inauthenticity. They know when someone is lying, instantly!

Imagine how difficult it is for these children to be in the current educational system, with much inauthenticity - such as, "Let's pretend that we like being here. Let's not discuss how unhappy we all are to be forced to come to this place and learn/teach things that we're unsure have any practical application in real life."

The Indigo Children have incarnated at this time for a very sacred reason: to usher in a new society based on honesty, cooperation and love. By the time they reach adulthood our world will be vastly different...We will remember our ability to manifest our needs, so there will be no need to compete with others. Since our natural telepathic skills will be rekindled, lying will be impossible. And because everyone will realize the oneness that exists between all living things, thoughtfulness will be the basis of society.

Lee Carroll & Jan Tober
The Indigo Children

This is a special opportunity for generations of Awakening parents, grandparents, extended family, to step into a New paradigm with these children, to actualize living the path of the Heart.

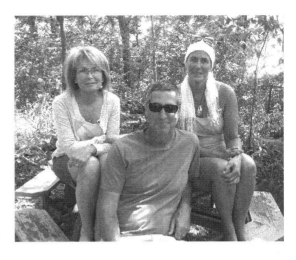

...Your children are not your children,They are the sons and daughters of Life's longing for itself. They came through you, not from you

And though they are with you, they belong not to you. You may give them your LOVE but not your thoughts, for they have their own thoughts.

You may house their bodies, but not their Souls.For their Souls dwell in the house of tomorrow, Which you cannot visit, not even in your dreams. You may strive to be like them, but seek not to make them like you...

Kahlil Gibran (1883-1931)
The Prophet

Children are awesome teachers! Reconnect through them with your innocence, Smile, Breathe, Laugh, Play, Be in the Moment, Flow with Life; rediscover Joy and Creativity! Children are naturals at this! They bring attitudes, resources and connection to Life that will allow them to take on our World in this Evolutionary Leap and beyond. We special adults have agreed to support them in discovering meaningful expression. Find New ways to communicate with these children, *always with positive reinforcement*. This may take re-educating *YOUR Mind!* These children resonate an entirely New societal model based in LOVE, encouraging in coming changes to magnetize Family-Community to do the same.

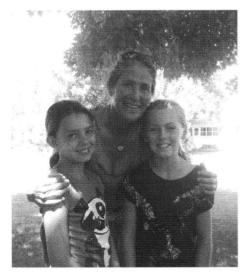

Preservation of a child's native esteem is far more important than acquisition of technical skills. Share with them knowledge they need, yet preserve their inherent confidence in themselves...

Honor and learn from Little Ones' intent to play. They teach us the innocence in their hearts that embraces unconditional love. They shall inherit the earth with this love.

...This is the Indigo's mission: to prepare humanity for the universal song of love...

See their hope and guide it, for this is the vision of tomorrow in the imaginations of today. Feel the playfulness of these imaginations. It is in this energy that we can find free choice... Understand their intentions and lead them to make choices that will help the planet grow toward peace. It is peace that they know. Through peace they are teaching us a greater understanding of humanity.

Lee Carroll & Jan Tober
The indigo Children

Children with advanced abilities and adults activating theirs, do better in creative learning environments, self-taught or in self-guided schools such as Waldorf or Montessori. These "Autodidactic" or self-learning styles have produced brilliant contributors such as Leonardo da Vinci, Frank Lloyd Wright, Thomas Edison, Buckminster Fuller, David Bowie, Ernest Hemingway and more. Tony Robbins told us, "More school dropouts achieved millionaire status, by thinking 'outside the box.'"

We are outgrowing old structures, that have suppressed the human spirit for too long. Trailblazers are breaking free to Live with Authentic self-expression. Younger generations and children are "teaching" parents, grandparents and caregivers who are teachable, with unbounded energy, high intelligence and desire to live beyond constraints. Many young people from infancy to mid-late twenties and early thirties do not fit current or old societal norms; they are seeking the path of expressing their *evolved DNA*.

I have discovered many Star-Children all over the world. The reason they are here is to act as conduits of energy needed in the evolution of Earth and to help raise human consciousness to a higher dimension.

Dolores Cannon
The Convoluted Universe

Those who support this younger generation on a creative and vital path, also mega-jump their own evolutionary process, shedding old ways like an ancient skin, celebrating New resonance of the Heart. For those with children in your Lives, read up on Indigo and Crystal children. Indigos began coming in 70 years ago so you may find *yourself* in descriptions of advanced and paranormal abilities!

You can discover more about a person in an hour of play
than in a year of conversation.

Plato

Anyone who has children or grandchildren of the one to twenty-something age, will notice most have essentially little interest in old 3-D pursuits, goals or expectations. They came to Planet Earth as 5-D Beings, and are in the midst of figuring out how to Live in this dynamic matrix. They are more advanced in many ways. They will be creating New paths.

Pressure from old paradigm family members pushing to join the ranks of the uninspired workforce leaves many in their twenties feeling disempowered yet still hopefully searching, perhaps confused. This generation leans toward Living with vivid self-expression, creativity and scintillating personality, naturally gathering together in Unity. This emerging Soul monad is demonstrated in a potent wave of yearly festivals Worldwide. Over a million attendees, unwinding from uninspired modern culture, seek their own radiant expression. [See The Bloom Series documentary].

These young souls inherit stewardship for our World, with ability to change the course of history in yet undreamed of ways. The thirty-something generation found ways to "fit in," however many of them are also 5-D souls as well, a transitional generation, rarely satisfied with jobs and roles in society, yet placeholders between the old and the new. As we begin to learn to live more multi-dimensionally, our culture will become more versatile, making room for native skills of these generations, suited to creative flowing expansive 4th and 5th dimensional pursuits. A new type of Earth community will emerge.

EXAMPLE: MY CHILD'S BEHAVIOR: One might ask, "How about my child's behavior, is even this a Mirroring of something inside me?" They and their behavior *or your perception of it* resonates into your "reality" as a magnetic match to *your* Attention on the *Field* as Observer-Creator. Whatever they are reflecting to you is a perfect opportunity to clear your own content, until you see only LOVE around you.

NOTE: As we are waking up to this process, there may be action to take to change situations, while at the same time becoming more aware of our own Mind-energy Not of LOVE is a good focus for clearing. *Include those involved if possible.* Find ways to receive and listen to your child's truth, honor it and support them in becoming Who they Are.

CLEARING SELF TO FLOW WITH CHILD: In the old paradigm, "my child" is outside myself, and they are to "blame," right or wrong. In this new paradigm of the Heart, I realize that what I believe I am seeing in them "Not of LOVE," is resonating from inside me! I get out *Ancient Aramaic Forgiveness Freedom Tools* [Part 2: MIND]. Going through the "goal canceling" process I discover *what is being brought up in me,* and what goal I need to cancel to clear, to live from my Heart of LOVE and Create a new "reality" from this space. As I do so, the situation changes and I Am better able to flow with my child.

What if I have family members who don't want to participate in this journey with me? Clear your own "corrupt-data" and restore your True Design LOVE. Breathe and Smile... This is the journey of "Waking Up." As you do so your energy will send new messages *and* situations *will change* around you. The more compassion you have for others, the quicker they change. Remember complimentary support and approval brings Healthy cooperation.

We ultimately realize we are ONE and heal all things, by taking Response-Ability for our own thought Creations, to restore LOVE, Compassion, Gratitude. Michael ryce says, "Did you ever notice the person who picks you up at the plane, finishes the sentence of the one who put you on it" *and you were the one there every time?* Teddi's friend Geoffrey Bullock said, *"We go from Loving arms to Loving arms, trusting the Universe is supporting us."*

My "reality" is my Response-Ability and comes from my personal and genetic Mind Energy. By taking time for Clearing, Meditation and Breathing we reset ourselves to Source-Energy. Do your best to return to this State. Teddi ♥

MR. EMOTO of *Messages from Water,* did a special experiment with beakers of rice. To the first beaker he said, "I hate you," which turned black and rotten. The second beaker he ignored completely; it soured. The third he said, "Thank you." It developed a sweet delicious fermentation. How simple. Even rice knows what energy is.

Our entire existence knows what energy is; our children, our families, our pets know. It can't be hidden. It emerges into "reality" as a PERFECT MIRROR of what's inside us. Simple enough to confound the wise, yet easy enough for a child to comprehend; caring for each other does matter! We are electromagnetic resonators. Creation can not be fooled.

Remember, *"there is no 'out there' out there."* What we experience or what is resonating in us, is initiated by the energy we carry inside. Those are old "tuning forks" as Jack White would say, "We draw others in with the magnets in our pockets!" When you meet someone and things get stirred up, it is Life *longing* to be set free. So set it free, by restoring your True Design LOVE. Then Shine!

That's what real LOVE amounts to - letting the other be what they really are.

Jim Morrison (1943-1971)
Lead Singer, The Doors, Rolling Stone's Top 100 Singers of All Time

This is the message the New children bring us. As long as we reflect in-Authenticity in our own Lives, as long as we resonate Ancient pain, they will call us on it, directly or indirectly. They come in with pure hearts, beyond the conditioning of thousands of generations that many of us carry. Freeing ourselves of this "old data," opens the doors to enlightening and mutually supportive relationships with the younger generations.

Cultivating the heart of compassion is what we're here to do.

Ram Dass
Polishing the Mirror

We are energy Beings, designed to thrive on LOVE. What else do we need to know? Thousands of years of blame-fear-hostility has had our "computer" operating with virus laden software programs. Let's practice True Forgiveness, removing our own "corrupt data," when we feel any issue with any family member. Invite Rookha d'Koodsha to clean out the virus and help cancel your goals. Use firewalls / filters Rakhma and Khooba for intentions and perceptions of LOVE. Clean out the virus, the system runs faster and better. LOVE Yourself, your children, your family, your pets. "The greatest of these is LOVE."

Pets and Animals

Animals carry the resonance of Pure Unconditional LOVE. They are here to share it with us, to Mirror us, to take on our pain, to LOVE us. Any animals' misery is the result of our Mind-energy. As Native Americans knew, our Hearts would be sad without animals.

They bring incredible joy, comfort and a wonderful invitation to open our Hearts. In the waking up process we learn to carry on telepathy with animals and build amazing bonds. Allow yourself to open more to the kind of Heart connection possible with your pets!

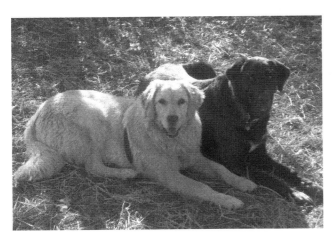

As animal Lovers know, there is a suffering epidemic of untold millions of stray and deserted cats, dogs and other pets, as well as devastating practices of factory farming. Animals express pure LOVE and bear the brunt of our suffering Mind-energy. Animal cruelty and killing to eat is left behind with choices in Higher Consciousness. Animals were given to be our friends and companions, yet it is a journey of waking up to come to a point where this is a Life-choice.

Nothing will benefit human health and increase the chances for survival of life on earth as much as the evolution to a vegetarian diet.

Our task must be to free ourselves from this prison by widening our circle of compassion to embrace all living creatures.

Albert Einstein (1879-1955)
General Theory of Relativity, Nobel Prize Physics 1921, Max Planck Medal 1929

Extinction and loss of species in our overly materialistic culture is rampant. Inhumane conditions or captivity bring up sorrow, rage, grief, fear, resistance, thought patterns that need to be removed from *our* unconscious (or we hold them in form). See Part 2: MIND to clear your "old data" to LOVE, Live with utmost Compassion and change this "reality!" An orca at Sea World killing a third trainer, sends a message that holding magnificent creatures in small spaces, must change to cultivate a World of Freedom for ALL. This may seem counterintuitive to our old way of thinking, yet it aligns with **Quantum Lifestyle**, where "reality" emerges from "Attention"upon the *Field*.

LOVE your animals, feed them healthy food - dogs are omnivores, may well have longer life as vegetarian. *AVOID or reduce* vaccinations. *(See our upcoming videos-ebooks for more on this)*. Natural organic food and Lifestyle is good for all pets and creatures in our care, as it is for us. Pet food can be homemade or supplemented with veggies, bit of green shake. We have much to learn about truly natural care for ourselves and these beloved creatures who grace our world as companions. Learn New *positive reinforcement training,* use tiny treats and enthusiastic voice to shape your pets' behavior with Joy and LOVE.

Through their bond with us pets and even plants experience Life in a more complex and rich way than they would alone, as we are multi-dimensional. Their connections with us enrich their journey here. It has been noted that pets often "look or act like" the humans they are with, as they absorb or harmonize with our frequencies. Additionally those awake tend to pull in Higher dimensional Beings to walk with them embodied as pet companions.

We awaken to Higher coexistence with family, children and pets in New *21st Century Superhuman* ways. Through these LOVING interrelationships, we deepen our connection to Self, to Source and to Living LOVE. In Heart-based Living we activate more DNA codons, extend Vitality and Life-expectancy, going beyond 3-D to express as multi-dimensional humans. It is a Living "reality," as we put it into practice, transforming self, family, friends and community.

> Be proud of who you are, where you come from and what you represent in this lifetime as it is so immensely important to love yourself by heart. It is your heart that is yearning for peace, understanding and allowance to move beyond concepts of time and illusion. You all are great bearers of Light and I AM so proud of you all and immensely grateful for your hearts
>
> *Lady Portia*
> *Méline Lafont*

Kirpal Singh, Indian guru and teacher of World peace, organized a World Conference on the Unity of Man over 40 years ago now in 1974, with over two thousand delegates, religious and political leaders from around the World and 100,000 attendees. He said then,

> We are *already One*, no proof is required. But we have forgotten that Unity...we are all children of Light. But we have forgotten ourselves....We have to realize Unity...
>
> They asked me in the West, "How can we evade the disaster of atomic war?" I told them, "When kings and presidents rise above and go beyond countries." ...They should not only tend their own garden, but help others to keep their gardens in full bloom... The basic purpose of this World Conference is to bring home to all the fact that we are already One... The highest knowledge is to realize Unity is innate in us... Know that we are all One.
>
> *Kirpal Singh (1894-1974)*
> *World Conference on the Unity of Man*

We are ALL better together. Whatever skills, vision and wisdom are yours, collaborate with those you are most closely connected with, family, extended family, friends, community and globally. Participate as a Conscious Creator of a Viable future. If you don't feel like you have family, join with others to share family-community. Let Children teach You. Enter into this mystical, magical Presence called LOVE to Live a New kind of *21st Century Superhuman* Life through the Heart. We are on a journey of Initiation, into a New paradigm of empowered *Quantum Lifestyle*, where we access Full Potential with Miracles, Wonder and Delight...*where Peace in Our Hearts IS Peace on Earth...* ♥

Part 3: SPIRIT

Chapter 13

One With Earth Mother Gaia

Humankind has not woven the web of Life.
We are but one thread within it.
Whatever we do to the web, we do to ourselves.
All things are bound together.

Chief Seattle (1780-1866)
Northwest Native American

The Gaia principle describes Earth as a sentient Being, integrated with all her organisms in a single well-orchestrated Living system. Gaia was first proposed by James Lovelock in 1965, while seeking to detect Life on Mars, perceiving Earth as a Living Being. His idea evolved into wise stewardship for Gaia based on conscientious living, while seeking viable solutions for climate and environmental change, birthing the thought: *"Let's acknowledge Earth as our Living Home."*

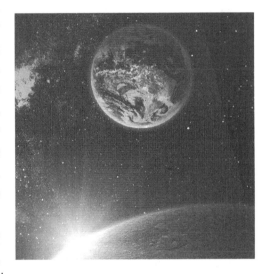

We are the intelligent elite among animal Life on earth and whatever our mistakes, [Earth] needs us. This may seem an odd statement after all that I have said about the way 20th century humans became almost a planetary dis-ease organism. But it has taken [Earth] 2.5 billion years to evolve an animal that can think and communicate its thoughts. If we become extinct she has small chance of evolving another.

James E. LOVElock
The Vanishing Face of Gaia: A Final Warning

Indigenous people of the Andes revered Pachamama as Earth Goddess, fearing her as a dragon who caused earthquakes, and requesting her blessings for fertility and harvest. Her self-sufficient power sustains Life on Earth. She is honored and appealed to regularly today, along with Earth elementals, Inti the Sun god and the Star People or quarks and electrons of the Source Field, as Andean shamans' insightful prayers appeal to the *Field*.

Earth emits low-frequency magnetic waves called the Schumann Resonance, after Winifried Otto Schumann (1888-1974) German physicist who first measured them in 1952. Earth's Schumann frequency can be likened to her "Heart-beat," the energy bouncing between Earth and her surrounding plasma layer, the ionosphere. Schumann Resonance is a pulse for Life on the Planet, setting tempo for health and well-being. Schumann Resonance is important to Well-Being of all Life on Earth, similar to brainwaves being subject to the Heart influencing the Body.

> Liquid crystals in DNA, brain ventricles, and cellular structures operate as antennae for detecting and decoding frequencies. Liquid crystals, an intrinsic part of cell membranes, act as a detector/amplifier/memory storage device for ELF EM patterns often around 10 Hz; a coherent wave-field may also emerge from the body's own liquid crystal matrix.

> *Schumann Resonance*
> *Excerpt from Nexus Magazine, Vol. 10, #3, April-May, 2003 by Iona Miller*

Gregg Braden discovered data from Norwegian and Russian researchers that Earth's electromagnetic frequency, pulse or "heartbeat," is on the increase, and has risen from 7.8 to 8.6 cycles per second related to shifting magnetics and weather patterns. Monitoring around 9/11 demonstrated that when humanity focuses with very strong common emotion, Earth's resonance responds.

> You are not separate from me, though you may think you are. Your mind and mine, the mind of the Earth, are One and the same.

> This One mind is called Noosphere – wrapped like an invisible mantle over the whole of my body, it penetrates every living thing, endowing each with a ray from the spectrum of living Consciousness spreading from the center of the galaxy to our sun to me and all of you who dwell on my surface.

> For those who have eyes to see, ears to hear, and Hearts that know from Within, Hear my manifesto for the Noosphere. Listen, and recite with me: I am One with the Earth. The Earth and mySelf are One mind...

> *Jose Arguelles (1939-2011)*
> *Organizer 1987 Harmonic Convergence*
> *The Mayan Factor: Path Beyond Technology*

We begin to comprehend, that our Planet Earth is not just a rock hurtling through space, that we happen to be riding on. She is a living organism; we are nourished by her and she by us. Being barefoot on the earth with head in the sky, produces an uplifting Life-giving electrical charge. Imagine yourself, a spark plug with this current of living electromagnetic energy passing through you, powering your Life Force. Synthetic footwear insulates us from this generative current, as does being inside most buildings and vehicles. *Find moments to go barefoot outdoors!* It's no wonder we LOVE being at the beach or being outside on the grass in the summertime. Make your yard organic. Enjoy Earth's Magic.

Our entire biological system, the brain and the Earth itself,
work on the same frequencies.

Nikola Tesla (1856-1943)
Inventor, physicist, and futurist
Designer of alternating current electricity and science for free energy

In essence, getting back to walking "barefoot" on Earth Mother Gaia is essential to obtaining Highest levels of Well-Being. Walk or do activities *with* shoes, *and then also* walk a few minutes in yard, park, beach or where you can *barefoot*. Being outdoors without glasses or sunglasses and minimal attire, also feeds us vital elements supplied by Solar rays within Earth's atmosphere, stimulating energy meridians and refreshing Body, Mind and Spirit. Walking barefoot on dew-laden grass (without chemicals) absorbs the fresh elixir of nature's purest distilled water with Living elements from grass and Earth. When you have a chance, go camping, sleep outdoors, open windows, sleep with windows open.

Merging with nature offers cooperation with Life and mutual aid for Well-Being. "Unnatural" cellphone and power grid networks on the other hand are disruptive to ours and Earth's magnetic field. These technologies put stress on our own natural energy systems, resulting in decreased Vitality. Studies show subjects living in isolation from Earth's geomagnetic rhythms over long periods, develop irregularities in psychobiology which is restored with introduction of a very weak 10Hz electrical field. Early astronauts suffered with this until resonance generators were installed in spacecraft. We discover that certain harmonic sound frequencies, also assist with restoring this balance, such as Kirtan and sacred chanting, Hemisync and other tonal frequencies that activate Alpha-Theta brain waves, restoring the 7.8-8.6 Hz. (recordings on YouTube).

Our exposure to radiation of man-made EMF (electric and magnetic *Fields*) has been shown to be as much as 100 million times more than simpler cultures had even 100 years ago. *Wow!* Research links EM (electromagnetic) radiation to increase cancer, Leukemia, Alzheimer's, Parkinson's and other degenerative conditions. *National Institute of Environmental Health Sciences* concludes that EMFs "should be regarded as possible carcinogens," after a review of 2,000+ studies.

Are we going to throw away our laptops, tablets, iPods, cell phones and other such devices? Probably not. These days even people in the furthest reaches of Africa and the Amazon rain forest are carrying cell phones as awesome communication devices. This wonderful "global brain" stimulates amazing progress, connection, development of ideas, vision and purpose, tools and resources, advancing human culture at an accelerated rate. Seek holistic solutions. Take a reprieve from electronic devices to integrate with Earth and restore balance. Find periods of each day where you can separate from phone/ computers / tv. Turn them off, leave them behind, go for a walk, Breathe the Earth. We are Now in early stages of harnessing "free energy" from the vacuum of space, soon to bring modern conveniences with clean environmentally harmonious natural energy systems.

Over thousands of years we've evolved with Gaia as our "Living Home." We are more healthy when harmoniously integrated with her Living Energy *Field*. Breathing fresh air, connecting with Earth balances our energy centers, nourishing vitality and Life. Make small changes to get out in nature for ideal self-care. A person who is glowing, vibrant, tan, fit is attractive because this is how we thrive, become more intelligent and are capable of our ultimate potential.

> Few people know how to take a walk. Qualifications are endurance, plain clothes, old shoes, an eye for nature, good humor, vast curiosity, good speech, good silence and nothing too much.
>
> *Ralph Waldo Emerson (1803-1882)*
> *Author, Transcendentalist, Self-Reliance*

We may think it difficult to change our Lives to get outdoors, however this is a critical piece of adapting ourselves to a more holistic, well-nourished **Quantum Lifestyle.** It is about *waking up*, and *knowing* tantalizing Cosmic influences are activating us. Body-Mind-Spirit request us to smuggle ourselves outdoors into natural Light and energy-fields.

> Numerous studies conducted by the Halberg Chronobiology Center at the University of Minnesota and others, have shown important links between Solar, Schumann and geomagnetic rhythms and a wide range of human and animal health and wellness indicators. Historical events such as war and social unrest have also been correlated with Solar cycles.
>
> *Dr. Rollin McCraty*
> *Global Coherence Initiative - Earth's Rhythms*

If you live in a major urban area with polluted air, consider the radical step of moving to where delicious air-quality exists. If you feel this is not an option, Create weekend escapes to more Vital natural environments to skyrocket your **Quantum Lifestyle.** Respond to cravings for "forbidden" juicy moments in nature, that activate, refresh and inspire!

Exposure to Solar rays and Schumann Resonance bouncing as harmonics between the Earth's magnetosphere and the Earth itself activate our pineal gland. Activate para-normal sensitivities by walking barefoot on the Earth, head in the sky, as Earth's resonant field activates transformative waking meditation in 7.82 8.6 Hz frequencies. We and Earth produce extra-low-frequency (ELF) electromagnetic *Fields* (EMFs) measured at 10 hertz, naturally harmonizing and mutually interactive.

> One of the affects of meditation is to "quiet the mind" as a method of allowing "free-run" (or silent deep thought immersion) to become entrained by natural geophysical rhythms. This form of tuning or "magnetoreception" is mediated by the pineal gland (30% of its cells are magnetically sensitive) and organic magnetite-containing tissues.
>
> *Magnetite in Human Tissues: A Mechanism for the Biological Effects of Weak ELF Magnetic Fields-*
> *Joseph L. Kirschvink, Atsuko Kobayashi-Kirschvink, Juan C. Diaz- Ricci, and Steven J. Kirschvink*

HEARTMATH INSTITUTE monitors effects of humans on Earth, and her's on us as well, revealing a deep and intrinsic connection between Sun, Earth and ALL people. Earth sensors reveal *Earth responds to Heart Coherence.* When a major event takes place that many are focused on, Earth's resonance spikes. Fluctuations of Earth's geomagnetic field also affects humanity. New Emerging thought is, as we attain Heart Coherence, we shift harmoniously with Gaia, our Solar system and the entire Universe. **ARC THE Hologram!**

• Earth's magnetic resonance matches heart rhythm and brainwave frequencies.

• Earth's varying electromagnetics affect health, feelings and behavior.

• When the Sun emits a 2.8 gigahertz radiowave frequency we feel better.

• Geomagnetic fluctuations disturb heart and nervous system.

• Prayers measure 8 Hz, matching the Earth's magnetic field of 8 Hz!

HeartMath's Global Coherence Initiative coordinates thousands around the World "...to unite in *Coherence*, where..increasing individual Coherence impacts the Whole."

Holographic consciousness provides for a change made anywhere in the system becoming a change everywhere in the system. Even with six billion plus people now sharing our world, we all benefit to some degree from the choices of peace and healing that are held by just a few.

Gregg Braden
The Divine Matrix

Our brain communicate with itself and the rest of the Body with Vibrational waveforms, easily measured by an EEG machine. These brainwave patterns are Beta (13 Hz), Alpha (7.8-12 Hz), Theta (3.5-7.8) and Delta (0.1 to 3.5 Hz), frequencies measured in cycles per second. Moments of genius flash in high electrical Gamma (25-40-100 Hz), common in Tibetan Buddhist monks in a transcendental state, with multiple brain wave frequencies operating simultaneously as right-left brain hemispheres communicate in a "diamond dance," bringing forth inspired vision, creativity and manifestation.

"Binaural beats" are used to synchronize brain frequencies: Play 2 tones the distance apart of the frequency you'd like to access (*i.e.* Alpha-Theta 7.8). The distance between the two tones will synchronize the brain to this frequency. Listen with headphones. (Do not use while operating machinery or driving). (Recordings on YouTube of various frequencies).

Researchers compared brain activity of Tibetan Buddhist monks to novice meditators (meditating one hour a day, one week prior). In a normal meditative state, both groups had similar brain activity. When the monks were told to generate an objective feeling of compassion during meditation, their brain activity began to fire in a rhythmic, coherent manner, suggesting neuronal structures were firing in harmony. This was observed at a frequency of 25–40 Hz, the rhythm of gamma waves. These gamma-band oscillations in the monk's brain signals were the largest seen in humans. *(Wikipedia)*

Gamma-band oscillations reflect in consciousness, bliss, and intellectual acuity after meditation. The Dalai Lama who meditates four hours each morning said that if there was an innovation to get him into this state rather than meditating four hours he would love to try it. Studies point to such possibilities.

PubMed September 2009 by JW Goethe University in Frankfort Germany; *Lucid dreaming: a state of consciousness with features of both waking and non-lucid dreaming* reported, "Lucid dreaming episodes tracked in Gamma bursts (40+ Hz) occurred as a result of pre-sleep autosuggestion. Meditation and or prayer/envisioning around LOVE, Compassion, Gratitude before going to sleep activates desires, ideas, visions and dreams on many levels.

Lucid dreaming constitutes a hybrid state of consciousness with definable and measurable differences from waking and REM sleep, particularly in frontal lobes of the brain with significant changes in electrophysiology." Collective-evolution.com offers this in October 18, 2013 article by Arjun Walia.

Research suggests that the existence of gamma brainwaves indicates a totally conscious experience, so the experience of being awake within a dream is a very real phenomenon. This begs the question, which state is actually real? Could what we perceive as being fully aware and awake be the real dream? Or are these just different aspects of reality that we are jumping to and from? Is our ability to Create our own reality easier in a state of lucid dreaming because our brain is functioning at a higher frequency?

What would we be capable of if we were able to attain that frequency without lucid dreaming? Would we be able to have instant manifestations like we do in our lucid dreams? Gamma brainwaves are involved in higher mental activity and consolidation of information. Operating from this frequency allows our brain to link and process information from multiple parts of the brain. We use more of our brain when we are experiencing lucid dreaming than we do when we are fully awake.

When doing your goal canceling process before going to sleep at night use *autosuggestion*. Breathing gently, call in *Rookha d'Koodsha*, Ancient Aramaic super-processor. Cancel goals bouncing around in your head - give them to the *Field*. Install your LOVE filters for *Rakhma* for perceptions and *Khooba* for intentions, focus around Heart Coherence - LOVE, Compassion, Gratitude. Say a prayer. Access your highest brain function and experience your Life changing as you give all this to the *Field*. Ask yourself, "Am I dreaming?" This will open up being more aware during lucid dream states to direct them

We transmit and receive extrasensory information through ELF electromagnetic frequencies more readily when synchronized with the Schumann Resonance. Healing and telepathic thought-forms of both sender and receiver are facilitated by entrainment with waveform patterns of the Earth environment.

Schumann's Resonances and Human Psychobiology (extended version)
Richard Alan Miller and Iona Miller Organization for the Advancement of Knowledge (O.A.K.), 2003

Theta is the deep meditation and light sleeping wave that includes REM dream state. This is the realm of the unconscious and stores our most deep seated programs, where we can reach a sense of Unity, connectedness and being at One with the Universe, with visualization, inspiration, profound creativity and exceptional insight. This is where Einstein used to go into 4 hour power naps with pencil and paper ready to jot down what came to him immediately upon awakening.

Over a decade of research on brain wave activity of healers from all cultures and religious backgrounds, psychics, shamans, dowsers, Christians, seers, ESP readers, kahuna, Santeria, Wicca and more...exhibited *"nearly identical EEG signatures"* during "healings:" 7.8-8Hz brainwaves lasting from one to several seconds, "phase and frequency-synchronized with Earth's geoelectric micropulses - Schumann Resonance. We harmonize with Earth outdoors, dropping into 7.8 - 8.6 Hz. This "sweet spot" accesses Alpha-Theta bringing vision, ideas and insights into Being

Delta is the slowest frequency, deep sleep, healing, regeneration, deep meditation, paranormal abilities. Tibetan Buddhist monks are known for going into Delta's deep states where awareness is detached and connection with paranormal is enhanced.

Beta (14040 Hz) is the wave of heightened awareness commonly used throughout the day "busy, coffee mind" where we can get stuck in worries, fears and rampant unconscious patterns that "drive the boat." Escaping outdoors is the certified way to clean up our Mind-Energy, to attain optimum harmonization with Earth Mother Gaia.

Beloved Brother, Earth Shaman Kailash plays didgeridoo, drum, flute, offering sacred ceremony connecting Heart with Earth. His didgeridoo backs the harmonic melody in this wonderful uplifting song (great for kids and adults). Listen with him leading this fantastic song-dance in Heidelberg, Germany on YouTube *Kailash Kokopelli WalkingTree Songdance.*

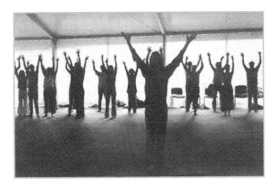

Walking Tree

I am a walking tree, You are a walking tree
Feet on the Earth - head in the sky
Heart joins together, the two to one to see
Bringing the light down, into the darkest ground
Releasing the dark side, into the light
I Breathe in what you Breathe out -
You Breathe in what I Breathe out
Breath is connecting us all
LOVE is connecting us all
Light is connecting us all

Kailash Kokopelli

Periods of immersing self in nature heightens and transforms telepathic, intuitive, creative and visionary abilities, aligning us Vibrantly with our true path and discovery of greater ways to express it. Ancient shamanic practices always included Vision Quests in natural places.A simple afternoon walk or a weekend or week(s) in forest, mountains, beach, river, jungle, ocean, drops us into miraculous Alpha-Theta brainwave state, where we deepen intuitive connection with Life and expression of our Greater Being.

> I went to the woods because I wished to live deliberately, to front only the essential facts of Life, and see if I could not learn what it had to teach and not when I came to die, discover that I had not lived.
>
> *Henry David Thoreau (1817-1862)*
> *American author of over 20 volumes poet, philosopher, abolitionist,*
> *naturalist, tax resister, surveyor, historian, and leading transcendentalist*

Whatever our every day Lifestyle, immersing in energies of Earth Mother Gaia and her Schumann Resonance, nourishes us with electromagnetic energies that benefit ALL we do. Get out for walks or bike rides and escape periodically to remote areas. Life becomes more *juicy* and vibrant when we are electromagnetically charged, with Vitality to fulfill our dreams.

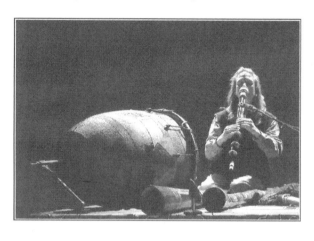

> If one advances confidently in the direction of his dreams, and endeavors to live the Life he has imagined, he will meet with success unexpected in common hours.
>
> *Henry David Thoreau (1817-1862)*
> *American author of over 20 volumes and leading Transcendentalist*

There can be many excuses: too busy, don't have "time," how do I fit this in with family, children, job, commitments? We tend to do what we're habituated to. We have in so many ways, pushed Mother Nature out the back door, while we recline in the comfort and luxury of couches, chairs, houses, carpets and cars, surrounded by all-absorbing technologies of computer, television, phone and other sundry things. *Make a date with Gaia!*

> Things do not change; we change.
>
> *Henry David Thoreau (1817-1862)*
> *Transcendentalist Author*

It may take commitment to cultivate taking regular walks, bike rides, getting out in yard or garden, *even just sitting* outdoors, harmonizing with resonance of the natural World, expressing primal aspects of who we are. Our natural instinct is to connect with Pachamama, even in modern Lifestyle. Let's shine a Light into those dark places and bring out the childlike part of us that enjoys movement and being out in the fresh air sunshine.

> What you get by achieving your goals is not as important as
> what you become by achieving your goals.

Henry David Thoreau (1817-1862)

Cultivate this **21st Century Superhuman** practice. Find a friend to walk or go on random jaunts with who relishes nature. If you're a paddler, hiker, camper, walker, kayaker, skier, snowboarder, outdoor activity LOVER, yeah a for you for being already integrated in one of the most thrilling, magnetic Joys of Life on Planet Earth!

The price of anything is the amount of Life you exchange for it.

Henry David Thoreau (1817-1862)

What is going on, on Planet Earth right Now? Let's put it into perspective. Earth is our Mother, our Home. Gaia is a Living resonant Being with whom we have an intrinsic deeply connected relationship, reflecting in our Life and hers. We are learning how to nourish and amplify our energies by connecting with her. *And* we are learning how to nourish her in return with our *Heart Coherence,* and to Live in more harmonious ways.

I believe the houses of the future will be...designed to welcome rather than to impress. People...will want homes in which every room is used every day and in which there are no wasted spaces--homes less like furniture stores or warehouses and more like nests.

John Robbins
The New Good Life: Living Better Than Ever in an Age of Less

This may give us an inkling of the possibilities of how we can change things on Planet Earth, simply by activating Heart Coherence. Once we LOVE the Earth, as Thoreau said, we shift our stance to, "Every creature is better alive than dead, men and moose and pine trees, and he who understands it aright will rather preserve its Life than destroy it."

The True Human tunes to the voice of the River to give it expression. The True Human tunes to the voice of the Wind and speaks the words the Wind cannot speak without human tongue. The True Human blends with the Essence of the Forest, Spirits of the Rain, the Spirit of every creeping, crawling living thing and represents them fairly, invoking from them the best they can be. The True Human is designed to aid the development of all Life–forms, drawing out their ever–expanding capacities to provide always fuller revelations of that which they were meant to be... Divine.   Teddi ♥

Richard Heinberg's, *The Party's Over,* offers an astute critical view of our current trajectory and its relationship with nature.

Humanity has reached a fundamental turning point in its economic [and technological] history. The expansionary trajectory of industrial civilization is colliding with non-negotiable natural limits.

Richard Heinberg
The Party's Over: : Oil, War & Fate of Industrialized Societies

To thrive on Planet Earth we must awaken to becoming a civilization abiding by Universal Law of Cause and Effect, founded in the Law of "ONE:" LOVE. Our thoughts are magnetic, they Create instantly and return in like-kind. Taking Response-Ability, we learn that the rules we play by have everything to do with the kind of future we and future generations inherit from our actions Now. *The greatest of these is LOVE.*

What we are doing to the forests of the world, is but a mirror reflection of what we are doing to ourselves and to one another.

Mahatma Gandhi (1969-1948)
Non-Violent Leader of India

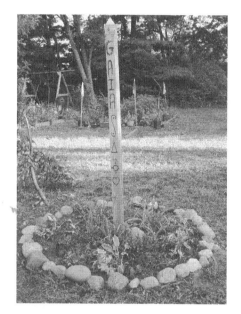

We stand at the bridge of Planetary crisis, both human and environmental. Our most compelling agenda as *21st Century Superhumans,* is to give our attention to shifting all things by clearing out our own Mind-Energy Not of LOVE. And then, rather than asking what this culture can give us, ask ourselves what we can do to bring forth a New Civilization based in LOVE, supportive of Mother Earth. We discover the answer in our Heart. Living from *Essence* we will be lead into New professions, careers and pastimes, from which will emerge an amazing New "reality."

I have no country to fight for; my country is the earth;
I am a citizen of the world.

Eugene Victor Debs, Orator (1855-1926)
American Labor Movement Leader, Ran for U.S. President 1912

As we make the *21st Century Superhuman* Leap, into Quantum "reality," it is as if we're adding two miles a day to our walk from a sedentary routine. So we add 1/4 mile each day, until heart, lungs, circulatory system, feet, legs, and muscles get used to added increments, and suddenly one day, two miles is easy. Integrating *Quantum Lifestyle,* thinking and Living is similar for the brain. From where we Now stand, trust us, it's worth it! Keep absorbing bit by bit, and as the brain and Being "chew on it," this new perceptual "reality" launches you *Lightyears* beyond where you've been!

We have emphasized...that the most natural means of doing so [activating DNA] is through the awareness of LOVE, both internally and externally. It is LOVE that activates the information within the recessive genes to Create the type of DNA advancement that you are seeking.

VogelCrystals dot net
DNA Activation Crystal

Fall in LOVE with Living Mother Gaia. Shift your Lifestyle to accommodate this Awakening. Notice in one dimension there is chaos and dissatisfying routine, in another uncensored peace. We're *aware* of incredible resources at our fingertips. We are learning to operate in our "New" *Quantum World,* leaving behind old beliefs that we are at the effect of what we see around us. We now know the atom that we were taught in school looked like a mini solar system, exists as a *Field* of *Infinite Possibilities,* awaiting our Attention upon it, to call *ANY* "reality" into being. Powerful reorganization and "times of great change" are born out of chaos. [Part 1: SHIFT OF THE AGES]

> As we get the mainstream scientific community to understand the theoretical function of [the idea, that we are all one], then we stand the chance to be able to apply it in the most powerful way to our society and move on to a New level of existence, which I call the Galactic Society.
>
> A society that is no longer confined to the surface of their planet, that has infinite amount of goods, infinite amount of power. A society that lives in abundance instead of scarcity, that has a concept that the value [of society] is only based on the creativity [that someone has]...
>
> *This is what I visualize when I see our future...*
>
> Nassim Haramein
The Resonance Project

Bigger glimpses into these concepts *tickle us,* our Hearts respond in New ways and we Smile! Shifting perception of our World, *it literally shifts* as a result of our Mind-energy upon it! *How cool is that?* Our white-knuckled grip is relaxing on the wheel, and rather than Being stressed by what we "see" around us, we recognize "reality" can and will change simply by us aligning with our Hearts and shifting the Vibration to LOVE! Breathe. Smile. Be Joyful! Twenty years from now we will have shifted timelines with thought, to where past darkness won't even be remembered. We will be in a Whole New World!

> When you, incarnate ...know that behind you is the same brilliance, light and warmth that expresses so passionately in the nuclear release of stars...the power of the creative, the power of the new, the balance, the synthesis, the power of truth... there is nothing to fear, for the immense powers of mother and father aspect of God – All that there is... have joined together in the creation of a material Universe designed for your support and flourishment.
>
> Ken Carey
Return of the Bird Tribes

Something emerges within us *hungering* to know our True expression, *itching* to *break free* from old boundaries that have held us encapsulated far too long (*unless just a blink of an eye*). Cosmic forces are acting upon us and we're understanding Quantum physics in everyday terms! *Just how great is this?* Thank *goodness* we are at the most amazing Evolutionary Leap in human history, *The Shift Of The Age*s. And it is a a game changer!

> Until the people of the world have embraced the fact that the world of the past no longer exists, and embrace solutions and ideas that support the new world, it's going to be very difficult to move into that world...people have put their lives on

hold, thinking it will go back to "normal." The way we live our lives is changing, the way we've thought of money in the past is changing, but nobody's told us that.

...Nature is based on harmony and mutual aid, not competition. What can we do when we wake up in the morning? We all ask ourselves a question...we look at the world and we say, "What can I get from the world that exists?" That's how we go about solving our problems, based upon false assumptions of science. New discoveries now give us a reason to change that question. The new question...is *"What can I share with the world that's emerging?* What can I contribute to the world that is emerging within my community, within my family, within myself?" The answer to that questions opens the door to powerful, powerful possibilities. New ways of sharing our passions and interests. Not just what we went to school to do,o or what our trade has trained us to do, but things that the world needs that we intuitively have picked up and learned on our own. And as we share those in a world that is now calling them forth, the flip side of that is that we are rewarded abundantly.

Gregg Braden
The Key to True Harmony

We the Beings from the Galactic OverSoul...The Center Heart of Prime Creator...volunteered to BE the Light and The Illumined Truth for Planet Earth. Our Sister Gaia put out a call, along with neighboring planets within her Galaxy, seeking assistance for her Ascension from a Planet of 3rd dimensional duality, into taking her place with planets of Higher Dimensional Oneness and Unity for All. We volunteer and hold the Frequency of Light with LOVE to assist every Man, Woman and Child to understand their Source of Origin, and to take their place in this Grand Shift of the Ages.

The Great Council: Lord Master Yeshua, Mary Magdalene, with Maitreya Master of the Blue Ray - Frequency of LOVE; Saint Germain - Violet Flame of Transmutation, Lady Portia - Grace - balances Mercy-Judgment; Arch-Angel Michael - Blue Flamed Sword of Truth; Lord Lanto-Innate Wisdom, Lao-Tsu-Tao, Quan-Yin-Compassion - Philosophy of Truth; Lord Kuthumi - Planetary LightCarrier, Recordkeeper; Lady Nada - Connecting with Essence, Unconditional LOVE.

We individualized our Soul's expressions into Human-Form, and have walked among our Sisters and Brothers with the Knowledge that we came here to serve. We have taken on "aspects" of the Great Council. We have woven ourselves through Many Star Systems to gain the necessary Alignment, Knowledge, Wisdom, Strength, Endurance to complete our Mission. The New Paradigm Grid is set in place around the Planet. We are All in our places, prepared, Body, Mind and Soul to continue to Educate, Demonstrate and Empower this Evolutionary Leap as Planned.

Teddi ♥

Part 3: SPIRIT

Chapter 14

Death The Great Mystery

It is not the end of the physical body that should worry us. Rather, our concern must be to live while we're alive - to release our inner selves from the spiritual death that comes with living behind a facade designed to conform to external definitions of who and what we are.

Elisabeth Kubler-Ross (1926-2004)
Pioneering work and author - On Death and Dying

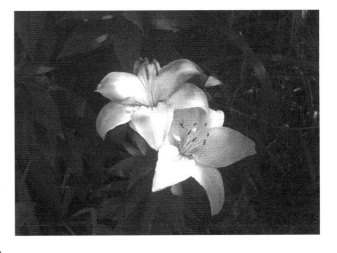

Emerging from the great sea of Infinite Consciousness, or Intelligence of Pure LOVE, we release our Greater Eternal Awareness to slip into an Earth Body, to grow in 3-4-D. An incredible opportunity to *choose* between good and evil, Light and dark, to remember Who We Are.

Recent images show a tiger bowing to a child, lion, tiger and bear beloved friends, elephants loving dogs, a woman scratching a deer's neck, a bear coming to play, all *sorts* of creatures who LOVE and LOVE one another, getting along, like the "lion and the lamb," when supported in the *Field of possibilities*, rather than the dishonoring that grows out of lower frequency Mind-Energy, of our soon to be distant past.

Evolving through playing in thought-forms outside of LOVE, for minimally up to 200,000 Earth years or more, "we" (humanity - our "blood line") immersed ourselves in "illusionary" culture based in Not of LOVE, so we could find our way back to the ONE. Materialistic Worldview and scientific elitism distanced us from our true nature, with mistaken beliefs that science and spirituality are incompatible. A*nything Not of LOVE is a result of playing in duality or the illusion.* **The only thing real is LOVE and it is magnificent!** Grasping this is *essential.* Then there's the **BIG QUESTION:** *What About Death?*

Death is Part of the Illusion...

Medical science has attempted to debunk glorious reports of dimensions of Light and LOVE, from those returning from death experiences with the idea they are a surge of "survival hormones." NDEs or Near Death Experiences have been widely documented for the past 4-5 decades, initially by Raymond Moody in *Life after Life,* when doctors began bringing cardiac patients "back from the dead" while maintaining oxygen levels in the brain. Elizabeth Kubler-Ross, Swiss psychiatrist, pioneered near-death studies and re-humanized the dying process with her groundbreaking book *On Death and Dying.*

Today there are *millions* of reports of being clinically dead, going to the "tunnel of light," visiting with Loved ones or Beings of Light on the "other side." Books on these deeply moving experiences can be helpful to read. In *Proof of Heaven: A Neurosurgeon's Journey into the Afterlife* Eben Alexander, M.D. relates his incredible recovery from 7 day coma (no neocortex activity), as a result of contracting a virulent unknown strain of meningitis from which statistically 97% would not have survived (and those who did would have had little likelihood of normal brain function thereafter).

Dr. Eban Alexander had amazingly speedy return of all faculties; surmising perhaps he was "given" this profound experience because of his unique ability as a neurosurgeon to relate it from a detailed scientific point of view. He was able to explain in depth "why his brain was incapable of fabricating this journey."

His awakening was profound, having previously been a "naysayer," who brushed aside numerous such stories from his patients as fantasy or hallucination. "He awoke certain of the infinite reach of the Soul. He was certain of a life *beyond* death." His personal experience and transformation is astounding, with the sobering severity of his coma, and brilliance of his experience "beyond." *The first comforting message given to him there was:*

> "You are loved and cherished, dearly, forever. You have nothing to fear. There is nothing you can do wrong." *The message flooded me with a vast and crazy sensation of relief. It was like being handed the rules to a game I'd been playing all my life without ever fully understanding it.*
>
> Eben Alexander III M.D.
Proof of Heaven: A Neurosurgeon's Journey into the Afterlife

He profoundly relates *"in limiting Earth language"* we are Beings of the most Infinite and All-encompassing LOVE; we emerge from an Immense Consciousness of Pure LOVE he calls God or *Om.* Without a doubt LOVE is the basis of everything, reality of realities, truth of truths, core of everything that exists or ever will. It is revealed in how we LOVE our Loved ones, spouse, children, parents and animals, a fully Unconditional LOVE. "...know this deep and comforting truth: our Eternal Spiritual Self is more real than anything we perceive in this physical realm, and has a divine connection to the Infinite Love of the Creator." Dr. Eban Alexander tells us:

The (false) suspicion that we can somehow be separated from God is the root of every form of anxiety in the universe, and the cure for it...

Evil was necessary because without it free will was impossible, and without free will there could be no growth...in the larger picture **Love** was overwhelmingly dominant, and it would ultimately be triumphant.

How do we get closer to this genuine spiritual self? By manifesting love and compassion. Why? Because love and compassion are far more than the abstractions many of us believe them to be. They are real. They are concrete. And they make up the very fabric of the spiritual realm...

...we have lost touch with the deep mystery at the center of existence— our consciousness...God is present in us at all times. Omniscient, omnipotent, personal - and loving us without conditions. We are connected as One through our divine link with God.

It is my belief that we are now facing a crucial time in our existence. We need to recover more of that larger knowledge while living here on earth, while our brains (including its left-side analytical parts) are fully functioning.

Eben Alexander III M.D.
Proof of Heaven: A Neurosurgeon's Journey into the Afterlife

We are eternal Beings - individualized whirlpools in the river of consciousness, *always One with the ONE,* in unbroken Union with the substance ALL that IS - LOVE. We may shed our Body in this Now, yet we do not "die." It is believed that within our junk DNA lies the capability of Living much longer, hundreds if not thousands of years, transitioning into ultimate immortality as we move into our crystalline 5th dimensional culture. Clearing lower frequency thought puts us in Heart Coherence, which shifts our endocrine system, adding more Light to the energy fields of the Body, increasing Life-span. This is true rejuvenation, clearing Mind-Heart-Body to LOVE, so we are producing youthful hormones.

For thousands of years we have believed that the "boogie man" death is real. This lie was fabricated for control, in power-over cultural dynamics, *and was believed.* "If you do or do not do such and such, you will be punished and go to___, or those who are *good* will get to go to ___." Terror grew up around these beliefs, developing into a cultural norm, growing denser and denser with Collective historical focus.

Vital mythologies about death carried deep truth in Ancient cultures, reminding of our True heritage from the Great Dimensions of LOVE. There were 3,000 years of teachings of how to dwell in *Divine Essence* as Creator-Beings. Then a great "forgetting" went on cultivating World systems outside of LOVE that are Now "crumbling." Science is Now helping us *remember* our Eternal State of Being and *unlimited Consciousness*.

Restoring our True Design LOVE and letting go deep Ancient fears, our Lives become abundant with Well-Being and fearless Action. Ultimately we will live in such High Frequency bodies with DNA codons turned on, that it may no longer be necessary to transition through the "death" portal. Are we ready to enter into the kind of "En-Light-enment" where we enter into Union with *Om* [God] Source here and Now, in a coherent state of LOVE? As we Live in LOVE, we become more acquainted with our "Eternalness" and the idea of whether we shed the Body or not.

Dr. Eban Alexander discovered Meditation and Brain-Heart Coherence assist us to access Universal Oneness experienced on the "other side." Ancient practices of Masters transcending physical with Breath to access Higher states, or Living without food and water also demonstrate capability of merging into less dense form.

To reborn into a new life, you have to die before dying.

Shams Tabrizi, Rumi's mentor

Tiniest particles, Light photons and electrons that make up Creation, ebb and flow through our presence, *and we thought we were solid and separate!* We are ALL intrinsically connected, in what Quantum mechanics calls "entanglement," *my thoughts, feelings, emotions and life influence yours.* The song, *"No man is an island, no man stands alone. Each man's joy is joy to me; each man's grief is my own..."* touches how deeply we affect one another. We are ONE. *At the level of Pure LOVE, death does not exist.*

You've heard it said, there's a window that opens from one mind to another.
If there's no wall, there's no need for fitting the window or the latch.

Rumi
13th Century Sufi Mystic, Poet

Caring for Loved ones in a gentle and respectful way as they near transition eases this change of form, by allowing a natural dying process, that we once insulated from. Dr. Dame Cicely Saunders worked with terminally ill, creating the first modern hospice in London in 1948. Dr. Elisabeth Kubler-Ross published her landmark best-seller, *On Death and Dying* in 1969 based on 500 interviews, identifying five stages through which terminally ill patients pass. She worked for acceptance of home care so patients could have death with dignity, resulting in wide acceptance of hospice. Thanks to these pioneers, resources Now support peaceful passing as has always been carried out in simpler cultures.

It may take shifting our thoughts, when a loved one "sheds the body," to embrace awareness that *there is no death,* for as Elizabeth Kubler-Ross says, "when one door closes behind us, another opens." Embracing Greater Existence beyond the body moves us into a New view of "death." Never-ending Creation nourishes us to connect more consciously with LOVE, our Eternal state-of-Being.

Establishing Life in Deep LOVE, Compassion and Gratitude, our Greatest possibilities emerge and our DNA codons are activated for rejuvenation and longer Life. This *Shift of the Ages* impels us into an unprecedented Evolutionary Leap, shifting the Collective to LOVE on Planet Earth, to Live in the Eternalness of our BEING. ♥ *As Osho says:*

The real question is not whether life exists after death.
The real question is whether you are alive before death.

Part 3: SPIRIT
Chapter 15
Amen - Namasté

The Beginning Is Near

Garret John LoPorto
Wayseer Manifesto

A s Teilhard de Chardin said, we are *spiritual beings having a human experience.* Most of us came into this Life adapting to what greeted us upon our arrival, and stepped in line to become part of the surrounding culture. The greatest aspect of "waking up," in this Now, initiated by powerful happenings during this *Shift Of The Ages,* is *remembering Who We Are.*

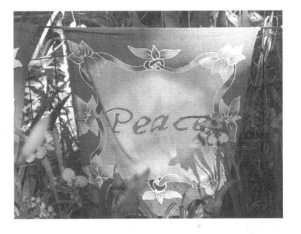

As Graham Hancock says, we are a civilization with amnesia, who will benefit from knowledge attained by peak civilizations, lost when Earth's cataclysms took them. Through modern instruments we see high speed photons of Light and Super Plasma Galactic Rays pouring through the extraordinary region of space we are Now transiting, activating this Awakening within us. Quantum physics and Ancient Texts focus our lens on how powerfully we can Create in this "reality," as we are now "surfing" this 9th wave of the Mayan Calendar.

> The dance goes from realizing that you're separate (which is the awakening) to then trying to find your way back into the totality of which you are not only a part, but of which you are."
>
> *Ram Dass*
> *Polishing the Mirror*

We poured ourselves from the Great Beyond, from the Unlimited, into this form in the Earth-plane, to Live the Journey of a Lifetime, to ultimately Wake Up and Remember. We are Abundant, and All That Ever Was or Will be is at our fingertips, once we remove the "filters" in our own Minds, that were "logjams: in Its flow.

When we're identified with Awareness, we're no longer living in a world of polarities. Everything is present at the same time.

Ram Dass
Polishing the Mirror

Plugging into *Essence* to Live as the Truly Incredible Beings we Are, we express our unique magnificence in the World. Reconnecting with our never ending Power Supply we access our own unlimitedness. This is the birthright of ALL, and as each of us steps up to Live and express it, we hold open the Vibrational doorway in this dimension for others to follow. Millions Worldwide are Now stepping through outmoded boundaries, to express True *Essence,* shifting the destiny of HUmanity.

Wayseers are the change agents of society. Wayseers are the ones who know first, who sense earliest the disturbances in the fabric of human affairs – the trends, the patterns, the fashions, the coming groundswells, the revolutions that are afoot.

Garret John LoPorto
The Wayseers

Become an agent for change in the World by doing something as simple and radical as following your Heart, finding your own True expression and a way to Live it. Moving beyond old programming that held you back in the past, takes a little inertia to get going, yet once rolling, *"...doors will open where there were only walls before."* You will be amazed, once you *break free,* to *Be Who You Truly ARE,* Life will take on an entirely new meaning, it will shine with Brightness Mirrored from your Heart. You will make an extraordinary difference in the World just by Being YOU.

What counts in life is not the mere fact we have lived it is what difference we have made in the lives of others that will determine the significance of the life we lead.

Nelson Mandela (1918-2013)
Nobel Peace Prize 1993, President S. Africa 1994-1999

What is your current job, profession or career? What direction is your Life taking you? Is it TRULY the direction you desire to go in your Heart of Hearts? Consider how you would engage with your skills in great or small World-changing enterprises if there were no limits. Your contribution to the Greater Good of humanity is just a few choices away.

We are moving away from living solely for the purpose of obtaining material goods, to fall asleep on the weekend and run the maze again the following week. Humanity and our future long to have YOUR Talents applied in more meaningful and creative ways. The energy of YOUR Life is extraordinary and extremely powerful. What YOU do with it is up to YOU. Your True expression in the World is irreplaceable

There is no passion to be found in playing small, in settling for a life that is less than the one you are capable of living.

Nelson Mandela (1918-2013)
Nobel Peace Prize 1993, President S. Africa 1994-1999

Millions around the World are stepping up Now, to represent True Human Life through the Heart, a New dawn of freedom is at hand. During a recent speech in Poland, former US National Security Advisor, Brzezinski said that the Worldwide "resistance" movement to "external control" driven by "populist activism" is threatening to derail the suppressive move towards a "new World order." (Reported by LiveFreeLiveNatural dot com Dec. 2013). Old domination and "power over" systems are proving to be unsustainable as more enter the Heart.

> Drop out – then let the world know you did and why. Courage is contagious and together we are strong. It's time to open our eyes to whatever corrupt institutions we may be supporting with our time, money or energy – and DROP OUT.
>
> *Garret John LoPorto*
> *The Wayseers*

As energies shift, suffering will be cleansed from the Planet. There will be no lack. As we change timelines with LOVE and move into "future" the old will be erased. Everything we need will be abundant in ways we have not yet imagined, as the Collective progresses into LOVE frequencies, *because YOU Are holding LOVE.*

In earlier chapters we discussed lowered Earth's magnetics and how Jesus and Buddha both incarnated during lower magnetics, when Minds are more open to New ideas. We are currently experiencing rock bottom levels of Earth's magnetic field, lowest since the 1600s. As Thich Nhat Hahn says, *"The next Buddha will be the Collective."* Many Ancient Texts carry a subtle message, that the next incarnation of *"Christed" or "Buddhic" Consciousness,* will emerge in thousands, millions then billions on Earth.

Change is going on all around us. As many old systems collapse, recognize this is a Transition. Anything lost will emerge into a Higher order, as we shed old forms into a more expansive culture of HU-Beings. As more move into and express their lives through our True Design LOVE, layers of distortion we had been programmed with long ago, fall away.

Although the natural instinct in the old paradigm was to keep the Heart closed; courageously opening the Heart Now to LOVE is the Key to shedding old Not of LOVE paradigms. As we experience change around us, Faith, Hope and Grace shift us into Higher Frequencies, while the New takes shape from the invisible into the visible. Be LOVE. Teach LOVE. Breathe. Smile. Play. Create.

> If someone thinks that peace and LOVE are just a cliche that must have been left behind in the 60s, that's a problem. Peace and LOVE are eternal.
>
> *John Lennon (1940-1980)*
> *Beatles, Singer, Songwriter, Activist*

The more we clear our "old data" to resonate from our True Design LOVE, we shift frequencies in the entire Planetary *Field.* All that exists in the outer, is Mirroring the resonance of Individuals and the World Community Collective. As we shift internally, we are part of a critical mass moving into LOVE to shift the entire Hologram.

> As long as you want power, you can't have it. The minute you don't want power,
> you'll have more than you ever dreamed possible...
>
> *Ram Dass*
> *Polishing the Mirror*

WHAT IS YOUR JOY? Consider what you would LOVE to be doing if the options were unlimited. Imagine what it would take to "make it so." For example, if you became an attorney to defend the innocent, but being an attorney in our current system has been draining the Life out of you, what if you helped the innocent more by Living Your Joy? Run a pre-school, write an ebook, work for Greenpeace, start a foundation to bring education to the 125 million uneducated women and children in the World. Raise Your flag.

> Every individual when honored, truly cared for, and empowered, becomes a
> valuable, contributing member to the whole community.
>
> *Stuart Royston*
> *Citizen of the Earth*

TED gave their first ever million dollar award, to two men who dug a hole in the ground in New Delhi, India near the dumps, and put a computer in it for impoverished children to play. The award is Now funding a globally accessible Cloud school for children.

> Educational researcher Dr. Sugata Mitra's "Hole in the Wall" experiments have shown that in the absence of supervision or formal teaching, children can teach themselves and each other, if they're motivated by curiosity and peer interest. In 1999, Mitra and his colleagues dug a hole in a wall bordering an urban slum in New Delhi, installed an Internet-connected PC, and left it there (with a hidden camera filming the area). What they saw was kids from the slum playing around with the computer and in the process learning how to use it and how to go online, and then teaching each other.
>
> The "Hole in the Wall" project demonstrates that, even in the absence of any direct input from a teacher, an environment that stimulates curiosity can cause learning through self-instruction and peer-shared knowledge. Mitra, who's now a professor of educational technology at Newcastle University (UK), calls it "minimally invasive education."
>
> *TED*

23 year old Maggie from New Jersey, went to hike in Nepal, became "mother" of thirty, and developed an orphanage that now houses and teaches 230 children. She is dedicated to finding a way to provide for the remaining 80 million orphaned children Worldwide. (23 Year Old Mother of 30 at KarmaTube dot com)

What if all those who "have," set out to Create *honest* programs, sharing resources with those who "have not," food, water, education, energy, housing. What if we used our intelligence to benefit ourselves and humanity, rather than submitting to bondage, drudgery, feudalism, serfdom, servitude, otherwise known as "work?" We are at a crisis on Earth, inviting us to change our ways and redistribute resources for ALL to thrive.

It seems impossible until it is done.

Nelson Mandela (1918-2013)
Nobel Peace Prize 1993, President S. Africa 1994-1999

As Einstein said, *"Problems cannot be solved at the level at which they were Created,"* It may seem like a difficult task to make a Leap from the traditional ideas, yet it is highly possible to use your old job or business to springboard you into more Soul-fulfilling enterprises. Breathe. Smile. Ask yourself how you would like to look back on your life when it is done; and what you would have liked to accomplish and who with. Start Now to get there...*"move into A Happy Dream..."*

Dr. Bruce Lipton, epigeneticist reminds us that simply by changing our perceptions we change our cells. We are conditioned to think that changing our Body or our Life happens from the outside, which can only be palliative. The Truth is, *all true change* happens from inside Mind-Heart. As we shift our beliefs and our perceptions, our "reality" shifts along with them. Entering into practices that restore our True Design LOVE, we literally shift our DNA, activating potential for Longer Life, Greater Well-Being and Supreme Happiness.

I am only one, but I am one. I cannot do everything, but I can do something. And because I cannot do everything, I will not refuse to do the something that I can do. What I can do, I should do. And what I should do, by the grace of God, I will do.

Edward Everett Hale (1882-1909)
Unity Minister, child prodigy, related to Helen Keller, Author "Man without a Country"

This is a Journey we will call an Evolutionary Leap of the human family, as we enter into an age established around our understanding through Quantum physics as the foundation of our existence, as creator-Beings of LOVE. We are in exciting times, we are in the *Shift of the Ages*. It behooves us to live in extraordinary ways.

Teilhard de Chardin saw societal problems of marginalization and isolation as huge inhibitors of evolution, as evolution requires unification of consciousness. "No evolutionary future awaits anyone except in association with everyone else."

Imagine no possessions, I wonder if you can, No need for greed or hunger,
A brotherhood of man. Imagine all the people, Sharing all the world...
You may say I'm a dreamer, But I'm not the only one
I hope someday you'll join us, And the world will live as one

John Lennon
Imagine Lyrics

"THE GREAT INVOCATION is a prayer of ancient origin--a mantric formula of tremendous potency that helps bring changes and readjustments within all aspects of our planetary life. It is a World prayer translated into 70 languages, used by all faiths." We have enjoyed it over many years, as recorded by Alice Bailey and Djwhal Khul. It has been used by the Findhorn in their Global "Network of Light meditations for peace" and widely used around the World.

THE GREAT INVOCATION *(adapted)*

From the point of light within the Mind of God
Let Light stream forth into our Minds
Let LIGHT descend on Earth.
From the point of LOVE within the Heart of God
Let LOVE stream forth into our Hearts
May LOVE increase on Earth.
From the center where the Will of God is known
Let purpose guide our wills

The PURPOSE which the Masters know and serve.

From the center which we call Humanity
Let the Plan of LOVE and Light work out
And may it seal the door where darkness dwells.

Let the Power of LOVE restore the Plan on Earth.

INCORPORATING REGULAR MEDITATION FOR TRANSFORMATION: Along with conscious beliefs and thought, it is essential to keep clearing the 95% old thought-emotion stored in the unconscious. [Part 2: MIND] Then combining our Newly-emerging clarity of LOVE-resonance with Life-enriching deep Meditation, we transform our Life to be filled with Pre-Cognizance, Synchronicities, Abundance, Vitality, Rewarding Productivity, Achievement, Great Relationships and Joy. *Because of its importance we will review here.*

A new study by researchers in Wisconsin, Spain, and France reports first evidence of molecular changes in the body following mindfulness practice.

The study investigated the effects of a day of intensive mindfulness practice in a group of experienced meditators, compared to a group of untrained control subjects who engaged in quiet non-meditative activities. After eight hours of mindfulness practice, the meditators showed a range of genetic and molecular differences, including altered levels of gene-regulating machinery and reduced levels of pro-inflammatory genes, which in turn correlated with faster physical recovery from a stressful situation.

"To the best of our knowledge, this is the first paper that shows rapid alterations in gene expression within subjects associated with meditation practice," says study author Richard J. Davidson, founder of the Center for Investigating Healthy Minds and the William James and Vilas Professor of Psychology and Psychiatry at University of Wisconsin-Madison.

Galactic Free Press
Sourced from Journal Psychoneuroendocrinology

Thousands of studies have Now been done on meditation by such as UCLA and Edgar Mitchell's IONS, demonstrating that alpha-theta brainwaves induced by typical meditation anyone can do, switch on paranormal abilities and a more flowing Life. From this state we have potential to shift events, matter, our health, influence others for the better and even affect the weather. Meditation in these brainwaves Creates brain coherence and accesses higher intelligence. Regular meditators report Lives flowing, things accomplished more easily, efficiently and successfully, with quicker recovery from challenges. 15-20 minutes of mediation once or twice daily super-powers any Lifestyle.

> Whenever you deeply accept this moment as it is..
> No matter what form it takes. You are still. You are at peace.
>
> *Eckhart Tolle, Power of Now*

PRACTICING HEART COHERENCE helps us replace perpetuated patterns we are "not." Research demonstrates Heart Coherence gives you *more of YOU!* Check out HeartMath®'s simple feedback tools for iPhone or computer, to become Heart Coherent in just a few weeks. Remember effective Heart Coherent emotions are LOVE, Compassion and Gratitude. Our final mediation process here includes Heart Coherence practices.

> If you want others to be happy, practice compassion.
> If you want to be happy, practice compassion.
>
> *The 14th Dalai Lama*

Global Heart Coherence Meditation

1. Sit or lie quietly 15-20 minutes a.m. / p.m. in a quiet place if possible
2. Relax completely, including jaw and mouth - Gently circular mouth-Breathe
3. Focus for a couple of minutes on Heart in center of chest. Breathe as if through Heart. Set your awareness to LOVE, Compassion or Gratitude.
4. Double-check body making sure all is relaxed
5. Say a short prayer of intention, protection and guidance to whom you are comfortable: God, Jesus, Angels, Higher Dimensional Beings of Light
6. Invite Rookha d'Koodsha to assist you with canceling all goals, conscious, subconsciousness, unconscious and incomplete
7. Reset Rakhma filter LOVE intentions / Khooba filter LOVE perceptions
8. Use your mantra (Sanskrit or Love, Peace, Compassion, Gratitude, or...) every time a thought comes up, allow the mantra to gently pull you back to quiet
9. As Quiet comes, know you are dropping into the *Infinite Field of Possibilities*
10. Release your cares, worries, visions and dreams to the *Field*
11. Know waves of the Ocean of existence carry them into New form with LOVE
12. Let yourself drop in deeper and deeper, gently becoming ONE with ALL
13. When you are finished gently stretch and re-engage with the outer peacefully
14. Breathe. Smile. LOVE.

Meditating regularly takes us into the *Divine Matrix* or *Field* from which all possibilities emerge. When consciousness becomes still it merges with the *Field*, and experiences its own experience of the illusion. With this awareness the consciousness can carry Visions, Desires and Dreams into the *Field,* to dance in it, developing greater and greater alignment with

Heart, Soul and Higher Frequencies of Life. Integrating meditation becomes a drawing force in our Lives, it pulls us in, to participate more actively in the miracle of Creation.

VIPASSANA MEDITATION used and taught by Buddha, acknowledges the fractals of Creation, tiniest particles passing by at trillions of times per second, awaiting our peaceful Attention to resonate into form. Upanishads, one of the oldest human records from Ancient India says, "Brahma the Creator, sitting on a lotus, opens his eyes and a World comes into being. Brahma closes his eyes, and a World goes out of being."

> The *Field* is not separate from you. It is you and you are it; it expresses through you. Creation expresses itself through you. When you wake up from the dream you see all the parts of the dream as you. Make it good dream. ♥

Well, *21st Century Superhumans*, thanks for Dreaming this Dream of making this Journey with us, and for expanding Mind-Heart into New dimensions. We trust you experience our favorite saying, *"I'm not the same person I was yesterday!"* Pass it on! Find companions of the Heart with whom you can share this adventure and accelerate to beyond where you would go singly, for *"where two or more are gathered"* incredible things occur... All it takes is ONE. Pass it on to ONE, and then Another, then Another. LOVE.

A Single Rose in My Garden.
A Single Friend in My World.

Danny Dieter (1947-1967)
Started meditating at 3 on his own ~

As our thoughts Create our world, we Create our own prophecies.

Teddi Mulder

We leave you *21st Century Superhumans* Now with wise words of Nelson Mandela, until we meet again in the great Rainbow of Light wrapping around this beautiful Planet waiting expectantly for us to Wake UP *fully, be at Peace, Breathe, Smile, and walk the talk...*

> ...A man of peace is not a pacifist; a man of peace is simply a pool of silence. He pulsates a new kind of energy into the world, he sings a new song. He lives in a totally new way. His very way of life is that of grace, that of prayer, that of compassion. Whomsoever he touches, he Creates more love-energy.
>
> The man of peace is creative. He is not against war, because to be against anything is to be at war. He is not against war, he simply understands why war exists. And out of that understanding he becomes peaceful. Only when there are many people who are pools of peace, silence, understanding, will war disappear...

♥ ♥ ♥

NEXT: **PART 4: BODY**
Rejuvenation & Growing Younger - Healthy Eating, Cleanse and Detox

Part 4 BODY

*Rejuvenation &
Growing Younger*

*with Healthy Eating,
Cleanse & Detox*

The joy is that we can take back our bodies,
reclaim our health,
and restore ourselves to balance.
We can take power over what and how we eat.
We can rejuvenate and recharge ourselves,
bringing healing
to the wounds we carry inside us,
and bringing to fuller life
the wonderful person
that each of us can be.

John Robbins
FoodRevolution dot org

Part 4 Body: Section 1
Back To The Garden

You may say I'm a dreamer, but I'm not the only one.
I hope someday you'll join us. And the world will live as one.

John Lennon
Imagine

Viktoras Kulvinskas published *Survival Into The 21st Century: Planetary Healers Manual* in 1972, and it came to us as a shining Light, guiding our way into greater awakening. Forerunner for our times, it held in-spiration and in-formation that helped us shape our lives. It pointed the way to learn and expand our horizons, resulting in many adventures in well-being and consciousness. I (Cary) had the great opportunity to spend time with Viktoras, living and learning on his Connecticut farm, which was wonderful and enlightening.

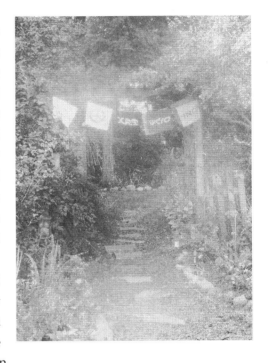

Seeking his own wellness Viktoras had discovered the natural path of fasting and raw foods, and in 1968 co-founded the Boston Hippocrates Institute with Dr. Ann Wigmore (1909-1993). His story of personal regeneration was ultimately inspiring. A pure mathematician and highly respected computer programmer, his book came forth as a brilliant detailed "data-dump" of his cosmic awakenings *and* recognition of what a truly healthy Life-path is. On the cover was hot pink Peter Max visionary art, with hand-done drawings throughout the book. Though the style was unconventional, it went out like wildfire *(still available online)*, as valuable a reference guide today as it was then. We *highly* recommend owning it, as it contains valuable details on thriving and surviving in our World, healthy concepts, wisdom-based tools, resources and foundational teachings around living foods, cleansing, regeneration and community.

Very rarely in Life does one encounter a book with the magnitude of Viktoras Kulvinskas' *Survival in the 21st Century*. Within it's pages, LOVE consciousness springs forth from a master of body ecology. Viktoras' pioneering work has touched so many people, it is considered by many as a "new age bible" in the holistic and health field. Few can resist the wisdom and experience this buried treasure shares and although Survival was written 27 years ago, one would be amazed at how time stands still within it's pages.

Darksunblade, Review at amazon.com

We initiate this part of our book with Viktoras, because *Survival into the 21st Century* was such a powerful springboard for us, landing us right where we are today. It is about vital connection with Earth, Sky and Heart. It inspires us to tap into *Essence* within ourselves, cultivating intelligent Survival, and beyond that our Thriving.

This place you are right now God circled on a map for you.

Hafiz, 14th Century Persian Mystic Poet

I NOW AFFIRM: I Am restoring my True Design LOVE and *Essence*. As I clear my Mind-Heart to Live this path, friends, family, community and relationships harmonize around my "reality." Synchronicities occur and doors open for the good of all.

You can survive. The spirit is timeless... I present ways to survive and prepare for the New World to come. Be not dismayed when you seem to be alone in the pursuit. Remember, "Few are chosen." Your close friends and members of your family may ridicule you. Let them not offend or provoke you. LOVE them just the same - do not fight back. Teach others by your example, not with empty words. "You shall know them by their deeds."

Viktoras Kulvinskas
Survival Into The 21st Century - Planetary Healers Manual (1975)

In 1969 at Yasgur's farm in upstate New York 32 bands and 400,000, "initiated" an "age" at *Woodstock,* opening Minds to a radical New way of Life. Crosby, Stills, Nash and Young prophetically sang, "We are caught in the devil's bargain," with unspoken hunger for that which seemed lost...

Well, then can I walk beside you? I have come here to lose the smog.
I feel like I am a cog in something turning.
And maybe it's the time of year, yes, maybe it's the time of man.
Got to get back to the land and set my Soul free
We are stardust, we are golden, we are billion year old carbon,
And we got to get ourselves back to the garden.

How we step into and express our Lives is critical to the Whole, for as Rumi says, *"Be relentless in your looking, because you are the one you seek."* In our deepest longings we discover vital keys to authentically reclaiming *SELF.* Taking clues we've been given, *21st Century Superhumans* enter a New way of Living, heightening self-expression and Well-Being. Ultimately we'll say, *"Thank you"* for this **Quantum Lifestyle** path laid out before us. You Now reading have begun to activate self-knowledge leading the way to En-Light-enment. Proper, natural care of the Body is foundational to this laudable Journey. ♥

378

Chapter 1

Choosing Your Approach to Wellness

All you need is LOVE. But a little
chocolate now and then doesn't hurt.

Charles M. Schulz (1992-2000)
Creator of" Peanuts"

How Body is nourished is one of the most nurturing and delicious topics to take place anywhere on Earth any day, despite the fact *some* know we *can* Live on *Prana* or Light. It is said we can get along for a week without laughter, yet if we were without food for that long most would grumble, though a short fast generally does us good. We may go days without laughter yet it is wonderfully beneficial. Robert T. Meuller PhD tells us, "The average

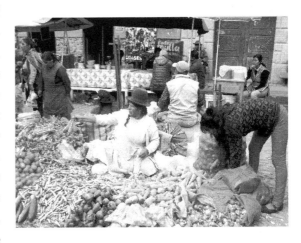

kindergartener laughs 300x/day, average adult 17." Let's laugh more! Choosing a healthy Lifestyle *through-time* is better than suddenly adopting it when things "go wrong."

We are moving beyond the belief that the only way the physical changes, is by changing the physical, which has been our working 3-D model. This is a "world is flat" philosophy. Bruce Lipton reminds us that Newtonian Physics says the World is made out of mechanical parts: the basis of medicine-when broken change the parts with chemicals, surgery and drugs. Quantum physics says everything is a *Field* in which we are immersed and the Field controls Biology. *The Field is the sole governing agency of the particle.* (Einstein)

> Quantum Reality: If everything we do and think is the byproduct of how we perceive the information (our reality bias) then it implies, that by adequately reordering our perceptions, we affect the outcome of everything in our lives.
>
> *Dr. Richard Bartlett*
> *Matrix Energetics.*

Studies Now show we can change the Body with thought. In his book, *Healing Back Pain: The Mind Body Connection,* back surgeon Dr. John Sarno tells us that *most back problems can be solved by clearing associated thought-emotional issues;* in 95% of cases, surgery is not required. The theory "if we 'eat right' we'll be healthy" is Newtonian. Physical is subject to thought resonating through the *Field*. Quantum physics tells us Life and Well-being emerge from Perception, Attitude and Belief. When these change, everything changes.

Powerful documentary *Water: The Great Mystery* by Les Sundeen, documents that water permeating our World has memory and carries thought. Shifting into LOVE, our thought-energy transmitted through water in the air and our Bodies, transforms us and our World. (Body 75-80% water, Earth's surface 70%). In 1472 a dedicated Abbott was imprisoned and given a crust of stale bread and dipper of stinking water daily. After 40 days he had gained health and strength. Extorted from him under *torture* he confessed he had "prayed over the water, giving thanks for what he had," and as he did so the water turned sweet and clear.

Thought links us to the fabric of Creation. We are the "pharmacist," instructing our endocrine system what chemicals to produce. As we operate in LOVE and Heart Coherence we change our internal chemistry, we awaken DNA, increase Longevity and Well-Being. Tibetan monks repeat prayers till water in the Body harmonizes to clear ailments. Prayers measure 7.8-8.6 Hz. matching Earth's resonance.

When dealing with illness in self or family members, adopting a healthy Quantum Lifestyle helps build a new foundation. Additionally benefits of modern medicine may assist to remedy a critical state, to give the Body a jump on recovery. Ultimately the wise human civilization will combine medical advancements with the amazing bounty of natural practices and remedies available, which we cover in this book. Such choices are personal and should be made with both research and listening to the Body and intuition. Leading example of combining holistic with the medical approach is the *Mercy Health Wege Institute for Mind, Body and Spirit* in Grand Rapids, Michigan, with the Mission:

> ...offering effective, individualized, patient care for mind, body and spirit, we both complete and enhance mainstream medical care by partnering progressive complementary therapies with mainstream medical services and practitioners.
>
> This integrative approach is a valuable resource for those who wish to increase self-awareness, enhance overall well being and prevent future health issues, as well as those who are chronically ill.

Coming chapters take us into Natural Body care. It *does* matter what we eat and how we nourish ourselves. It also matters what kind of Mind-energy we hold around water, food and Life, for in so doing we are literally creating the substance of our Body and our World, our state of well-being and our relationship with the Web of Life. ♥

> Your Life does matter. It always matters whether you reach out in friendship or lash out in anger. It always matters whether you live with compassion and awareness or whether you succumb to distractions and trivia. It always matters how you treat other people, how you treat animals, and how you treat yourself. It always matters what you do. It always matters what you say. And it always matters what you eat.
>
> John Robbins
> *The Food Revolution: How Your Diet Can Help Save Your Life and Our World*

Chapter 2

How Thought Affects The Body

Your health is what you make of it. Everything you do and think either adds to the vitality, energy and spirit you possess, or takes away from it.

Dr. Ann Wigmore (1909-1993)
"Grandmother" of Wheatgrass - Living Foods

T ibetan Monks of the Dalai Lama's lineage followed detailed Ancient Traditions over thousands of years, perfecting mantras to influence weather and World conditions. They report that "When we have a pure heart and sound our mantras correctly, the 'Lord of the water' brings us rain." They are living repositories of very specific Ancient knowledge of the science of how we operate in this World. Accessing Heart Coherence through deep Compassion without judgment, their sacred, effective mantra-prayer is based in Quantum physics!

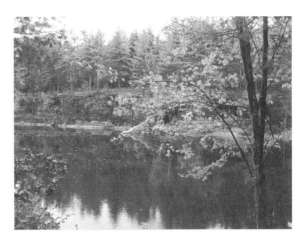

Another example of Ancient knowledge offers affects of prayer on the physical. In 1991 in a desperate two year drought, Israel's only freshwater lake was critically low. So 10,000 Israelis gathered at the Wailing Wall, *chanted and prayed rain;* within 3 days rain came in torrents. A rabbi explained their religion's traditions are designed *to affect the outcome;* and those who call this "coincidence" are not interested in Living True Response-Ability.

Not a single scientist who is familiar with systems theory doubts [shifting the physical with prayer]. It is entirely a question of waiting for a moment when the system is in a state of instability. In a phase of instability, the motion of thought alone is sufficient for the system to start to change.

Gerbert Klima, Professor of Inst. Nuclear Physics, Vienna Austria
Water: The Great Mystery by Les Sundeen

We've experienced affirming the sky is clear and blue on a day when "chemtrails" were filling the sky, and within minutes the sky was perfectly clear. Alternate reality?

HeartMath® research reveals that a person in *Heart Coherence* literally turns on codons in their own and others DNA, offering powerful insight into the Evolutionary Leap in which we are Now engaged. HeartMath® finds measurable Heart Coherence is Created by Deep LOVE, Compassion and Gratitude. Literally in simple terms, *all* that is needed to shift health, well-being, and our World, is clearing Not of LOVE thought-emotional patterns, to our True Design LOVE (covered in detail Part 2: MIND). Clearing Now. Breathe. Smile.

> Beautify your thoughts. Thoughts are the headwaters
> of action, life and manifestation.
>
> David Wolfe
> *The Sunfood Diet Success System*

It's amazing we Now have the understanding of exactly how these powerful keys work to transform us as **21st Century Superhumans** and our World! It's not rocket science, yet it is a complete turnaround from how we've been thinking and Living the last many thousand years! The instant we change, *everything* changes. This is Universal Law number two – Law of Correspondence, *"As above, so below, as below, so above"* - the same pattern expresses on all planes of existence from the smallest electron to the largest star and vice versa. Shift ourselves - shift the entire Hologram. *Arc the Hologram Now with LOVE.*

> We live at the threshold of Universal recognition
> that the human being is not mere matter,
> but a potent, energetic, field of consciousness.
>
> Michael Beckwith, New Thought Minister
> *Founder Agape International Spiritual Center, 8,000 members*

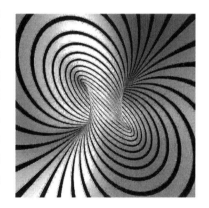

Energy pattern found throughout Creation called a torus field, recorded in Ancient petroglyphs and described in Sacred Geometry promises to be our source of infinitely abundant, clean, free energy based on today's cutting edge innovations. The doughnut shaped torus field spins and implodes in on itself continuously, creating a gravity vortex. Quantum physicist Nassim Haramein hints that within the gravity of black holes we actually may discover LOVE or Source, holding Creation in form.

Our HEART is located in the central vortex of our own torus field. As we resonate LOVE, Compassion and Gratitude into the World through the Heart, our spinning torus field expands, sending our resonance powerfully into our cells and the surrounding field. It shrinks when relating with Not of LOVE thoughts or emotions, and it can extend out to 8-12' to *miles* when we resonate Deep LOVE, Compassion and Gratitude. As we tune our Heart with coherent emotions, we, our bodies and our World emerge into New regenerative form.

Dr. Berrenda Fox, naturopath and holistic practitioner at Avalon Wellness Centre in Mt. Shasta, California and advisor for television shows about UFO contact, works with children born with additionally activated DNA strands, which she says is becoming quite common. "These children can move objects across the room just by concentrating on them and can fill a glass of water just by looking at it." This type of DNA change is also happening in adults Now moving into in LOVE.

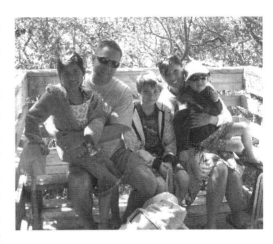

These extraordinary children show New potential with more DNA activated. They tend to be able to instantly correct issues that may have previously seemed "unsolvable." They naturally shift self and World in extraordinary ways, easily solving *seemingly* overwhelming "problems" with Mind and Heart. These children bear witness to higher potentials, already within *us* for self-healing, regeneration and radiant Living. Be sure to learn how to fully activate these levels in yourself, throughout all 4 Parts of this *21st Century Superhuman* series, videos and more at our website.

Dr. Fox tells us we are transitioning from a carbon based body structure that we've had for thousands of years, to a crystalline structure, to easily navigate and adapt to Higher dimensions. Some are beginning to exhibit this New Light Body. Remember, Not of LOVE Mind-energy is like a "logjam," that solidifies or crystalizes in the body, slowing down Life-force. Dissolving this density, first we shed water-tears, then vapor. As we increase our capacity to resonate LOVE, Gratitude, Compassion in ALL situations, ALL that is Not of LOVE vaporizes, and we and our entire World move into frequencies of higher dimensional existence. Heeding our language is highly critical in to our DNA. Words carry vibrational resonance, shaping us and our "reality." *Speak every word as Conscious Creator.* Vibrational resonance of every word matters.

..how many DNA strands are we capable of possessing? Some geneticists are claiming humans will one day have 12 strands.

Dr. Fox says, "There are major changes and mutations occurring in our DNA. We are evolving. "We will be developing twelve helixes. During this time, which seems to have started 5 to 20 years ago, we have been mutating...into something for which the end result is not yet known."

...DNA holds genetic codes for physical and emotional evolution through frequency held in languages we speak....Russian linguists found that the genetic code, especially in the apparently useless junk DNA, follows the same rules as all our human language...our DNA follows a regular grammar...like our languages. So human languages did not appear coincidentally but are a reflection of our inherent DNA [and vice versa].

Russian biophysicist and molecular biologist Pjotr Garjajev...explored Vibrational behavior of DNA. "Living chromosomes function just like solitonic/ holographic computers..." This explains why affirmations, autogenous training [such as our upcoming goal canceling] and hypnosis have such strong effects on humans and our bodies. *It is entirely normal and natural for our DNA to react to language....*

During this time in the 75,000 year cycle, we are now exposed to the most torsion energy waves, affecting our DNA, reorganizing the 97% "junk" DNA from 2-strand double helix to a 12-strand helix, advancing humanity in a leap of evolution.

Marco Torres
Scientists Finally Present Evidence On Expanding DNA Strands

Heart Coherence, based in the state of Deep LOVE, Compassion , Gratitude is one of the single most effective keys for **21st Century Superhumans** to implement! [Discussed at length in Part 2: MIND]. As we clear the unconscious, activating this state, we establish new neurological pathways transforming our entire Vibrational context to LOVE. HeartMath® offers an app with sensory-feedback unit for iPhone and computer. Users report use for 15-20 minutes a day for 2-3 weeks achieves Heart Coherence. This is an easy tool to use, share with friends, family or organization, to transform Life with simple Heart Coherence.

Our Heart's torus field sends out a more expansive resonance when Coherent in LOVE, Compassion, Gratitude. Heart Coherence hugely shifts personal issues and energies, as a result shifts the entire collective. Focusing Mind-Energy in LOVE, turns on DNA codons and empowers our visions and dreams. Accessing Heart Coherence "changes our World," *Arc the Hologram with LOVE!*

We do not experience things as they really are! We experience them only through a filter, which determines what information will enter our awareness and what will be rejected. If we change the filter [our content or belief system], we automatically experience the world in a completely different way.

David Wolfe
The Sunfood Diet Success System

When *fear* and *hostility* bathe our cells with their chemicals, unless we shift this resonance, acidity, inflammation and circulating sticky material called fibrins eventually cause toxemia that results in dis-ease and death. It is essential to clear our thought-emotional patterns in order to restore Heart Coherence. Our Emotional Tone Scale in Part 3: SPIRIT, is of great assistance to keep us moving upscale toward Joy and Enthusiasm.

Even our WORDS Create a Living resonance in our World. The Original Language, called the Language of Light, contained literally vibrational patterns that called Creation into Being. Ancient Languages such as Aramaic, Sanskrit, Hebrew, Lakota and others contain much of this original resonance, some of which has been lost in our modern languaging. However, nevertheless, Every Word We Speak sends its resonance into the World whether to Create or destroy. Language has also been made confusing with too many meaningless words such as "the" to remove us from flowing with Creation.

BEING AWARE OF EVERY WORD is a powerful *21st Century Superhuman* trait. We KNOW Every Word carries creative thought resonance, holding Attention on the *Field*. Choosing our Words well is a *VITAL PRACTICE*, supporting clearing of old data [Part 2: MIND] to change our "reality" Now. Besides the obvious hurtful words, weed out those such as but, might, must, can, could would, wish, time and hope. Cultivate thought and Words along the lines of "I Am," aligned with continual flow of Creation from the *Field*.

Powerful resources are readily available to re-tool our thought pathways. If you have not already done this vital personal realignment of your Words, grab some books or audios and zip through them to ground your Vital Positively Productive Mind-Heart-Voice. Our all time favorites include Godfrey Ray King's *I Am Discourses* from the 1930s. Louise Hay's *You Can Heal Your Life* and many more, with thoughts and affirmations for Positive Creation. The *Abraham* work of Jerry and Esther Hicks has also opened up profound ideas.

Learn to clarify how to use your Words, to assist with clearing old data from the unconscious, to present the powerful energy of your Mind-Heart to the *Field* to Create in New ways! Proper use of Words supports removing our old data or content Not of LOVE from the unconscious, using our *Ancient Aramaic* clearing techniques. Another excellent supportive tool is EFT-tapping, which helps ground in our neurobiology this work we are doing. Be sure to read Part 2: MIND to fully grasp what we are discussing here.

Now, Ideal Nutrition and physical Cleanse and Detox, along with clearing Mind-Heart, totally shifts our internal chemistry with renewed focus on LOVE. This complete-person "waking up" is a Journey of the *21st Century Superhuman.* As we enter this clearing it's common to have all-encompassing waves of Not of LOVE offload from thousands of generations. Dredging up old layers stored in "carbon-based-memory" of the unconscious, we are Now installing a new "operating system" founded in our True Design LOVE.

Now, Rather than going in to old reactive patterns or suppressing what's uncomfortable, our New way of Being in the World, notices what comes up, clears it on the spot, and we go right back into our natural state of Pure LOVE, Breathing and Smiling. Those on the cutting edge of "food and consciousness," know that True High Frequency Living incorporates Food and Cleansing, and equally essential Mind-Heart. "Rock star of the superfood World," David Wolfe says:

> The world we think we see is only a view, a collective description of the world that we Create through our belief systems. Accepting this fact seems to be one of the most empowering things one can do.

David Wolfe
Sunfood Diet Success System

Always vigilant, we recognize the dominant role thought-emotion plays a in what Creates our state of Being. Tony Robbins taught us *everything is about "State."* It determines what kind of fluids our body's cells are bathed in, how we make food and life choices, and whether our Life is in a chronic state of covering up what bothers us, or opening to Greater LOVE, *Essence* and Well-Being. Our state of Mind-Heart is a key determinant to well-being.

> It's not correct to see yourself as an isolated organism in time and space, occupying 6 ft.³ of volume, lasting seven or eight decades. Rather, you are one cell in the cosmic body entitled to all privileges of cosmic status including perfect health. Nature made us thinkers so we could realize this truth.
>
> *Deepak Chopra MD*
> *Perfect Health*

In the beginning we approach "getting what we desire" from the "outside:" "I'd like to heal ___, or I'd like to look better___, there's an area I'd like to improve, have a better relationship, more money, be more healthy." We plead, affirm, cajole, command, wish, hope with our 5% conscious thought (Harvard studies). The amazing thing is, once we go *deeper "inside,"* we discover that the entire World around us emanates from *within,* based on state of Mind-Heart (conscious-unconscious). Once we use our tools to go *inside* Mind-Heart, to view and alter things from *this* vantage point, we discover and align with how our resonance shapes what comes into Being around us. *[Covered extensively in Part 2: MIND]*

Much as we desire to send "healthy, productive" messages to our body, we still must clear our 95% unconscious thought so messages get to our body in the form we truly desire. Becoming Beings of LOVE, Compassion and Gratitude with every Breath, every Word, every Thought, every Action...ups the ante for ultimate well-being. So where is the *power* when we would like to "lose" weight, or "heal" from a dis-ease? Is it in the *food? Is it in how and when we eat? Healing methods?* It all *begins* with Mind-Heart Energy (conscious-unconscious), and how these qualify Creation of our "reality," as even physical choices emerge from it.

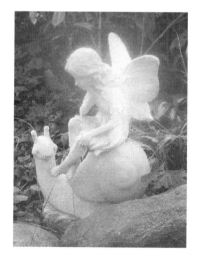

At the current vibrational state of our Body, water is a key thought transmitter that permeates our World. Centered in LOVE, more Light shows up in reflecting off of moisture surrounding us (as in image above). As we "cleanse and feed our our Living house" and settle into knowing ourselves as Divine Creator Beings of LOVE, Compassion and Gratitude Living in Truth and Authenticity, ALL in our World and our Body transforms. Thus the **21st Century Superhuman**, with Power of Coherent thought, activates our Evolving DNA in this Evolutionary Leap called *Shift of the Ages.* [Part 1] ♥

Chapter 3

What Is Ideal Nutrition?

Every aspect of our lives is, in a sense,
a vote for the kind of world we want to live in.

Frances Moore Lappé
Diet for A Small Planet

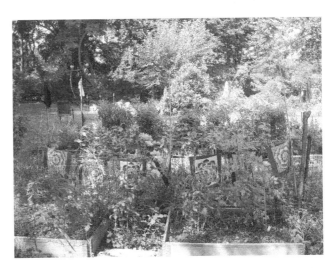

Vegan, Vegetarian, Lacto-Vegetarian, Ovo-Vegetarian, Lacto-Ovo-Vegetarian, Omnivore, Paleo, Carnivore, Pescetarian, Flexitarian, Eat for Your Blood Type, Macrobiotic, Fruitarian, Breatharian, confused? Rather than saying exactly what the *right* diet *is*, let's review cutting edge data for you to make your own educated choices. It's easy to be attached to familiar habits, caught between old conditioning and New ideas so let's consider current research. Choices they can be gradual, unless recovery from illness is at hand.

The 4th Universal Law of Polarity, states that two opposites are different Vibrational frequencies of the same energy, "all truths are but half-truths, all paradoxes may be reconciled." A Master changes the form of opposites, by changing Mind-Energy to achieve balance. We've observed that exploring the opposite is a way of discovering balance, which often is part of the learning curve. [*Universal Laws Part 1: SHIFT OF THE AGES*]

An alchemist is one who transforms everything with LOVE.

Emmanuel Dagher
Co-Creating Miracles

Based on the Law of Cause and Effect, we might call habits enhancing vitality within the body systems a *live-it,* and habits that reduce flow of energy within body systems a *die-it.* Even so, the live-it or die-it we choose, is going to be a product of our Mind-energy.

It is no secret that most chronic dis-eases result from high-fat, sugar and over-processed foods of the standard American diet or SAD, consumed in most developed nations. A glance at statistics causes us to wonder why anyone would continue following this diet, however based on advertising of food production industry and pharmaceutical companies, many are obviously convinced that it's okay to over-consume, then medicate, that one can circumvent nature and get "fixed" when something goes amiss.

The food you eat can be either the safest and most powerful form of medicine or the slowest form of poison.

Ann Wigmore
Founder Original Hippocrates Health Institute-Wheatgrass and Living Foods

The Center for Dis-Ease Control reported out of 2.5 million deaths in the U.S. in 2010 almost half were caused by heart dis-ease and cancer. Heart dis-ease is the leading cause, though both are very close. *Here are statistics per year:*

- Heart dis-ease: 597,689
- Cancer: 574,743
- Chronic lower respiratory dis-eases: 138,080
- Stroke (cerebrovascular dis-eases): 129,476
- Accidents (unintentional injuries): 120,859
- Alzheimer's dis-ease: 83,494
- Diabetes: 69,071
- Nephritis, nephrotic syndrome, and nephrosis: 50,476
- Influenza and Pneumonia: 50,097

The World Health Organization reported in 2011 that *two thirds* of 55 million deaths Globally were due to non-communicable dis-eases, cardiovascular, cancer, diabetes and chronic lung dis-ease; with 87% of deaths in high income countries attributed to cardiovascular issues, including stroke and heart attack.

The beef industry has contributed to more American deaths than all the wars of this century, all natural disasters, and all automobile accidents combined.

Dr. Neal Barnard
Go Healthy Go Vegan Cookbook

USDA reports 62% of Americans are overweight, 27% classified as obese (30 pounds overweight), with an alarming trend toward obesity in children. Convenience foods increased cheese consumption from 7.7 pounds per person per year in the 1950s to 29.8 pounds in 2000; meat consumption 195 pounds in 2,000, up from 57 pounds per year during the 1950s. Might we call this "slow suicide"?

If beef is your idea of 'real food for real people,'
you'd better live real close to a real good hospital.

Dr. Neal Barnard
Prevent and Reverse Heart Disease

Fast Food Statistics website reports 160,000 fast food restaurants in America with 50 million served daily (2012). Annual North American fast food revenue, $110 *Billion*. Fast food contains more fat, calories, sugar, sodium, and less nutrition and vitamins.

> Chicken fat, beef fat, fish fat, fried foods - these are the foods that fuel our fat genes by giving them raw materials for building body fat.
>
> *Dr. Neal Barnard*
> *Author of Turn Off the Fat Genes*

With a glance at statistics above and what follows, we might wonder why we don't run the other way as fast as we can? What suppressive Mind-Energy perpetuates this cycle? Let's familiarize ourselves with landmark research of the last quarter-century, on prevention and reversal of degenerative conditions as a product of dietary choices. In Part 2: MIND we covered in detail how thoughts play an intrinsic role in wellness and illness.

> I believe that coronary artery dis-ease is preventable and that even after it is underway, its progress can be stopped, its insidious effects reversed. I believe, and my work over the past twenty years has demonstrated that all this can be accomplished without expensive mechanical intervention and with minimal use of drugs. The key lies in nutrition - specifically, in abandoning the toxic American diet and maintaining cholesterol levels well below those historically recommended by health policy experts.
>
> *Dr. Caldwell Esselstyn*
> *Prevent and Reverse Heart Disease*

Internationally known surgeon, researcher, and former clinician at the Cleveland Clinic, Dr. Caldwell Esselstyn put patients who had less than a year to live on a plant-based, fat-free diet. He prevented and reversed progression of heart dis-ease. Patients who stuck with the program improved dramatically, twenty years later remaining symptom-free. For those ready to to change Lifestyle habits, it's documented in his NY Times bestseller, *Prevent and Reverse Heart Disease,* with recipes for heart-healthy plant-based diet.

> Every mouthful of oils and animal products, including dairy foods, initiates an assault on these [cell] membranes and, therefore, on the cells they protect. These foods produce a cascade of free radicals in our bodies - especially harmful chemical substances that induce metabolic injuries from which there is only a partial recovery. Year after year, the effects accumulate. And eventually, the cumulative cell injury is great enough to become obvious, to express itself as what physicians define as dis-ease.
>
> Plants and grains do not induce the deadly cascade of free radicals. In fact, they carry an antidote. Unlike oils and animal products, they contain antioxidants, which help to neutralize the free radicals and also, recent research suggests, may provide considerable protection against cancer.
>
> *Dr. Caldwell Esselstyn*
> *Prevent and Reverse Heart Disease*

Dr. Esselstyn is a featured expert in the acclaimed documentary *Forks Over Knives*. His work has helped thousands, with his book behind Bill Clinton's Life-changing vegan diet. His book *Prevent and Reverse Heart Dis-Ease* explains the science behind the simple plan that changed the lives of his heart dis-ease patients forever, empowering readers with tools to take control of their Heart health.

> And it's not just a matter of bad information. The truth is that we are addicted to fat - literally. Receptors in our brains account for our addiction to nicotine, heroin, and cocaine, and similar cravings have been identified for fat and sugars as well.
>
> *Dr. Caldwell Esselstyn*
> *Prevent and Reverse Heart Disease*

Reading Dr. Caldwell's book encouraged *us* to take a look at consumption of healthy free fats and oils (refined-extracted not a whole food), minimizing olive and coconut oils, instead to good benefit, relying on *whole raw* nuts, seeds, avocado. For vegans and vegetarians whole food with a little healthy fat is okay. Soaking nuts and seeds starts sprouting and brings them to Life. Westin Price discovered healing elements in certain fats such as butter and cod liver oil, as he traveled the World searching for secrets to good health. He found nothing replaces natural unprocessed foods (Price-Pottenger Foundation).

> ...[oils] are not heart healthy. Between 14 and 17 percent of olive oil is saturated, artery-clogging fat - every bit as aggressive in promoting heart dis-ease as the saturated fat in roast beef. And even though a Mediterranean-style diet that allows such oils may slow the rate of progression of coronary heart dis-ease, when compared with diets even higher in saturated fat, it does not arrest the dis-ease and reverse its effects.
>
> *Dr. Caldwell Esselstyn*
> *Prevent and Reverse Heart Disease*

Reversing bodily health conditions that are products of how we Eat, Think and Live, may require letting go social customs established by commercialism in the blame-fear-hostility culture, plus clearing out old thought-emotional content still driving the boat. Taking a couple of weeks at a Cleansing, Detox, Nutritional and Mind-changing program can help ground new habits *(check our website)*. Developing consistency at home with New shopping list, food and recipes establishes good routines. Clearing old habitual thought patterns from conscious-unconscious Mind is necessary also to clearly invoke new habits

> When it comes to food choices, habit is stupendously powerful. Our familiar foods give us comfort, reassurance, and a sense of identity. They are there for us when the world may not be... On the other hand, it does take effort to question whether our conventional ways of thinking and acting truly serve us.
>
> *John Robbins*
> *Diet for a New America*

Time-honored instruction on "our ideal nutrition" is vegan fare though later instruction revolved around that people *were* consuming meat, most likely after survival of an ice age.

> Then God said, "I give you every seed-bearing plant on the face of the whole earth and every tree that has fruit with seed in it. They will be yours for food.
>
> *Genesis 1:29*

Another physician offering tremendous model for prevention and longevity, Dr. Neal Barnard, recommends low-fat vegan diet for maintenance of good health and reversal of heart dis-ease and diabetes. He is currently doing research to demonstrate that this regimen also reverses cancer. Dr. Barnard is founding president of the Physicians Committee for Responsible Medicine, an international network of physicians, scientists, and laypeople promoting preventive medicine.

> In my own Life, I decided to leave meat off my plate in medical school, but was a bit slow to realize dairy products and eggs are not health foods either.
>
> *Dr. Neal Barnard*
> *Get Healthy, Go Vegan Cookbook*

Dr. Barnard's advocacy of a low-fat, whole food, plant-based diet is presented for anyone to follow in his 15+ books that have sold over 2 million copies, including *Power Foods for the Brain* (prevention for Alzheimer's); *The 21-Day Weight Loss Kickstart*; *Dr. Neal Barnard's Program for Reversing Diabetes* (remove animal products; minimize vegetable oils, stick to low glycemic index); *Breaking the Food Seduction*. His *Get Healthy, Go Vegan Cookbook* and *Foods that Cause You to Lose Weight* have great recipes to help any of us get started, get inspired and change our Lives forever!

Dean Ornish says about Barnard, "[He is] a leading pioneer in educating the public about the healing power of diet and nutrition." Dr. Henry Heimlich (of the Heimlich maneuver and progressive treatments for malaria) says, "Barnard's tremendous influence on dietary practices and promotion of a vegan diet is done with such eloquence as to make the proposition sound almost inviting."

> We help people to begin truly healthful diets, and it is absolutely wonderful to see not only their success, but also their delight at their ability to break old habits and feel really healthy for a change.
>
> *Dr. Neal Barnard*
> *The 21-Day Weight Loss Kickstart*

Another landmark study was done by Dr. Colin Campbell, over 20 years with 3,700 adults in 65 counties in China. Dr. Campbell was professor of nutritional biochemistry at Cornell. He went to the China Study as top protein researcher and came back vegetarian.

His book, *The China Study: The Most Comprehensive Study of Nutrition Ever Conducted And the Startling Implications for Diet, Weight Loss, And Long-term Health,* has sold over 500,000 copies; reporting that all degenerative conditions are prevented and reversed with a mostly vegetarian whole foods diet (max 7% animal products). This book is bound to have long range ramifications and huge impact on our "scientific proof oriented" society. Here's what is being said about *The China Study*:

> Today AICR [American Institute for Cancer Research] advocates a predominantly plant-based diet for lower cancer risk because of the great work of Dr. Campbell and a few other visionaries, beginning around 25 years ago.
>
> *Marilyn Gentry*
> *President, AICR*

> [These] findings from the most comprehensive large study ever undertaken on relationship between diet and risk of developing dis-ease, are challenging much of American dietary dogma.
>
> *New York Times*

> The most important book on health, diet and nutrition ever written. Its impact will only grow over time and it will ultimately improve the health and longevity of tens of millions of people around the world.
>
> *John Mackey, CEO Whole Foods*

> This is one of the most important books about nutrition ever written—reading it may save your Life.
>
> *Dean Ornish, MD*
> *Dr. Dean Ornish's Program for Reversing Heart Dis-Ease*

Another vegan advocate, John Robbins, groomed as heir to the Baskin and Robbins family ice cream business, chose to walk away from Baskin-Robbins and immense wealth it represented to "...pursue the deeper American Dream, ...of a society at peace with its conscience because it respects and lives in harmony with all Life forms...a society that is truly healthy, practicing wise and compassionate stewardship of a balanced ecosystem."

> Few of us are aware that the act of eating can be a powerful statement of commitment to our own well-being, and at the same time the creation of a healthier habitat. Your health, happiness, and the future of Life on earth are rarely so much in your own hands as when you sit down to eat.
>
> *John Robbins*
> *Diet for a New America*

John Robbins became aware at a young age of the devastating effects of animal-based diet on humans, animals and the eco-system. He became a vegan activist and thought-leader with numerous best-selling books that offer a wealth of information about better food choices: *Voices of the Food Revolution, No Happy Cows, Diet for a new America*, and more. John is Founder of EarthSave International, co-founder and co-host 100,000+ member Food Revolution Network *foodrevolution.org*. Books also include *THE new GOOD Life: Living Better Than Ever in an Age of Less; HEALTHY AT 100: Scientifically Proven Secrets of the World's Healthiest and Longest-Lived Peoples; THE AWAKENED HEART: Meditations on Finding Harmony in a Changing World; RECLAIMING OUR HEALTH: Exploding Medical Myth.*

John Robbins' Life along with wife Deo and son Ocean, has been dedicated to living wisely on Planet Earth. His widespread impact resulting from a Life well-lived, is an example of walking away from societal promises of safety and security, and dedicating Life and talents to Heart-inspired Vision and Purpose. *Wow!*

When I walked away from Baskin-Robbins and the money it represented, I did so because I knew there was a deeper dream. I did it because I knew that with all the reasons that each of us has to despair and become cynical, there still beats in our common heart our deepest prayers for a better Life and a more loving world.

John Robbins
Diet for a New America

I (Cary) was privileged to work with John Robbins, his family and co-author Jia Patton for a short time in Santa Cruz, California in early 1990s, which was inspirational and heartwarming. His work has been subject of cover stories and feature articles in San Francisco Chronicle, Los Angeles Times, Chicago Life, Washington Post and New York Times. His Life and work have also been featured in PBS special, *Diet For A new America*.

You see the changes in many places. You see people refusing to buy shampoos or other body care products from companies that test on animals, and instead buying cosmetics and other household products that are made without cruelty. We're learning to see what we didn't see before, and then, when we have the courage, creating the changes that make our lives congruent with what we know.

John Robbins
Healthy at 100

John Robbins work in *Diet For A new America* brought to the forefront, how inhumane and environmentally damaging commercial animal food production is. Most factory farming practices are unbelievably horrendously destructive to Life, with animals injuriously imprisoned, piled on top of one another, rarely getting a minute of "real" Life.

Animals do not 'give' their life to us, as the sugar-coated lie would have it. No, we take their lives. They struggle and fight to the last breath, just as we would do if we were in their place.

John Robbins

If it is an individual's choice to consume meat, it is one thing to find a local producer who is raising animals organically and humanely, and another to just pick up a neatly wrapped package in the meat department at your grocery store, with little thought as to what that animal went through in its Life for that package of meat to be there in your hands. It's essential we wake up to the implications of our actions. Pigs are the 4th most intelligent animal known, and what most know them for is bacon or ham. Devastating.

Rather than closed eyes, do your research, watch films, visit animal food production, and then consider vegan or vegetarianism. Watch: *Fast food Nation, Supersize Me* and *Forks*

Over Knives, others recommended by PETA (people for ethical treatment of animals). Respect Universal Law, use Mind-Energy and choose your Vibration wisely.

> Once you start to notice the surging interest in compassion toward animals, you find it's everywhere...
>
> Although extreme crowding of animals greatly increases rates of animals' illness and death, it nevertheless also raises profits. Even when more than 20 percent of pigs and chickens die prematurely in today's intensive husbandry systems for instance, producers find their profits increased by such practices.
>
> Overcrowding that's typical today would once have been unthinkable, because animals kept in such conditions would have been decimated by dis-ease. Now, with antibiotics mixed into every meal, with widespread use of hormones, drugs, and biocides, enough animals are kept alive so overcrowding becomes cost-effective...
>
> Layer hens, meanwhile, are crammed together in cages so tiny that they do not have enough space even to begin to lift a single wing...More than 99 percent of the hens who lay eggs eaten in the United States are debeaked and kept in cages where the excrement from the birds in the upper tiers collects above them, often falling through onto their heads.'
>
> *John Robbins*
> *Diet for a new America*

It's easy to say, "Oh these choices would be difficult to make because of my husband, wife, family, or what my neighbors and friends might think," or "I might have to learn something New." Or if you're a confirmed meat, egg and dairy eater, one good option is to find a humane local producer, and buy from them rather than abusive mass production. And yes, this kind of awareness may stimulate changes, yet it can also be easy and fun. As we continue to develop Mastery, such food choices become a matter of Awareness.

> There are people in the world so hungry,
> that God cannot appear to them except in the form of bread.
>
> *Mahatma Gandhi (1969-1948)*
> *Non-Violent Leader of India*

Outside health of our body, and health and welfare of hundreds of millions of animals suffering today, the ecology of our Planet is also at stake. New York Times Week In Review reported in Jan. 2008, "Rethinking the Meat Guzzler," "Just this week, the president of Brazil announced emergency measures to halt burning and cutting of rain forest for crop-grazing land [by such as McDonalds]. In the last five months alone, the government says, 1,250 square miles were lost."

> ...The real cause of hunger is a scarcity of justice, not a scarcity of food. Enough grain is squandered every day in raising American livestock for meat to provide every human being on earth with two loaves of bread.
>
> John Robbins, *Diet for a new America:*
> *How Your Food Choices Affect Your Health,*
> *Happiness and the Future of Life on Earth*

This is a Mind-full to consider. If you are not vegan or vegetarian, there is wisdom in considering this "path" for your body, the environment and all creatures. Daniel of the Old Testament and his men, on a diet of "pulse" (peas and beans) were "fairer and fatter than all the kings men." If you are of the mindset that you *must have* animal products, accessing those produced in a humane manner, to bring a different kind of resonance through you.

> The ancient Greeks told of a philosopher eating bread and lentils for dinner. He was approached by another man, who lived sumptuously by flattering the king. Said the flatterer, "If you would learn to be subservient to the king, you would not have to live on lentils." The philosopher replied, "If you would learn to live on lentils, you would not have to give up your independence in order to be docile and acquiescent to the king.
>
> *John Robbins*
> *The new Good Life: Living Better Than Ever in an Age of Less*

Teddi suggests to her clients, "Only eat it if it's a whole food, not processed and picked as it grew." Cary's philosophy has been, *"Whole foods in as close to their simple and natural form as possible."* Cary's book **Super Immunity Secrets,** available on Amazon and Kindle, is a great guide, with 50 easy basic everyday vegan-vegetarian recipes, belongs in every kitchen *(check our website).* Also look for Food Prep videos at our website and Youtube.

One of the most empowering solutions to many issues we face today includes growing a garden, or buying from local growers. One man in Los Angeles featured on TED startted "Guerrilla Gardens" on median strips and any open soil in L.A., giving birth to neighborhood access to free fresh food. Barbara Kingsolver's *Animal, Vegetable, Miracle: A Year of Food Life,* is a wonderful story of a family who ate only what was obtainable locally for a year! inspirational! Another family lived *Trash Free* for a Year, blogging about this New way to Live, ending up with only one tiny ziplock of trash at the end! We can do it!

A clean body supports clear Mind-Energy. Now popular Raw Food movement and Juicing, cleanses, alkalizes and brings the Body into harmonious function; it is easier than ever to get on a "cleanup program." Enzymes and Life-force of Raw-Living Foods-Juices restore Life-giving elements to cells. Dr. Gabriel Cousens, MD author of *Conscious Eating,* who established Tree of Life rejuvenation and learning center near Patagonia, Arizona says:

> A live-food diet has been used with great success to heal...degenerative dis-eases or poor states of health, such as arthritis, high blood pressure, menstrual difficulties, obesity, allergies, diabetes, ulcers, heart and other circulatory dis-eases, hormone disturbances, diverticulosis, anemia, weak immune system, and other poor states of health. Many people have found a live-food diet an excellent aid for improving brain/mind function...a high percentage of live food in the diet plays an important part in creating healthful longevity.

So is there a black-and-white answer as to what is the best *live-it* or *die-it?* The truth is, we choose our food based on where we are in Awareness. As we clear unconscious content, live in the Heart and focus in LOVE, we are most likely moving toward Lighter, rejuvenating, kind, organic nutrition and Lifestyle, based around *ahimsa,* ancient practice of harmlessness. Honor others' choices, Live with Joy on your own path.

It seems the whole works of humankind are backwards. Most are trying to convince, instruct, and purify everyone else - without first purifying themselves. To enlighten others we have to enlighten ourselves.

David Wolfe
Sunfood Diet Success System

Whatever our choices, it's important to Live without judgment. The the more present we are, the more clear it becomes how we affect the whole. The more Awake we are, the more we consider every action to be an act of consciousness, ruled by the Universal Law of Cause and Affect. Becoming vegan or vegetarian, obtaining our food in ecological holistic ways emanates from the Heart. As "fear-hostility" clear from our Vibration we naturally shift to kinder choices. Everything that manifests is a result of Vibrational cause. Let go of fear about whatever you choose. The biggest cause to act from, is our True Design, LOVE.

Vegetarianism preserves Life, health, peace and ecology, Creates a more equitable distribution of resources, helps feed the hungry, encourages nonviolence for animal and human members of the planet, and is a powerful aid for spiritual transformation of body, emotions, mind and spirit.

Gabriel Cousens
Conscious Eating

Foods and beverages can be used as "drugs" to numb us. It may take choice of will to remove ourselves from surrounding temptations. It requires sincere dedication and effort to exit social inertia, and instead set ourselves up with nourishing food and beverages. Layers of belief systems we grew up with and cultural programming can be "sticky wickets" to move beyond. Be patient with the process, LOVE self and let go all judgment. Empower yourself with your deep Heart-felt Desire to Live with Health and Vibrancy.

Instead of doing battle with inner struggles, use our essential tools [Part 2: MIND], to clear resonance from the unconscious. Align with Universal Laws 1 & 3 Mind-Energy, Vibration. As we release and let go blame-fear-hostility, food choices naturally Lighten up.

Deepening Heart connection we find our way, discovering we Know that we Know, based on Eternal connection with the Innate. We enter a chrysalis like the caterpillar, unwinding the old paradigm through deep transformative darkness and chaos of Mirrored shadows, emerging finally into our True Design LOVE, stretching our New wings to fly.

This genius is inside you, a part of your inner blueprint that cannot be erased..."The inner intelligence of the body is the ultimate and supreme genius in nature. It mirrors the wisdom of the cosmos." (Vedic text)... At the Quantum mechanical level, there is no sharp boundary dividing you from the rest of the Universe.

Deepak Chopra M
Perfect Health: A Complete Mind-Body Guide

Frequencies of foods below measured with a radionics machine demonstrate how much they raised body vitality. Those at top #1 raised it most. This basic awareness of energies and frequencies of foods was mapped by Margueritte Weippers, who used radionics to consistently grow incredibly extraordinary organic blueberries.

ELECTROVIBRATORY RATE OF NOURISHMENT OF FOODS

1. Chelated Colloidal Mineral Water
2. Fresh Pressed Greens - Wheatgrass, Spirulina, Chlorella
3. Sprouts
4. Fresh Pressed Fruits & Vegetables (juiced or blended)
5. Raw Salads
6. Raw Fruits
7. Sprouted Seeds and Nuts
8. Sprouted Grains - Essene Bread
9. Highly Mineralized Herbs
10. Bee Pollen
11. Raw Honey

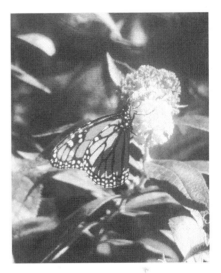

1. Legumes cooked with spices
2. Seeds & Nuts (ground and soaked)
3. Steamed Veggies
4. Baked Potatoes or Yams
5. Brown Rice and Whole Grains, cooked
6. Natural Sweet Treats - carob, seeds, fruit, raw honey

Do not live in the body alone; live in consciousness. Be aware of your progress. Know your destiny. Meaning will become clear. Seek gratefully, ask reverently...knock humbly. And above all have faith, you will receive!

Margueritte Weippers
Radionics Master

NUTRITION LEVELS LIST

Use upper 3 categories below to "Lighten up." A common option is to cleanse one day per week and have a salad daily, it depends on you. Variety is important. Listen to YOUR body & intuition; get organic-naturally grown, local whenever possible.

CLEANSING

Fasting - water, fresh air, sunshine, gentle movement, Breathing, rest

Beverages - water; water with lemon, herbal tea, pinch baking soda

Juices - fresh only, dilute with water 1/5th - excellent for cleansing & nourishing

Cleanses - (homemade or purchased) eliminative herbs, psyllium, flax

REGENERATIVE - ALL RAW

Green Shakes /Smoothies water /vegan milk, fruit fresh-frozen, green powders, algae, grasses, seaweeds, superfoods, soaked seeds & nuts, hemp, flax, greens

Fruits - ripe, in season, eat only with light foods for best digestion

Veggies- ripe, in season - raw in salads

Sprouts - alfalfa, clover, radish, broccoli, peas, adzuki beans, mung, sunnies

Fermented Foods - raw: sauerkraut, kimchee, rejuvelac

Nuts and Seeds - soaked overnight, then refrigerate

Dried Fruit (no sulphur or sugar) rehydrated

Essene Bread - sprouted grains - very low temp or dehydrate

Seasonings - Herbs, Spices. Lemon, sm. amt. olive/coconut oil, cayenne, Celtic, Himalayan or sea salt, dulse & seaweeds, garlic, onion, nutritional yeast

MAINTENANCE - COOKED VEGAN *(recipes at our website)*

Fruits - ripe, in season, (separate from veggies) raw or simple pies/jams

Veggies- baked, steamed, sautéed

Soups - veggies, moderate grains, beans, herbs

Legumes - soak 12-24 hrs, pour off water, sprout and/or simmer

Grains - lean toward non-gluten such as rice, quinoa, amaranth, oats

Nuts & Seeds, Nut Butters - great oil source, whole raw, not sprouted

Ezekiel or Essene Sprouted Grain Bread - sprouted grains, seeds, veggies

Whole Grain Preparations (sprouted preferred) tortillas, bread, crackers, pasta

Seasoning - see list above

LACTO-OVO VEGETARIAN All of above plus Healthy, Organic, Humanely, Kindly Farm Produced Eggs & Dairy. Generous foods from all previous categories

FISH - MEAT Reduce quantity, organic, have less often, obtain only humanely raised, increase foods from all above categories. HUMANE CARE: Temple Grandin's work listed in *Time's 100 Most Influential People: Heroes*, documentary "The Woman Who Thinks Like A Cow." *"Nature is cruel but we don't have to be; we owe them some respect."*

REMOVE White flour, white sugar, excesses, processed, fast and fried foods

GREAT RECIPES - Cary's book, **Super Immunity Secrets,** quick, easy, delicious, vegan-vegetarian w/shopping list. *(See our website for more books and videos)*

Climb the Transitional Ladder Chart chart by Cary Ellis. *(check our website)*

FOOD FOR THOUGHT: Mind-Energy covers *everything:* we may seek health due to our of fear of death. Or we may say, "Live for today," and do whatever we feel like. As we let go fear, clearing unconscious content, we choose to be healthy, embracing Life. Genetic patterns often trigger food choices. These shift as we clear our unconscious data and integrate Higher Frequency dynamics, from choice point of Now. *Choosing a healthy path requires dedication and commitment, yet bears fruit in results that uplift the entire Life.*

CAUSE & EFFECT Universal Law: How does this work with food? Just ask yourself, "Did this food come from the Earth Mother, in a natural wholesome form, in Vibrational harmony and Coherence with my body?" If the answer is Yes, then enjoy it with LOVE and Gratitude. If its production is based on refinement or suffering to get it to your table, seek other choices and consider *effect* manifested from *cause*. *[Universal Laws Part 2: MIND]*

> So the question that remains is: Why does the live-food diet give us the best effect in terms of decreasing our caloric intake and maximizing the quality of our food intake? The point from basic nutrient mathematics is that by eating live foods, we get complete nutrition by eating 50 to 80 percent less food.
>
> *Dr. Gabriel Cousens*
> *Spiritual Nutrition*

WEIGHT LOSS AND HEALTHY WEIGHT MAINTENANCE: Many yo-yo with dietary confusion. The most vital solution is to remove all animal products and refined foods; follow *Daily Cleansing: Simple Rules* in our *Cleanse and Detox* chapter. Find Cary's books at Amazon: *Why Become a Vegetarian?* and *Truth About Weight Loss* and more at our website.

DAILY REGENERATIVE REGIMEN
Adapt and apply to what fits for you! (visit our website for more)

These Lifestyle Habits bring Vitality and Clarity to our Mind-Energy. Masters of all ages have harmonized body and spirit with simple high-frequency nourishment. RULES: 4-5 hrs. btw. meals; 12 hrs. at night empty stomach; moderate meal size. Choose from suggested foods suitable to your path.

UPON ARISING

❑ Stretch, Breathe, notice what is bubbling up, note dreams, or "worries" to clear with quick goal canceling or tapping - give them to the *Field*. (see Part 2: MIND)

❑ You are rising from fasting all night. Honor this - rooted in the 5th Universal Law (Mutable) of Rhythm. During morning routine, to flush elimination from night's fast from cells, organs, tissues, DRINK *1 quart warm:*
   • water or water water with a wedge of lemon or lime
   • or water with lemon-lime and a pinch of baking soda *(alkalizing)*
   • herbal tea *(no caffeine for cleansing, then regular tea or coffee after)*

❑ **GREEN SHAKE** Pre mixed green powder or Create your own combo *including*: grass powders, chlorella, Spirulina, blue-green algae, golden flax (ground-soaked), fresh or frozen fruit, water, nut-seed milk, vegan protein powder, chia, hemp

❑ **BREAKFAST** - The Lighter we become, the more the above is sufficient. For more, let the above settle then have your choice from list

- Smoothies, Raw nuts, Fruit
- Ezekiel or Essene bread-toast, plain, w/nut butter (opt.)
- Muesli cereal raw - oats, nuts, dried fruit - soaked overnight
- Potatoes, tofu, toast, or *choice of above list based on current Lifestyle*

☐ **LUNCH** - drink water or beverage on empty stomach 1/2 hr before meal

- Raw salad, veggies, sprouts, sprouted seeds, dress with All Raw Seasonings list above. Once a habit these become good craving!
- Sandwich or roll up made with sprouts, veggies (your pick on list above)
- Ezekiel or Essene bread-toast, plain, w/nut butter (opt.)
- Cooked veggies or Soup (homemade when possible - make on weekend to have during week)
- If animal products desired: *quantity size of palm of hand*

☐ **DINNER** - drink beverages on empty stomach 1/2 hr before meal

- Raw salad, veggies, sprouts, sprouted seeds, dress with All Raw Seasonings list above. Once a habit salads become a good craving!
- Ezekiel or Essene bread-toast, plain, w/nut butter (opt.)
- Cooked, baked, steamed veggies
- Soup - one of our mainstays - especially in chilly weather, a great Light, hearty nourishment with veggies, herbs, spices, a little grain, legume - so easy to prepare - throw everything in pot and let simmer when home to have later in week if it lasts!
- If you desire animal products, *quantity size of palm of hand*

> It's not what goes into your mouth that defiles you;
> you are defiled by the words that come out of your mouth.
>
> *Matthew 15:11*

Mind-Energy or Vibration within us calls Creation into being, thus determining the state of our physical body and our "reality." Establishing LOVING family and community we find support for better choices, as "no one is an island." Joining others who share Visions and Dreams carries us a long way toward well-being. *[Part 3: SPIRIT]*

Over the years we have followed healthy lifestyle practices, both Teddi and I (Cary) have found our own paths become simpler and simpler. We have learned to have a deep gratitude for that which is given us, as Sun Bear taught, and to encompass the prayer that all may be fed, and we may give our Lives to service that brings well-being to ALL.

After breathing, we smile...Contemplating our food for a few seconds before eating, and eating in mindfulness, can bring us much happiness...Having the opportunity to sit with family and friends and enjoy wonderful food is something precious, something not everyone has. Many people in the world are hungry. When I hold a bowl of rice or a piece of bread, I know that I am fortunate, and I feel compassion for all those who have no food to eat and are without friends or family. This is a very deep practice...Mindful eating can cultivate seeds of compassion and understanding that will strengthen us to do something to help hungry and lonely people to be nourished.

John Robbins
Diet for a New World

CARY'S LIFESTYLE JOURNEY: I was lucky enough to grow up in the midst of gardens and an orchard, with wonderful produce that fed us and others all year. Our Mediterranean diet with small amounts of meat and abundant fruit and vegetables was quite healthy. I went to the West Coast from Michigan at age 18, where my World opened up to new ideas including becoming vegetarian.

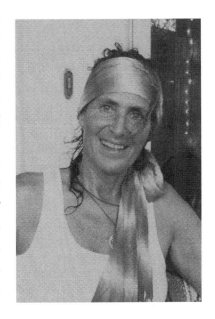

So for 40+ years I have been various forms of vegan, vegetarian, occasionally a tiny bit of fish or dairy, with longest periods on mostly Raw and Living Foods. My current Lifestyle is 65%-95% Raw depending upon season, location, availability; Green Shakes, salads, herbs, spices, juice, Essene or Ezekiel bread, nuts, seeds, legumes, quinoa, amaranth or rice mostly in winter soups and salads. Simple. Simple.

I met Teddi with her then husband Lou in 1980, when they visited the Wheatgrass Institute in Michigan where I was co-director. This center was a most significant and enjoyable experience of my Life: great community, crew, gardens, and many attendees learning to Live Lifestyle-changes. Consuming large amounts of wheatgrass juice, sprouting, fasting, cleansing, juices, banquets of Living food, Life supporting rejuvenation. I encourage anyone seeking higher levels of Vitality to experience such an immersion in cleansing and high frequency nutrition to accelerate your Journey.

EVERYTHING we share here is a result of having seen thousands of lives change over many years. We have both always sought simple, practical, effective answers that individuals can carry out themselves. Being Healthy is not complicated, yet takes re-education. It is easy to feel like you're stuck, or to think you can't do it, yet the reason we are here with you is because we LOVE what we're doing and know you can change too. It's easier than you think, and we're here to guide you!

Much on this journey of Life inspired me to question more deeply, such as being around hunting and extreme winters in the Colorado Rocky Mountains for 16 years; deciding whether to feed my dogs meat and when they died of cancer, questioning whether they really were carnivorous, wishing I'd been knowledgeable enough not to vaccinate; watching many friends who had been vegetarian go back to meat eating; watching some people die of cancer and other degenerative conditions and others get well, always seeking to know why. Reflecting on my own experiences of Mind-Energy and Body, I've always searched for answers to such deep and probing questions.

My sweetest discoveries revolve around how physical health is a result of so much more than physical habits. I flow more Freely these days, with simple gratitude for what IS, knowing many in the World do not currently have choices available that I do. My Life is dedicated to practical solutions now on a Globally scale, initiating a New Civilization based in LOVE. Most important for me these days, is following my Heart of Hearts to Live Authentically from Essence... ♥ *Cary*

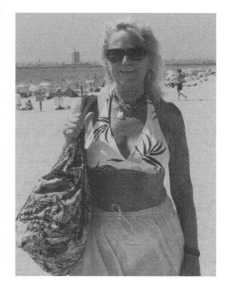

TEDDI'S LIFESTYLE JOURNEY: *As a child I had a natural aversion to dairy products. My parents couldn't get me to eat an egg, even if they disguised it or scrambled it. And as for anything like meat, beef or chicken, if I saw the bones, that was it for me! I am so thankful that my parents gave me the opportunity to choose what my Body-Mind-Spirit told me to eat!*

So you might ask, why was a child like me so filled with food dislikes? The one answer is this, my grandfather lived on a farm a few miles from our house... and we visited often. So I knew what the barn and the chicken coop smelled like. Milk came into our house warm and smelled like the cows, eggs came into our house dirty and had to be cleaned or sandpapered before they were put into the fridge. Because I was brought up with a truck farm nearby, and we had large gardens, I always knew there was plenty of food to choose from and unlimited fresh fruit and vegetables, making healthy food choices easy.

Needless to say when I had my four children, I listened to their individual choices. I continue to know that gardening is a way of Life for me wherever I am. I am fully aware of the Food Pyramids, the Whole Foods Ladder, the Maker's Diet, Eating Right for Your Blood Type, and the list goes on and on, and still I like the gentle "middle path," based in a variety of good, natural, organic, unprocessed, fresh and simply prepared whole foods..

Thirty years of client services working directly with Dr. Stone's environmentally sensitive clients and nutritional soundness with Dr. Versendaal, gave me depth of insight on advice focused around individual needs, which I have come to understand is ultimately important. Reminding people to listen to their own intuition and get to know their body offers a primary key to wellness.

I have had a simple approach to living healthfully. I listen to my body. I make good natural, whole food choices, and I leave a little wiggle room for picnics, parties and play. Do your best to keep fear out of your food or the food of others; bless what you do have, and eat as close to nature as possible. ♥ *Teddi*

Part 4: BODY

Chapter 4

Superior Supplements: *Superfoods*

Superfoods represent a uniquely promising piece of the nutrition puzzle, as they are great sources of clean protein, vitamins, minerals, enzymes, antioxidants, good fats and oils, nutrients, essential fatty and amino acids.

David Wolfe
Superfoods: The Food and Medicine of the Future

Our favorite way of buffing-out nutrition, providing the Body "super" nutrients on which to thrive, is with powerful whole "Superfoods," the most nutrient dense foods on the Planet. They increase vital force, boost the immune system, elevate serotonin production, enhance sexuality and alkalize. Mother Nature contains within her bounty an amazing array of super-nutrients not found in your local grocery store. Our first LOVE of Superfoods is grasses, algae and other greens.

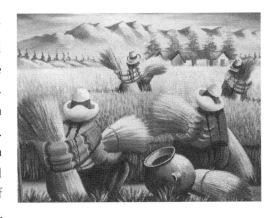

We consider them *Essential* to high-quality nutrition.

Many Superfoods have been used in Ancient cultures for thousands of years, to promote longevity and vitality. Incorporating Superfoods into our Lifestyle may take a little research, as some are shipped from faraway, though Now so popular, many can be easily ordered online or purchased at your local health food store.

Once you become involved in the Superfoods "community" you are likely to meet interesting people, and change your Life as a result. Superfoods tap us into Ancient roots of natural Wisdom, activating latent elements in our consciousness. They carry in their cellular memory millennia of "plant knowing" and Living elements. Viewed with Kirlian photography superfoods have large vibrant, radiant auras, electromagnetic or pranic *Fields*. This super vital Life force is transmitted to us, as we use them with LOVE and Gratitude.

In ancient Egypt green was used for healing, and this has proves itself out over and over through various programs. Powerful foods for regeneration are grasses and algae. Observing the regenerative condition of people in our circles over many years, daily consumption of these foods seems to make the biggest difference. When I (Cary) look around at other people my age and I ask myself the difference between them and what I have done for so long, my conclusion has been that daily for 40 over years I have consumed a green shake of some sort or green drinks with grasses, living green leaves and algae for protein consistently.

Participating in wheatgrass and living foods institutes proved this out, watching hundreds of people transform their bodies in just a manner of weeks. Also, working with Gerson Cancer Therapy Institute where 13 juices per day produced amazing results.

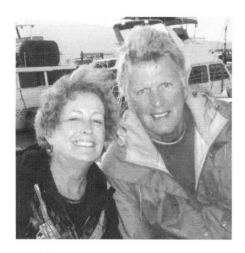

I have been in dialogue with close friend Dennis since early 1980s, who consistently included endurance in his regimens. He participated in numerous hundred mile ultramarathons, through-hiked Appalachian Trail in five months, and over many years has consistently been a high-level athlete as a mostly Raw Vegan - Vegetarian, and "O" blood type.

At the time of this writing he is 70 years young, and one of the most vital bright people I know. He and his wife Wendy live authentic, "present" lives filled with the kind of vitality most people dream of yet think may be out of reach. They would like others to know this is attainable, though requires commitment to Lifestyle changes. One of their secrets to operating at this level of well-being is dedication to expressing True *Essence*, Living for the betterment for humanity and participating in service to others.

> To me conscious living means I'm aware of each and everything that I do in terms of my thoughts, what I put into my body and the ways I keep my body fit and whole. This translates into how I make choices about everything I think, say and do.
>
> *Dennis Shackley*
> *Leader The Mankind Project, Raw Food Vegan*

In a culture where a majority have long been caught in poor nutritional practices, it's awesome to have a circle of friends modeling excellence, as this is how we learn and grow, by associating with others dedicated to Mastery. In our ongoing dialogs with one another Dennis and I have concluded, observing our lives, that consistency with grasses, greens and algae, with salads and other Raw foods, is an *essential* piece that has helped us both stay consistently vital and regenerative. This is a Life-path commitment! What Dennis and I would like others to know, is that this is within reach for ANYONE. It simply requires dedication to get and stay on the path of Awakened Living.

There is Now a cultural wave going on, including younger generations and and all ages getting into juicing and raw foods. This is very exciting! When a person cultivates desire, they can also find companionship, inspiration, support and community. We acknowledge friendships over many years, are one of biggest support for each of us to stay with our chosen path, with dialogue, encouragement, and space held without judgement to look deeper into unraveling our own shadows. The Buddy System works! Find friends and community of matching Vibration to inspire you to live *Lightly* today!

We find the most regenerative *Live-it* foods are concentrated green powders containing grasses and algae along with fresh greens such as kale or spinach and more. Moving away from traditional Lifestyle, using greens daily is a big habit to incorporate. This single simple habit heightens our potential for well-being and vitality, and gets us on a track for revitalized living. Daily greens keep us resilient, chase away illness, with clarity of Mind-Energy, higher Vibrational frequency and positive effect on the Whole. Change yourself, change the World. *Arc the Hologram Now with LOVE!*

Concentrated Green Superfoods

Most below are available at local health food store or ordered easily online. Wheatgrass is easy and inexpensive to grow at home. Some adventurous Souls are learning aquaculture to grow algae, very exciting as Dr. Christopher Hills taught that we could completely feed ALL with this single regenerative food. These are some of the most basic and concentrated foods on the Planet, best to be enjoyed in shakes or can alternatively be taken in capsules or bars on the go.

WHEATGRASS & BARLEY GRASS [grasses of grains gluten free at this stage of development] harvested within first 7-14 days are a rich chlorophyll source, very alkalizing, aid in cell detoxification, internal cleansing, cleanse and rebuild, improv energy and mental clarity by oxygenating blood, improve digestion, contain concentrated nutrients, iron, calcium, magnesium, amino acids, vitamins A, C, K, E; are 22% protein. Grasses are potent antioxidants, reducing Body stress by neutralizing toxins. Grass powder is good, *juice powder* is even more potent and excellent to use on a daily basis!

ORMUS SUPERGREENS by Sunwarrior are grown in volcanic soil; highly mineralized it is loaded with micro amounts of platinum, gold and silver. These ORMUS trace minerals instill the greens with a magnetic Life force property, raising Vibrational frequency for those consuming it. Use of such potent greens can activate higher energetic frequencies in the Body, so better to increase slowly with this Ancient Alchemy. *Ormus Supergreens* also contain oat grass, barley and wheatgrass alfalfa, yucca, stevia parsley, spinach, probiotic, peppermint.

SPIRULINA an algae, is 60% complete protein and contains important vitamins and minerals, B complex, vitamin E, carotenoids, iodine, iron, manganese, zinc, essential fatty acids such as gamma-Linolenic acid (found in mother's milk), more beta carotene than carrots! Plant source B12.

CHLORELLA is high in chlorophyll. Raw, broken-cell walled chlorella is deep green in color, is considered to enhance immune system, increases growth of "friendly" bacteria, lowers blood pressure and cholesterol, promotes healing of intestinal issues, "cleanses" blood and liver; is protective against cancer, diabetes and other degenerative conditions. Chlorella attracts and cleanse the Body of toxins and heavy metals; it is particularly useful in clearing mercury exposure commonly resulting from old dental fillings and coal burning power plants.

BLUE-GREEN ALGAE Algae first appeared on the planet over 3.5 billion years ago. As one of the first Life forms capable of photosynthesis, it quickly became a primary foundation food for all Life on the planet. During photosynthesis, sunlight transforms water and carbon dioxide in algae into oxygen, essential nutrients, elemental compounds and vibrant Life-energy. As a result, algae is responsible for an astonishing 80% of the global oxygen supply and provides vital nourishment for every species that consumes it. It is a valuable phytonutrient considered by many to be one of nature's most cleansing and regenerating substances.

It provides a highly bioavailable protein that is 80% assimilated in our bodies (compared to meat protein, which is only 20% assimilated). Blue-green algae's amino acid profile is optimal for humans; and it contains the world's most concentrated source of chlorophyll.

The Toltec, Aztec and Mayan Indians so prized algae for its powerful, Life-sustaining qualities that they cultivated it in carefully built aqueducts. The Kanembu people of Saharan Africa continue the ancient tradition of annual pilgrimages to Lake Johann to gather the vital wild algae blooming in its waters for nourishment and food throughout the coming year. Today, scientific research has confirmed what traditional cultures always knew - algae is one of the most nutrient-dense and restorative whole foods available to humankind. Many scientists and nutritionists expect the extraordinary properties of edible algae to play a substantial role in feeding and healing people of the 21st century.

GREEN POWDER BLENDS - Many awesome blends are now available that containing greens to seaweed, mushrooms and high frequency superfoods. One of these is a great way to get started, rather than multiple bags or bottles. There are only four or five different organizations that actually make greens Blends so what you will start noticing Read labels and you will learn to recognize the various blends, try them out and discover which you like best.

There are numerous excellent resources online and at your local health food store to obtain these items; try a few things till you become familiar with what works for you and what you like. It's always good when starting out with concentrated green powders, to start with a small amount such as 1/4 teaspoon of each, gradually increase, as they can initiate cleansing. Gradually increase to larger amounts, blending them into green shakes every morning; so nutritious these are sustaining for much of the day. Using a mix of grasses and algae it is amazing how well nutritional needs are met with added protein of the algae; we find these green shakes a mainstay.

> When you are young and healthy, it never occurs to you
> that in a single second your whole Life could change.
>
> *Annette Funicello (1942-2013)*
> *Actress, Singer, Mouseketeer*

We have seen much recovery from dis-ease and access to wellness over many years, by those committed to transforming their Lives with these concentrated green Superfoods, clearly showing their value. While running the wheatgrass institute one man with leukemia who had a blood count so low he should have been dead, after using wheatgrass juice for one week achieved a normal blood count. Composition of hemoglobin and chlorophyll are identical except hemoglobin has iron at its nucleus and and chlorophyll has magnesium. As a result chlorophyll rebuilds the blood and tissues very quickly.

> To keep the body in good health is a duty...
> otherwise we shall not be able to keep our mind strong and clear.
>
> *Buddha*

I (Cary) observed a client at Gerson Cancer Institute eliminate a grapefruit-sized tumor through his chest wall. This is the power of aligning with Life in *harmony* with nature, clearing Mind and Heart. This is the power of rightly lived Cause and Effect, resulting in manifestation transforming from the inside out. To accomplish such required commitment to grow beyond societal and personal conditioning. This is an elite visionary, who recognized the value of regenerative Lifestyle to sustain, maintain, regain optimum health and clarity of Body-Mind-Spirit. Superfoods hold a cellular dynamic that plays a key role in such recoveries, empowering restoration of a living clean vital body.

> The way you think, the way you behave,
> the way you eat, can influence your Life-span by 30 to 50 years.
>
> *Deepak Chopra MD*
> *Natural Physician, New Thought Author*

After a near-fatal car crash, Mitchell May was told he would never walk again. Thanks to his dedication to heal and support of his medically oriented family who went beyond their conditioning, he made medical history by regenerating nerve, bone, muscle and organ tissue, after his Body was almost totally crushed. On this extraordinary healing journey, he learned the art of non-traditional self-healing. He developed a powerful Superfood blend, *Pure Synergy*, which was all he consumed for a year, recovering use of bone, muscle and nerve thought beyond hope. Pure Synergy has since, offered healing Lifestyle to others.

> A wise man should consider that health is the greatest of human blessings, and
> learn how by his own thought to derive benefit from his illnesses.
>
> *Hippocrates (460 B.C.- 367 B.C.)*
> *Father of Modern Medicine*

These stories and more, assist us to realize it is never too late to heal, to make the choice to be well, to change the course or direction our Body is headed. It is always a choice of Mind-Heart based Action. The Body is an amazing miraculous mechanism, *whose pure drive is toward Life.* As we remove toxins blocking Life-force from poor habits, and provide high-frequency Superfoods, the body moves diligently toward wholeness and wellness. This is how we access brightness of Mind and Spirit and give our best to Life.

Many unhealthy Lifestyle habits are perpetuated when we suppress expression of Truth and Authenticity, or carry around pain that is a resonance we must remove from the unconscious. Utilizing tools in other parts of this series: Part 2: MIND and Part 3: SPIRIT, are essential for ultimate well-being, as Body-Mind-Spirit are infinitely connected.

Freeing ourselves from a false sense of obligation and duty developed in the blame-fear-hostility culture, and bringing forth the creative Being that Lives within us, vital Superfoods *accelerate* the process. Even working through a residual of old suppressive habits, adding Superfoods such as a green shake daily strengthens Mind and Heart to assist us in releasing these old cycles.

This is LOVING self. Superfood nutrition helps bring clarity to Mind and Heart to LOVE more and let go suppressive habits, because it feels so good to be clear! It provides clarity of Mind to bring inspired Dreams into being, strengthening us to courageously find the way on our own path of Living Authentically from *Essence.* Seeking to know and express the depths of who we are, is ultimately the driving force in finding peace.

Before we take a look at the more exotic Superfoods, let's dig a little deeper into why we're hungry for them, which returns us to lack of mineralization in declining soils. We *can* get Super-nutrients from organically grown produce in our back yards; however most soils are so depleted, nutrient value they ought to have is not there. If you are lucky enough to have garden rich soil, you're an "exclusive clubber," and you have one of the best foundations possible, deeply harmonious with Pachamama or Mother Earth. Adding rock dust to your garden soil is a huge bonus, to increase longevity and resistance to dis-ease.

> Our immune system and even our physical structure, is a reflection of the foods we have eaten from either toxic and nutrient depleted soils, or wonderfully fertile soils.
>
> Eryn Paige
> *How to Grow Glorious Wheatgrass at Home Tutorial - With Salty Sea Mineral Eco-Fertilization*

If you are an avid organic gardener, you know that vegetables grown in your garden taste infinitely better than grocery store produce and are Worlds apart. In fact, delicious, sweet and "addicting" food grows in highly mineralized soils. This is why we have a natural hunger for sweetness, and why sweetness is addicting, because our bodies are looking for sweetness that is naturally occurring in foods grown in highly mineralized soil.

Our psychobiology *knows* highly mineralized foods are the best thing possible for us to consume. To optimally improve soil at home in your garden, obtain rock dust at your local gravel pit where rock is sorted, and incorporate it into your soil with humus, compost and other organic matter. This remineralization is essential, as we are about to learn. The land of the Hunzas in the Himalayas and Villacamba Valley in Ecuador, both are examples of highly mineralized soil from glacial runoff, boasting many centenarians.

> The soil is the great connector of lives, the source and destination of all. It is the healer and restorer and resurrector, by which dis-ease passes into health, age into youth, death into Life. Without proper care for it we can have no community, because without proper care for it we can have no Life.
>
> *Wendell Berry, Author, Farmer, Activist*
> *The Unsettling of America: Culture and Agriculture*

Mineralization is one of the most critical needs of our bodies, which must be supplied through organic plant matter or in fulvic (organic easy to absorb) form to be assimilated. We were at one time instrumental in discovering a rich source of fulvic minerals, which friends now distribute. We consider these a first line of defense for the body for superior mineralization, and will have a special offer for them at our website. First we can use such a resource to mineralize ourselves; next we'll look at how to mineralize the Planet.

Let's take a look at why mineralizing the soil with rock dust offers a critical key to our very survival. John D. Haymaker was a talented mechanical engineer, ecologist, and researcher in soil remineralization, rock dust, mineral cycles, climate cycles and glaciology. He made the important correlation that our global climate issues are a result of soil demineralization, and highly at cause in global warming. He came up with a brilliant plan to remineralize soil with rock dust, by mimicking what a glacier does, without us having to go through hundreds of years in an Ice Age to get the same results.

In 1982 Haymaker wrote an extremely important book in conjunction with California ecologist Donald A. Weaver, called *The Survival Of Civilization* (accessible free online); please pass it on into millions of hands. This work inspired a growing movement toward natural remineralization of soil. Findings were corroborated by scientists in the UK. Haymaker appeared on Ted Turner's Atlanta Superstation, and Scripps Institute of Oceanography. *Scientific American* also published articles backing his work.

Haymaker pointed out that we face the threat of an imminent ice age, and how this can be averted by remineralizing with rock dust and reforestation to restore CO_2 levels by propagating "carbon sinks" (carbon lost through deforestation) for climatic stability, *which would result in two moderate seasons each year. How wonderful is this?*

Though Haymaker has departed this World, Don Weaver continues this important work with his latest book, *Regenerate the Earth*. These two became catalysts for the founding of a great organization, Remineralize The Earth, Now doing projects Worldwide. Besides mineralizing soils for better nutrition, they are using rock dust to bioremediate oil spills on farm lands and in waterways, restoring soil fertility and carbon sequestration. They are a great organization to volunteer with. Remineralize dot org Stepping out of "normal" routines to volunteer or participate in such work can help build a highly sustainable future!

Weaver and Haymaker are adamant on critical need for soil mineralization in regard to health, stating that food without mineralization has greatly reduced nutritional value, and mineralized food supports supreme well-being and longevity.

Virtually all subsoil and most topsoil of the world have been stripped of all but a small quantity of elements [primarily by agriculture]. So it is not surprising that the chemical-grown corn had substantially less mineral content than the 1963 corn described in the USDA Handbook of the Nutritional Contents of Food..

As elements have been used up in the soil a poor food supply in 1963 turned into a 100 percent junk food supply in 1978. There has been a corresponding increase in dis-ease and medical costs. Essentially, dis-ease means that enzyme systems are malfunctioning for lack of the elements required to make the enzymes.

Hunza is a small country in a high Himalayan mountain valley. Health, strength and longevity of the Hunzacuts is legendary. A key factor is irrigation of valley soils with a milky-colored stream from the meltwater of the Ultar glacier. The color comes from the mixed rock ground beneath the glacier. The people are virtually never sick. They do not develop cancer. Many are active workers at 90; some live to be 120. These facts are well documented, yet the world's "health professionals" ignore them while continuing the hopeless search for man-made "cures."

John D. Haymaker (1914-1994) & Don Weaver
The Survival Of Civilization: Carbon Dioxide, Investment Money, Population –
Three Problems Threatening Our Existence

What do we think exotic Superfoods will do for us? Our hope is they will help us be less tired, have more energy, be more beautiful, sexy, vital, handsome, slimmer, fit, beautiful skin thicker hair Right? ...the external "fix." Even if they give us such results, the reason is because they are providing high frequency mineralized nourishment to our cells inducing electromagnetics that support flow of Life-force. Exotic Superfoods are wonderful, delicious, fun and excellent for the Body. They give us the boost to live more vital Lives, because they have evolved harmoniously with our Earth Mother.

Our commercial food supply is literally "foodless," profoundly lacking mineralization that Creates Life-force. In this case, ignorance is not bliss; if we keep running like lemmings toward this cliff, humanity may have to start over again. This is a less than happy future for for our children, grandchildren, great grandchildren, their children's children, and a sad ending for a very bright civilization. A critical move toward a viable future requires stepping out of this old "dying" system, growing a home garden in highly mineralized soil, and/or participating in the global movement to remineralize soils for our future survival as a species. Find a way to contribute or volunteer at Remineralize dot org

Does the average person realize, when eating a "cheap" hamburger at McDonald's, deforestation of rainforest to grow the beef they're eating is driving us toward another Ice

Age and potential extinction? Ignorance is not bliss. We are living unsustainably and must change to move toward a viable future, how cool that we are educated enough to understand this. A small movement of the rudder will land us at a different place on the shore. Our individual choices are critical to where we land as a civilization of the future.

Although you may have lived most of your Life this way, we encourage you to wake up out of the mindset that there must be an instant cure for everything. Marketing and our societal mindset would like us to think so; this is exactly how billions are made off pain and suffering. Foundational Living in harmony with Nature and Mother Earth are critical to our very survival itself. Perhaps it might be worthwhile to consider selling your business or moving away from your current Life, and immersing yourself and family into a viable Planetary future. Believe it or not, EVERY PERSON makes a huge difference!

The truest answer is that we Wake Up. The true solution, the true magic pill, is dedication to higher ideals and practices, and the path of the Heart, harmonizing with Earth Mother Gaia. Cultivating Lifestyle to nourish Well-Being, we gradually open the door within, to be proactive in our Life and the World. Meanwhile, consuming Superfoods can help us have the regenerative energy, ability and power to do it!

> Man cannot discover new oceans unless he has the
> courage to lose sight of the shore.
>
> *Andre Gide (1869-1951) Nobel Prize Literature, 1947*
> *Wrote on freedom and empowerment in the face of moralistic and puritanical constraints*

Walking in balance with our Earth Mother, learning to harmonize our lives with our amazing ecosystem, Living at Cause rather than Effect is the prime objective of *21st Century Superhumans*. Here are more of John Haymaker and Don Weaver's reminders about *real* secrets to good health, well-being and our very survival itself:

Ten thousand years ago the Mississippi Valley was fed and built up by runoff from the glaciers. The deep deposit of organically-enriched alluvial soil in Illinois attests to a long period of luxuriant plant growth. Yet, when the settlers plowed the valley, they did not find topsoil that would give the health record of the Hunzacuts. Ten thousand years of leaching by a 30-inch annual rainfall is the difference. Man can stay on this Earth only if the glacial periods come every 100,000 years to replenish the mineral supply—or man gets bright enough to grind the rock himself.

There are several other places in the world similar to Hunza, such as the Caucasus Mountains in Russia where 10 percent of the people are centenarians. There are glaciers in the mountains. Regardless of where it is that people attain excellent health and maximum Life, it can be traced to a continual supply of fresh-ground mixed rocks flowing to the soil where their crops are grown.

Thus the secret of good health and long Life lies not in the fountain of youth or in a chemical company's laboratory, but in the acceleration of the natural biological processes.Failure to remineralize the soil will not just cause a continued mental and physical degeneration of humanity but will quickly bring famine, death, and glaciation in that order. Glaciation is nature's way of remineralizing the soil.

Doesn't this make you want to go out and grow your own or neighborhood garden, enrich the soil with rock dust and other organic matter, envision yourself, family, friends and community with juicy gardens and orchards, healthier and more vital, supporting remineralization of the Planet? Our minds are even brighter, when we are well nourished and mineralized; and again this is the cycle of Cause and Effect as we learn to understand and harmonize our lives with the natural ecosystem in which we are designed to Live.

Odd as I am sure it will appear to some, I can think of no better form of personal involvement in the cure of the environment than that of gardening. A person who is growing a garden, if growing it organically, is improving a piece of the world. They are producing something to eat, which makes them somewhat independent of the grocery business, and they are also enlarging for themselves and others, the meaning of food and the pleasure of eating.

Wendell Berry , Author, Activist, Farmer
The Art of the Commonplace: The Agrarian Essays

Do you know what makes a Superfood a Superfood? Many of them are from plants going back thousands of years, surviving natural selection. This means the strongest and healthiest traits are carried on from generation to generation, making the food source within the plant of exceptional quality. In addition many super foods tend to have evolved in a naturalized setting within a forest or ecosystem. Again this means they have picked up minerals and natural elements that more cultivated varieties may not contain. Similar benefits exist with wild foods and foraging.

Superfood guru, David Wolfe maintains, "Superfoods are an essential part of a balanced diet and allow us to get more nutrition with less eating."

Superfoods comprise a specific set of edible nutritious plants that cannot be classified as foods or medicines, because they combine positive aspects of both.

David Wolfe
Superfoods: The Food and Medicine of the Future

Drop down into the Heart with Deep Gratitude, aligning frequency, when taking in Raw Superfoods. These High Vibrational foods become alchemically One with the body and raise our Frequency. As we Lighten up our Being with Superfoods, with Gratitude to Pachamama, the Earth Mother, we make a difference by Living inspired energized lives as *21st Century Superhumans*!

Following is a partial list of exotic Superfoods now popularly available, delicious added to smoothies and green shakes, eaten alone or added to raw Creations.

GOGI BERRY is a sweet red fruit native to Asia, and has been used as a medicinal food for thousands of years. It is s a noted food of many centurians living active lives to well-over 100. With high protein, 21 essential minerals, and 18 amino acids, the goji berry is a nutrient-dense superfood in a class all its own; once you get started on it, you'll be hooked.

CACAO obtained raw, dried at low temperature, is a completely different food then the processed chocolate with which we are familiar. The crunchy "nibs" can be chewed whole, or added ground to shakes and sweet treats. Cacao is super-high in antioxidants, contains magnesium, sulfur, benefits cardio, skin, hair and immune systems. Cacao increases endorphins and has been used ceremonially for thousands of years in South America to open the Heart. Native to central and South America, the cacao is delightful when picked fresh, commonly made into a beverage including it's natural cocoa butter, without theobromine of the seeds.

HEMPSEED comes from the Cannabis plant, a different variety than the "herb." Hempseed is an amazing food, containing all essential amino acids and fatty acids necessary to maintain Life, with close to complete amino acid profile. 30-35% weight of hempseed is hemp oil, 80% essential fatty acids (EFAs) more balanced than flax, (which can Create a deficiency in GLA). Hemp farming is a great way to go. It is fast growing, renewable, sustainable, and can replace much of what we use trees (producing fiber for cloth and rope, building materials, paper, and high quality oil, protein and herb).

MACA was revered by the Incas for endurance and to increase stamina; they also used it to recover from illness as it is an adaptogen. According to folk belief, it has a legendary ability to deliver energy, mental clarity and enhance sex drive. It contains sterols (can have similar effects), should be used in small quantities and off and on rather than daily.

SALT - unpolluted salts from the sea and ancient sea beds contain full mineral complexes that are preferable to commercial salt. Real Salt and Sea Salt particularly Celtic are some of the best. Himalayan contains many minerals too. Variety is good to access various mineral complexes. Westin Price found that when people in primitive cultures accessed greens, they did not travel as much for salt. This is good advice to us. A high frequency salt in small amounts can add mineralization to our food, and optimum is developing highly mineralized soil and eating fresh greens grown in it.

OTHER SUPERFOODS include numerous exotic and delicious fruits, berries, nuts, seeds, herbs and spices. Get to know them and how they feel to your Body, gradually incorporate and enjoy the benefits of these Light filled nutrition sources.

Life-Force is the greatest "Superfood nutrient." We can measure protein, fat, carbohydrates, vitamins and minerals, yet if the food is "low frequency," it depletes Life rather than supporting it. It is important to become aware that most commercially available food has *little* Life-Force. This is one reason we have become addicted to caffeine and other stimulants, because we're missing natural vitality that comes from Live foods. Dead processed foods require enzymes to digest and assimilate, robbing them from vital bodily functions, diminishing Life force. Change your Life Now, adopt a Superfoods *Live-it!*

Dr. Edward Howell's book *Enzyme Nutrition* from 1898 is a *classic* essential reference for understanding enzymes as spark plugs of Life. Distinction between Raw and Living foods is based on enzyme content and Life Force. *Raw food* is "mature," such as apples or lettuce picked from garden or orchard when ripe. *Living food* such as sprouts and grasses, are harvested in the first seven days of Life after the seeds sprout. During this first 7 days cells rapidly multiply and enzymes are far more abundant than they will be at any other time in the Life of the plant. Sprouts and young grasses regenerate the body; wheatgrass and sprouted/Living Food programs work well to reverse degenerative conditions for vitality and regeneration. Powerful Lifestyle choices incorporate these elements.

Seeds contain enzyme inhibitors to keep them dormant until the next growing season. When we eat wheat ground to flour, it contains enzyme inhibitors designed to protect the dormant seed. Once soaked in water and sprouting beings, enzyme inhibitors are washed away, the seed becomes a Living sprout, and is much more nutritious. This is why we suggest sprouted grain or Ezekiel bread as a first choice for breads, tortillas, crackers, etc.

Fresh, Raw, Living Foods transmit Life and are ultra-easy to digest. Their enzymes contribute to cellular Life-force rather than taking from it. When nutrition is at least 50% Raw and Living Food, it is of **huge benefit**; we are leaner with more energy and youthfulness. Fresh salads, sprouts, green shakes, vegetables, fresh fruit, juices and Superfoods are a daily mainstay for greater vitality. Integrating Raw and Living foods into our *Live-it*, is essential to Well-Being, a must for **21st Century Superhumans**.

Every long-lived culture around the World has some sort of fermented or cultured food such as sauerkraut, kimchee, yogurt, kombucha, miso or tamari as part of their everyday cuisine. Always include fermented foods in your *Live-it*. They contain beneficial enzymes, probiotics and Life force that assist digestion, small and large intestine and body enzymes.

Having used regenerative foods for many years, we notice the difference in just a day or two of heavier foods when visiting or traveling. It is super-fun to eat, Live and think Lightly, bringing energy and vitality to Life of self, family and friends! Lifestyle habits are either adding to Life or taking it away. *You pick!* It may require major Lifestyle changes to implement these things, yet worth it! Be sure to check out our website and videos for tips and quick, easy support of these Lifestyle habits! ♥

Part 4: BODY

Chapter 5

Naturally Attractive Hair, Skin, Body

To LOVE beauty is to see LIGHT.

Victor Hugo (1802-1885)
Writer, Artist, Statesman
Les Miserables, Hunchback of Notre-Dame

I t's exciting we are moving toward self-acceptance with natural hair, skin and Body styles. Being fit with glowing skin and hair and a bright Smile from the Heart is Always "In." We encourage moving this direction! The closer you get to "natural," the more you will LOVE it!

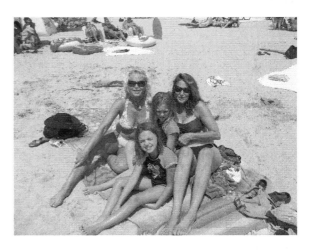

BODY: LOVE yours! Commit to Being naturally healthy and attractive from inside-out. Implement *21st Century Superhuman Quantum Lifestyle!*

Follow instructions in all Chapters on cleansing, detox and nutrition. Be sure to include time outdoors, and if living in a winter climate or indoors a lot, Vitamins D3 & K2. *Check out our additional books and videos on weight loss, recipes, fitness, radiance and more.* Smile.

NOTE: **Whatever we put on skin or hair appears in the organs within 56 seconds!** Healthy Lifestyle with high frequency nutrition and cleansing makes skin and hair radiant! Reduce use of products containing items you wouldn't eat. Experiment till you find what works best for you.

    HAIR PURPOSE: Our hair is our antenna, receiving electromagnetic Cosmic waves and energies, emitting our neurological signals to our surroundings. Hair is an extension of the nervous system, transmitting our energy from the brain into the outer environment, so when hair is cut, receiving and sending transmissions are dampened. One story reports the US military enrolled Native American trackers who lost psychic and tracking ability when hair was cut. Sikhs and many "masters" such as Moses, Buddha, Jesus, Shiva had long hair.

HAIR CARE: The first rule for healthy hair is a *Live-it*, rich in micro-nutrients and high frequency foods. Hair can be washed-rinsed with water containing a dash of vinegar for dark hair or a dash of lemon-lime juice for light. Gently clean hair and scalp with fingertips and rinse. It is amazing how healthy and vibrant hair becomes doing this a short time, without any commercial products! Cultivate a hair style requiring minimal cuts and products that suits you and your Lifestyle. It may take a few weeks for your hair to adjust.

Commercial products rob hair of it's natural beauty. Even healthy shampoo strips hair of natural oils, "healthy" conditioners contain polymers, silicones (plastics). If using get sulphur-free shampoo & polymer free conditioner, and give hair a rest as often as possible.

Nourish hair with avocado, leave in 1/2 hour and rinse; or apply a *tiny* bit of edible oil such as olive or coconut rubbed on palms of hands smoothed lightly through hair while wet during quiet time. Rub a bit of favorite essential oils into scalp and hair, rosemary excellent (good for memory). Comb or pic gently in shower to detangle. *Take a month to test it out. See if hair feels like the magnetic extension of your Higher senses it was designed to be.*

SKIN PURPOSE: The skin is the largest eliminative organ of the body. When overloaded the skin takes over. Toxins show up as oil, acne, blemishes or dry. First rule of healthy skin is cleanse and detox internally, and high frequency living foods. Good elimination is essential for smooth, alive skin. A simple first step is to add ground golden flaxseed to your *Live-it.* Follow instructions in chapters on cleansing, detox and nutrition. Check our videos.

SKIN CARE: Natural skin brush wet or dry. Reduce or eliminate use of soap except when dirty or to clean odor. Best to put on skin a light amount of olive oil or coconut oil. If skin is oily, clean with *dilute* hydrogen peroxide, vinegar or witch hazel. If desiring products, only use most natural, with organic, wildcrafted ingredients, such as *Annmarie Gianni.*

SUNSCREEN: We are solar Beings. Vitamin D is made in our Body by exposure to the sun, and is more than a vitamin, it is a hormone precursor. Without proper amounts of solar exposure and vitamin D3, our genetic structure becomes destabilized, as D3 is involved in regulation of over 2,000 genes. Getting outdoors in the sun increases longevity and vitality. Learn how to use Vitamins D & K2 (Read: *The Miraculous Results of Extremely High Doses of Sunshine Hormone* by Jeff Boles). If sunscreen is desired, find products with edible ingredients - make your own mixture with these Oils & SPFs: Coconut 2-8, Olive 2-8, Avocado 4-15, Raspberry Seed Oil 28-50, Almond 5, Jojoba 4, Shea Butter 3-6, Macadamia 6, Carrot Seed Oil 38-40. Include vinegar with the oil to protect and balance skin's pH. Add a little carrot seed oil for natural protection 38-40. Use SPF clothing and hat to shade body.

TEETH: Brush-floss regularly. Rather than fluoridated toothpaste, use one or more: baking soda, diluted hydrogen peroxide, occasional sea salt. *Oil pulling* is an excellent Ayurvedic technique, to whiten and clean teeth and detoxify body. Swish 1 T sesame or coconut oil in a.m. 15-20 min. Spit out. Brush w/above. *More in our videos and at our website!* LOVE U! ♥

Part 4 Body: Section 2
How To Cleanse And Detox

My body is a projection of my consciousness.

Deepak Chopra MD
Natural Physician, New Thought Author

It is amazing to recognize that our body reflects our consciousness; that all dis-comfort, dis-ease, illness and mental or physical pain is Vibrational expression of thought-emotion Not of LOVE. This may take a little practice to decipher, so use our tools from Part 2: MIND to assist with clarity. Quantum Lifestyle of the *21st Century Superhuman* integrates cleansing and detox habits into daily Life to clear old toxins (a product of

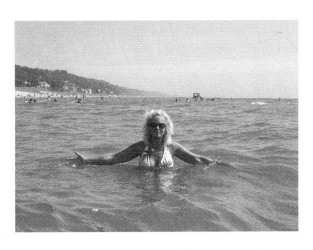

Mind-energy in the physical), to support restoring well-being.

A Clean Body harmonizes and brightens the Radiance of our Being, to reflect more Light, which can be observed in images of the the human aura. Get more effective physical cleanses, by also resolving root cause by clearing thought-emotion coming up from the unconscious. Physical cleansing *combined* with mental clearing offers deeper, more productive and lasting results. As Dr. John Ray used to tell us, *"Our Perfect Electronic Blueprint already exists, all we have to do is step into it."* Cultivating a clean system, allows us to merge easily with our perfect blueprint resonating from LOVE.

Integrate habits of cleansing, detox and nutrition. Harmonize Body for optimum Well-Being in sync with 5th Universal Law of Rhythm, as waves go in and out from the shore:
- Sleep at night provides opportunity for digestive system to rest. Sleep on empty stomach, allow organs to rest in nightly "mini-fast."
- Upon arising *flush* what the body eliminated at a cellular level during the night. Have 1 qt. warm water plain, with lemon or pinch baking soda (to alkalize).
- Daylight Body energy supports digestion, assimilation, burning of energy; earlier is better for taking in nutrition, 3-5 hrs before bed, so Body can cleanse at night.
- Longer fasts or cleanses harmonize with yearly cycles such as spring/fall.

Incorporate cleansing and detox into your daily routine to *feel Lighter*. Most healthy nourishment is also cleansing. Remember the 6th Universal Law *Cause and Effect:*

Chance is but a name for Law not recognized; there are many planes of causation, but nothing escapes the Law. Every thought-emotion, word and action sets in motion an effect that materializes.

J.H. Tilden M.D. wrote *Toxemia Explained: The True Interpretation of The Cause of All Dis-Ease* in the 1800s. His key principle true then and now was that the body must run as a "clean machine." Our cells, bloodstream, organs and glands, take in nourishment and eliminate waste. When any of these systems are overloaded, acute conditions result such as exhaustion, cold, flu or fever Body's supreme efforts to detox.

Even epidemics are representative of a toxic cultural condition from predominant habits such as excessive meat consumption and refined foods, with perhaps cultural thought patterns thrown in. Pharmaceutical companies may take advantage of this offering the "next great vaccine," when better results would be obtained by teaching the culture to cleanse, detox and use high frequency nutrition.

Excess toxicity and repeated acute conditions continued over years, result in "organic damage" known as chronic degenerative conditions such as cancer, heart dis-ease, arthritis and others. Tilden's statement in review:

So-called dis-ease was a toxemic crisis, and when toxins were eliminated below the toleration point, the sickness passed - automatically health returned. But the dis-ease was not cured; for if cause is continued, toxins still accumulate, and in due time another crisis appears. Unless the cause is discovered and removed, crises will recur until functional derangements give way to organic dis-ease.

J.H. Tilden MD (1851-1940)
Toxemia Explained: The True Interpretation of The Cause of All Dis-Ease

There is one way, and one way alone to get and keep the Body well. Once you know this secret, you will be able to *stay* well, *avoid* illness being "passed around," escape and evade degenerative conditions *and* enter a state of youthful regeneration! As Tilden says, "The true interpretation of the cause of dis-ease and how to cure is an obvious sequence, the antidote to fear, frenzy and the popular mad chasing after so-called cures." It requires dedication, self-education and discipline in Lifestyle patterns to establish long lasting Vitality and Well-Being, that sustain us throughout Life in extraordinary ways.

This venerable secret is *"keep your "house" clean!"* Unless our Body is clean and well-nourished it cannot do the job it is designed to do. All its energy goes into efforts to cleanse and restore balance. Every illness is simply the body's attempt to "clean house" of old residue. Today's buzzwords for toxemia are *inflammation* and *acidity.* We are about to learn how to use a super cleansing system to clean the "house we live in" for lasting regenerative effects, with tricks easy to implement in busy Lives. ♥

Part 4: BODY
Chapter 6
"7 Days" To A new YOU!

Whether we acknowledge it or not, we all have a choice to be either accomplices in the status quo or everyday revolutionaries. We have a choice whether to succumb to the cultural trance, eat fast food, and race by each other in the night, or to build lives of caring, substance, and healing. So much depends on that choice.

John Robbins
Founder EarthSave, Diet for a new America

Our most productive energy flows through the creative *Essence* of our True Being LOVE, embodied best in a detoxified Body and Mind. Physical and mental cleansing brings clarity to Body-Mind, more easily transmitting Heart Coherence, Smile, Breathing, and High-Frequency thought-emotional patterns of LOVE.

HOW TO CHANGE A HABIT! EASY PEASY: Research shows that in just a few days we develop *new neurological pathways, becoming very strong by day 7.* Within 4 weeks or 28 days *entirely new habits* have formed *Neurologically.* Old less-used pathways atrophy, and a New bump forms so the distance the tiny "electric shock" jumps to send the new message is shorter than the old. *So the new habit literally encodes into our physiology.* Yes there is

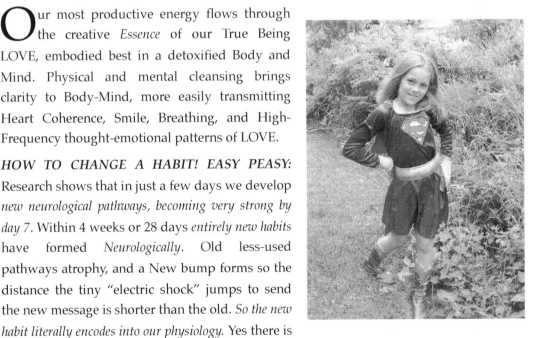

great potential even for those with long ingrained habits to make real changes in lifetime pattern. It is just a matter of staying in the new routine long enough for neurology to shift.

Our brain and nervous system continually update perceptions about our current "reality," interpreting it for survival. There is no need to be "stuck in the past" (including yesterday or five minutes ago), as New neurological pathways for processing our "reality" are continuously developing. With every override of old responses and habit patterns, we Create New neural pathways, thus our clearing and goal canceling is also important.

There is no mental event that does not have a neural correlate.

Deepak Chopra MD
Natural Physician, New Thought Author

Repetition develops larger neurons and new branches or synapses like twigs on a tree. As old neurological pathways are less used, they shrink and disappear with non-use. When we change our kitchen set-up and food availability, cultivate a new social circle or put ourselves into a fresh environment such as a live-in education program, we offer ourselves the best opportunity to fire New signals in our neurobiology, and *consistently* embed the New "code." Such change of environment is a Mind-choice that integrates physiologically.

There is a difference between knowing
the path and walking the path.

Morpheus, The Matrix

Every experience is for our learning and should not be judged as success or failure, it is simply helping us discover how to steer our course. Be loving, patient and kind both with others and self, while integrating these concepts into Life. Cultivate the image that we each already exist in our "Perfect Blueprint", and we are simply on a journey of discovering alignment with it. There is no such thing as a mistake! It is all just learning along the way.

If you can dream—and not make dreams your master
If you can think—and not make thoughts your aim
If you can meet with Triumph and Disaster
And treat those two impostors just the same

Rudyard Kipling (1835-1936)
First and Youngest recipient of Nobel Prize Literature 1907

Taking good care of ourselves, then *going back* to old habits gives us contrast to make better choices next time. We may bounce around like this at first, but stay with it. Staying "neutral," Loving ourselves and the Truth of our experience, being at peace with the choices we make ultimately empower us to a new path, as we go through the learning curve of changing our patterns. Freeing ourselves from old paradigm ways of thinking, it is LOVE, not punishment or judgment that instills a New path. Positive reinforcement works best with pets, and us too!

It's important to learn to not give up when we "fall or fail" – to learn from our experience, LOVE ourselves, pick up and go on. It requires much more than just a passing interest to find vitality and well-being. It requires commitment of Lifestyle and habit. These traits begin with dedication and commitment to choosing what we've discovered is best for us. We will do more out of LOVE than anything else. LOVING Self, LOVING our process, LOVING our New choices; Breathing, Smiling.

What we "do" day-in and day-out is cumulative and adds up over time, so the highest % of our regular habits becomes our central theme. We like the 80/20 rule: if we do what's "best" 80% of the time, the other 20% takes care of itself. Repetition develops New neuro-receptors, integrating patterns in brain and nervous system. The more often we make a desired choice the more easily it happens the next time. As we participate in our own journey of cultivating healthy habits, it eventually emerges as our own personalized, miraculous way of Living, reflecting our radiance and well-being in the World. Remember, laugh, play and have fun with it!

Loving and accepting ourselves just as we are, is the most important habit to cultivate, for it helps us flow from what's truly inside us rather than responding to external pressure. By accepting, trusting, allowing and Loving ourselves and our process as it occurs, we eventually come to the point where new habits result from authentic desire flowing from within because we LOVE it! Loving Ourselves, Honoring Ourselves and every choice is the Quickest Way to Success...

> It's of no use walking anywhere to preach
> unless our walking is our preaching.
>
> *St. Francis of Assisi (1182-1226)*
> *Order of St. Francis*

Most of us, even those somewhat Awake, have spent much of our lives overcoming deficits we have blamed on parents, circumstances or genes. At this point we are learning they were not at fault, perhaps acting out their own deep pain, suffering and "Power Person Dynamic." *AND we drew them in and they us,* because of "matching resonance or Vibration for us to Mirror to one another what needed to be cleared from the unconscious and restored to LOVE.

Historian and Author of *Fingerprints of the Gods,* Graham Hancock, calls us a civilization with cultural *amnesia,* as we are missing critical records from advanced civilizations in antiquity who left us important clues. Within our DNA is the gene potential to operate as highly intelligent, creative Beings of LOVE and Light. *We are now learning* how to switch on our dormant 97% "junk" DNA. If we suddenly become curious as to why we have only 3% operational DNA, when a tree frog has 17% active DNA, answers lie in pre-historical accounts, Now becoming available thanks to modern technology.

Michael Tellinger's research and documented theories in *Adam's Calendar* and *Slave Species of the Gods* suggest a strong probability that we, like *Sleeping Beauty,* fell into a deep sleep long ago, with some of our DNA *turned off* so we would perform as an "obedient and hard working race." We are just now waking up to our true potential as Creator Beings, which we are stepping into very likely for the first time in history of humankind. We might imagine our DNA like Legos, lying in a pile, waiting for us to pick them up and put them back together.

The only currently known method for turning on our dormant DNA, was established by HeartMath®'s progressive research, showing that in Heart Coherence: LOVE,

Compassion, Gratitude, non-judgement, Unity, Oneness, we restructure and activate more DNA codons. We are called forth as *21st Century Superhumans* to embrace this state of being, based 100% in our True Design LOVE. This is *the resonance* that increases our well-being and vitality, and activates our 97% "sleeping" DNA. *Wow! Get ready because here we come!*

Turning on our 97% dormant DNA:

• *We activate our DNA by integrating Heart Coherence as our "normal state,"* and being fully present in Heart Coherence at all times. This is True Science of Higher Living, where LOVE, Compassion and Gratitude are the most powerful 3 words or states of BEING we ever embrace!!! Make them part of every Now Moment. This means integrating new perceptions when we see horrible things still going on in the World (rather than hatred). This is what Yeshua-Jesus meant about "turning the other cheek." As we shift our resonance to LOVE and inspire others to do the same all residual of darkness will fade. As we enter the future together in Pure LOVE, we will not even have memory of these things, because they will be erased from all timelines as LOVE was held for them. Breathe. Smile.

• Prime objective for *EVERY* **21st Century Superhuman:** *Restore our True Design, LOVE.* This is the path to Genius, Creativity, Productivity, and *the most powerful tool to change the Structure of our "Reality."* Change yourself. Change the Whole. *Arc the Hologram NOW!!!*

• *Cleansing the Body* assists us to hold High Vibrational Frequencies of LOVE, Light and Heart Coherence. Our Body is the Vehicle for our neurobiology, our biocomputer, our Mind-Energy, and Coherent Heart torus-field to resonate into the World with *our Greatest Creative Potential.*

• Releasing, *letting go old thought-emotional energy* carried in the unconscious (lower part of the iceberg) and conscious (tip of the iceberg), removes Vibrations Not of LOVE, so our *Attention in the Field manifests through our True Design LOVE. Yeshua-Jesus came to Earth to get us going this direction, with the Ancient Aramaic Forgiveness process.* If it had been understood in the culture of the day, we would be Living in a different World Now. Critical key to accessing our higher potential is *clearing our unconscious* of any and all resonance Not of LOVE with *Ancient Aramaic Forgiveness Freedom Tools* and Goal Canceling process [Part 2: MIND].

One man tells his amazing story of being infected with one of the most virulent forms of HIV as a hospital medical lab tech. He took the recommended medications, became extremely emaciated, and did not feel there was any reason to go on living. He was led to an *ayahuasca* shamanistic ceremony at a church in the Netherlands, which activated his DMT, taking him on an amazing inward "journey." He saw his DNA as curled and disconnected segments; in his "journey" he was directed to straighten out and reconnect it, which he did. From that day forward he began to get well, and lives to tell about it nine years later. We are *so much more* that just physical devices, it is critical that we grasp this, Activating Body-Mind-Heart with LOVE.

We are getting to the core, the bottom root level of why we express dis-ease and discomfort in Mind-Body. We are *Breaking Free* from a thought-emotional imprisonment, robbing us of our birthright of regenerative vitality and long Life. It is suggested by Michael Tellinger that in our non-functioning DNA, we have potential for continual physical regeneration and either much longer Lives or some sort of physical immortality.

As we release Not of LOVE thought-emotion our human bio-computer is *upgrading its program.* This natural Evolutionary process merges with a New holographic "reality," tuning us to Higher frequencies of Light and LOVE. Flowing aspects of self activate this shift. Examples are demonstrated in new children born with more codons already turned on in their DNA, resulting in 30% higher intelligence, telepathic skills and greater self-actualization at a young age. Even adults shifting to non-judgement, Unity and LOVE are having *their* DNA restructure.

> Then they found another kid with these codons turned on...then 10,000, then 100,000, then a million...UCLA, by watching world-wide DNA testing, estimates that 1% of the world has this new DNA. That breaks down to approximately 60 million people who are not human by the old criteria.
>
> *Drunvalo Melchizedek*
> *Ancient Secret of the Flower of Life Vol. 1*

Parents, grandparents and extended family have the opportunity to nurture this Higher intelligence and advanced DNA. It activates us to "wake up," as we adapt to and Create a hospitable environment for these young carriers of more advanced and awakened DNA to grow and develop. They will inherit the path that carried humanity into the future. The more we adjust our lives to support this evolving consciousness, the greater gifts there will be for us and those who come after.

Since the 1980s a new wave of humans have been arriving on Earth, with more codons turned on in their DNA (24 as opposed to the usual 20). UCLA's studies have found over a million with this advanced DNA, children all over the World who have paranormal abilities, including resistance to all disease including HIV/AIDS and Cancer. Drunvalo Melchizedek reports in an interview, that this seems to be spreading like a wave through our culture, with the expanded DNA even activating in adults.

> It is a very specific emotional, mental body response – a waveform coming off the body that is causing the DNA to mutate in a certain way. I've sat with Gregg Braden who was one of the first persons to write about this and what we believe is that there are 3 parts to this phenomenon. The first part is the mind that sees Unity. It sees the Flower of Life. It sees everything interconnected in all ways. It doesn't see anything as separate.
>
> And the second part is being centered in the heart – to be Loving.

And the third thing is to step out of polarity – to no longer judge the world. As long as we are judging the world as good or bad, then we are inside polarity and remain in the fallen state. I believe these people (with the new DNA) have somehow stepped out of judging and are in a state where they see everything as one and feeling LOVE.

Whatever they are doing within themselves is producing a waveform that when seen on computer screens looks almost identical to the DNA molecule. So the researchers think that by the very expression of their Life that these people are mapping with the DNA – resonating it – and are changing these 4 codons and in so doing become immune to the dis-ease.

Interview by Diane with Drunvalo Melchizedek

By Enoch Tan, new Earth Daily #1 Source for Positive News

We have this amazing piece of research done by HeartMath Institute, that when a person is in Heart Coherence, based in LOVE-Compassion-Gratitude, they literally straighten out curves in their own DNA and that of others! This essentially leads us to the conclusion that we have the amazing capacity to reactivate nonfunctioning portions of our 97% "junk" DNA *when in Heart Coherence.* During this research they found that a person *not* in Heart Coherence could *not* straighten out the DNA.

Grasping and understanding this single idea is a critically powerful tool for changing ourselves, our World and all of humanity, Now and into past and future of the 'No - Time' Continuum to shift all timelines. We have just barely tapped into our potential in this area. We activate more of our DNA potential as we integrate Heart Coherence more deeply and it becomes our natural, consistent mode of operation. *Integrating Heart Coherence is a primary practice* of **21st Century Superhumans**, similar to martial arts, meditation, chanting and prayer used by "Great Masters" of the ages.

During these Cosmic Activations, we are being inspired to Lighten up the physical Body-Mind also. As we clear old thought-emotional patterns to LOVE, and Lighten up physical habits, we increase our capacity to Live Joyful, Fulfilling Masterful Lives. Shedding physical toxicity, we also shed toxic Mind-Energy as we give Attention to our focus, Breathing, Smiling and canceling goals [Part 2: MIND].

We encourage you to enter this powerful planetary Ascension wave, by adopting **Quantum Lifestyle** habits to upgrade YOU energetically. YOU will be able to let go of shadows of victim mentality, and gain the resilience to Master YOUR existence. At this point YOU will be fully able to shape YOUR "reality" by choice.

In this fast paced world it is too frequently the case that people accept what society, family members and the authorities, whom nobody ever seems to question, believe regarding how to live their lives. And yet, the happiest people I know have been those who have accepted the primary responsibility for their own spiritual and physical well-being - those who have inner strength, courage, determination, common sense and faith in the process of creating more balanced and satisfying lives for themselves.

Dr. Ann Wigmore (1909-1993)
"Grandmother" Founder of Wheatgrass and Living Foods programs

Along with restructuring physical habits we integrate our Quantum knowing and change history, simply by upgrading our Mind-Energy about ourselves in our Newly formed "reality." This means if we've thought of ourselves as being a particular way (*i.e.* weight, smoking, dis-ease, drugs, poverty) for a long "time," we will get over it, shift the Hologram, transform our history and "Create" a New state of Being.

When you identify and hold your thought purely, on any topic for 17 seconds, it is enough to set the Universe into motion, and the Universe which has Infinite ability and resources to match the Vibration of your being, will do so.

Esther Hicks
The Teachings of Abraham, 17 Seconds

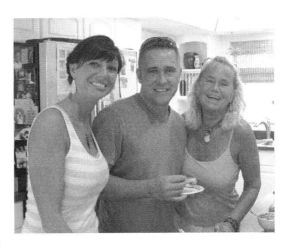

Once we incorporate our new patterns we become an example to others - not so much by what we speak - by our Vibrational presence that surrounds how we Live. Respect each person's journey, allowing his/her perfect process of choice and discovery. We cannot know the path of another unless we "walk in their shoes;" so making our own choices without control or judgment, allowing others their growth process, releases us from worrying about what someone else does or does not do. Even if it seems like the "ship" of someone close to us "may be sinking," we still allow them their perfect journey of unfolding, reminding them that we LOVE and care, while honoring their choices! Breathe. Smile. Laugh. Release and let go, and ALL will change.

Years ago, when I was first changing my Lifestyle around age 18-20, making different choices than most, my rambunctious friend, J.B., harassed me continually about what I was doing. Ten years later, I ran into him after a long absence and he said, "I know I gave you a hard time back then because I wanted to see what you were made of. You Living what you believed completely changed my Life. I now live and teach similarly to you." Wow! What a great lesson on how we may not know the effect we have on others! Recently I saw my brother after months apart, and he had switched from coffee in the a.m. to Greenshakes. I was amazed at the wonderful rosy color on his face and how great he looked! Live Your Joy and Keep Sharing! ♥ Cary

We may never know how we affect another, yet we can trust that our influence goes out into the *Field* surrounding us and by virtue of our Vibration, our resonance is experienced by those around us. No one likes to be criticized or told what they *ought* to be doing. When we live our truth and follow our path Joyfully, we can count on the fact, that deep inside most peoples' Hearts are hungry for authenticity, vitality and well-being, and somewhere along the way a bit is likely to rub off. As the old saying goes, *most would rather see a sermon than hear one...Just Live your best and Be Happy!*

The lives of those who "walk their talk" have great impact in this World. Often not saying a thing, just BEING what we KNOW is the best "teaching" we can generate. After all, everything in Life is based on Vibration and frequency. Our Life resonates through the Field, entraining others to it, and magnetizing that which is like itself.

> Life is actually a circle, for a vibrant body begets well mind and emotions, and healthy mind and emotions contribute to a vibrant body.

Folk Saying

It is a discipline, a practice and an art of the highest order, to naturally cultivate our daily Life and habits around well-being of Mind and Body; this is a Sacred Journey embracing Contentment, Vitality, Youthfulness, Peace, Longevity, Resilience and the ability to Contribute our best to Life and the Future of Humanity. With each Breath and Choice we make, we hold our Attention on the *Field of Possibilities*, and resonate our Creative presence into the World. *Let's get going on this Adventure!*

7 Days To A new YOU!

(1) KNOW YOU Create YOUR "REALITY" ♥ your Vibrational Presence and Attention on the *Field of Possibilities* calls your "reality" into form. Know you are establishing new neurological pathways and diminishing the old.

(2) PRINT 50 COPIES *ARAMAIC FORGIVENESS Freedom Tool* [Part 2: MIND]

(3) DO 1-5 WORKSHEETS NOW (from #2) on the issue(s) you would like to shift your Vibration in regard to during the next 7 days, and then the following 3 weeks. *Do your best.* Listen to Mindshifter radio for guidance *whyagain.org*

(4) 2-5 WORKSHEETS DAILY (from #2) *each day for the next 7 days!* Do them as quickly as possible, without laboring too much over whether "right or wrong." They will gradually get easier. Keep track of how many you do. Throw them away. You are done with this energy.

(5) MEAL PLAN Chapter 49, *Ideal Nutrition*, look at *LIVE-IT NUTRITION* list. Jot down your meal plan for the week, Breakfast, Lunch, Dinner, snacks, based on high frequency whole foods. Commit to following your meal plan. Whether you make your own food or eat out, Create a meal plan, based around your favorite whole natural foods.

(6) DRINK UPON ARISING DAILY warm 1/2-1 quart warm water, water with a pinch of baking soda and a wedge of lemon to alkalize and cleanse; can also add a pinch of cayenne if desired for deeper cleansing. AFTER water; tea if desired. Eliminate coffee if possible; otherwise have decaf.

(7) CANCEL GOALS each evening when you go to bed; lie flat, use gentle circular mouth Breath to keep energy open and flowing. Relax jaw. invite *Rookha d'Koodsha* (Aramaic), elemental aspect of our Being, the super-processor, to help cancel your goals. Mentally cancel goals for all thoughts causing stress, or that you're thinking about doing or accomplishing. Say to yourself, "I now cancel all my goals, conscious, subconscious, unconscious and incomplete." Choose 1 thing to accomplish in the next 24 hours and set that as your goal for the following day. You may also do this exercise in the a.m. before arising.

(8) RESET PROCESS - do this process as you start your week, and every time you feel you need a "reset" of integration with your purpose for the week. Sit, close eyes, Breathe gently, relax. You may meditate, pray, listen to music - get yourself our of "monkey mind" and into **Heart -Compassion without Judgment.** Marry Mind and Heart. Envision and experience within your week the way you would like it to unfold, all happening beautifully. Experience it as "it already IS so." Focus 17 seconds. Give it to the *Field*. Breathe. Smile.

(9) Do several quick rounds of *EFT tapping* (find our videos or FastEFT)

(10) REPEAT Reset Process again. If you feel you stumble at any time.

(11) HEART COHERENCE Focus in LOVE, COMPASSION, GRATITUDE

(12) LOVE YOURSELF. SMILE, Breathe. Flow, express your joy, creativity, and your True Design, LOVE.

(13) HONOR YOURSELF that you are building and establishing new neural pathways, that with use, become better established than the old.

The world is a mirror,
forever reflecting what you see inside yourself.
Neville Goddard (1905-1972)
Manifestation, the Promise & the Law

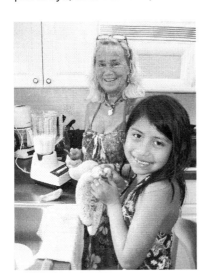

Suggestions - 7 Day Meal Plan

Eliminate white sugar, white flour, refined foods. Use sprouted grain bread or crackers. Reduce or eliminate meat, other animal products and most fats. Add fiber, enjoy freely fresh raw fruits and vegetables, juices, soups. Include raw fermented foods daily to boost enzymes, immune system and cleansing.

For Quick Easy Recipes get - **Super Immunity**

Secrets by Cary Ellis [app coming soon!]

(1) *Morning Flush:* 1 qt. warm water with pinch Bob's Baking Soda (non-aluminum), wedge fresh lemon or lime; or plain warm water; or plain w/lemon

(2) Tea or decaf coffee - optional

(3) *Green Shake or Smoothie* - recipe next chapter, or raw meuseli type cereal with vegan milk

(4) *Between Meals:* Allow stomach to empty. Good to have 4-5 hours between meals. Allow body to restore "fasting" equilibrium. Have only water or plain tea. (If you choose to have coffee decaf is better, as is espresso or cold pressed as they reduce acid. Coffee has a tendency to irritate liver and stomach, so can activate cravings. Reduce use if possible.)

(5) *Lunch*: Raw Juices; Salad - fresh veggies, sprouts, beans, tofu, lemon juice-olive oil, pinch earth salt, herbs. Soups - homemade, fresh veggies, quinoa, sprouted beans. Sandwich or roll-up (sprouted grain bread); veggies, tahini, almond butter.

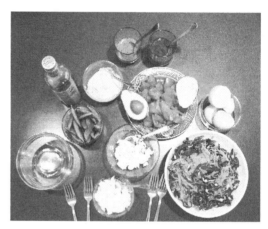

(6) *Dinner:* Juice; Salad - fresh veggies, sprouts, beans, tofu, lemon juice-olive oil, pinch earth salt, herbs. Soup - homemade, fresh veggies, quinoa, sprouted beans. Sprouted grain bread or crackers. Rice or quinoa. Healthy international foods.

(7) *Dessert:* There are amazing, wonderful and delicious deserts available to buy at health food store or make at home using natural sweeteners.

(8) *Snacks:* Fresh fruit or veggies, juices, tea

(9) *Bedtime:* Allow 2-4 hours after dinner with stomach empty before going to bed. This gives digestive organs a well-needed rest while you sleep.

First commit. Then follow up, putting into practice New foods and habits. Enjoy!

Giving yourself just seven days to experiment with this kind of easy Cleansing Nutrition can provide such energy and Lightness of Being, that you may choose to incorporate these Quantum Lifestyle habits on an everyday basis. The ***21st Century Superhuman*** Journey is an exploration of our own Body-Mind, and how to optimize care and feeding for Authentic self-expression, achievement and accomplishing what we came into this World to do! ♥

Chapter 7

Cleanse & Detox: 3 - 7 - 30 Day Cleanses

A fast, rest in bed, and the giving up of enervating habits, mental and physical will allow nature to eliminate the accumulated toxin; then if enervating habits are given up, and rational living habits adopted, health will come back to stay.

Dr. J. H. Tilden
Toxemia Explained, the True Interpretation of the Cause of Dis-Ease

Have you done a cleanse or detox? This is an opportunity to give the body a rest from dense food, increase fluids, add herbs, lighten nutrition, and use essential oils, massage or energy work to free things up and get the body flowing. It is one of the most liberating things we can do, and the feeling of "Lightness of Being" it brings is extraordinary!

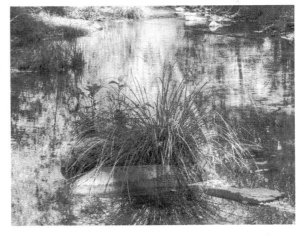

Cleanses have gained popularity in recent years, as our culture is on almost continual overload, from lower frequency and excessive food, beverages and mental stress that exhaust and devitalize the system. Cleanse and detox are relatively interchangeable, and may be directed at the entire body as we are here, or organ specific *(more at our website)*. *Enervating habits* in quote above means, "To weaken or destroy the" strength or vitality of;" such as luxury or excess that destroys health.

Cleansing and detox help us recover from excesses of modern Lifestyle, and "Clean the House We Live In," to restore connection with *the sacred within*. Sun Bear was a gifted Native American medicine man and shaman, with whom Teddi, her then partner and four year old daughter were invited to spend the summer with at *Vision Mountain* retreat in Ford, Washington near Spokane 1983. Their experience with him deepened their understanding of cleansing on many levels.

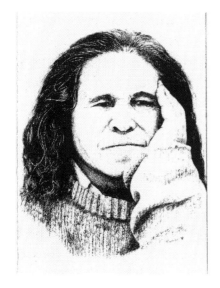

We met Sun bear at a Medicine Wheel gathering in Gainesville, Florida, where we were attracted to his teaching, 'Walking in Balance on Mother Earth.' He invited us to come to Spokane, as apprentices and to assist with his vision quests. Every two weeks new apprentices arrived, and Sunday evening Sun Bear instructed them to to go up on the Mountain and cry for their vision. He told them not to come down till they knew what they had come to Earth to do, for without a mission they would walk through Life empty. "What did you come here to do? It's inside of you..."

Grandfather, look upon our brokenness... We know that in all Creation, only the Human Family has strayed from the Sacred Way. We are the ones who must come back together to walk in the Sacred Way. Grandfather, Sacred One, teach us LOVE, Compassion and Honor, that we may heal the Earth Mother Gaia and heal each other from separateness.

Sun Bear's Ojibwe Prayer

*People came from California, Germany, Mexico, Florida, Montana, all over the World, drawn by his workshops and books. Most well known was, **Walk in Balance on the Earth Mother**. This was a self-reliance retreat where participants learned gardening, food preservation and building root cellars. He taught a sacred way to take the Life of an animal if needed to be self-reliant. At the root of everything he taught was recognition of the sacred in connecting with the Earth Mother Gaia, and the importance of everyone finding their own path.*

As visitors arrived at the longhouse on Vision Mountain, Sun Bear walked among them, taking out compost, feeding chickens, chopping wood for sweat lodges, carrying water to the chicken coop. He walked among the people all day, and no one recognized him. Then at six o'clock, after the evening meal, Sun Bear changed into his medicine attire; black fringed shirt and hat, medicine beads, sacred objects, sacred rattle, sacred pipe. When he walked down the stairs, a whisper went through the room. He had walked among them all day and they had not noticed, as was his plan - teaching them to treat everyone as a sacred medicine person.

He told them to go out and find their places on the mountain for three days, draw an eight foot circle around themselves, not leave the circle and cry for their vision. He had them make their own sacred space on Mother Earth, dig a hole and empty their emotions, pain, suffering and their past into the Earth, then cry out to the their 'brothers and sisters the Stars,' until they were empty of that which did not belong, and reconnected with their True Spirit; so when they came down off the mountain they were a True Human Being...

In gentleness there is great strength, power can be a very quiet thing.

Sun Bear
Native American Shaman, Medicine Man

During the next few days, we set water and herbal tea outside each circle for the apprentices and heard their primal shouts on the wind, as they connected with Great Spirit. Sun Bear would say, 'You can call me Medicine Man, you can call me Shaman; what I'm here to do is instruct you in the ways of Great Spirit, to 'Walk in Balance on Our Earth Mother. We are ALL the Rainbow Nation. Nataqua Assay'* ♥ *Teddi*

CLEARING WHAT DRIVES OUR HABITS: "Why do we perpetuate habits that require cleansing and detoxification? What is it that causes us to eat too much, heavy greasy foods, excessive animal products, beverages containing sugar, stimulants or alcohol, drugs and pharmaceuticals; consuming destructive unnatural substances to such an extent that 60 to 70% are dying of de-generative conditions?? *AND* offloading our dis-harmony to pets, with 60 to 70% of them dying of de-generative illness?? We are *regenerative* if we choose to be. It is our choice - *it takes clearing out our unconscious container of our "old pain-data-base" to access our regenerative potential.*

The deepest, most Innate aspect of our Being is constantly moving toward Union with our True Nature LOVE. Habits blocking Life Force are uncomfortable for good reason! They point to our generational and historical database, to clear it, run the anti-virus in our "computer system," remove the old thought-emotion inharmonious with Source, stored in our unconscious container, causing PAIN! When we are ready to "wake up" we release habits causing physical pain, Mirroring our shadows!

Understood by few throughout the ages, dis-comfort is an opportunity to remove old "corrupt data." It resonates louder and louder with our pain from the shadows of our personal and collective unconscious, till we notice and clear it. We are in a time of crisis for all systems surrounding us, our self-expression, our bodies, our ecosystem, governments, banking systems, our Planet and her creatures. Pain and discomfort Mirrored thought-emotion in personal and collective "realities" asks to be set Free.

THE SOLUTION is to clear all Not of LOVE thought-emotion from OURSELVES, buried in the unconscious, our *unaware* Vibration in our World. Finally, with Quantum physics, we understand what this is and *HOW* it works.

> ...referring to the multi-generational database stored in our carbon based memory; when it fires, takes over or is resonated with enough amplitude, it robs us of our awareness that we were Created by creator to act as the Active Presence of LOVE.
>
> *dr. michael ryce, whyagain.org*

Have you done a cleanse or detox, and done it again a few months later? Our objective is to clean "our house" or Body-Mind, and use habits that nourish and cleanse everyday. A periodic cleanse or detox can then be used to Lighten things up. Successful cleansing removes Body-Mind toxemia. Habits clogging our system at the root of dis-ease, are a result of Not of LOVE Mind-Energy, getting our Attention through pain, to restore LOVE.

When we are awake enough to remove remove the shadow-pain within us, we restore the ever-flowing state of Vibrancy and Vitality that is our natural birthright. Check the list below for what might be hidden in your historical memory banks; or perhaps find evidence recognizable in your bloodline. Any such issues can also be at the root of physical discomfort, illness, pain, imbalanced weight, even colds and flu.

☐ Beloved friend, relative or pet died; grief, sorrow, rage or guilt about it
☐ Adopted, do or do not know who your parents were
☐ Still blaming your parents for your issues
☐ Sexual abuse somewhere in the family
☐ Rage, fear or shame as a child
☐ Rage, fear or shame as an adult
☐ Panic attacks
☐ Don't like your body, hair or face
☐ Punished as a child
☐ Guilt or shame
☐ War or some other traumatic societal event (or someone close to you)
☐ Would like to fix the World
☐ Anesthetic during medical or dental procedure
☐ Near death experience NDE (we like to call near Life experience:)
☐ Drugs and or alcohol regular use or to unconsciousness
☐ Smoking
☐ Low frequency foods
☐ Terror or rage history in bloodline
☐ Can't stand to see someone or something suffer
☐ Rage or fear at all the terrible things going on around us
☐ Don't like job
☐ Don't like how government or economic system handling things
☐ Have aches, pains, illness, dis-ease
☐ Afraid won't be able to pay bills
☐ Work out of necessity or obligation with little joy
☐ In relationship, don't feel understood, cared for or appreciated
☐ Would like to have a relationship yet don't
☐ Strongly dislike some people
☐ Feel -felt abandoned
☐ Dreams hope to do "someday"
☐ Don't know if will ever do what really good at
☐ Other _____

Okay, did you check some boxes? *Right, not a fun list.* Many of us have trained ourselves to *not* dwell on such things. What's valuable is to bring them up from our unconscious, do goal canceling processes until the charge is gone, so they can discharge while we're also physically cleansing. The old resonance will dissolve from us and Planet Earth, as we "clean house," remembering *there is no 'out there' out there*, moving into LOVE.

Clearing thought-emotion Not of LOVE, *along with* physical cleansing and detox removes it from Body-Mind. *Thought-data crystalized in the physical structure, slows energy flow and accumulates toxins, so clearing the two together is imperative!* Dr. Wayne Dyer says,

The unconscious is a machine,
it replays the program unless you change it.

Clearing thought-emotion along with Body addresses toxemia at its root. If it's been there for years, it's not likely to go away on its own. This primary teaching Yeshua brought forth in Ancient Aramaic for "forgiveness" was to remove the thought-resonance from within ourselves. [Part 2: MIND] He knew it was crucial for humanity to progress, as is Now confirmed by Quantum physics and Attention on the *Field!* We are reversing a lifetime of thinking that our "misery" originates outside of us, discovering it comes from within.

EXAMPLES: Teddi comes from a family where at least five known generations of women have had the "LOVE of their life" die unexpectedly, in an unfortunate accident or war at a young age. As mysterious as it is to untangle, do you think there might be a genetic Mind-Energy holding resonance for this pattern to continue through these generations?

Teddi worked on her own process to clear shadow thoughts in her subconscious, so that this pattern would not have to carry forward in her bloodline energetically. Here are her thoughts on how this has been transformed within her, by doing her inner clearing.

When I met up with Dr. John Ray, and I was on the Body Electronics point holding table, my issues from these ongoing family circumstances arose. It was amazing how a flood of memories came up, around loss of a beloved and being left alone, not just from myself, also from my great-grandmother, grandmother, mother and daughter. It became very clear how this genetic heritage played a role in what occurred in my own life, both through subtle thoughts I had experienced and unconscious patterns "driving the boat," energetically.

As I went into the pain that came up and brought it to the conscious mental level for clearing while my points were held on the table, these energetic patterns brought to conscious awareness began to clear from my field. I was able to go forward from those sessions with a New level of freedom from things layered in my genetic past; I was able to end that genetic dysfunction. We know the World has upside down energy patterns. It is up to us to live consciously and enter into consciously creating. It is by doing this personal inner work, that we are able to change the World around us, beginning first with self and our family history past, present and future - and cleaning up our manifestation filters, resonating to others. ♥ *Teddi*

Here is how my (Cary's) genetic history has played into what I've been clearing: *I know where I get my fiery spirit and intelligence; and I also know where I got rage and terror; as my genetic heritage is partially Middle Eastern with European and a little Jewish thrown in. Over a couple of years of doing several thousand of dr. michael ryce's "goal canceling" worksheets, the more I discovered the roots of terror and rage within me. Because of what was surfacing, michael encouraged me to watch the movie* **The Stoning of Soraya M***. It took me a long time, because I don't commonly watch things "upsetting." However when I finally did, it was one of the most powerful, life-changing experiences ever, because I did it along* **with numerous Ancient Aramaic True Forgiveness "goal canceling" worksheets***; diffusing energetic patterns from my genetic databank, hidden there for millennia. After the movie and clearing intensely related layers, I was able to step more powerfully into my own path and actually Create this book! [Details in Part 2: MIND]*

I also discovered that stoning and executing those who don't abide by strict religious standards still "to my horror" exist today in some places; residual from an ignorant history, seeds of which were in my unconscious container. **The only way we will remove such things from our World, is to remove them from our own unconscious.** *I have been in spiritual circles for years, and enjoy a gentle way of being; yet I learned when we are willing to step into the depths of our pain to remove the old thought-emotion holding resonance, we free these frequencies forever.*

Millions yet unborn will benefit from the work you do.

dr. michael ryce's comment
A Course In Miracles

Although I had read Zecharia Sitchin years ago, Michael Tellinger's "Slave Species of the Gods" has Now shed a bright Light on the same pre-history from Ancient tablets of Sumer; my Mind has been jostled to a deeper awareness of "stories" of why there is such suffering on Earth and within us. We are Now letting thousands of years of oppression and suffering go from within us. It is Mind-Energy. "There is no 'out there' out there." As we clear anything in the way projecting into our World, our connection with Source, LOVE shines through. ♥ *Cary [For complete understanding be sure to read Part 1: SHIFT OF THE AGES, Part 2: MIND, Part 3: SPIRIT].*

As we release "old data" from the unconscious that has been driving behavior, neurobiology and Body-Mind restructure. We see toxin patterns show up in the iris of the eye similarly in families (learn more about Iridology at our website). We bring true desires into Creation by removing these inhibiting frequencies and our bodies become Lighter!

Make your requests, concerns and desires in the language of fun...
the Universe will be quicker to respond to your needs.

Dr. Richard Bartlett
Matrix Energetics

ALL Not of LOVE, stored in the unconscious also "crystalizes" in the physical structure. We use open mouthed Breathing to assist with releasing this "old data," the physical "crystals" dissolve into water (tears), then vapor. Keep Breathing (beyond crying) through the layers to transmute ALL, release, let go and surrender. *Meditation* in Part 2 offers excellent daily clearing processes. Breathe. Smile.

Suffering comes from holding on to what does not serve our personal evolution. We let it go to make room for the new Life emerging within us. As we prepare for a cleanse or detox we "let go" on many levels. Once we clear ourselves and enter Heart Coherence with Pure LOVE, Compassion and Gratitude, we no longer accumulate "layers," and clear ourselves to Live in Pure LOVE!

> The only devil you need to be concerned about
> is the one running around in your own heart.
>
> *Mahatma Gandhi (1969-1948)*
> *Non-Violent Leader of India*

Note areas you would like to clear during your cleanse or detox. Our teachers and mentors guiding *us* on the path, taught us that once we learn to cleanse and detox, it becomes an integral part of our daily Lives. Occasionally a more in-depth retreat deepens our experience in clearing, using these experiences to go inward and achieve deeper clarity. Check our website for retreats and gatherings; also those by dr. michael ryce. We invite you to incorporate these foundational practices into your everyday Life. Live from your Heart. Live Authentically expressing True *Essence,* beyond old layers or external expectation. Breathe. Smile.

> Even a Vessel of Gold needs polishing occasionally.
>
> *Jack White (1934-1998)*
> *God's Game of Life*

CLEANSING OUR VESSEL - DAILY PRACTICES - MIND & HEART

1. *First thing in morning connect with the Circle of Life.* Express gratitude; Breathe and Smile your prayers or meditation forward into your day. Walk outside to commune with and receive gifts of nature in your surroundings, gardens, plants, flowers, trees, water, Sun, Earth, Sky. It already knows you are coming. Feel your Oneness with everything, during your walk and putting out your prayers.

   a. Teddi says, *"First thing in the morning as the sun was coming up, Sun Bear would get me from the kitchen to take a walk and get our daily vegetables. As we walked to the garden path he would already start talking to the vegetables in the garden and say they knew we were coming. I believe he shared this with me so I would learn to feel Oneness with everything; with the onions, carrots, sorrel, anything we needed for our sustenance that day, we were*

435

already One with it. That's the kind of thought he gave his day. He knew how his whole day would unfold by doing this process."

b. We pray from the moment we wake up. Pray it forward. Unfold your day with prayer, thought, vision, intention. This is mastery. In our consciousness we're sitting in the Himalayas or Andes, walking the Earth plane, blessing every moment.

Ask and it will be given to you, search and you will find, knock and the door will be opened for you. For everyone who asks, receives, and everyone who searches finds, and for everyone who knocks the door will be opened.

Matthew 7:7-8

2. *Clearing ripples and bubbles.* Notice energy that is stuck, repetitive or not moving easily. Breathe into it with open mouth, smile, release and let it go. Prayers, giving it to the *Field* help clear. EFT tapping is useful here. If you are consistent with these practices, one day you will wake up and you will have shifted to a New neurobiology. Here is an example of using Light for clearing.

Honor your Inner feelings - ...feel in every moment the energies that overlay them. Keep your Heart in a rhythm that welcomes those feelings, and deepen them with total Compassion. Compassion is the knowing impetus and the platform for connecting with all interdimensional realms.

Unconditional Loving Compassion heals and reactivates the natural *Essence* of all original cellular lifeforms. Use the Violet Flame to transmute all incongruent feelings and follow with waves of Gold and White Light flowing over and purifying all in the Earth Plane. Thank you Divine Spirit.

Sharon Hall
Meditative Thoughts

3. *"Go into the pain."* [Dr. John Ray] Whatever comes up Not of LOVE go into it, allow it to surface until dissolves. Notice if you are feeling something about what "someone else did or is doing," remove blame, clear your thought. Cancel goals that have not been met. *"I now invite Aramaic - Rookha d'koodsha (my Divine super-processor) to help me cancel all my goals, conscious, unconscious, subconscious and incomplete."* [Part 2: MIND] With this we clear away mind-clutter that takes away from Higher focus or is based on shadow content. Notice your belief system adjusting to knowing you Create your "reality." Breathe. Smile. Welcome response from the *Field of Possibilities*, beyond your imagining. Early in this process there may be catharsis, as when Sun Bear sent apprentices to the mountain to cry for their vision, releasing all falsely programmed belief systems. We are releasing generational constructs and false expectations we believed were real.

4. *Seek your own vision. Seek your deeper mission. Seek your True Self, your Authenticity.* Your expression in this World will always feel lacking until you do this. Give up all falsehoods perpetuated in you to get along with partner, friends, society, family. Every

part of our Journey has value, even when we're not living our Truth, its one of the ways we get to find out what we *desire* that is our Truth and how to Live it.

"My" Perfect LOVE for you is your perfect freedom.

Jack White (1934-1998)
God's Game of Life

5. ***Fast and pray. Cleanse and detox.*** *'Follow the yellow brick road.'* Adopt Lifestyle habits that include these things *Everyday.* Do them out of LOVE. Life is a journey. *Remember, journey of a thousand miles begins with the first step...*

    a. Take note of your words and how are you are expressing your creative thought through your words. Use only positive creative words both audibly and in thought. Remember, *Yoda said, "There is no try, it is do or do not."*

6. To integrate into your being, speak it out loud or share with someone. ***Where two or more are gathered...*** Write down or share with a friend what you learned about your mission and what Great Spirit has shared with you. Always heed your inner voice.

    a. Breathe into and imagine your Life flowing with your own purpose, your own "river." Experience it "IS" in the "Now," expressing your best talents, doing things you LOVE. "I Am Now _____..."

        ii. From a Quantum perspective Dr. Richard Bartlett of Matrix Energetics emphasizes that left brain holds particles in form, and right brain entertains Quantum potential that can shift things in an instant. *Trust whatever shows up in your awareness, even if it doesn't make any sense or appear to be useful in the moment. You have a potentially infinite set of possibilities within the morphic grid of what can manifest in the very next moment. The Field is continually moving into New Creation!*

By cultivating the habit of asking powerful mind altering questions, you are training your right brain to respond to the signals from your unconscious.

Dr. Richard Bartlett
Matrix Energetics

CLEANSING OUR VESSEL - DAILY PRACTICES - BODY

INTEGRATING CLEANSING into our daily routine is a ***21st Century Superhuman Quantum Lifestyle*** tool for excellence! Set up daily rituals similar to brushing teeth, for example:

- Begin each day with 1 quart warm water (lemon, cayenne, opt.)
- Begin each day with lighting a candle, doing a short meditation-clearing
- Green Shake for breakfast or blended raw soup
- 2 more meals - 5 hrs. apart / vegetable based

BATHING: If you live in an area where chlorine or fluoride is added to the water, get a filter for your shower. Take a shower or bath daily. Use as few man-made shampoos, soaps, conditioners as possible. Experiment with a little vinegar in water for hair. Discover favorite essential oils for during or after bathing. Put in hair or dilute with carrier oil and use on skin. Use a skin brush to freshen and clean skin, stimulating healthy circulation. Final rinse with cool water if comfortable, to close pores and stimulate blood. Epsom Salts, Baking Soda or Magnesium Chloride can be used in soaks for good benefit.

Cleansing is part of daily routine in *Quantum Lifestyle*. Basic practices integrated over many years build a foundation for sustainable good health. A clean body, mind, spirit lays foundation for Well-Being and Vitality.

Toxemia at a cellular level lays foundation for illness. Much of our modern Lifestyle contributes to overloading the body, from overeating, excessive fats, sugars, and proteins, lack of exercise, pesticides, polluted water, chlorinated and fluoridated water, environmental toxins, vaccinations, pharmaceuticals, silver-mercury dental fillings, food additives, GMOs, negative thought and emotion, stress. So whatever we do on a regular basis to "keep our house clean" is very worthwhile.

> One of my goals each day is to fully embody the "new Way of Life" and teach by example the higher spiritual principles, which will transform this world into Light. I am constantly checking every area of my Life, in an effort to fine-tune and upgrade all my methods and perceptions.
>
> *Bryan de Flores*
> *Lightquest International*

Detoxing and cleansing have become so popular they're mainstream, even promoted by Dr. Oz, with millions of cleanses offered online, and instructions anyone can follow. Going to a natural healing center to learn how to detox or cleanse, is a great way to experience the basics, yet it can also be learned at home. Don't make cleansing "just another way to purge" or "self-punishment for overdoing." Modern civilization is built on a house of cards with constant running after illusory satisfaction to "look or feel better."

A healthy routine we can live with on a daily basis is easier than extremes for Body-Mind to restore Energy and Vitality. Set up your home as a wonderful nucleus, where Healthy Foods you Love, and routine aimed at Vitality and Inner Peace support your Journey. *21st Century Superhuman* Cleanse and Detox is about shedding false layers, finding and expressing our True Spirit and discovering our own Authentic Expression. Recovering True sense of purpose takes courage and perhaps "going against" the cultural flow. However once we reclaim this Birthright, Vitality returns!

> Take therefore no thought for the morrow:
> for the morrow shall take thought for the things of itself.
>
> *Matthew 6:34*

Play with what's here and cultivate your own routine; do what works with your Lifestyle, your personal tastes and what you discover raises *your* Vitality. Remember, once vitality increases from physical-thought-emotional cleansing, New layers are likely to surface to clear! [Part 3: SPIRIT]

It's important for each individual to seek their own path, listen to their Body and learn what is most appropriate for them at each stage. If operating from "old data" suppressed in the unconscious, suppressive foods may be chosen. This is a good area to us Aramaic Forgiveness Freedom Tools *[Part 2: MIND]* to move toward Lightening up. Listen to your Body-Mind, keep clearing out old content and toxins that want to "run the show" to discover a Lighter, more resilient you!

NOTE ON COFFEE AND STIMULANTS: Let's face it, as a modern culture we have a "coffee habit" difficult to walk away from. One reason coffee and cola beverages are so prevalent in our daily routine, is because high fat, high animal protein diet eventually destroys our natural enzymes needed for digestion, and we crave the acidity in these beverages to make digestion work. In this sense they are actually "medicinal." "Old thought data" that suppresses Life-force also invites stimulants. Wellness requires an alkaline Body, yet these beverages set up chronic acidity that can precede degeneration.

Coffee and cola beverages "push" our hormonal systems and Create acidity aggravating to the liver, making it difficult to stick with a raw, living foods or vegan diet. To enjoy a continually regenerative Lifestyle, commit to gradually withdrawing from anything but occasional coffee, benefits when eating heavier food. Decaf, espresso, French and cold pressed coffees are less acidic; also those produced without mold, organic and free-trade are "karma free." Even killing animals for food is a product of shadow blame-fear-hostility in the unconscious. Craving acidity and heavy foods expresses our burden of rage-fear-blame still in the suppressed in the unconscious causing acidic emotions.

Check our website for our additional books, videos, recipes, dietary transition chart *Climb the Transitional Ladder* and further accomplishing your Journey into greater Well-Being. It's nice to have guidance when we're getting started. For additional support, currently available on Amazon and Kindle by Cary Ellis: *Super Immunity Secrets - Fifty Vegan-Vegetarian Recipes & Immune Protective Herbs; Why Become a Vegetarian? Benefits for Health and Longevity; Truth About Weight Loss.*

DAILY CLEANSING ROUTINE - "SIMPLE RULES"

These "simple rules" are based on recovering healthy "leptin," the master hormone of the body that manages fat burning and keeping a lean, healthy metabolism.

1. BETWEEN MEALS - water - up to 4 quarts / day. Tea (coffee-min) - nothing added.

    a. Do not drink water at meals, instead drink 2 glasses 1/2 hour before meals. Studies have shown this helps with staying lean.

2. 3 MODERATE SIZE MEALS PER DAY (stomach size of two palms cupped)

3. 4-5 HRS. BETWEEN MEALS

4. 3 HRS. BETWEEN DINNER AND BED - NO FOOD

   a. If you feel the need to have something, make it a whole food. Herbal tea.

5. BREAKFAST CONTAINING PROTEIN or Low Glycemic foods

6. AVOID REFINED FOODS, WHITE FLOUR, WHITE SUGAR

7. LEAVE SOME WIGGLE ROOM 80/20 RULE - a "treat" now and then OK.

8. STICK WITH LOW GLYCEMIC FOODS (UNDER 55) [lists can be found online]

a. Examples

Low GI, 55 or less Examples include: legumes such as kidney, white, black, pink, soybeans; nuts (almonds, peanuts, walnuts, chickpeas), and Seeds (sunflower, flax, pumpkin, poppy, sesame); most fruits (peaches, strawberries, mangos), most vegetables (beets, squash, parsnips); most whole intact grains (durum, spelt, kamut wheat, millet, oat, rye, rice, barley).

Medium GI, 56–69 Examples include: pita bread, basmati rice, potato, grape juice, raisins, prunes, pumpernickel bread, cranberry juice, regular ice cream, sucrose, and banana.

High GI, 70 and above Examples include: white bread, most white rice, corn flakes, most breakfast cereals, potato, and pretzels.

drpielet.com/3-things-you-can-do-today-to-start-losing-weight/

DAILY CLEANSING ROUTINE - BREAKFAST

1. **1 Qt. Warm Water a.m.** - Upon arising - warm or body temp water assists body
   1. plain or add a wedge or squeeze of fresh lemon or lime, or to alkalize - wedge of lime/lemon with pinch of baking soda (non-aluminum *Bob's*)

2. **TEA** (opt.) Herbal, black, green or white tea (no sweetener) Organic.

3. **COFFEE** Eliminate or reduce. If you're really hooked on coffee - have it after the above, try to stick to one cup per day or less. First Decaf then Espresso (home machine great) or cold press better than brewed - reduces acid; decaf also better. Organic. Fair Trade. Mold-free. Become a tea drinker!

NOTE: Yogic tradition of ***cleansing the stomach and intestines on awakening*** is long honored and beneficial. During the night we fast., after moderate dinner the evening before preferably 2-4 hrs before bed. During the night the stomach is empty, and by morning the body is ready to flush out waste products the organs and cells eliminated during the night. Up to a quart of warm water plain or with lemon-lime, is a wonderful routine first thing a.m.! :) It Lightens the body; clean feeling.

Daily practices clear Body-Mind-Spirit (previous section), burn incense, uplifting music, focus, meditate, pray in preparation for the Day; or as our Native American brother, John Woolf does, express three things you are Grateful for; as Ram Dass said, "Be Here Now..." connect with unlimited Creation from the *Field*.

LIGHT SUSTENANCE: We've supported our cleanse of the night with a Morning Flush. Our body appreciates us being gentle on our digestive system, breaking our night's "fast" with lighter fare, such as Smoothie or Green Shake. These are so popular they are available almost anywhere. Be sure to check ingredients to avoid refined sugar. Make at home with fresh ingredients (below), a great habit to cultivate; potent, regenerative Light nourishment! Making your own ensures your Smoothie or Green Shake is made from the best ingredients, and just right for you. Blend or shake, or just stir in a cup when traveling.

1. Smoothie or Green Shake - Light Sustenance (Recipe at end of chapter)
2. Follow with or have on alternate days heavier breakfast of choice
    a. Essene or Sprouted Grain Bread - Toast - Coconut Oil or avocado (opt.)
    b. Whole or sprouted grain tortilla - nut butter
    c. Raw Meuseli Cereal (rolled oats, raisins, nuts, coconut, nut milk) soak
    d. Potatoes / toast - If eating eggs or tofu - option

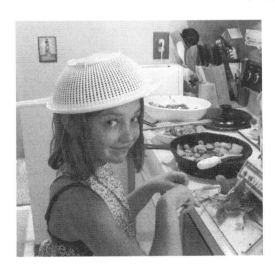

DAILY CLEANSING ROUTINE - LUNCH

Experiment with wholesome light Recipes at our site SuperImmunitySecrets.com

• Soups
• Salads
• Sandwiches, Sprouted Grain Breads or Tortillas
• Favorite PROTEINS

Francis Moore Lappé's 1971 bestselling *Diet for a Small Planet* and her subsequent books are foundational resources for how to meet protein needs on a vegan-vegetarian diet. Another tremendous resource is John Robbins (author of *Diet for a new America* and many more) *May All Be Fed: a Diet For A new World : Including Recipes By Jia Patton And Friends* with 200 awesome recipes. *(Cary worked a little with Jia Patton and EarthSave years ago in early stages of this book).*

• Beans and Peas such as black, great northern, white, navy, lentils, garbanzos, mung, adzuki *(sprout or soak and cook)*
• Grains such as quinoa and amaranth for balanced high protein
• Decrease animal products to less days per week or smaller quantities

- Fermented foods such as Kimchee or Raw Sauerkraut keep enzyme levels up
- Baked or stir-fried veggies
- International foods often contain great combinations of legumes and grains with vegetables and choice of no animal protein: Chinese, Mexican, Vietnamese, Mediterranean, Middle Eastern, Ethiopian, Thai and more...

DAILY CLEANSING ROUTINE - DINNER

Similar pattern to Lunch - with your (and your family's) favorite combos. Make dinner either same size or smaller than lunch; based on the principle that we cleanse overnight, allowing the system to rest. Our stomach is about the same size as our two palms cupped together; this is accurate for any size person or pet - based on their hands (or paws) and how much food intake is appropriate.

DAILY CLEANSING ROUTINE - 1 DAY FAST/week

It has been a practice of many we know on the path, to go without food or switch to Juices or All Raw one day per week. Whatever current Lifestyle style habits, it's a great experience to spend one day a week with Lighter intake, and also dedicate this day to thought-emotional clearing and "goal canceling;" framing new and realistic goals, developing our "purpose;" reading or dr. michael ryce video-audio (whyagain.org) or our videos, deepen the Journey, "develop new brain cells."

DAILY CLEANSING ROUTINE - NOTES

1. Yes you may make more trips to the bathroom. Be thankful that which no longer belongs is leaving. Drink less in evening. Keep water next to bed in case thirsty.

2. Bowel movements should occur at least once every 24 hours, supported by water drinking and fiber. Become familiar with your own bowel "transit time:" Eat beets or take charcoal tablets, which show up in stools as red or black. Support your Body rhythms, using the following to support healthy transit time and easy elimination.

- 1-2 tsp/day ground or soaked flax, psyllium husks, chia seed (rotate flax as it is a healthy food, thought daily use can Create GLA deficiency) good in shake

- Herbal Laxative - prefer blend with *cascara sagrada* over *senna* when needed

- Healthy gut bacteria is super-important, destroyed by antibiotics and meds. Restore w/probiotics (health food store), and regular use of raw cultured foods.

NOTE ON CLEANSES: Below are outlines of cleanses. Do your research, listen to your body. A cleanse is a personal choice. Consider weight, toxicity, how current habits differ from cleanse protocol. *Middle path is wisdom*; moderation in all things. Mix-and-match routines. These basics have worked for us well over many years (videos at our website).

DETOX: Add herbs, essential oils, with special focus and bodywork to cleanse/detox a particular organ/ tissue, or remove residues from the body.

GUIDED CLEANSES: It is good to have a buddy with whom you can exchange notes with who is familiar with cleansing. If you have not done a cleanse or feel you have an overload of toxins, seek out practitioners or a residential program to experience a cleanse the first time. Many programs such as wheatgrass institutes teach how to use enemas, colonics and wheatgrass implants, which can accelerate the body's cleansing process.

3 DAY CLEANSE (1x/month or every other)

TRUE ARAMAIC FORGIVENESS - Freedom Tool [Part 2: MIND] 3-5/day

Follow instructions (this chapter):
CLEANSING OUR VESSEL - DAILY PRACTICES FOR MIND & HEART

DAILY ROUTINE

"1 Qt. Warm Water a.m." instructions under *Daily Cleansing Routine Breakfast*

    a. warm water with pinch of baking soda and wedge of lemon

    b. enjoy tea - let go of coffee for these 3 days

    c. drink 2-4 qts water and/or herbal tea during day between meals

DAY 1:

    a. Green Shake or Smoothie - Breakfast

    b. Salad with Steamed or Baked Veggies Lunch

    c. Fresh, Raw Vegetable Juices or Raw Blended Veggie Soup - Dinner

    d. Herbal Laxative, 1 tsp Ground Golden Flax or Psyllium Husks in glass water

DAY 2:

    a. Green Shake or Smoothie -Breakfast

    b. Fresh, Raw Vegetable Juices or Raw Blended Veggie Soup - Lunch

    c.Raw Salad - Dinner

    d. Herbal Laxative, 1 tsp Ground Golden Flax or Psyllium Husks in glass water

DAY 3:

    a. Fresh, Raw Vegetable Juices or Raw Blended Veggie Soup - Bkfst

    b. Fresh, Raw Vegetable Juices or Raw Blended Veggie Soup - Lunch

    c. Raw Salad and Vegan Soup cooked or raw - Dinner

    d. Herbal Laxative, 1 tsp Ground Golden Flax or Psyllium Husks in glass water

    Yay! You did it! Enjoy your Lightness and sticking to Lighter foods!

7 DAY CLEANSE (1x spring- 1x fall)

TRUE ARAMAIC FORGIVENESS - Freedom Tool [Part 2: MIND] 3-5/day

Follow instructions daily (this chapter):
CLEANSING OUR VESSEL - DAILY PRACTICES FOR MIND & HEART

DAILY ROUTINE

"1 Qt. Warm Water a.m." instructions under *Daily Cleansing Routine Breakfast*

    a. warm water with pinch of baking soda and wedge of lemon

    b. enjoy tea - let go of coffee for these 3 days

    c. drink 2-4 qts water and/or herbal tea during day between meals

DAY 1: Same as DAY 1 - 3 Day Cleanse

DAY 2: Same as DAY 2 - 3 Day Cleanse

DAYS 3-4:

    a. Green Shake or Smoothie - Breakfast

    b.Fresh, Raw Vegetable Juices or Raw Blended Veggie Soup - Lunch

    c.Fresh, Raw Vegetable Juices - Dinner 1-3 cups

    d.Herbal Laxative, 1 tsp Ground Golden Flax or Psyllium Husks in glass water

DAY 5: *(trade shake or smoothie for 1 juice meal)*

    a.Fresh, Raw Vegetable Juices - Breakfast 1-3 cups

    b.Fresh, Raw Vegetable Juices - or Raw Blended Veggie Soup - Lunch

    c.Fresh, Raw Vegetable Juices - Dinner 1-3 cups

    d.Herbal Laxative, 1 tsp Ground Golden Flax or Psyllium Husks in glass water

DAY 7:

    a. Same as DAY 2 - 3 Day Cleanse

DAY 7:

    a. Green Shake or Smoothie -Breakfast

    b. Salad with Steamed or Baked Veggies Lunch

    c. Raw Salad and Vegan Soup - Dinner

    d. Herbal Laxative, 1 tsp Ground Golden Flax or Psyllium Husks in glass water

30 DAY CLEANSE (opt. 1x/yr)

TRUE ARAMAIC FORGIVENESS - Freedom Tool [Part 2: MIND] 3-5/day

Follow instructions daily (this chapter):

CLEANSING OUR VESSEL - DAILY PRACTICES FOR MIND & HEART

DAILY ROUTINE

"1 Qt. Warm Water a.m." instructions under *Daily Cleansing Routine Breakfast*

    e. warm water with pinch of baking soda and wedge of lemon

    f. enjoy tea - let go of coffee for these 3 days

    g. drink 2-4 qts water and/or herbal tea during day between meals

DAYS 1-30:

    a. Adapt patterns established in 3 DAY and 7 DAY Cleanses. Create your own "mix-and-match" based on:

        a. current lifestyle

b. whether you have time to "retreat" or are doing this during normal work - home week

c. if current nutrition has been a bit heavy or if dealing with illness, disease, or sensitivities - go gently

d. One option is to do several repeats of the 7DAY and end with the 3 DAY, or whatever adaptation fits.

21st Century Superhuman
GREEN SHAKE & SMOOTHIE RECIPES
more recipes at SuperImmunitySecrets.com

SMOOTHIES AND GREEN 98SHAKES: Mix and match from this general list, based on what you have available and suits your taste and phase of dietary transition. Shop at your local health food store, natural foods section at your grocery store, local organic grower or order online. There are awesome online and offline resources for live Superfoods. Measurements are for 1 shake. All ingredients and measurements are variable to taste. GENERAL RECIPE:

LIQUID 2 cups Water with Nut, Coconut, Rice Milk. If you buy pre-made, get without sugar. Make your own, blend soaked nuts-seeds with water.

GREENS - 1-2 Tbs Wheatgrass, Barleygrass, Other Mixed Grass Powders; Spirulina - Excellent Protein Source; Chlorella - a must for detoxing mercury; Blue Green Algae; Supergreen Blends (several excellent available); Ormus Supergreens (Sunwarrior)

FIBER 1-3 tsp
Psyllium Husks, Ground Flax - golden (preferable), Soaked Whole Flax

PROTEIN 1-2 T Vegan Protein Powder; raw soaked nuts-seed

FRUIT Fresh, Frozen, Dried, preferably organic; Frozen bananas thicken

SUPERFOODS Many popular exotic - try out different things and find out what you like Cacao, Carob, Maca, Gogi Berry, Ginseng, Bilberry, Bee Pollen

NUTS OR SEEDS Chia Seed, Hemp Seed, Coconut, Raw Nuts or Seeds (soaked)
Soak overnight to start sprouting process and make "living food"

SPICES: Cinnamon. Coriander, Ginger

FRESH GREENS & VEGGIES: Kale, cucumber, apple, ginger, broccoli, spinach, etc.

21st Century Superhuman GREEN SHAKE

NOTE: Rotate items for variety. Enjoy in a.m. & save in fridg for later, or make more and share with household. NOTE: Can also be savory shake without fruit. Blend in blender with 2-4 cups water:

•1/2 cup Frozen Organic fruit, 1/2 banana, 1/2-1 fresh apple (choice or blend)

• 1/2-1 tsp. Spirulina; 1/2-1 tsp. Chlorella; 1/2-1 tsp. blue-green algae (choice or blend)

•1-2 tsp Ormus Supergreens (build up to it); 2 tsp Wheatgrass/Barleygrass Powder

•1 T Supergreen Powder Blend: *Pure Synergy* , *Vitamineral Green* or blend with probiotics
• 1 T Hemp Seed (whole); 1 T Chia Seed (whole) - can soak overnight
• 2 T Soaked (whole) or ground Golden Flaxseed (include walnuts or hemp for Omega 6)
• 1 T Vegan Protein Powder (opt) favorites: Sunwarrior & Garden of Life
• Fresh organic greens such as spinach or kale; Moranga powder (40% protein leaf)
      With veggies and no fruit: opt. cayenne, ginger, garlic, cumin, curry

21st Century Superhuman SMOOTHIE

A Smoothie provides quick, easy nutritious, delicious substantive meal that can carry us for hours.
Fun and delicious!   Blend in blender:

• 2 cups favorite Milk Alternative (nut, seed, coconut, almond, hemp, hazelnut, soy)
• Dilute with a little water (opt). Can make own nut/seed milk w/water & flavor.
• 1/2 cup Frozen Fruit / frozen banana with other fruit thickens (or use no fruit)
• If sweeter desired, add a couple of dates or dash maple syrup
• 1-2 T Vegan Protein Powder - favorites: Sunwarrior, Garden of Life, Ultimate Meal

Optional additions:
• 1 tsp green powder blend (see Green Shake - any combo)
• 1/2 tsp cacao, vanilla, cinnamon, ginger, coriander, carob
• gogi berries, maca or other favorite superfood
• 1 tsp hempseed, chia seed, flaxseed (soaked or ground)
• (include walnuts or hemp for Omega 6 to balance flax)

RAW BLENDED VEGGIE SOUP: 2-3 cups water, cut up raw organic veggies seasonal, greens, tomatoes, cucumbers, garlic, cruciferous, lemon juice, sea salt, cayenne herbs, spices, tamari, umeboshi plum.

THINK GREEN: In Ancient Egypt Green was used for healing. Chlorophyll and hemoglobin are identical, except hemoglobin has iron at the center of the molecule, and chlorophyll has magnesium. Blood cleanses and rebuilds quickly with dark green. Wheatgrass juice has many testimonials to this. Wheatgrass juice and green powders purify the blood, and clean out eliminative organs, open channels of elimination. If flu-like symptoms occur, increase fluids and support better elimination (enemas, herbs, implants).

WHEATGRASS: Without having to grow your own wheatgrass, stir into water daily excellent dehydrated wheatgrass juice powders.

CATCH OUR VIDEOS - at YouTube and at our website easy cleansing-detox "how to's."

Chapter 8

Nature's Simplest Remedies

Deprive a cell of 35% of its oxygen for 48 hours and it may become cancerous.

Dr. Otto H. Warburg (1883-1970)
Nobel Prize Medicine 1931, Nominated Nobel Prize Physiology 1944

Mother Nature is simple; when we understand how she works and plays, we align with the grandest, most Innate power there is. Simple basic principles and practices hold the *Field* for health, well-being and vitality. There is peace in knowing we are One with All That Is. Aligning Mind-Heart with LOVE and clearing ALL thought-emotion Not of LOVE, is our first step, then according to Universal Law we discover resources within nature that kindly nurture and help correct our imbalances.

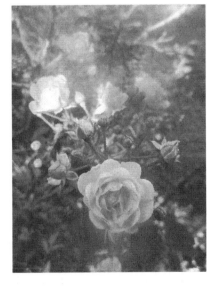

> Everything is energy and that's all there is to it. Match the frequency of the reality you want and you cannot help but get that reality. It can be no other way. This is not philosophy. This is physics.
>
> *Albert Einstein (1879-1955)*
> *Theory or Relativity, Nobel Prize Physics 1921, Max Planck Medal 1929*

It is amazing how once we become confident of the direction we are going, how much our Lifestyle changes, and just a few simple remedies can give us a feeling of comfort and relief. Remember: the body's movement is *always* toward wellness. Any typical symptom that might be considered cold, flu, coughing, sneezing, nausea, vomiting, diarrhea, and even degenerative conditions, are generally efforts of the body to cleanse and Lighten up!

Critical to physical well-being is that cells and tissues require oxygen, as demonstrated by Nobel Laureate Dr. Otto Warburg in 1924. Simplest natural remedies help clear away acidity, inflammation and toxicity, restoring oxygenation to the cells. When access to oxygen is blocked because of cellular congestion, cells become anaerobic and fermentation occurs. Nature uses her best efforts to clean-up where the flow of Life Force is blocked, with these typical acute symptoms of cleansing.

> Cancer, above all other diseases, has countless secondary causes. But, even for cancer, there is only one prime cause. Summarized in a few words, the prime cause of cancer is the replacement of the respiration of oxygen in normal body cells by a fermentation of sugar [or anaerobic condition].

Dr. Otto H. Warburg (1883-1970)
Nobel Prize Medicine 1931, Nominated Nobel Prize Physiology 1944

Health, holy, holistic and whole come from the same Indo-European root word (6-7,000 years ago), to be healthy is to be whole is to be holy. When Life Force flows to us continually from the ever-creating *Field* we are well and whole. If this flow of Life Energy and oxygen is blocked dis-ease results.

Where does this flow being blocked begin? Mind-Energy Not of LOVE. As a result of this thought-emotion the the system becomes overloaded with too much, too heavy, too rich, toxic substances, and the flow of Life Force slows. Toxins crystalize in tissues and cells, acidity, inflammation, fibrins and free radicals reduce oxygen levels and stimulate development of layers of mucous for buffering. So toxemia begins. Fasting, cleansing and goal canceling remove unconscious Mind-Energy. This is when it's nice to have simple remedies to assist.

When we have accumulated enough toxic waste in our system and eliminative organs from heavier and richer foods, in greater quantity than the body needs, it has no choice but to cleanse, which we call illness. Statistically those who become vegan, vegetarian and eat lightly, are much less prone to illness. The fastest, most efficient and lasting way to remove symptoms when they do show up, is by changing our internal ecosystem; juicing, fasting, cleansing and restoring balance to the gut with probiotics.

FURTHER READING: Dr. Sircus.com: on baking soda, magnesium chloride and iodine is very informative. Founder, International Medical Veritas Association (IMVA), he cites these remedies as primary to keep us well in today's World; *excellent resource.*

Baking Soda - Best Friend

Optimally we maintain healthy alkalinity through low-fat, high percentage raw, vegan-vegetarian foods, green shakes, juices, water, cleansing and clear Mind-Heart. However modern lifestyle results in inflammation due to stress and poor diet, with resulting acidity and overload of toxemia, laying the foundation for degenerative dis-ease.

Our body is like an alkaline battery, much more power, endurance and running best when it is in alkaline balance. Oxygen to the cells is a critical factor. So if our bodies are in overload, in order to relieve our discomfort we seek cleansing and alkalization. The long term answer builds this into our Lifestyle. Alkalizing water machines can also support alkalinity. Primary is learning about alkaline lifestyle from foods, soil and incorporating.

Regular small pinches of baking soda in water can assist in restoring alkaline pH to the body, while at the same time we clear thoughts, cleanse and detox, while transitioning to more alkaline nutrition. A tiny pinch of (non-aluminum such as Bob's) baking soda in water in the morning assists with neutralizing acidity.

Teddi's experience with Dr. Stone: Teddi spent many years taking environmentally sensitive clients for treatment with Dr. Stone. A client going through a panic attack when they walked in the door, was handed a small cup half-full of a clear liquid. The client drank it down with symptoms of panic or allergy instantly relieved. "What was it?" they asked. It was "baking soda and water." Powerful, simple support for many "crisis" situations.

Testing pH: For accuracy, one can obtain pH test paper at a pharmacy. Optimal pH range is 6.5 to 7.2. Test saliva or clean stream of urine first thing in a.m. Baking soda more or less often can help maintain ph level. Eventually you will learn what it feels like to be alkaline.

First aid: In the case of anything that itches or burns, where the body is activating a histamine reaction, such as stings, bites or poison ivy or oak, a sip of baking soda internally and application externally support the body in relief of symptoms.

Baking Soda for cancer: Dr. Simoncini oncologist in Italy uses sodium bicarbonate intravenously to reverse cancer successfully. Dr. Sircus relates that taking baking soda internally and soaking in baths is equal to Dr. Simoncini's IV treatments.

Stories of cancer reversal with Baking Soda (online): One man cured himself of cancer by using baking soda with molasses. The sweetness carries the baking soda into the cell and helps the cell become alkaline, acting like a Trojan horse. Another young woman who had four sisters who died of breast cancer, when questioned as to what she thought was different about herself, said she sipped on water with baking soda and maple syrup daily; similarly to gentleman above. (See his videos online "Run From the Cure")

Colds -Flu: Dr. Sircus encourages a daily combination of baking soda, magnesium chloride and iodine to prevent any symptoms of cold of flu during winter seasons. We include with that the benefits of cleansing and Living on Lighter nutrition to Create a foundational clean Body honored as the *"House We Live In."* Food grown in mineralized soils does a great deal to keep us more alkaline.

Magnesium Chloride

Magnesium deficiency is rampant in the modern diet, with excess refined grains and sugars. Demineralization of soils and non-organic foods have also greatly reduced magnesium levels in foods. Common Epsom Salts boost magnesium levels, though does not last long. Dr. Sircus recommends the use of transdermal magnesium chloride as the most effective way to improve magnesium levels quickly.

Magnesium is an Essential Mineral used for hundreds of biochemical reactions, making it crucial for health. Massive magnesium deficiencies in the general population have led to a tidal wave of sudden coronary deaths, diabetes, strokes and cancer. Even a mild deficiency of magnesium can cause increased sensitivity to noise, nervousness, irritability, mental depression, confusion, twitching, trembling, apprehension, and insomnia.

Dr. Sircus, Dr Sircus.com

We use his recommended magnesium chloride from an ancient seabed, just a pinch in our water in the morning, and foot soaks with excellent results. Dr. Sircus suggests use of these 3 inexpensive, self-treatable natural substances, for supporting renewal of equilibrium of the body; baking soda, magnesium chloride and transdermal iodine. He suggests a high quality iodine - easily rub a bit into skin of forearm rather than internally.

Epsom Salts

Readily available: Epsom salts can be easily and inexpensively found at any pharmacy. S form of magnesium obtainable if a person does not have access to Ancient seabed magnesium chloride. Used externally for foot soaks and baths, Epsom salts assist the body to shift to an alkaline state and can relieve tension and cramping. Dr. Sircus recommends both baking soda and magnesium for cardio and cancer, two leading de-generative conditions in the modern World. Epsom salt soak or foot soak when feeling stressed, over-tired or toxic can be beneficial, however the magnesium is not retained long in this form.

Hydrotherapy: Simply getting into a tub of warm water is an old form of hydrotherapy, drawing congestion from the trunk of the body, rebalancing the body's energy flows in a gentle way. Using Epsom salts along with a warm bath can be very supportive of improving one's state of well-being, or simply a warm-hot bath alone assists body balance.

Diatomaceous Earth

A fossil of ancient algae: Diatomaceous earth is a naturally occurring fossilized rock that crumbles into a fine white powder, called "fossil shell flour." It can be slightly abrasive and is highly porous. It is commonly used for filtration, in gardens, sometimes in toothpaste, and is a mechanical insecticide, shredding the gut of the insect that ingests it. Engineer, Wilhelm Berkefeld recognized its ability to filter, and developed tubular filters (known as filter candles) fired from diatomaceous earth, successfully used in the1892 cholera epidemic in Germany.

Because diatomaceous earth occurs naturally in various deposits, different "mines" contain various minerals not for internal consumption. Perma-guard, mines and seels "animal food grade" diatomaceous earth, approved for the consumption of animals. Diatomaceous earth is hollow with negatively charged spaces that draw toxins or positively charged ions such as heavy metals out of the body.

Founder and former president of Perma-Guard, Wally Tharp passed away at the ripe age of 89, after 52 years of spreading information about use of diatomaceous earth. When I (Cary) met him he was 80, with a spring in his step and the brightest blue eyes I had ever seen. He told me he been taking a teaspoon a day of diatomaceous earth for 30 years, besides which he lived a committed healthy Lifestyle. I've always attributed the brightness of his eyes to the regular pulling of toxins with the diatomaceous earth.

Perma-guard diatomaceous earth is a great non-toxic insecticide, for home, garden and on pets for fleas. Internally for animals it has been found to do no harm and in tests run where animals took it for five years it kept away bacteria and parasites. Wally told a story of two sheep with brucellosis a serious bacterial illness, next to each other; one was given diatomaceous earth in its food and was alive the next morning, the other did not survive.

Diatomaceous earth is used for filtering pool water, this one could be used for filtering water on camping trips or outside the normal system. It is it an excellent resource to replace insecticides that might be used around home, pets or garden, with a non-toxic substance supportive of human health. The greatest precaution, as Wally used to tell us, is just to be careful not to inhale it! I like carrying a supply on camping trips and into the wilderness.

Activated Charcoal

Activated Charcoal is an old-time remedy: It probably goes back to the stone age. We've never tried chewing on a stick of wood burned to black char out of the fire pit, but the right wood would do, in an emergency. Videos online explain how to make your own charcoal with traditional time-honored methods, going back historically in many cultures. It would be fun and useful to try out and make homemade charcoal.

We generally purchase what is called activated (oxygen added) charcoal tablets or capsules at the health food store, considering it an important item for our *"natural first aid kit."* Charcoal is commonly used for poisoning or snake venom because it draws or *adsorbs* hundreds of times its volume, meaning it attracts or magnetizes particles holding them like a magnet to be carried away.

Activated charcoal tablets or caps are an excellent resource, commonly used for stomach gas or indigestion, and have been shown to reduce diarrhea in cancer patients. Charcoal biscuits were sold in England in the early 19th century for gas and stomach troubles. Activated charcoal is used in acute poisoning, and has also been found to remove pesticide residue from the body. It is a great addition to a cleanse for elimination of heavy metals, mercury and pesticides. Carbon removes chlorine and other impurities in home water filtration, but does not remove fluoride. (Do NOT use prepared charcoal for the grill internally, as it often contains chemicals).

Flower Remedies

Flower Remedies are low potency homeopathic solutions made from flowers and plants, to harmonize and balance the emotional body. Edward Bach had a gift for developing these gentle flower remedies, by putting blossoms in a clean glass bowl in water in the sunlight to extract their essence. "...They cure not by attacking the dis-ease, but by flooding our bodies with beautiful Vibrations of our higher nature, in the presence of which disease melts away as snow in the sunshine. There is no true healing unless there is a change in outlook, peace of mind, and inner happiness."

All fear must be cast out; it should never exist in the human mind...The cause of all our troubles is self and separateness, and this vanishes as soon as LOVE and the knowledge of the great Unity become part of our natures. ... A person's body is the objective manifestation of his internal nature; he is the expression of himself, the materialization of the qualities of his consciousness.

Edward Bach 1886-1936
The Bach Flower Remedies

Flower essences can be obtained from natural health suppliers or online, with books available, and numerous flower essences produced by gifted Beings. Enjoy Lightening Body-Mind-Heart, support your movement into Higher thought-emotional Frequencies with emotional clearing. RESOURCES: The Bach Centre, La Vie de la Rose Flower Essences

Essential Oils

In Ancient times Essential Oils were valued as it takes much of a natural substance to produce the oils. Several companies make high quality oils and offer amazing combinations anti viral-fungal-bacterial and supportive of Well-Being. This is an entire field of study, so do your research, learn which ones you are drawn to and use regularly. They're addicting!

Herbs and Spices - Super Immunity Secrets

We LOVE herbs and spices fresh and dried! Senses respond in a kitchen where food is being prepared with herbs and spices. We hunger for scents, frequencies and energies that herbs and spices bring into our lives. It's easy to learn how to add herbs and spices to dishes both hot and cold, saturating the dish with super micro-nutrients and subtle miraculous, nurturing, healing qualities. It is said that plants foods when taken into the body actually communicate with and harmonize energy in the cells.

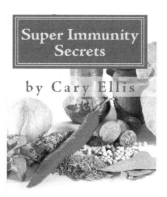

Cary's book, *Super Immunity Secrets*, available on Amazon and Kindle, contains 175 clinical references on herbs and spices, and 50 vegan-vegetarian recipes enriched by these nourishing elements. Once you have a few herbs blessing your kitchen, you won't ever be without them. Growing them in your garden, or in pots around the house is a wonderful addition to a healthy home, as are the fresh supplies of dried bulk herbs and spices obtainable at your local health food store or co-op.

Herbs and spices contain some of the deepest neurological links for our DNA coding, connecting us to literally thousands of years of humanity walking in Earth-Wisdom, flowing with the seasons living in harmony with the natural World. Herbs bring us subtle messages through energies of nature, Earth Mother Gaia and plant elementals.

Spices and herbs contain micronutrients, and even their scents offer gifts to the body. They evolved through natural selection over thousands of years. They offer potentized intrinsic Life elements, that cannot be identified in a laboratory. They bring eternal gifts for the Body when they bless us with their presence. Treasure your sources, your plant cuttings, seeds and starts to be shared with friends, family and community.

Here is a quick sampling:

Cilantro *detoxes mercury* - add to soups, salads. Cilantro Pesto - grind together in food processor: 1 bunch cilantro, 1 bunch parsley, 5-6 cloves garlic, salt, lemon, 1/-2 - 1 cup walnuts or pine nuts, 1/2 cup olive oil, dash lemon or lime juice. Yum! Have on toast, sandwiches, salads or by the spoon. Great detoxifier.

Garlic *natural anti-biotic, contains allicin* - very similar to Penicillin. Use in soups, salads, sandwiches and salad dressings. Teddi's grandkids love slices of raw garlic on crackers during "cold" season. Chlorophyll or parsley helps take away the garlic smell, as does peppermint. As a more "sociable" resort, garlic capsules offer some of the elements of raw garlic.

Garlic is high in selenium: decreases toxic affects of fluoride and mercury binds with them; assists with glutathione production and the conversion of T4 to T3 supporting healthy thyroid function. Selenium supports healthy DNA, keeps unhealthy molecules from reproducing, inhibits tumor growth and causes death of cancerous and precancerous cells. Positive effects increase when taken with iodine. Metal Detox: garlic-cilantro juice with chlorella

Ginger - Supports digestion, add fresh to soups, stir-fry, smoothies, juices

Turmeric - Shown to be as *effective anti-inflammatory* as Hydrocortisone. Warm up in almond or coconut milk for an evening beverage.

Medical Marijuana - Successfully used in cancer treatment pets and people

ACTIVATE NEW FREQUENCIES: Herbs and spices subtly help remove layering, and bring Higher Frequencies to our physical vehicle with micro-nutrition. These are true gifts of the natural World, that smooth out our neurobiological response to Life, making our transit through things that come up happen with greater ease.

Probiotics

Probiotics are essential microorganisms, naturally found in a healthy intestinal track. Once we have taken antibiotics (against life) even once, we kill off the most beneficial, and it is important to repopulate them. Bifidus is the bacteria found in the gut in infancy, killed off when a first antibiotic is taken. Get to know and use raw cultured foods such as sauerkraut, kimchee, miso, yogurt, kombucha, natural pickles and more; also capsules and liquids can be found at health food suppliers. Repopulate healthy bacteria in the gut for wellness and protection of well-being. The are a key subtle factor within the body that assists us to fight illness and stay well. One young mother we know keeps probiotics capsules in the house, and when anyone in her family is fighting off a cold or sickness, she loads them up with probiotics, supporting the body's natural immunity.

Food Grade Hydrogen Peroxide, MMS, Colloidal Silver

Food grade hydrogen peroxide was first used in 1920 by IV to successfully treat a pneumonia epidemic. In the 1940's Father Richard Willhelm, pioneer in promoting peroxide use, reported on it being used to treat everything from bacterial-related mental illness to skin disease and polio. It has been used successfully for cancer and a list of other illness. Its effectiveness has to do with its extra molecule of oxygen.

Food grade hydrogen peroxide 10-35% is purchased from health food suppliers. ALWAYS dilute before using as this concentration is dangerous. (Do not use drug store type as it contains additives not to be taken internally. Do not use hair products). Look up proper dilutions. Once diluted it can be used to support internal and external cleansing. Do your research before use. It is also used for disinfecting externally. Much information is available at numerous sites.

MMS is chlorine dioxide. Drops are mixed with citric acid to activate and diluted in water to drink. It has been used now to cure hundreds of cases of HIV, malaria, parasites and more. Jim Humble has spent many years working to educate on the value of MMS. His educational materials are very informative. MMS generally needs to be purchased in the U.S. as a water purifier. Do your research. This is a great and useful item to have on hand, excellent for traveling with exposure to microorganisms.

Colloidal silver is water that has been exposed to silver so retains the memory, frequency or small amount of silver in it. It is taken internally as an antibiotic, and is so potent it was used by the military to clean wounds in Afghanistan. Can be made o bought.

Restructuring Water

Natural water carries great Life-force for the body. This is a great way to restore charge to water that has traveled through pipes. Use a short piece of PVC pipe 8-12." Add another piece of pipe to cup over end, with added piece on bottom to Create a smaller outlet. Get non-toxic clear glass marbles and fill the pipe. This will allow the water to flow in vortex motions like eddies in current, mimic flow of nature through the marbles, creating a natural charge. Simply pour water through marbles in pipe into cup. Drink.

Sunshine, Solar Rays, Vitamin D3, Fresh Air

Who loves to be outdoors? We Are Solar Earth Beings. Get inspired to be outside whenever you can. Escape the indoor prison of our modern Lifestyle. If you live in a winter climate learn about and use Vitamins D3 and K2 (Jeff Bowles books), take a trip to warmer climes; photosynthesis with your skin. Solar energies on our bodies play a profound role in rejuvenating glandular function, supporting youthfulness and vitality. Raise your frequency with Solar Energy Now! Be Radiant! Smile! ♥

Chapter 9

Supportive Modalities

*Once the power of frequency is understood,
it's easy to bring the body back to balance.
Happy cells are the body's equivalent to bliss.*

Thomas Stone M.D.
Environmental Medicine

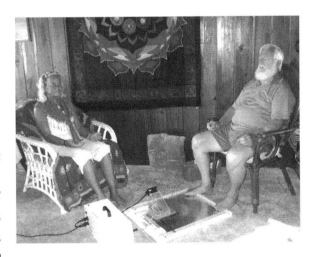

Do we understand yet that we are energy beings? It is a very big leap after so many eons of living and believing our World is simply mechanical parts, Now revealing we are made of energy. Even our bodies are made up of fast moving particles, our senses interpret as solid form yet constantly in motion.

As matter emerges from the *Field of Possibilities* it forms spinning atoms made of protons neutrons, electrons and smaller particles, leptons and quarks. As comprehension grows we view our World in an expanded way. Exciting remedial measures are emerging that support the Body by reading, engaging, adjusting and balancing its natural energetic electromagnetic systems.

These systems measure what is inhibiting or over-amping natural energy flow. Thinking we have an illness or that an illness is incurable, is a mis-understanding of how our Body operates. The question is, "How much are we willing to shift our thoughts and Lifestyle, and use supportive modalities to restore flow of Innate Creative energy without interruption, gifting us with wellness and vitality as our reward!

What we can Be, experience and do is slowed only by lingering old programs within us and associated habits. We are entering a new paradigm of human existence, breaking free from old conditioning, and growing into our potential to operate without limits forever! Our favorite *Remedial Measures* help us refresh our neurobiology, as we shed old layers of inhibiting thought-emotion. The first thing to ask ourselves when we're feeling sick, unwell, un-comfortable, or that dis-ease or de-generation is brewing, is to Leap into our "Greater Self," and ask self, "Self, where am I "shut down" on a physical, thought or emotional level? And how can I clear it quickly, easily?

> Between stimulus and response there is a space... In that space is our power to choose our response. In our response lies our growth and our freedom.
>
> *Dr. Viktor Frankl (1905-1997)*
> *Auschwitz Survivor, "Man's Search for Meaning"*

This can be a scary question (this is why we're dis-eased, because this information was so painful we shut it away in the first place), and we might not know how to unravel it. For this reason, wonderful remedial measures can help us regain and keep balance in our organism, while we're learning to clean out deeper content at cause. Old "corrupt data," carbon-based thought-emotion crystallizes in the body creating dis-comfort and dis-ease as a feedback mechanism. To dissolve the crystallization and free ourselves from its associated data we move through things we've likely been "stuck" in for years.

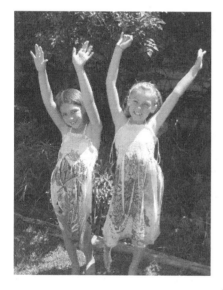

Tony Robbins taught us to use Pattern Interrupts to get out of being *Stuck!* This means exploring new ways to move out of "normal" mode. Surprise yourself, jump up-and-down or just Smile to access a new state of Being! As our physiology changes, our thought-emotional content shifts. Get out of being STUCK Now!!! Move! Breathe! Smile! Play with a friend, *Leap for Joy! Laugh!*

As we move out of our old "stuck" states, we can access greater clarity. We have the option to shape ourselves anew and choose to open up! It's vitally important to LOVE ourselves without judgment or expectation, with full self-acceptance just as we are. As William Shakespeare said, *"There is nothing good or bad but our thinking makes it so."* Upcoming remedial measures are of great assistance to move forward with deep clearing to bring Wellness and Vitality, shedding dis-integrative old patterns.

> I was very afraid at the beginning, until Master told me that pain isn't the truth; it's what you have to get through in order to find the truth.
>
> Deepak Chopra MD
> *The Return of Merlin*

There is no dark or light, no good or evil; *all there is is energy* and how we qualify it with our thought-emotion, conscious-unconscious Mind-Energy. We have the opportunity every moment, to step into a self healing, regenerative mode, where our cells wake up, spin faster and take out the "garbage" for vitality and well-being! *"Tell the truth quicker, have more fun per hour!"*

As long as we carry fear and hostility in Mind-Body structure, we crave things and express thoughts that bathe our tissues in acidic fluids, sustaining the state of fear or hostility crystallized in our cellular structure. It takes choice of "will" to to follow a "higher path" to let go ten thousand generations of blame-fear-hostility. The purpose of remedial measures is to ease and accelerate our restorative process.

Each individual practitioner has their own belief and method of expressing their craft. They may or may not fully "get" what you are learning here or they may (you can always introduce them to it). Seek out those who harmonize with your objectives. Learn what modalities work best for you. Different practitioners and methodologies will serve you better at different times, depending on your level of density or Lightness of Being. We offer short definitions here to assist you in finding helpful services to meet your needs. Do your own research of practitioners in your area to find those who are most supportive.

Breath Work

Conscious use of the Breath has been an active part of healing techniques for thousands of years. Simple relaxation and focusing on the Breath as a meditation in and of itself, gradually shifts us internally. During the last century Rebirthing and Holotropic Breath work were developed and became popular. They are most often practiced with a facilitator, to release holding patterns in Body-Mind.

Holding the Breath is a residual of blame-fear-hostility mode, usually learned in childhood, continuing until Attention is brought to it. dr. michael ryce developed Stillpoint which we do a version of in our programs, and he and his instructors do as well. Releasing through Breath with Stillpoint detaches layers of "corrupt data" from Body-Mind, conscious-unconscious, and supports us in entering an expanded state.

Placing Attention on clearing thought-emotion with our "goal canceling" processes, we Breathe through whatever comes up. It's important to note thought crystalized in Body goes through 3 stages while releasing: 1. solid crystals, 2. liquid - tears, 3 vapor - dissipates. Breathing through, rather than getting "stuck" in crying is helpful to move layers of old pain to be transmuted into vapor.

Breathing through the layers moves us through them much more quickly, rather than crying, which is a way to hold onto our resistance. Breathing helps us keep clearing the old "data banks" of the unconscious. In the Ancient Aramaic it says that when Yeshua-Jesus was with a crowd, he "Breathed them." With no context for what that meant, it was translated in the Bible as he "Breathed on them." dr. michael ryce's work with the Aramaic brings forward that Yeshua-Jesus "Breathed them," or taught them to Breathe, to release unconscious data in the true Aramaic Forgiveness process.

Breathe. Breathe. Breathe. Breathe...

Find a friend to support you in Breathing through things as they come up with your "goal canceling process," when layers surface. Breathing activates *Khooba* LOVE filter in the brain for *Perceptions*; Smiling activates *Rakhma* LOVE filter in the brain for our *Intentions*; important neurobiological reasons to Breathe and SMILE. [Part 2: MIND]

EFT - Emotional Freedom Technique or Tapping

EFT tapping is a very simple and effective method of rewiring our neurobiology, by tapping lightly with one's own fingertips on meridian points on head, face and more, while issues clear and new thoughts replace them. It's easy to learn how to do tapping on yourself, and it is also done by practitioners.

EFT tapping is beneficial to incorporate for anyone desiring greater clarity, well-being and empowerment. We make the biggest changes when we "free the resistance." This "rewiring" is important for the **21st Century Superhuman** toolbox to transform stored trauma and drama into positive and productive states.

This is an extremely powerful technology to utilize along with the Ancient Aramaic Forgiveness goal canceling processes to literally remove thousands of generations of "corrupt data," and then support re-wiring of our neural systems. As we clear our unconscious container of "old data" EFT tapping helps establish and sustain our new state of Being; beneficial to integrate into daily routine.

EFT has become very popular, with many easy tutorials online. Gary Craig developed EFT in the early 90's. A Stanford engineer, he trained in Dr. Roger Callahan's Thought Field Therapy or TFT, which became the father of EFT. They worked together with a woman client who was terrified of water. After doing tapping with her, she was instantly so unafraid she was willing to go swimming.

At www.emofree.com Gary (the originator's) free tutorials show how to do tapping yourself, with many other videos available as well such as Nick Ortner's Tapping Summit. Over five years of working with clients, Gary discovered that the sequence of tapping was basically irrelevant. He says, "Memories buried alive never die, they just show up in a bigger, uglier way." Robert Smith's FastEFT is also excellent, with instructions on YouTube.

Essential Oils and Aromatherapy

Essential oils and combinations are a fabulous addition to Healthy Lifestyle. Recent studies show that plant essences communicate with the cells of the body, interacting with them with Innate wisdom. Using essential oils on a regular basis is powerfully protective and beneficial. Also called Aromatherapy, essential oils shift body frequencies and assist it to clear, passing the blood-brain barrier and interacting with the body at subtle levels. Essential oils have been used for thousands of years as medicines, incense, insect repellent, perfume, antiseptic, anti-inflammatory, analgesic - pain relief, much proven scientifically in recent years. Undiluted oils are known as therapeutic grade and should be diluted with carrier oils. Dilute essential oils have been rubbed on baby's spines as young as a day old, and on mama's tummies before birth.

Aerial diffusion: fragrance; aerial disinfection; Vibrational clearing

Direct inhalation of scent: respiratory disinfection, decongestion, expectoration; psychological and neurobiological clearing and balancing

Topically in carrier oil: massage, body and energy work; baths, foot soaks, compresses and therapeutic skin care

Crystals, Gemstones, Gem Elixirs,

Once exposed to natural essential oils and their combinations, they become a fantastic addition to h

Bodywork: Massage, Feldenkrais, Rolfing, Reflexology, Point Holding, Acupressure, Hot Stone Massage, and more

In our modern culture it's easy to lose touch with the Body. Touch, and the comfort of bodywork can play an intrinsic role to restore health and well being. Good bodywork is extremely healing, and most of us could give and receive more. The soothing comfort of touch from friend, family member or practitioner, can assist with letting go of layers with ease, through both bodywork and energy work.

Wonderful styles of body work have evolved, that help restore balance, equilibrium and connectedness within the Body. Some swear by "their form of bodywork," which just shows the difference between bodies and individual needs. If you are drawn to a practitioner and a particular style of massage or bodywork, and can afford it, enjoy the regular therapy of receiving; in fact signing up for regular sessions or a series can produce deep and long-lasting results.

There are great techniques to good massage, yet most of us have an innate sense of the Body, when we allow ourselves. Access your sensitivity by working on someone else and letting intuition direct. Trading with a friend and giving each other feedback assists us to grow in this important art. Massage and energy work do not necessarily have a sexual connotation although they are used with Ancient Tantra. They are wonderful tools through which we assist one another in our personal, physical-spiritual Evolution, removing old layers that no longer serve and vitalizing Joyful Being.

Owning a massage table shared between several, is a fine resource for exchanging bodywork and energy balancing. Learning as you go is supportive of inner healing for both giver and receiver. Add essential oils, Breathwork and energy balancing for an extraordinary experience. This is also a wonderful nurturing exchange between partners in a relationship, with agreement as to what focus to take. Massage and energy work can easily be done as an exchange between friends. There are hundreds of types of massage, descriptions available online. To become a practitioner be sure to check with regulations in your area.

"Energy Medicine:" Acupuncture, Reiki, Polarity, Crystals, Qi-Gong, Chakra Balancing, Meridian Healing, Matrix Energetics, Sound Healing, Crystal Bowls, Gongs, Tai Chi, Martial Arts and more

"Energy Medicine" emerged with the Indus Valley civilization around 3,500 B.C. and fed out into many cultures and practices in the Eastern World, China, India, Japan, Asia, Tibet and more. Acupuncture, Vedic system, Qi-Gong, Chakras, Gongs, Chanting, Reiki and other energy balancing practices care for the body as an energy vehicle, with energetic pathways not perceived by modern medicine in the West.

The various arts of energy medicine are extremely effective, non-invasive, supporting the body in regaining balance so it can continue with its movement towards wellness. Most of them include dietary practices predominantly toward vegetarian. Several recognize emotions being stored in the unconscious with practices for clearing.

Certain forms of energy work are done with hands off the body or lightly touching to activate, balance, energize, shift and move energy *Fields*. Again, we all have the ability to sense energy *Fields* in and around the body and can learn to support them, by working on one another, apprenticing or following our intuition.

In Lynn McTaggart's book, *"The Field"* she reminds us that *everyone*, even those who don't think they do, have intuitive sensitivities. As we learn to exchange healing touch and support, it can be bonding among community, friends or family, and nurturing and healing to all.

It is relatively easy these days to locate practitioners or teachers of Acupuncture, Qi-gong, Reiki, Crystal Bowls and more. Participating in groups who use gongs chanting and movement is a great way to cultivate energy enhancing practices.

Yoga - Hatha, Kundalini, Ashtanga, Bikram, Hot, Iyengar, Vinyasa, more

Although physical yoga popularized in the modern World, might be "exercise," it is also essentially a therapeutic blending of Body-Mind-Heart-Spirit with the goal of raising consciousness, emerging from thousands of years of highly evolved Ancient Tradition. Indus Valley Civilization dating to 3,500 B.C.E. depicted figures in yoga or meditation poses on clay tablets. Emerging current views on "reality," align with more with these inherited Ancient Teachings than with recent science.

Yoga is designed to keep Body and Breath flowing, activating energy pathways, glands and chakras, by objectifying Enlightenment, through clarifying the physical form to reflect more Light. Many yogic traditions range from hatha yoga, often taught to beginners and accessible to seniors, though it also ranges to powerful disciplines along with others such as kundalini and ashtanga.

Yoga is inherited from Ancient Vedic teachings of 7000 years ago, a practice associated with attaining a state of "permanent peace or bliss." Yoga is a Sanskrit word meaning union, interpreted as union with the divine. Later ideas associate it with samadhi or concentration leading to union with the divine, and another to yoke. Someone who practices yoga or follows the yogic philosophy with a high level of commitment, is called a Masculine yogi or Feminine yogini. The ultimate goal of Yoga is "liberation."

Incorporating yoga at any age, is fun and of great benefit to creating a flowing connection with Body, Mind and Heart. Attention to Breath and stretching movements bring the focus inward, like a moving meditation. Most classes are set up so one can progress at their own pace. Attending classes until developing our own routine is an optimum way to learn and integrate this Ancient Art into the Life. *For those so drawn, yoga is a wonderful addition to the self-healing awakening journey!!!*

Naturopathy

Naturopathy, or naturopathic medicine, is a form of alternative medicine supporting vital energy or vital force of the bodily processes such as metabolism, reproduction, growth, and adaptation. Naturopathy favors a holistic approach with non-invasive treatment and generally avoids the use of surgery and drugs. Among naturopaths, there is a broad range of treatment and support for wellness.

NAET

This is another brilliant, gentle effective method to rewire the neurobiology, from which we have seen profound results. NAET uses a gentle systematized approach to remove sensitivities, pain, allergies, vaccination residual, through a combination of meridian stimulation and homeopathic doses of allergens.

> According to Oriental medical principles, "when the body is in perfect balance, no disease is possible." Any disturbance in the homeostasis can cause disease. Any allergen capable of producing a weakening muscular effect in the body can cause disturbance in homeostasis. Hence, diseases can be prevented and cured by maintaining homeostasis. According to acupuncture theory, acupuncture and/or Acupressure...is capable of bringing the body to...homeostasis by removing...blockages from energy pathways known as meridians. When the blockages are removed, energy can flow freely through the energy meridians, bringing the body in perfect balance.
>
> *NAET, naet.com*

"NAET® was discovered by Dr. Devi S. Nambudripad in 1983. Nambudripad's Allergy Elimination Techniques, also known as NAET, are a non-invasive, drug free, natural solution to alleviate allergies of all types and intensities, using a blend of selective energy balancing, testing and treatments...from acupuncture/acupressure, allopathy, chiropractic, nutrition, kinesiology.." Over 12,000 practitioners Worldwide. www. naet.com This type of "rewiring" is very helpful for the *21st Century Superhuman, Quantum Lifestyle* toolbox for clearing and creating balance, so that we can continue unwinding our self-healing journey gently and with ease.

Chiropractic

Chiropractic is a familiar methodology, yet a broad range of practices are embraced by many chiropractors supporting wellness. Thought of as regarding the spine, yet broadly it is about balancing energy channels of the body. There are many excellent chiropractors and a broad range of methodologies. When seeking a practitioner, find one whose work is particularly effective for *you*.

CRA - Contact Reflex Analysis

CRA®, a focused type of "muscle testing" scores the body's reflexes to determine what the body needs to operate at the greatest vitality in all situations. It is practiced by chiropractors and other practitioners trained in it, can be found by searching online. It is an excellent, non-invasive system using the body's bioelectricity to determine how to achieve optimal function.

Contact Reflex Analysis was developed by Dr. Dick Versendaal, D.C. with whom Teddi had the good fortune of interning and sharing clients with for over twenty years. Dr. Versendaal said, "It's about connecting the Brain and the Heart which is where the Soul resides;" and quoted DD Palmer, founder of chiropractic, "Too much or too little energy is disease." Several of his books are available online with details.

When you're right with Innate, Innate is right with you.

D.A. Versendaal D.C.
Founder, Contact Reflex Analysis

Dr. Versendaal describes how CRA® works, "Research has proven the human body to be like a computer, made of the brain (electrical generator and memory bank) and thousands of miles of...nerves, connecting every organ, gland and tissue of the body. They also connect with "breaker switches" called contact reflexes. By contacting these reflexes, using the body's muscular system as an indicator, we are able to monitor function of body systems." *Standard Process* products often used with CRA®.

Homeopathy

Homeopathy began with the work of Dr. Samuel Hahnemann (1755-1843) who as a physician was disillusioned with medical treatment of the day. He developed a system of taking energetic doses of substances to remove the same symptoms they caused in physical doses. He developed the philosophy, "Let like be cured by like."

A homeopathic remedy is made by diluting the substance into potencies shaken in water hundreds of times until there is no physical substance left, only the energetic frequency of the substance that Creates the symptoms. When ingested or even sniffed by the "patient" it can negate symptoms and participant moves toward wellness.

Homeopathy is noninvasive, can provide amazing results, yet is a bit complex with thousands of remedies. Homeopaths take a case history to determine a remedy to help restore vital force, assisting the body to move into its own healing process.

HOMEOPATHIC FIRST AID KIT: A homeopathic first aide kit, with low potency remedies 30c can be used in everyday situations with outstanding results. Most come with a small description sheet covering main symptoms of each remedy with with which one can easily work through symptoms that arise of cold, flu, insect bites, wounds and other everyday occurrences. A simple book and first aid kit is a great way to learn and use homeopathy at home. For more in-depth situations it's best to consult a practitioner who is familiar with remedies.

I had a brown recluse bite on my foot and was able to take homeopathic remedies from my first aid kit and work through the symptoms as each new symptom emerged, I would take another remedy for that symptom and within two weeks the bite was gone. ♥ *Cary*

Radionics

Radionics uses a non-traditional form of homeopathy. A small machine measures electromagnetic *Fields* through meridians or energy pathways of the body, providing a readout that can then be fed through a plate or device into water. The water becomes potentized with these energetic frequencies that when taken then assist to neutralize those patterns in the body. Such a process is a gentle powerful support for moving into greater balance. Radionics is supportive of stronger Life-Force for plants, pets and people.

I have known excellent practitioners over the years who use radionics machines. These simply require a photo, hair or some representation of the person, in order to determine correct frequencies to potentize a bottle of water to be a matching energetic signature or imprint, for the symptoms the person, pet or plant has. A traditional homeopath would consider this a transgression, however I have seen profound results with this science also. Radionics machines work with rates and frequencies, and Create a homeopathic response to eliminate the pattern of the dis-order or dis-ease from the body. ♥ *Teddi*

Electromagnetic Frequency Machines

Numerous sophisticated energy machines are leading us into our future of healing, with energy frequencies and waves. Energy healing is Now suggested by the American Cancer Society: "Electromagnetic therapy involves the use of electromagnetic energy to diagnose or treat disease...low-voltage electricity, magnetic *Fields*, radio waves, electromagnetic energy generated for this purpose. Some systems: BioResonance Tumor Therapy, Rife machine, Zapper...and more."

Electromagnetic therapy, lasers, light, electromagnetic resonance biofeedback, and pulsed electromagnetic *Fields* are available, some developed by NASA and Russian space programs, now found in private sector around the World.

Two types systems exist: Some test the body's meridians for weakness or blockages, returning a homeopathic signal to neutralize or equalize the energy patterns. Others emit frequencies, light or wave patterns, also effective. *What we come back to is this:* use all these wonderful tools to assist the body back on track; *AND* there is only one *"cure all:"* clean cells and oxygen respiration; restoring alkalinity with baking soda, simple natural foods and cleansing of Body-Mind.

One of the greatest scientists in history much of whose work around healing and free energy was destroyed was Nicola Tesla. His brilliant inventions of radio, remote control, alternating current, induction motors and more paved the way for modern society. Royal Rife (1888-1971) developed the Rife healing technology, with the ability to cure cancer, suppressed by the establishment. Rife machines are available today, and emit frequencies to negate cancer, herpes and other disorders. There is a resurgence of healing tools with Teslas' energy discoveries.

> The day Science begins to study nonphysical phenomena, it will make more progress in one decade than in all previous centuries of its existence.
>
> Nikola Tesla (1856-1943)

Nikola Tesla and Royal Rife's work are closely related in the field of Bioelectromagnetic Healing. For a person interested in using these devices further research is suggested to discover possibilities available in this field.

Many astounding inventions have been suppressed by "powers that be" during the last few centuries, (Now diminishing in power as we shift into Heart frequencies where they can no longer exist). As we Live in Joy as free sovereign creative beings, we change our global culture, based in our own true value and well-being for all. Old paradigm systems will no longer hold frequency in our World, as we *shift our resonance* from blame-fear-hostility to embrace our True Design LOVE.

Ralph Ring Natural Scientist worked with Otis Carr (Tesla Prodigy) on Alternative Technologies and Teleportation. He was One of three to pilot a Man-Made Spaceship, the OTC-X1. Ralph works on producing advanced technologies based on Tesla's work at BlueStarEnterprise.com, reminding us that Tesla said our greatest scientific developments will come when we understand them in light of Consciousness.

Our quest on the Earth-plane, is to reopen to the totality of the Heart. *Quantum Lifestyle* claims Health and Longevity as our birthright, using advanced science to Create balance, as we free ourselves from old Vibrational content, shifting our "reality" Now. Doing so frees us to choose wiser, more sovereign Lifestyle practices for ourselves and Loved ones, restoring a Truly Healthy Planetary Earth Community, founded in our True Design, LOVE. ♥

Part 4 Body: Section 3

Dis-Ease The Illusion

God implanted in your mind neural structures which will guide you when they are active. If they are active, you who follow these instructions will come into conscious possession of and be able to use this latent guidance system, designed to make available thoughts and actions that will increase your happiness and well-being.

Yeshua (Jesus)
Aramaic translation of TOUVEYHOUN - Begins each Beatitude, dr. michael ryce

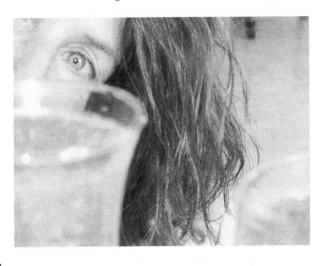

What lens are we looking through? Is the glass half empty or half full? Are you on the way *up* the spiral, or you are you on the way down? A young friend once said "if we're on the Titanic, and it's going down, we might as well party," which many in World have adopted as their philosophy. Based on Sir Isaac Newton's Mechanical Law of Inertia, we know it takes effort to get moving new directions beyond the status quo surrounding us. Let's Be inspired to get our inertia going, as it is so worth it!

Health, Well-Being, Vitality and reversal of dis-ease begin in Mind-Heart. Dis-ease is a *learning tool,* Mirroring to us where we are disconnected from Source - our True Power Supply, where there's a "logjam in the river," or where we still carry thought Not of LOVE. Tools in Part 2: MIND teach us very specific skills to remove this old content.

Learning through pain and suffering "sandpapers us," removing rough edges. Awakening teaches us, *"I'm not my Mind, I'm not my Body, Immortal Self I Am,"* yet it is a Journey to bring this in to focus. Our commercialized culture lures us with every "cure-all" imaginable, take this or that to lose weight, get rid of symptoms or feel good, promising to solve ALL our problems from the outer. The only way these things will truly change is to address the Vibration *inside* us of old thought-emotional energy, holding them in form.

Once we change our Mind-energy we are more willing to implement Healthy Lifestyle habits, such as natural healthy foods, cleansing and detox, to assist the body to move up in frequency, so that old thought-emotional content will surface and be released. Tools and habits harmonize with the Law of Cause and Effect, powerful when rightly understood.

Dr. Esselstyn, Dr. Barnard and Dr. Campbell all demonstrated over 20-30 years, dramatic reversal of potentially *ALL* degenerative conditions in weeks, with vegan low-fat diet. This is also confirmed by *Electrovibratory Rate of Nourishment of Foods* chart in Nutrition chapter. Adopting vegan-vegetarian Lifestyle may seem like a big step right Now, however bless where you are on the path and your own growth process, and consider these steps for Healing, Well-Being and Longevity. As Sun Bear would say, *"The Highest Gift you can give yourself is to Bless Everything and Live as a Blessing to the World."*

Physical detox and clearing of self-destructive thought and habits land us in support of Vitality and Well-Being. Claiming this birthright is one of the greatest steps we will ever take, toward sovereignty and freeing ourselves from self-serving systems. Rewards are Abundance, LOVE, Intelligence and capability to bring our Gifts into the World.

Burdens from past generations' imprints and our early environment are catalogued in our body structure as "crystals" [Dr. John Whitman Ray] or "carbon based data" [dr. michael ryce.] Body and Mind are intertwined, so clearing must happen both from unconscious thought and Body.

If we are stuck in old patterns and covering them up with Life's "obligations," disconnected from the Heart, it's critical to get moving into clearing, releasing, letting go to restore *Essence*. We've developed the cultural idea that if we just "do what's healthy" we'll be fine, yet removing our unconscious "old corrupt data" *is essential*. "Not of LOVE" thought-emotion expresses through eating and living habits that Create a "logjam in the river," which adds up to toxemia in the Body.

> So-called dis-ease is a toxemic crisis. When toxins are eliminated...the sickness passes - automatically health returns. But the dis-ease was not cured; for if the cause is continued, toxins still accumulate, and in due course of time another crisis appears. Unless the cause is discovered and removed, crises will recur until functional derangements will give way to organic dis-ease.
>
> *J.H. Tilden MD (1851-1940)*
> *Toxemia Explained: The True Interpretation of The Cause of All Dis-Ease*

Develop your own pattern of unique healthy habits, shaped around *your* Body-Mind and personal place on the path. Participating from the standpoint of *knowing ourselves,* we use cleansing, mineralization and whole organic foods, superfoods and thought to raise cellular vitality, to assist "corrupt data" to surface and be cleared with LOVE.

High-Frequency Nutrition with hands-on Energy-Balancing by friend or energy worker, opens energy pathways to move out old thought-emotional content. As we remove "corrupt data," we open energy pathways with **21st Century Superhuman Quantum Lifestyle** Habits, inspired by our Newfound vitality. Then our enthusiastic high-frequency Body-Mind-Heart is truly supported in Vitality and Well-Being, and we are on the *Path*, to Living our full Authenticity from the Heart and *Essence*, also known as En-Light-enment. ♥

Chapter 10

Toxemia The Cause Of Dis-Ease

I shall recognize all dis-ease as the result of my transgressions against health laws and I shall undo it with right eating, less eating, fasting, more exercise and right thinking.

Paramhansa Yogananda (1893-1952)
Founder Self-Realization Fellowship, "Autobiography of a Yogi"

During the last century excellent foundational principles were developed for reversing and preventing disease, that still hold true today. They taught how design of our body requires cleansing and Light nutrition to prevent and recover from dis-ease or i-llness.

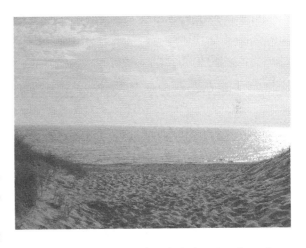

Every so-called dis-ease is a crisis of Toxemia; which means that toxin has accumulated in the blood above the toleration-point, and the crisis, the so-called dis-ease—is a vicarious elimination. Nature is endeavoring to rid the body of toxins. Any treatment that obstructs this effort at elimination baffles nature in her effort at self-curing.

J.H. Tilden MD (1851-1940)
Toxemia Explained: The True Interpretation of The Cause of All Dis-Ease

These valuable principles were described by JH Tilden MD, in his 1926 book, *Toxemia Explained: The True Interpretation of The Cause of All Dis-Ease,* a classic worth reading, available free online. Tilden's foundational principles were adopted by the Natural Hygiene Society and widely used with great success. Retreat centers grew up around these principles of fasting, cleansing, raw and foods and juices, similar to European sanitariums where Tilden gained his early ideas.

To do nothing is also a good remedy.

Hippocrates
Father of Modern Medicine

Foundational principle taught by Tilden is that the Body must be restored to run as a "clean machine." Our cells, bloodstream, organs and glands take in nourishment and eliminate waste. When the system gets overloaded with waste products at cellular, blood and organ level faster than it can eliminate them, "acute" conditions arise, such as stress, exhaustion, cold, flu and fever, as attempts of the body to cleanse and restore balance. Understanding this one principle and how to implement it is *the* Key.

The old saying commonly misinterpreted *"starve a cold, feed a fever,"* actually evolved from this Tilden philosophy, which stated correctly says, *"starve a cold LEST you feed a fever."* This means that ALL illness is the body requesting us to reduce food consumption and support it in cleansing through fasting, juices, living foods and light nutrition. This is what we call a "Healing Crisis." The body is requesting lightening foods, increased fluids, *and* clearing of all Not of LOVE thought (conscious-unconscious).

When confronted with illness, it is helpful to learn to say, "I am cleansing," or "I'm in a detox," rather than saying, "I am sick" (because otherwise this is what we're creating). Follow-up with physical-mental cleansing and detox of Body-Mind. Clearing the unconscious with *Freedom Tools* [Part 2: MIND] addresses how we got "overloaded" or "toxic" in the first place. Then support with Cleansing and Detox, juices, fasting, Ideal Nutrition and Superfoods, with nurturing from natural practitioners, friends and self-care.

Tilden's principles, still true today, are foundational to restoring well-being.

Every so called dis-ease is a crisis of Toxemia; meaning toxins have accumulated in the blood beyond a toleration-point, and the crisis, the so-called dis-ease - call it cold, flu, pneumonia, headache, or typhoid fever - is a vicarious elimination. Nature is endeavoring to rid the body of toxin. Any treatment obstructing this effort baffles nature in her effort at self-curing.

J.H. Tilden MD (1851-1940)
Toxemia Explained: The True Interpretation of The Cause of All Dis-Ease

Repeated overloading the system accumulates toxins and initiates chronic conditions. Cumulative "toxemia" causes suppression of Life-force throughout the Body, resulting in degenerative conditions such as cancer, heart and cardiovascular dis-ease, arthritis, diabetes and numerous other dis-orders. The moment we make different choices with Cleansing and Detoxing Body-Mind, Regeneration kicks in!

Remember, we are *Energy Beings*. Becoming involved in taking care of our own Living vehicle is one of the most exciting, productive actions we ever take, and has been a basic aspect of "waking up," in ALL true spiritual traditions throughout history. We either bemoan our miseries, or engage as Master or Mistress of our Destiny. The *moment* we let go of suppressive habits and clarify thought, nutrition, action and focus, our Life process shifts to move in a *positive direction*. Breathe and Smile.

Taking Health into our own hands by living Response-Ably is one of the most Freeing and self-empowering things we do. It requires awakening from the slumber of television, advertising and general brainwashing common in today's World. Creating alliances with Healthcare practitioners, Naturally and traditionally aligned with us can be helpful.

A physician, naturopath or holistic practitioner can assist with gradually withdrawing from drugs. Natural supplements can assist with this transition, turning suppression into support of Life-force. Modern medicine may "save a Life" to give us "another chance," then practitioners can help restore connection to Life Flow. Interview practitioners to find those harmonious with your philosophy. Find a massage therapist, energy worker, acupuncturist, electro-Vibrational practitioner, chiropractor or medical practitioner comfortable for you, who supports you in Your Journey. LOVE yourself.

True interpretation of cause of dis-ease, and how to cure is an obvious sequence; an antidote to fear, frenzy and the popular mad chasing after so-called cures.

J.H. Tilden MD (1851-1940)
Toxemia Explained: The True Interpretation of The Cause of All Dis-Ease

Pursue your own regenerative process, rather than perpetuating the old "patch it up and get rid of my symptoms" philosophy. Obtain support, nurturing, nourishment and regeneration with well-chosen practitioners, friends and self. *Do your goal canceling process* to remove unconscious thought-emotional content, that Created these blocks in the first place. You may find yourself feeling *TIRED* while in phases of clearing. This is natural as we go through unconscious layers. No matter how deep dark and scary they are, you will never be free until you do your clearing of "old corrupt data." Utilizing numerous resources recommended in this book, we invite you to nourish and cleanse Body-Mind with *LOVE and JOY*. Breathe. Smile. Feeling better is an inside job. Self-LOVE is important.

Every time we align with a "feeling better" thought-emotion, we move in the right direction. We improve, vitality increases, and a sense of well-being takes over as we clear "old data," and take a pro-active role in our self-care. We may hit a "conditional ceiling," where we get to a level of feeling good, yet once there, an old voice inside us says, "I can't do it, or I want to quit." Make this a squeaky or sexy voice just to disempower it! We find the level we're at on the Emotional Tone Scale [Part 3: Spirit] and do more clearing of "old data," [Part 2: MIND] to move beyond tendencies to fall into depressive or suppressed coping. Higher LOVE, extra rest and self-nurturing move us into Enthusiasm! We are here to be Joyful, Creative LOVING Beings. This Journey is about restoring our Authentic Self.

At first to go past a "ceiling" may mean expressing anger or frustration. Share with family and friends you need to do this for your healing, and ask them not to take it personally. Tell them you're having a "clear the shadows moment." Use Goal Canceling to clear items peeking out of your unconscious. Know you may end up doing a "medusa" of worksheets - where one leads into another and you empty the "can of worms," to remove this old thought-emotional toxemia.[Part 2: MIND] Guaranteed, as your Vitality goes up, you *will* access new levels to clear. Be excited as you move past what used to be a "ceiling" and keep moving upscale. This trail leads us to the 6th UNIVERSAL LAW of Cause and Effect, which describes for us how the ever-flowing, Living *Field* of Creation operates:

Chance is but a name for Law not recognized; there are many planes of causation, but nothing escapes the Law." Every thought-emotion, word and action sets in motion an effect that materializes.

What materializes is a direct result of Vibration within us of LOVE or Not of LOVE *Mind-Energy* [Harvard studies - 5% conscious, 95% unconscious]. Simple. We are not used to thinking about dis-ease and illness this way, so it is a learning process to free ourselves from a system that makes *billions off of our deepest fear and ignorance about laws of Life.* Assist your body with its natural process of clearing thoughts not of LOVE, cleansing, healing nourishment, herbs, oils and connecting with nature's energetic Vibrations. Establish a True Path to Wellness with *self-empowering Commitment to your journey* above ALL else.

This helps us get, Be and stay well. When we Live these secrets, vitality goes up, making it easier to *avoid* what's "going around" and avoid future degenerative conditions by establishing Cleanse and Detox habits of Mind-Body on a daily basis. The secret is *"Keep your house clean!"*...Keep Body-Mind clean. Nourish with cleansing, good food, and energy channels kept open with High Frequency thoughts. *Start today!* Start your day with a quart of warm plain or lemon water to cleanse every day! Simple.

Today's buzzwords for **toxemia** are **inflammation** and **acidity**. **When we are on overload, first comes acidity, then irritation, then inflammation, then fibrins (as seen in Live Blood Analysis) then degenerative illness and death.** Each of these strategies is the body's attempt to cleanse and restore alkalinity. The fibrin stage is the body's attempt to make small fibers to cover up tissues at risk, thus fibrous tumors often precede cancerous conditions. Andrew Weil has written excellent current material on inflammation.

Our nutritional and cleansing programs are ALL designed to alkalize the body, reduce inflammation, and support a clean, healing vibratory condition for all around well-being. Juicing or blending raw vegetable soups, great ways to alkalize the body, have now gone mainstream, with these wonderful methods and how to do them, easily accessible to anyone. Natural programs for reducing inflammation and acidity are popular for a good reason, **they work!** You no longer have to be the "odd person out," or do it on your own. Upscale your Life with friends of common interest and share the journey of renewal.

We won't beat cancer by any one approach. I believe it must be multifocal. In other words, beef up the immune system, detoxify, eliminate dental infections and toxic dental materials, alkalinize your body, oxidize the body with oxidation therapy, and give specific nutrients to throw a monkey wrench into cancer's peculiar metabolic pathways.

Robert J. Rowen, MD
Bitter Melon Article, Second Opinion Newsletter

Toxemia seen through a modern lens, is well handled with regular habits of cleansing and detox, part of an everyday routine. Habits to include for an everyday approach of detoxifying and cleansing include:

- water, tea, fresh juices, fasting
- fresh air, natural environments - earth, air, water, sky, sunlight, moonlight, starlight
- walking, running, swimming, yoga, movement , barefoot
- rest, naps, lucid dreaming, deep sleep, introspection, Breathing
- clear thought, prayer, chanting, gongs, bowls, music, meditation [Part 2: MIND]
- Letting go all old thought-emotion Not of LOVE, clearing-unconscious,
    "goal canceling" [Part 2: MIND]
- I Am Creator: Attention on the *Field* is *always* creating [Part 1: SHIFT OF THE AGES]
- Creativity, flowing, allowing, "going general," releasing to the *Field*
- Joyful Enthusiasm! Laughter, Smiling, Breathing
- Heart Coherence through Deep LOVE, COMPASSION, GRATITUDE
- High-frequency foods and beverages, Superfoods, Water
- Herbs and Extracts, Essential Oils, Homeopathy, Acupuncture, Massage
- Knowing "I Am Creative Being of LOVE," flowing from me to ALL

Doesn't it increase your Energy, just reading this list? When these elements are integrated into the Life, we call it *Quantum Lifestyle!*

Though there are many sincere medical professionals, pharmaceutical companies owned by petroleum companies have hijacked health freedom and knowledge through greed. In hot pursuit of profits their high-dollar lobbying, has instigated laws making it difficult (or illegal) to easily choose the Natural path to Wellness.

Insiders have reported ad campaigns describing dis-ease symptoms 1-3 years prior to release of a drug, so by the time the drug is developed, viewers are convinced they have the symptoms and "must have" the "miracle drug" to "get better." Overuse of prescription drugs is at epidemic proportions, perpetuated by patients *fearfully* desiring instant relief and doctors obliging.

Medical intervention is of benefit, particularly when natural laws of nutrition, cleanse and detox have been ignored. There are many *good* people in medical professions whose greatest interest is well-being of others; yet the system is built around the drug industry's practices of *suppressing symptoms,* rather than encouraging wellness through harmony with Nature. Desire for profit to the detriment of humanity is unsustainable and will not long survive. The more individuals who learn and choose habits supporting Well-Being and we expand our Knowledge and Wisdom, the faster our culture will move beyond this .

If mammograms were really finding deadly cancers sooner (as suggested by the rise in early detection), then cases of advanced cancer should have been reduced in kind. But that didn't happen. In other words, the researchers concluded, mammograms didn't work.

New York Times

Think Progress (online magazine) reports that the megalithic pharmaceutical industry reaped *$84 Billion* in 2012, and *$711 Billion* in the last decade. They continue to shape our medical system into what it is today. NPR's *Talk of the Nation*, Sept. 2011 reported, "Pro Publica investigation shows that many doctors are being paid [to do training, presentation and use equipment] by the same drug companies whose medicines they prescribe." It's easy to take a pill every time we feel bad because our system supports it.

To be well, energized and vital, foundational health requires a clean running body, that establishes its own inner strength. Cleansing and Lightening up nourishment are best resources when sniffles and dis-comforts come around, which also sets us up to avoid later degeneration. This requires self-education and Lifestyle commitment to remove ourselves from the greed-based pharmaceutical system that has dominated our health care industry.

Findings...reveal doctors prescribed antibiotics to 60% of sore throat patients - despite that drugs are only thought to be necessary in about 10% of cases...

Another interesting finding: growing popularity of expensive, broad-spectrum antibiotics such as *Azithromycin,* over tried-and-true drugs like *Penicillin.* Last year the *new York Times* noted that *Azithromycin* "may increase likelihood of sudden death" in adults at risk for heart dis-ease.

Dr. John G. Bartlett, a professor of medicine at Johns Hopkins University School of Medicine, told *the Times* that he believed that overprescription of *Azithromycin* could also contribute to antibiotic resistance. "We use *Azithromycin* for an awful lot of things, and we abuse it terribly," he said. "It's very convenient. Patients LOVE it. 'Give me the *Z-Pak.*' For most of where we use it, the best option is not to give an antibiotic, quite frankly."

If the looming threat of antibiotic resistance isn't reason enough for concern about doctors' free-hand with antibiotics, there's also the considerable cost to our health care system—an estimated $500 million for antibiotics prescribed unnecessarily for sore throat alone between 1997 and 2010. If you include cost of treating side effects of unnecessary antibiotics such as diarrhea and yeast infections, the study's authors estimate costs would increase 40-fold.

Mother Jones
The Scary Truth About Antibiotic Overprescription

Anti-biotic means "against Life." Although there may be times a life is saved by an anti-biotic, they are taken far too often, and kill off healthy microorganisms that belong in the gut. Learning how to Live a healthy *Quantum Lifestyle*, with use of Herbs, Cleansing, Nutrition and Thought fortifies body and immune system, so such drugs are not needed.

One geriatric nurse observing greater confusion and hallucinations with prescribed meds for Alzheimer's said, "Prognosis is the same for patients who take medication and those who don't, the drugs have such terrible side effects I don't know why they are given...." Regular intake of coconut, coconut oil and external use of rosemary oil have been shown to prevent and diminish Alzheimer's and dementia symptoms.

What is average cost for treatment of cancer for one person? $300,000. For the same person to pursue natural treatment to regain wellness, rough estimate is $10,000. Most treatments have been ostracized by the legal-medical system (pushed by big Pharma), to take refuge in less developed countries, and thus difficult to access, yet doable with desire.

What will it take for our "medical" system to be built around cleansing, nutrition and we-llness? Much is up to us. Clear out our blame-fear-hostility from old "corrupt data" stored in our unconscious. LOVE ourselves! Step into self-empowerment. Take Response-Ability for and Live *Quantum Lifestyle* habits to cultivate Wellness. Choose Health practitioners capable of supporting us in this process.

Fidelity oversees 12 million 401K accounts; they reported in 2012 that a retiring person needs $240,000 for out of pocket medical expenses later in Life. Who are they kidding? Shall we wake up to awareness that big business reaps billions from *fear; bringing home necessity* to harmonize our Lives with Well-Being through Natural means?

These examples expose how out of balance these systems are, to which most subject themselves. *As there is no 'out there' out there, we have Created this* in Quantum "reality," and we Create change by waking up and changing ourselves. Thanks to the Natural Health movement of the last 50 years many are Now aware. We know fruits and vegetables are good for us, we know Organic is better. Popularity of juicing, cleansing and detoxing has educated many to lighten up. Herbs and essential oils are now familiar and widely used.

We are understanding cause and meaning of dis-ease, and how to take charge of our Health Destiny. Eternal Flow of Life is toward Health and Well-Being, opened with *Quantum Lifestyle* through Nutrition, Thought clearing, Cleansing and Detox. Once eour connection with Natural habits is understood, we are better able to make choices when and if medical intervention can be beneficial or is needed, thus we access Best of both Worlds.

In developed countries 2/3 deaths are from degenerative illness

- one out of five cancer,
- one out of five heart dis-ease
- one out of 6 diabetic related illness.

Is this *"natural?"* Do we even know what *"natural"* is? How far off track from wholesome Natural Life are we? Does this concern us? Modern or SAD (Standard American Diet common in developed countries) is refined, fried, contains fats, sugars, and large amounts of inhumanely raised animal protein, and has been shown to play a pivotal role in this high preponderance of degenerative i-llness.

ALL degenerative and acute conditions reverse when dietary habits are upscaled to whole food, primarily low-fat, vegan-vegetarian nutrition. ALL choices in this direction have been shown to decrease susceptibility to degenerative conditions. Thoughts also play a role in vitality and choice of habits. Old Fear and Hostility are the greatest toxemia, buried in the 95% unconscious, hidden by denial, and root cause of ALL pain and i-llness.

Next time something is "going around," a cold, congestion, cough, sneeze, digestive upset, or just feeling poorly, Cleanse. Drink warm lemon water. Juice. Make sure colon is clean and support with probiotics. Consume Light raw foods, blended soups, fruit and veggies, juices and water. Detoxify and cleanse to support healthy Body ecology. Cleansing clears out mucous in which bacteria and viruses like to grow, activating Healthy immune response. Remove their habitat. Changing Body's ecology in this way increases immune capability and reduces need for anti-biotics! Clear Mind-Heart.

Clearing Ancient pain (generations) assists us to resolve issues at root cause, opening us to greater flow of Life-force. Rather than asking how to "fix me" or get rid of my symptoms with suppressive medication, I clear my thoughts and adopt a Natural progression to healthier Lifestyle Habits. Are you living Authentically or conforming to fit in? Is there a pull between Innate longing to Create and express *Essence*, yet suppressing self to fit into society, causing lowered Life-force resulting in potential for eventual "sickness.?" How many have lived entire lives doing what they're "supposed" to do...dreaming of the real "me" inside, that might express someday? *There is only ONE YOU! That someday is here, Now!* Imagine the possibilities! Breathe and Smile.

> There is a vitality, a life force, an energy, a quickening that is translated through you into action, and because there is only one of you in all of time, this expression is unique. And if you block it, it will never exist through any other medium and it will be lost. The world will not have it.
>
> *Martha Graham (1894-1991)*
> *Influential Modern Dancer, Presidential Medal of Freedom (1976)*

- When we feel good it's easier to be Happy and attain our dreams.

- Vitality, Health of Body-Mind, and habits of Well-Being are products of Thought

- It's easier to feel good when we let go of toxins in Mind and Body.

- How are you doing with adopting high frequency *Quantum Lifestyle* habits?

- *Journey of a thousand miles begins with the first step. And then the next...*

- Our future civilization and even sustainability on Earth, depend upon us reclaiming Ourselves as Creative, Joyful, Beings we are designed to BE!

- *We are Now Waking Up!*

What Vibrational energy is holding resonance in your World? Are there things you can clear? Are there changes you can make in your Lifestyle to be more Vital, Lean, Fit, Healthy, Clear and Radiant in Body and Mind? Contemplate your answers. Activate new "tuning forks" based in LOVE, Heart, *Essence*, Cleansing, Detox High Frequency Nutrition and *21st Century Superhuman Quantum Lifestyle habits!*

Breathe. Smile. LOVE. ♥

Chapter 11

The Curse Causeless
Shall Not Come

(Proverbs 26:2)

When diet is wrong medicine is of no use.
When diet is correct medicine is of no need.

Ayurvedic Proverb

A Course In Miracles tells us anything Not of LOVE is *part of the illusion*.

Nothing real can be threatened.
Nothing unreal exists.
Herein lies the peace of God.

We merge this with our understanding that the *Infinite Field of Possibilities* is an Eternal sea of *LOVE*, constantly creating, surrounding us, bathing and nourishing us, bringing us Life. It can only Mirror our thought as our "reality," for us to

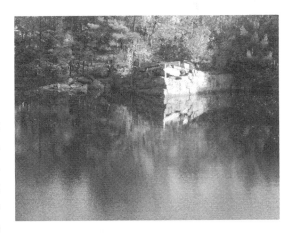

determine whether we have thoughts to clear, to align with our True Design. Anything we experience painful or Not of LOVE is showing us what needs to change *in us*!

Illness, sickness, dis-ease, dis-comfort, pain, war, death, loss, suffering, bothersome things in our day, and *even Joy and Happiness* are a product of our own Mind-energy. It is an amazing *Leap* to embrace and absorb. Clearing our thought-content, our "reality" shifts, and Vibration of our New thought is Mirrored around us by the *Field*. This is an endless feedback loop, letting us know whether or not we have cleared everything to LOVE.

One of the first questions that pops up around this is, "What about my 'Loved One or pet or whoever,' is it my *fault* they are sick, died, etc? These things are not "our *fault*." If we carry a certain Vibrational content in our unconscious, it is simply a law of the Universe that we are will magnetically draw in someone with matching resonance in their genetic or thought history, stored in the unconscious. It is the "hope of the soul" or the nature of the *Field*, that we will go through a process or event with this other Being that plays out this

475

resonance, so both have opportunity to become aware of these issues and clear them with LOVE. It is simple, yet can take a bit of getting used to, as this is the Quantum view of Life.

How much *"blame-fear-hostility-judgment-control"* is in us? Are we ready to let it go? Our genetic, experiential and historical memories, with coded thought-forms (conscious-unconscious), tend to run our Lives from the unconscious. We are Now shedding this dis-integrative energy Forever, for self and future generations. Are you ready to Live as a Joyful Being of LOVE, shifting inside so much that all you experience in the world is LOVE for all things, situations and people? Breathe. Smile. LOVE Yourself.

> Millions of people live a one-sided Life and pass on in incompleteness. God has given each of us a Soul, a mind, and a body, which we should try to develop uniformly. If you have led a Life dominated by worldly influences, do not let the world impose its delusions on you any longer. Control your own Life henceforth; become the ruler of your own mental kingdom. Fears, worries, discontent, and unhappiness all result from a Life uncontrolled by wisdom.
>
> *Paramhansa Yogananda (1893-1952)*
> *Founder Self-Realization Fellowship, "Autobiography of a Yogi"*

Do you get a dose of traditional News on tel-lie-vision? How do you feel about severe weather patterns, bombing, war, nuclear plants at risk? Do you wonder what is happening to your food supply, air and water? How do you feel when a terrorist attack, random shooting or sexual affront is broadcast on the News? Dwelling in fear holds such fearful things in form, as our Attention on the *Field*. [Part 1: SHIFT OF THE AGES] Are you ready to reframe and release this *Creation from within YOU so New can form in LOVE?*

You are most likely in a wonderful place, with a wonderful friends, family, relatively comfortable by global standards; yet *what is buried in your unconscious resonating subtly "Not of LOVE," (worries, dis-comforts, news)?* **What is your most productive self-inquiry, that will allow you to shift awareness to change your "reality" and World NOW?**

> The mark of your ignorance is the depth of your belief in injustice and tragedy. What the caterpillar calls the end of the world, the master calls a butterfly.
>
> *Richard Bach*
> *Illusions, The Adventures of a Reluctant Messiah 1977*

Our Health, Well-Being, Relationships, Abundance, Vitality and even Physical World change, as we clear our "old data" and thus clean up our Vibration. Pollution, Chemtrails, GMO's, leaky nuclear power plants, Love and bank accounts, all change the instant we cancel, release, let go Ancient corrupt Mind-energy (conscious-unconscious-generational-environmental) and step into our *True Design LOVE*. There is more to our existence than meets the eye or has been commonly given credit for; *play with it and let it work for you...*

> Biology is the feedback mechanism
> for the universe to learn more about itself.
>
> *Nassim Haramein*
> *Transformational Physicist, Founder, The Resonance Project*

ALL experienced in Body-Mind: pain, pleasure, well-being, dis-ease, are feedback of our thought resonance. It is a puzzle, unwinding what is at cause. How do we do this? We start with what is closest at hand. Whatever issues are up in Mind-Body are revealed by what *WE FEEL.* This is our point of focus, which we use for doing worksheets, the *Ancient Aramaic Forgiveness* freedom tools, to clear issues surfacing. [Part 2: MIND]

The further we dig down, the more we offload "old data," surfacing in the situation. If you have a child or partner with issues, work on *your own stuff. This is the only place you can change it.* **Doing the process reveals the process. Committing to actually doing 3-5 worksheets per day, will teach you more about your own internal content than anything else in this experience!** There is no 'out there' out there (no one else). "Cleanup" happens within. Others Mirror what lies in the shadows of our unconscious. At first this is difficult, yet as we unravel these threads they make more sense, and the Lights go On!

Dissolving false premises we have surrounded ourselves with in this modern culture, we recognize how our thoughts "Not of LOVE," hold dis-harmonious Vibration expressing in our Bodies and our World. We begin to recognize, "The curse causeless does not come." ALL the *Field* or *Divine Matrix* returns to us is based on resonance within us. ALL "Not of LOVE" within us, is part of the illusion in which we've been playing. We learn to see truth of our thought being revealed in interactions between self and others. This removes any need for judgment or control, as we take Response-Ability for our own Mind-energy.

> To extend is a fundamental aspect of God... In the creation, God extended Himself to His creations and imbued them with the same loving Will to Create. You have not only been fully Created, but have also been Created perfect. There is no emptiness in you. Because of your likeness to your Creator you are creative. No child of God can lose this ability because it is inherent in what he is, but he can use it inappropriately by projecting. The inappropriate use of extension, or projection, occurs when you believe that some emptiness or lack exists in you [or another], and that you can fill it with your own ideas instead of truth. [LOVE]

> *A Course In Miracles*
> *Chapter 2 T T-2.I.1., 1-10*

A Course In Miracles tells us that we are "creators," that thought projections Not of LOVE are inappropriate projecting. When aligned with Source, we Live in a state in which nothing is needed and ALL is continually supplied. The moment we stop believing illusionary projections, they perfectly disappear, replaced by our restored Vibration in the *Field* of LOVE and its continual supply of LOVE, Abundance, Health, Success and Relationships flowing to us from Source.

> You do not have to continue to believe what is not true unless you choose to...All that can literally disappear in the twinkling of an eye because it is merely a misperception. What is seen in dreams seems to be very real...The world has not yet experienced any comprehensive reawakening or rebirth. Such a rebirth is

impossible as long as you continue to project or mis-Create. It still remains within you however, to extend as God extended His Spirit to you. In reality this is your only choice, because your free will was given you for your joy in creating the perfect.

A Course In Miracles
Chapter 2 T-2.I.3., 1-10

Most on the path of Healthy Lifestyle are aware of good nutrition. We cleanse, detox, go organic, get outdoors, clear Mind-Heart-Body, enjoy movement and implement natural remedial measures when needed. We recognize that *our unconscious "old data,"* is Mirrored in *our "reality,"* by our Attention or "projection" on the *Field.* As we clear "old data" thought-emotion, and purify our vehicle, we return to our resonance of LOVE.

It's far more important to know what person
the dis-ease has than what dis-ease the person has.

Hippocrates

Health and Well-Being are based on higher Mind-Energy, from which productive Life flows. When we feel LOVE and contentment, the body releases "LOVE" hormones that make us feel good, such as oxytocin, dopamine, serotonin and opiates. These make us "feel good" and they bring Healthy balance to Body systems, support vital immune response and develop **21st Century Superhuman** state of Heart Coherence! Sadness, anger, fear, worry and negative emotions produce stress hormones, adrenaline and cortisol, weaken immune system, elevate blood pressure and Heart-rate, make platelets sticky, disrupt the body and take us out of Heart Coherence.

Cellular resonance: it's like when you pluck one string in on two different guitars in the same room - one will resonate with the other, both striking the same note. This Creates a force of attraction, so the peptides resonate with their receptors and come together to strike the emotional chord as they bind.

Dr. Candace Pert
Discovered Opiate Receptors; "Your Body Is Your Unconscious Mind" Audio

Studies reveal that thinking a thought produces a neuropeptide, which travels through the Body to land on a cell activating matching energy. This thought chemistry bathes us internally, so if we're carrying fear or anger inside, we live with the chemistry of fear or anger. If we're attuned clearly to LOVE, Compassion, Gratitude, we are bathed internally with those "chemicals." We are powerfully affected by whatever thought-emotional energy is carried in the unconscious. *Laughter brings more well-being to our Lives than anything.*

Flow of Life pushes us to move beyond self-limiting energies of anger, fear, guilt, self-doubt or sadness. Pain is our awakener. Like bumping a splinter we draw the *perfect person, event or situation* into our "reality," to "Mirror" our own inharmonious Mind-energy. This offers opportunity to clear, cancel, get rid of, release, let go the old thought buried in the dungeon of our unconscious from genetics and early imprints. It requires strong self discipline to actually do the work to remove our unconscious content in every situation. This is the New "aikido" or "dance" of Life. [Part 2: MIND]

Ouch! Our old response might have been to point a finger at "them" and say, "They are to 'blame,' it's their fault." *Now we know better.* Realizing how essential it is to clear these energies from *our* Being, establishes a new Response-Ability pattern. When the situation arises again with a different person or situation, our Life force offers us "pain," asking us to recognize and clear our own blocked energy, to move toward greater clarity and energy. As we utilize tools in Part 2: MIND and Part 1: SHIFT OF THE AGES, we become proficient at this process, and we shift so much internally we discover we have entered an entirely New perspective of Living.

Even choices to use medications, drugs, vaccinations, alcohol, heavy foods and other suppressive substances come from cover-up or denial of inner fear, driving us to conform to societal norms without heeding the voice of our own Wisdom, Heart and Inner Spirit. It takes amazing courage and commitment to address this inner conflict and unwind it. This is why Sun Bear said, *"Only when we LOVE someone or something enough, do we get the lesson."* So pain comes as our great teacher, directing us into clearing to LOVE.

It is our deep LOVE that drives us beyond our ancient fears. It is our deep LOVE that heals us and our Loved ones. Embracing Deep LOVE, Compassion and Gratitude in all situations helps us to choose higher frequency actions. Integrating work and family with Lives based in *Essence* and connection with Heart, our body produces "happy chemicals" making us and all around us Healthier and Happier. Thus we access our True Gifts.

Consider moving beyond a meaningless job. Groom a path for yourself to make changes in a Healthy way. Seek out others ready to share a home, either blood-family or community. By doing so you assist one another to access more LOVE. Discover a way to support yourself that brings Joy to your life. Break out of traditional molds to cultivate this in your Life, restore Health and Vitality to Mind-Body-Spirit. Give thanks. [Part 3: SPIRIT]

★ *Choose Others to Be with who are choosing to learn and practice these qualities...*
 • *What does Unconditional LOVE look, feel, sound like?*
 • *How do we Live True Peace and Harmony?*
★ *The Path of En-Light-enment is Truly A Lifestyle - choose to be with others who:*
 • *Practice the Art of Heart-Centered Living, Meditation and Mindful Speaking*
 • *Be around Others who practice the Art of Living Consciously & Breathing*
★ *Discover Others who Mirror Ways of Living Consciously*
 • *We are ALL Aspects of God Consciousness...*
 • *Choose those who demonstrate Oneness rather than separation...*
★ *Enjoy Alone-Time & Together-Time*
 • *Seek those who understand the flow of Life and are willing to Flow with You*

Teddi ♥

Our current Acceleration or Ascension activated by where we are in the Cosmos [Part 1: SHIFT OF THE AGES] takes us into Awareness or En-Light-enment (to transmit more Light), waking up from the "dream" of our projections, knowing our Immutable Presence is ONE with ALL THAT IS. Here are "two realities" in Quantum terms:

(1)   The zero Point *Field of Possibilities* or *The Divine Matrix* is continually emerging Creation, ever flowing anew from Source.

(2) We are intrinsically One with this *Field*, with All That Is, *"I Am not just the drop within the ocean, but the ocean within the drop." Sufi.* Torus field within Torus field, connects us through our Heart with LOVE.

(3) The *second* "reality" is Illusion, or duality we have chosen to "play" in to rediscover our Oneness. It is our Not of LOVE Mind-Energy, Mirrored from the *Field*, appearing as our "reality." This "reality" is a dream world. The "dream world" of Illusion outside of LOVE, is only escaped by releasing, letting go, clearing, canceling all "old data" Not of LOVE hidden within the unconscious, to restore our True Resonance LOVE. [Part 2: MIND] *True Aramaic Forgiveness*

(4) As we do this inner personal work, we restore connection with our Heart and begin Living from *Essence*. Authenticity is the New En-Light-enment.

An infinitely important concept we are integrating, is that of *two* "Worlds" or levels of "reality;" one is Immutable, Eternal, an ever flowing sea of LOVE, of which our individualized consciousness and Being is an intrinsic part and continually emerging.

The second is like an overlay over the first; our *projections,* our experiments in playing in and focusing around *Not of LOVE* Mind-Energy, exploring duality outside of Oneness. We choose between these two parallel Worlds with self-awareness and reflection; within us is always choice, whether to nourish thoughts of unlimited Health, Abundance and Well-Being or participate in the worry and illusion of dis-comfort, pain, blame and illness.

Anything we experience Not of LOVE is of the Illusion. *Period. Beneath it is the Perfect Blueprint of Pure LOVE, Immortal, Eternal, Ever Flowing with opportunity of continual Creation; into which we reintegrate fully, at ANY MOMENT we choose.*

A Course in Miracles describes these two realities this way:

(1) Knowledge is truth, under one law, the law of LOVE or God. Truth is unalterable, eternal and unambiguous. It can be unrecognized, but it cannot be changed. It applies to everything that [All ONE] God Created, and only what He Created is real. It is beyond learning because it is beyond time and process. It has no opposite; no beginning and no end. It merely is.

(2) The world of perception, on the other hand, is the world of time, of change, of beginnings and endings. It is based on interpretation, not on facts. It is the world of birth and death, founded on the belief in scarcity, loss, separation and death. It is

learned rather than given, selective in its perceptual emphases, unstable in its functioning, and inaccurate in its interpretations.

How this *Field of LOVE* operates with Truth immutable and unchangeable, is the teaching of *Universal Laws.*[Part 2: MIND] Awakening to a new Experience of Life, we discover Creation based in pure LOVE is True and Real. Beyond it is the World of perceptions populated by Not of LOVE, called Illusion - which dissolves the instant we shift into LOVE.

Pain is a sign illusion reigns in place of truth.

A Course In Miracles

We are asking ourselves to bite off a big piece here. To see ourselves and our World in completely New ways than we have for thousands of years. Excitingly Quantum physics scientifically grounds this New perception of "reality" in a very practical way, which spiritual traditions throughout the ages have attempted to transmit. *TODAY* we have capacity to take this all in, even if it *STRETCHES US!* Be patient with yourself and others opening to these new ideas. Let them settle in and take root. Remember there is no time, there is no pressure. *Be LOVE. Smile. Breathe. Grow into this at your own pace.*

Our "reality filter" is the lens through which we view our World. Many learned to view the World through negative filters, associated with Not of LOVE perceptions within the illusion. This negative thought process ties into timelines (marking movement of consciousness). [Part 2: MIND] When we dwell upon this Mind-Energy long enough it becomes our "reality."

This is how "viruses" *begin, in the mind.* We think of a virus as a live thing outside ourselves, yet a virus is a perpetuated negative thought-form, beginning with our choice of how we use our Mind-Energy. Clearing negative thoughts, removes Vibrational frequency in which a virus can live. Even children benefit from gentle support in removing old and genetic thought-forms, to enter more fully into LOVE and keep thought viruses away.

Negative filters are most always the byproduct of a thought virus. Thought viruses are thoughtforms that seek to enslave us [our choice]. When we look through a negative lens, we believe we are victims, that others have negative opinions of us and that we have limited capabilities. A negative filter will in time transfer you to the timeline where the negative reality is manifested.

We are just as able to choose positive filters that empower us and help us live our highest visions, seen in our sleeping and waking dreams. Whereas a negative filter is centered on what you don't want, a positive filter focuses your energy and attention on what you do want. In creating a positive filter, look at your strengths, talents, potentials and desires and forge a new lens of perception that allows you to strengthen your talents, abilities and cultivate new experiences that you desire.

Regardless of what lens or belief you hold about reality, you will find validation in the outer world... Often people are indoctrinated into negative filters as children.

After a negative lens is implanted, thought viruses keep people from developing the emotional freedom and spiritual awareness to allow them to see through the viruses's fear loop.

When you begin to live life as you see it through your positive lenses, your mind and Soul become harmonized. From this place of inner peace, you naturally make decisions and choices that help you realize your highest visions and find your place in the new timeline.

Wes Annac, Aquarius Paradigm
DL Zeta: Upgrading our Lens of Perception Shifts us to Fifth-Dimensional Timelines

Becoming aware we are continually creating "reality," we *release focus* from a negative lens, shifting into positive, powerful Creation of LOVE, becoming unstoppable and radiant. We are *transforming* an entire cultural paradigm as *21st Century Superhumans*, by activating DNA codons, with prime focus on our Authenticity, Living in LOVE.

Information is the resolution of uncertainty.

Deepak Chopra MD
Natural Physician, New Thought Author

LOVE is the One Law superseding all laws. LOVE is the energy behind all Creation. We activate continual *REGENERATION* when we center Life in LOVE. Thus the amazing and beautiful becomes the everyday "norm," in our *21st Century Superhuman Journey*.

We Now express LOVE thought-emotion within and through the Vibrational resonance of our Lives. We affirm and call in: *Deep LOVE, COMPASSION, GRATITUDE, Breathing, Smiling, Laughter, Vitality, Well-Being, Health, Joyous Relationship, Living from the Heart, Loving Friendship and Companionship, Expressing from Essence Pure Self-Expression, Service to others, walking Gently on Earth Mother Gaia or Pachamama, Veganism-Vegetarianism, Breatharianism, Dreaming Peacefully, Naturally Flowing Abundance, Happy Children, Loving Families, Communities, Pets, Comfort, Food, Water, Sanitation, Shelter and Needs Met for ALL, Organic Gardening, Nurturing Wild Places, Living Harmoniously with the Earth, Mineralized Soil, ALL Creatures Free, Biocompatible Free Energy Planet-wide, Teleportation, Communication Technologies Furthering Global Mind, Education Expanding ALL Human-Huwom Intelligence and Creativity, Knowledge, Information Shared Freely, Ideas and Creativity of the Many Feeding into an ever Escalating Spiral Positive Evolution for Humanity-Huwomity, each person born with Intrinsic Value Beyond Measure, ALL organization emerges out of Movement Toward the Common Good, peaceful Solutions Honoring Sovereignty of ALL with LOVE.* ♥

Chapter 12

Enviro Toxins

The best way to detoxify is to stop putting toxic things into the body and depend upon it's own mechanisms.

Dr. Andrew Weil
Founder, Professor and Director of Arizona Center for Integrative Medicine at U of A

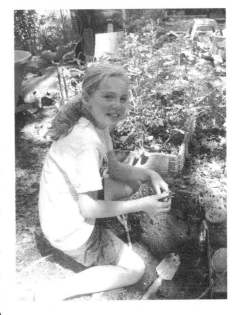

We all have a good idea that in today's World we have relatively high exposure to toxins in our environment. First let us say, this is a product of Mind-Energy. No matter how long you've been an environmentalist, no matter how hard you've been fighting for good, no matter how convinced you are, it's something 'out there' and "the bad guys" are creating this, no matter how "mad" you are at "them," environmental toxins are a product of the thought-emotional toxicity vibrating within us as a Collective creating this "reality." *Wow! Okay, let's reflect on that...ha!*

We've Lived for thousands of years in blame-fear-hostility culture with Mind-Energy resonating from this focus, rather than our True Design LOVE. We are *Observer-Creators*; our *Attention* upon the *Field of Possibilities*, calls our *"reality"* into being personally and in our World! Vibrations of anger, hurt or sadness about what appears to be going on in the World, holds it in form, until we cancel our goals and clear, release, let it go. Simple, just say, "I cancel my goals that the world be a safe place, that there be no war, etc." [Part2: MIND] We powerfully change what appears around us the instant we change the resonance within us. Removing all "corrupt data" from our unconscious "operating system," focusing Mind and Heart in LOVE, everything in our World changes form molecularly to match our resonance.

Every conscious thought you have, every moment you spend on an idea, is a commitment to be stuck with that idea and with aspects of that level of thinking, for the rest of your life [until you change it]. Spending just 10 seconds focusing on a topic that does not serve your interests, is to invest your energy along a path that will continue to draw from you and define you.

Kevin Michel
Moving Through Parallel Worlds To Achieve Your Dreams

The 6th Universal Mutable Law of Cause and Effect teaches us balance out such exposures in the physical World, avoiding substances, removing them and using chelating substances to remove them. Hold the creative thought potential, envisioning our *Field* and our existence as operating as a healthy and beautiful environment for all, "mud between the toes." Let's review environmental toxins we are exposed to in the current state of our World, while we are changing our thinking as a collective Now!

It is an unnatural stress to counterbalance when we are exposed to pesticides, herbicides, household and chemical cleaners, synthetic air fresheners, radiation and metals that disturb the immune system, causing irritation, acidity, inflammation and fibrins. As we detoxify and clear Mind and Heart,we are able to transform results of Not of LOVE "realities" in our bodies and in our World. We offer key points toward further research, pro-action and resources to clear or counterbalance such deviations.

DENTAL: SILVER MERCURY, METAL & ROOT CANALS

Great teeth are awesomely wonderful, and as continual regeneration is our birthright, it will be exciting one day, to align with regeneration and perfect teeth! The greatest challenge today is severe demineralization of soils. If possible, live where you can eat produce grown in soil enriched with rock dust or is naturally mineralized. Thought patterns associated with teeth connect with the throat chakra and our ability to speak Truth. Loss of teeth and dental suppression come with generational waves around karmic suppression of individual voice, left from the blame-fear-hostility culture.

We are now in the midst of releasing this old paradigm, healing ourselves by getting the metal out of our mouths, and allowing the body to open up to higher frequencies. Mercury is the metal of the mind. It is also a potent neuro-toxin, and as long as we carry it in our teeth, tends to suppress Mind-Body, sending the mind in endless loops.

Dan Dieska, DDS, a close friend trained in Higher Teachings, shortened his own life in service to remove this toxic substance. A rare dentist, he said, "My mission is to free people from the illusion of thinking that silver-mercury is beneficial; the best thing for health is to remove it," and he probably gave his life in this service, departing at a young age.

Younger generations who have had only white fillings or none, and/or preventive coating in childhood to prevent decay, congratulations! You are of the lucky ones. You also "came in" as a Soul with less "karma" to clear, easily sharing your voice in the World. Those who have had your silver-mercury fillings removed, congratulations!!! This is not an easy process. Sometimes teeth are lost as a result, yet a preferable foundation for vitality and well-being.

1. Mercury is a potent neurotoxin and does not belong in a healthy body

2. Mixes with mouth vapor and saliva; has galvanic reactions with other metals

3. Chewing, mixed with saliva and heat it becomes methyl-mercury (more toxic)

4. In the brain it suppresses clear thought and is a contributor to degenerative neurological disorders such as Alzheimer's, Dementia, MS, Lou Gehrig's

5. Accumulates in brain, thyroid, spine, kidneys, liver, lungs, glands

6. Found to be precursor to cancer and other degenerative illness; as a toxin it causes inflammation in the body, removal of which supports remission

7. Mind and conversation tend to stay in endless loops rather than resolution

CILANTRO NATURAL CHELATOR: A Japanese dentist ran a urine test with each patient after removing silver fillings. He discovered by chance that those who had soup for lunch with cilantro, excreted more mercury in their urine, cultivating awareness of this easy "poor man's" chelation for mercury, freeing mercury from the tissues. Once mercury is pulled into solution with cilantro or cilantro extract, it is best to combine with carrier to remove it such as chlorella and food grade diatomaceous earth. We have noticed many who still have silver fillings tend to dislike cilantro, because it pulls the mercury into solution. It is good *not* to use cilantro until silver fillings are removed; meanwhile chlorella is helpful to carry away residue.

All metals in the mouth gradually slough tiny particles into the body, affecting brain, neurobiology and overall well-being. Root canals can be a source of chronic low grade bacterial discharge. All of this is outside conventional dental practices, however there is a growing field of dentists dedicated to overall well-being through non-toxic dentistry. Educate yourself. If cost is an issue there are now great resources in foreign countries. For longevity of body and mind, removal of metals is a must! Even gold and gold alloys in fillings and crowns have a suppressive effect.

RESTORING NATURAL BALANCE: Use cilantro and cilantro extract to chelate once fillings have been removed; Pesto made with cilantro instead of basil; add cilantro to soups. Chlorella regular ingredient in Green Shakes. Chlorella and food grade diatomaceous earth (PermaGuard brand) absorb and carry away residue.

RESOURCES:

• International Academy of Oral Medicine Toxicology IAOMT iaomt dot org

• Hal Huggins DDS HugginsAppliedHealing dot com

• Books by Sam and Michael Ziff

• Rescued by My Dentist DentistryHealth dot com

FLUORIDE

Fluoride defenders offer the story that when fluoride is added to public water supplies it improves dental well-being. They originally used a widely publicized two-year study from the 1940s that showed Hereford, Texas to have the lowest tooth decay rate among schoolchildren of any city in the US. What is left out of that story, is that Hereford, Texas is a town in Deaf Smith County, where is found the richest mineralized soil anywhere in the US, left from from ancient seabeds. Primary cause for dental issues: *you got it -* demineralization of soil. Want to fix it? Follow Haymaker's advice and remineralize gardens, agricultural land and the Earth with rock dust, before it requires another ice age to put things right. Anyone who deals with organic whole grains knows Deaf Smith County produces highest quality organic grains and beans as a result of its mineralized soil. Thus evolved a story that Hereford had high fluorine levels in their soil, when actually they had a composite of mineralization that resulted in their good dental record.

Blog.Fluoride-Free Austin tells how this whole story got started. In 1941, the year the US entered World War II, the war machine was gearing up, and fluoride, vital byproduct of wartime production of metals and enriched uranium was acquiring an unsavory reputation for its high toxicity; while government and industry-sponsored scientists were frantically looking for ways to rehabilitate it. A "researcher" reported to the research section of the American Dental Association, that fluoride added to water based on dental history of Hereford, TX, might prove to be "one of the most important discoveries in dental history."

It carried on from there, as fluoride is a byproduct of the aluminum and chemical fertilizer industries. Piles of this waste to be gotten rid of are now sold to cities for their water systems and dental hygiene manufacturers. Most tests run on cities with fluoridated water show that teeth of children drinking fluoridated water are no better than those in the cities that don't, and in fact even in cities with fluoridated water decay continues to increase. Harvard's School of Public Health reported studies showed fluoride may decrease cognitive ability in children.

> July 25, 2012 — For years health experts have been unable to agree on whether fluoride in the drinking water may be toxic to the developing human brain. Extremely high levels of fluoride are known to cause neurotoxicity in adults, and negative impacts on memory and learning have been reported in rodent studies, but little is known about the substance's impact on children's neurodevelopment. In a meta-analysis, researchers from Harvard School of Public Health (HSPH) and China Medical University in Shenyang for the first time combined 27 studies and found strong indications that fluoride may adversely affect cognitive development in children. Based on the findings, the authors say that this risk should not be ignored, and that more research on fluoride's impact on the developing brain is warranted.
>
> *HSPH - Harvard School of Public Health News*
> *Impact of fluoride on neurological development in children*

Fluoride was used in Nazi Concentration camps and the gulags in Siberia to make prisoners docile and controllable. At the end of the war the Allies discovered tons of fluoride piled it in concentration camps. When it's added to city water the entire population is dosed with what is considered a "medication," without consent and one dose for everyone - depending of course on how much water they drink. It is also absorbed through the skin while bathing and showering, absorbed through tissues of mouth when brushing teeth. You don't have to swallow it: cooking with fluoride in water concentrates in food and beverages; it doesn't cook out. Only 50% is excreted by the body, so it is a cumulative toxin leading to many health problems. It is not a nutrient; it damages bones.

Have some fluoride in your toothpaste?

In 1991, the Akron (Ohio) Regional Poison Center reported that "death has been reported following ingestion of 16mg/kg of fluoride. Only 1/10 of an ounce of fluoride can kill a 100 pound adult. According to the Center, "fluoride toothpaste contains up to 1mg/gram of fluoride." Even Proctor and Gamble, the makers of Crest, acknowledge that a family-sized tube "theoretically contains enough fluoride to kill a small child."

FLUORIDE FACTS

1. Fluoride - main ingredient in rat poison.

2. Fluoride - main ingredient in Sarin nerve gas.

3. Fluoride - main ingredient in Prozak, and cancer and HIV meds.

4. Fluoride - destroys brain function, accumulates in pineal, bones organs and causes cancer. (inflammation)

5. Hitler and Stalin used it in concentration camps and gulags as a mass control instrument to make prisoners docile.

6. Guess why fluoride is added to drinking water? What in us accepts this?

7. Over 170 million people, or 67% of the US population drink fluoridated water. 43 of the 50 largest cities in the country are fluoridated.

8. What do you think fluoridated water and antidepressants such as Prozak are all about?

9. Fluoride damages DNA.

10. Is it worth drinking filtered water, filtering shower, moving to the country?

Three types of filters that remove fluoride are reverse osmosis, deionization (ion-exchange resins), and activated alumina. Each removes about 90% of fluoride. "Activated carbon" filters (e.g., Brita & Pur) do not remove fluoride.

Let's clear our unconscious data banks of all thought-emotion that gives up our own Life to a suppressive, oppressive culture. Lies told about these things are told so big industry can control the wealth of the World and drain Life out of its citizens. It takes a valiant effort to wake up and make waves; to walk a different path than lemmings running toward a cliff. Let's wake up and fly!

RESOURCES:

• Fluoride Action Network fluoridealert.org

• *An Inconvenient TOOTH* - fluoride documentary (currently YouTube)

• Shower Filter plus drink reverse osmosis or filtered water

• Move to the country and drink natural well or spring water

• Get large water jugs, fill with reverse osmosis water (grocery store)

• Personal water container. Plastic trash is epidemic (no small bottles).

• *Iodine Protects Against Fluoride Toxicity* article DrSircus.com

CHLORINE

Disinfecting water with chlorine began in the 1800s when there weren't many choices; today there are alternatives much more supportive of LIFE to be used. It's like a little poison daily with a dash of "chlorine bleach," drink filtered or natural water if possible.

Dr. Joseph Price wrote a controversial book in the '60s, *Coronaries/Cholesterol/Chlorine*, showing that coronary heart disease increased in subjects drinking chlorinated water. He later headed up a study demonstrating chickens fed chlorine-free water were healthier than those given chlorinated water, still used today by poultry farmers. Global Healing Center's blog, Natural Health and Organic Living reports in *Chlorine, Cancer and Heart Disease*:

> There is well-founded concern about chlorine. When added to our water, it combines with other natural compounds to form Trihalomethanes (chlorination byproducts), or THMs. These chlorine byproducts trigger the production of free radicals in the body, causing cell damage, and are highly carcinogenic. The Environmental Defense Fund warns that, "Although concentrations of these carcinogens (THMs) are low, it is precisely these low levels that cancer scientists believe are responsible for a majority of human cancers in the United States."

Dr. Robert Carlson, a highly respected University of Minnesota researcher whose work is sponsored by the Federal Environmental Protection Agency, sums it up, "the chlorine problem is similar to that of air pollution" and adds that "chlorine is the greatest crippler and killer of modern times!" It is just simple wisdom to avoid chlorine if you can. There are more healthy ways to Create sanitary water.

> We are quite convinced, based on this study, that there is an association between cancer and chlorinated water.
>
> *Medical College Of Wisconsin*

RESOURCES:

• Minimally charcoal filter for tap and shower

- Hydrogen Peroxide - for disinfecting (10 min application kills HIV)
- Move to the country and drink natural well or spring water
- Get large water jugs, fill with reverse osmosis water (grocery store)
- Personal water container. Plastic trash is epidemic (no small bottles).

RADIATION

One day rather than clean power inventions being suppressed by those making billions in the petrochemical industry, we will break free, and use free clean power on Earth. We envision this day coming soon. (mud between the toes!) In one cubic foot of space there is enough energy to run everything on Planet Earth for 100 years!!!

Meanwhile (due to rage and fear in the collective unconscious that is Now leaving...) we still use nuclear plants with leaking radiation and radioactive waste. Japan's Fukushima plant, damaged by 2011 earthquake is leaking contaminated water at 1 million times normal levels, says Japanese News. There is wisdom today in being aware and protecting from radiation. Hiroshima survivors ate miso soup with seaweed daily; which is basically a daily dose of iodine, minerals and enzymes.

A favorite resource, Dr. Sircus of International Medical Veritas Association, offers information on iodine as protective against radiation, mercury and other environmental toxins. This is an essential resource for today, especially as it's a common deficiency. Consumption of seaweeds has been proven historically beneficial, as is red marine algae. High quality liquid iodine is best,used transdermally (applied to the skin - forearm good). Caution some have sensitivities.

Additionally we are now exposed to a great deal of electromagnetic radiation with barely a person without a cell phone, cell phone towers and networks around the World, computers, baby monitors, portable phones and electricity itself. Leaving behind electromagnetic devices and reconnecting with the Earth is the best solution to restore our natural electromagnetic frequencies. New protective devices are being developed such as holographic stickers. Do your research. Be aware. RESOURCES:

- International Medial Veritas Association IMVA dot info
- Dr. Sircus (founder IMVA) articles and great iodine source
- Miso and seaweed proved protective in Hiroshima (iodine, enzymes)
- Radiationnetwork.com
- Article: Iodine Supplementation HealthWyze dot org

VACCINATIONS

Self-education is essential, rather than yielding to a system that does not have well-being of adults, children or pets at heart. Pharmaceutical companies make billions from vaccinations, which weaken the immune system and are aimed at global population reduction. Waking up to the truth, and taking a stand for health and well-being is critical.

We have absorbed the "fix me" mentality, "just give me a shot and I won't have to take Response-Ability for my own habits and how they affect my body." The theory of toxemia is more accurate than the germ theory. Yes germs grow in a toxic organism; *cleaning up the body keeps us well*, and has long-lasting benefits.

Multiply $35, $45, $65, $95 by millions-billions made by pharmaceutical giants; only by keeping people in the dark (ignorant to the ill-effects of vaccines) can vaccination profit-levels be kept high. Records show a list of 30 people in political positions with the federal government who also work for pharmaceutical companies. Proponent of healthy lifestyle Dr. Mercola, offers *Vaccination Statistics* at mercola.com.

Pro-vaccination is all that is offered in the media, schools, doctor's offices, PHS, and all government publications. This is a biased one-sided view of vaccinations based much on manufacturer's studies and writings.

Extreme pressures placed on parents to signing permission and accept all responsibility for toxic vaccines. Yet, doctors cannot guarantee safety of vaccines.... Many vaccinations fail to achieve intended immunity and many cause horrible complications (including death)... trade-off not worth the risk.

• 1992 - American Journal of Epidemiology...children die 8 times rate of normal within three days of DPT vaccination.

• Center for Disease Control (CDC) - children who received HiB vaccine ... were **5 times more likely** to contract the disease than children who had not.

• new England Journal of Medicine July 1994 - 80% of children under 5, who had whooping cough had been **fully vaccinated.**

• 1977 Dr Jonas Salk (inventor polio vaccine) testified that 87% polio cases in US since 1970 were by-product of polio vaccine.

• Sabin oral polio vaccine (OPV) is **only known cause of polio** in US today.

• February 1981- AMA Journal found 90% obstetricians, 66% pediatricians **refused** to take rubella vaccine.

Mercury in vaccines has been shown to cause excessive free radicals, found to cause autism. However coming to the forefront now, with understanding of inflammation and fibrin development, due to repeated vaccine failure manufactures attempt to make them more potent by adding immune stimulators, adjuvants. With an injection, a vaccination bypasses the body's natural protective systems, mouth, skin, nose, and gut. Vaccination's also bypass protective mechanism of the brain called the blood-brain barrier causing chronic inflammation. By 7-8 children have been given up to 30 vaccines, when their immune systems are just developing and they are overridden by this massive dumping of foreign substances through the blood-brain barrier from which many never recover.

The brain's immune cells move through the nervous system, secreting numerous immune chemicals, pouring out an enormous amount of free radicals to fight the invading organism. The problem is there is no invading organism, the brain has been tricked by the vaccine to believe there is resulting over-reaction of the immune system, inflammation, acidity and fibrin development. This rush of free radicals created by the body to protect itself against the vaccine creates additional pieces of tissue in the body called fibrins. This is what makes up a fibroid tumor; it is excess tissue that the body creates to *protect itself* from invasion of some sort, such as free radicals caused by the vaccine. A state of inflammation or acidity is being artificially created, resulting in asbestos-like fibers floating through the system, visible in dark-field live blood cell analysis.

Mercola article, *Vaccination Dangers Can Kill You or Ruin Your Life,* reports syndromes known to result from vaccines, obviously a product of this assault on the brain, and its fight to protect itself, resulting in fibrin development are Autism, ADD, ADHD, Gulf War Syndrome, More common neurodegenerative diseases, Parkinson's, Alzheimer's, dementia and ALS. Studies at the University of Wisconsin in Madison are now proving repeated rabies and other vaccines for dogs are equally damaging, causing chronic inflammation, potentially highly at cause in the 60-70% rate of dogs dying from cancer. Nov. 2013, 19 year old Utah boy died of flu vaccine.

Mercola's article answers the question, *what about flu vaccines?* "A recent study by World-renowned immunologist Dr. H. Hugh Fudenberg found that adults vaccinated yearly for five years in a row with the flu vaccine had a 10-fold increased risk of developing Alzheimer's. He attributes this to the mercury and aluminum in the vaccine. Interestingly, both of these metals have been shown to activate microglia and *increase excitotoxicity (inflammation=fibrins)* in the brain. Basically what we're doing with vaccines is initiating chronic brain and body degenerative inflammation .

Once this over-reaction begins in the brain, it does not stop, affecting individuals differently; a severe example is autism, with ADD, ADHD and Alzheimer's run a close second, with more pharmaceuticals used to feed the drug industry. On top of all this billions has been spent by the Gates Foundation to develop RFID tracking chips to be used in vaccines. Sunday, March 21, 2010 Senate Healthcare Bill HR3200 requiring implantation of radio chips to transmit health and banking information with Obamacare chip implants.

Teddi tells the story of her little grandson, one of the brightest children she had seen, and after returning from getting a vaccination with his parents lost that sparkle, which took him a long time to regain with remedial measures. What residual Mind-Energy is limiting Life force culturally? Educating with Truth we make better choices, to exit the *statistical path*. It takes courage to step out of the traces, educating ourselves, and holding hands around a circle of Truth; a circle connecting us with Natural Law, rather than coffers of the "power-over" greed driven machine. *APPLY Ancient Aramaic Forgiveness goal canceling here! LOVE.*

No parent purposely harms their child. No pet owner purposely harms their pet. We do not purposely harm ourselves. However we must *"awaken from our slumber;"* of generations of subjugation to debilitating and dehumanizing systems and habits.

We are Free Beings. We are Free to Choose. Inspiration comes from gathering in community with like-minded individuals, expanding knowledge for well-being, sovereign in our expression of Life. This requires the effort of taking care of ourselves self-responsibly; changing Lifestyle to that of *21st Century Superhumans* who understand Quantum principles, that we are "creators" of our "reality;" and good health is as close as choosing *Quantum Lifestyle* habits of thought Mind-Body-Heart.

In many chilling ways, drug companies promise us a utopian future without pain, without disease and illness, thanks to prescription drugs. But is the cost more than we bargained for?

Ray Williams in Wired for Success
How the Drug Companies Are Controlling Our Lives Part 1, Psychology Today, May 23,2011

Are we ready to wake up? To make choices to protect our brains, our health and our Lives, those of our children's and pets; and learn how to detoxify our Mind-Energy and our Bodies? Reclaiming our greatest possibilities, rather than submitting to a money-hungry pharmaceutical system, that emerged from the Vibration of blame-fear-hostility in our unconscious thought-emotional container takes courage, commitment and education around natural wellness methods. *Let's restore our True Design LOVE, and Live as vital regenerative Beings.* **Arc the Hologram with LOVE!**

RESOURCES:

• long term recovery - alkalize, NAET, EFT (next chapter)
• NIVC.org, MCIR.org, vaclib.org, knowthelies.com, know-vaccines.org
• articles.mercola.com Legal Vaccine Exemptions (more articles)
• healthypets.mercola.com, truth4pets.org, dogs4dogs.com, synbiotics.com

GMOs

One of the most amazing things about Living on Planet Earth is the millions of species of plants, insects, water creatures and animals that grow naturally, in an incredibly rich and beautiful ecosystem. The modern developed World has built up an artificial lifestyle contained in cities and suburbs, that largely cut off this natural flow of life. Pavement, city buildings, suburban neighborhoods, manicured lawns, pesticides and weedkillers of the insulate us from nature, and push her away.

Have you heard of *SELF-SUFFICIENCY?* Do you consider yourself to be so? What would happen if there were no food in the grocery store? Do you and your neighbors have gardens so you could share food with one another? Or are there growers nearby? Will seeds you bought at the hardware store grow plants again next year? Or are they hybrid?

Hybrid means that two plants have been cross pollinated, to bear bigger-better fruit, but the seeds from that plant will not produce the same as the parent plant. This means you have to go back and buy seeds from the big company that manufactured them. *This ensures they stay in business.*

To grow plants that produce food and save seeds, and produce true to the parent plant the following year, you must start with open pollinated or Heirloom (over 50 year old variety) seeds. Many reading this book today, have likely never grown a garden to produce their own food, though certainly some have. And likely, many may not *want* to produce their own food. Bill Mollison, father of Permaculture, described perfect cities and towns in an amoeba shape; where developed areas, ebb and flow with U-shaped areas of farms, gardens and farm markets, *an ideal symbiosis.* We might imagine this is a wonderful way to *re-Create cities and towns.*

Healthiest foods for our bodies are those that have grown and evolved naturally with the Earth, so *it benefits us to maintain open pollinated or Heirloom seeds.* Heirloom or open pollinated seeds are those plants that have evolved by natural selection as the healthiest over time. They produce the *BEST TASTING* and most nourishing vegetables and fruits. Whether we are growing a garden ourselves, or supporting growers in our community, obtain foods a grown from Organic, Heirloom or open pollinated seeds. Cultivating neighborhoods and communities, where this is the type of food produced and shared is an essential type of *Self-Sufficiency* we benefit ourselves by returning to.

When exposed to hybrid or GMO pollen, open pollinated or Heirloom seeds become corrupt, and are unable to pass on their genetic heritage of a pure healthy plant that evolved with Earth Mother Gaia to their offspring. Enter GMOs, which we've figured out are causing health problems.

WHAT ARE GMOs? " Genetically modified organisms" are plants and animals that have been engineered with DNA from bacteria, viruses or other plants and animals, with sophisticated technologies such as retroviruses and gene guns, combining genes from different species that cannot occur in nature. GMOs have the capability of destroying all natural food production, eventually leading to total reduction of food sources. Corporations pushing this "cloning" are unthinking of anything but their own profit. *APPLY Ancient Aramaic Forgiveness goal canceling here!*

Virtually all commercial GMOs are engineered to withstand direct application of herbicide and/or to produce an insecticide. Despite biotech industry promises, none of the GMO traits currently on the market offer increased yield, drought tolerance, enhanced nutrition, or any other consumer benefit. A growing body of evidence connects GMOs with health problems, environmental damage and violation of farmers' and consumers' rights. Bt GMO corn, designed by Monsanto to kill corn borers by perforating its gut, has now been found in the guts of humans, causing sensitivities and new illnesses. Monsanto's global efforts to take over food production with GMO seeds in undeveloped countries are relentless. A friend from the Philippines tells of growers bringing in hybridized rice to plant. Local farmers planted the modern seeds on the front edge of the rice paddies, as they knew inspectors wouldn't walk into the paddy. They planted traditional seeds in the back.

Far beyond hybridization is a no man's land of GMOs, experiment in the unnatural, that cannot bode well for the health and well-being of living things. The problem is it that GMOs do not stay put, they infect nearby *Fields* polluting with Frankenstein-like qualities, incapable of producing young.

A Global leader on open pollinated seeds is Vandana Shiva, E. Indian environmental activist and anti-globalization author who has written over 20 books. Time Magazine identified Dr. Shiva as an *environmental "hero"* in 2003. She has been awarded the *Right Livelihood Award, Sydney Peace Prize* and *Fukuoka Asian Culture Prize;* in good company with Nelson Mandela and the Dalai Lama having been one of the few recipients of the *Gold Medal for Peace with Justice.*

Internationally known for encouraging, teaching and promoting seed saving to eradicate poverty, Create self-sufficiency and independence, she has initiated a national movement to protect the diversity and integrity of living resources, especially native seed, promotion of organic farming and fair trade. *She is in a 3 year project with Bhutan to become the first 100% organic sovereign country.*

GROW YOUR OWN GARDEN WITH HEIRLOOM SEEDS: If you have a yard and can grow a garden, grow your own food with heirloom seeds. The next best thing is to support growers in your neighborhood or area by buying local organic food. Creating a viable future means participating in critical choices about where our food comes from, how it is grown, and what its actual nutritional quality. Sept. 2013 UN report, "Wake Up Before It's Too Late links global security and escalating conflicts with the urgent need to transform agriculture toward what it calls "ecological intensification" with local small gardens.

Remineralized soil, open pollinated heirloom, organic, every little choice makes a big difference. Participate in getting us back on track rather than derailed as a modern culture.

YOUR FOOD CHOICE MAKE A HUGE DIFFERENCE: Growing food in your yard makes a huge stand for the future, with Organic, Heirloom, Open Pollinated, Locally Grown food sources. Teach others the same; Neighborhood gardens, seed exchange.

Holding LOVE, Breathing, Smiling. No GMO. And YES many good things! It is our choice. Make the choice rather than leaving it to chance. Live organically with LOVE on Earth. Change our Vibration - change the World. *Arc the Hologram Now with LOVE!* ♥

• Non-GMO Project nongmoproject.org • Permaculture Magazine • Urban Farm

• Heirloom, Open Pollinated Seeds • LAGuerillaGardening.org

• peakprosperity.com • Baker Creek Heirloom Seeds rareseeds.com

Part 4: BODY

Chapter 13

Miraculous Tales

*If we are creating ourselves all the time, then it is never too late
to begin creating the bodies we want instead of the ones
we mistakenly assume we are stuck with.*

Deepak Chopra MD
Natural Physician, New Thought Author

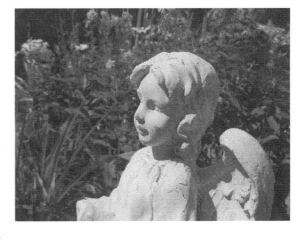

*T*he biggest gift I ever got, was when I was holding points on this man, and he was yelling, "Stop it, stop it, you're hurting me, get your elbow off my backside you @*%^!!! John Ray walked over to me, and looked at me with those big blue eyes and said, "Stop resisting his resistance." It was like a giant light bulb went on in my head!" ♥ Teddi

Most importantly what we learned over may years from Dr. John Ray, dr. michael ryce, Tony Robbins and others was "Go into the pain," "move through it with tools and focus." Any area we are uncomfortable in Life or "suffering" physically, mentally, emotionally, our pain shows us where the "logjam" is in the river of Creative flow from Source, where old thought-emotion blocks our Life from being vibrantly well. Elevating Vibrational rate of nourishment, using remedial measures to strengthen Mind-Body to enter its full regenerative capacity are Vital Keys to generate greater Life-Force.

'Wizards? Do you mean they do things a different way?' 'No, just the way we do,' Merlin replied. With a flick of his finger he lit the soggy heap of kindling that Arthur had gathered... A blaze leapt up on the instant. Merlin then opened his hands and produced food out of thin air."

Deepak Chopra M
The Way of the Wizard: Twenty Spiritual Lessons for Creating the Life You Want

The secret to becoming a "wizard," or bringing forth our natural capability to produce miracles, lies within regular practice of moving beyond any tendency to go into denial with food, drugs, alcohol, rage, busyness, and fine tune our ability to clear conscious-unconscious content Not of LOVE.

We must practice peace, harmony, individuality and firmness of purpose and increasingly develop the knowledge that in essence we are of Divine origin, children of the Creator, and thus have within us, if we will but develop it, as in time we surely must, the power to attain perfection. And this reality must increase within us until it becomes the most outstanding feature of our existence.

We must steadfastly practice peace, imagining our minds as a lake ever to be kept calm, without waves, or even ripples, to disturb its tranquility, and gradually develop this state of peace until no event of life, no circumstance, no other personality is able under any condition to ruffle the surface of that lake or raise within us, any feelings of irritability, depression or doubt.

It will materially help to set apart a short time each day to think quietly of the beauty of peace and the benefits of calmness, and to realize that it is neither by worrying nor hurrying that we accomplish most, but by calm, quiet thought and action become more efficient in all we undertake.

To harmonize our conduct in this life in accordance with the wishes of our own Soul, and to remain in such a state of peace that the trials and disturbances of the world leave us unruffled, is great attainment indeed and brings us that Peace which passeth understanding; and though at first it may seem beyond our dreams, it is in reality, with patience and perseverance, within the reach of us all.

Edward Bach M.D. and F.J. Wheeler M.D.
The Bach Flower Remedies

Lynn McTaggart, British investigative journalist noted in her book the *Field*, that *everyone*, even those who don't think they do, have "paranormal" abilities including telepathy and remote viewing. We barely grasp the full extent of possibility of using these subtler abilities, as for centuries superstition has held us back from these Innate talents. Whether we recognize it or not, we have Infinite access to the miraculous.

Just as one person may be able to wiggle an ear or an eyebrow and another read minds, we each have special skills or "super" abilities if you will. Leaving behind limiting beliefs from "the World is flat" mentality, we open ourselves to access these "paranormal" abilities dormant within us, just waiting for us to practice and add them to our repertoire, as we expand into who we are becoming and what is emerging within us, during this Evolutionary Leap the *Shift of the Ages*. [Part 1: SHIFT OF THE AGES]

CATCH YOUR DREAMS: Routinely note your stream of consciousness. Prime time is on awakening or just after focus, meditation, goal canceling or any awareness practice. Lucid dreaming flashes of genius have been measured at 40 Ghz Gamma brain waves, tapping into our "paranormal" abilities. To capture more awareness in this zone, when you are awake during the day, ask the question, "Am I awake"? When you become aware in lucid dreaming you may be cognitive to ask the same question, and then direct your lucid dream! Record your notes without judgment! Enjoy what comes forth as messages from your super-conscious!

Spontaneous Remission

In 1993 the Institute of Noetic Sciences IONS, founded by Astronaut Ed Mitchell, published *Spontaneous Remission: An Annotated Bibliography* at their website. It is the largest database of spontaneous remissions in the World, containing 3,500 cases from 800 journals in 20 languages. This phenomenon may not be as rare as was once thought, as reported cases have increased in recent decades. Embracing this concept assists us to recognize the continual process toward wellness flowing into our Being. If spontaneous remission is so possible, some may ask, "then why did my Loved One die," addressed in various ways throughout the book.

Spontaneous remission generally reported as a rare occurrence, is actually readily available to us. It is supported by clearing Not of LOVE content from our Being, then accessing Light or ever flowing Source *Field* energy, opening pathways for Higher Frequencies to flow. In spontaneous remission, an individual enters into their *Essence* as Light, connection to God, Source *Field,* continuous Creation or Eternal flow of Being, accessing a state where their Body instantly restructures. Our "Light Body" amplifies when our attention is focused in this way.

Highest, Healthiest Intention is LOVE

Marcel Vogel, was born in San Francisco in 1917. At age six he was pronounced dead from pneumonia, yet within a couple of hours to everyone's surprise, had come back to Life. In his early teens he was so dedicated to serious pursuits, he walked to mass daily and was "told" he would bring forth progressive books and inventions, which he did. He spent 27 years as top scientist for IBM and developed 150 patents, among which was technology that evolved into today's computer hard drives.

Marcel's greatest legacy was that he devised ways to measure energy emanating from thoughts and emotions. He developed the Vogel Cut for crystals, with a 51 degree angle matching the Great Pyramid in Egypt, and researched the *Secret Life of Plants*. His crystal cut is still legendary. He also demonstrated that quartz crystals send out frequencies and amplify thought. [Tree of Life Tech carries on his work today.]

Vogel showed the world scientifically *(those who would listen)*, that a person's highest and healthiest intention is LOVE. He found that...any intention is amplified and transmitted with phenomenal change happening to the energy of that intention. This he clearly showed *(for all who would see)* that this is a little understood yet perfect, and perfectly manifesting Life-giving energy force. ...He found and showed others how to connect to themselves and their higher selves with a simple tool. Therefore connecting through themselves to the energy that makes them.

Tree of Life Tech on Dr. Marcel Vogel (1917-1991)
Energy Scientists and Developer of Vogel Crystals

Recall Generational Memory In Utero

Our powerful thoughts emerge into words and deeds, affecting seven generations, though literally to infinity. Our gene pool is run by and inherits the resonance, programmed by our thoughts-emotions and those of our generations. Clearing thought stored in unconscious Not of LOVE, we clear timelines, offering better "realities" to future generations. This generational story fascinatingly demonstrates how thought is passed on from one generation to the next, a favorite from our Body Electronics point-holding days.

A friend participating with us at Health and the Human Mind with Dr. John Whitman Ray, had a 3 year-old daughter with a fever, sleeping on on a pallet on the floor. Our friend K and her then partner B were gently "holding points" on the little girl as she slept. Suddenly the little girl tossed and turned, muttering in her sleep, "Oh no, not now...Oh no, not now..."

K looked at B aghast! "That is exactly what I said the moment I realized I was pregnant with her!!" This amazing example brought home to us and our classmates, how specifically thoughts, words and emotions are stored in the Body-Mind continuum; passed on for each generation to sort out and re-live, unless brought into consciousness to be cleared!

It is amazing that we can access parents, grandparents and 10,000 generations of thought resonating within us, handed down through family dynamics. Wherever we have resistance (old energy Not of LOVE), thoughts-emotions are Vibrationally stored until removed. If we have *any kind of physical ailment or condition*, handed down to us from our family line, we absolutely *must* clear the Mind-energy related to this, to accomplish wellness. We've heard many stories over the years, too numerous to count, of families playing out unmistakable patterns from former generations or bloodline idiosyncrasies. Think of what your family physical and behavioral patterns are.

Young children, barely old enough to understand, recount stories from in utero and of past generations or past lives, that can be traced back to accurate historical records! The wonder of the "holographic mind" shows through its Vibrational patterns and memories so perfectly how we can both imprint and clear past and future generations by clearing ourselves. Historical resonance of thought-emotion imprints on timespace or the 'No - Time' continuum. As we shed old thought patterns we participate with Greater Awareness in this connected Life-process, changing history with clearing, cleansing and LOVE.

In every deliberation, we must consider the impact
on the seventh generation...

Great Law of the Native American Iroquois Nation

As we clear unconscious Vibrational content from generational dynamics, we open ourselves to greater healing potential. Whether or not we have biological children our entire gene pool shifts as we do our clearing, through timespace like dominoes. Ultimately we all are related, and there is no time or space, for we are One and *we are our own ancestors...* We emerge as the miraculous beings we were designed to be, supporting ALL on this Journey of returning to *Essence*! Breathing, Smiling, Changing ourselves, changing the Whole. *Arcing the Hologram Now with LOVE!*

> We should seek not so much to pray
> but to become prayer.
>
> *St. Francis of Assisi (1182-1226)*
> *Order of St. Francis*

Activation from Celestial events in our Cosmos immerses us in an entirely New energetic matrix in the Earth-plane, opening us to a New perceptions of Being. Deep adaptation is taking place within each of us, activated to heightened states of Awareness, triggered through exposure to Greater Light in this Evolutionary shift. As we open our Hearts to creative aspects of our *Essence*, we also open to our miraculous healing potential.

> Once we learn to LOVE everyone unconditionally, releasing need to judge others and self, learning to use the Light of the Creator, we will be able to manifest everything we need to live in harmony and in the new World. We then become Masters, helping others in their spiritual ascension process.
>
> *Cynthia T. Crawford, sculptor*
> *Working with the Star Beings to Awaken Humanity*

Miraculous Messages for Healing

Anya Petrovic received a "message" from Sai Baba (1926-2011), "Pranic Energy in the Ionosphere, as you call it, will soon solve the issue of the shortage of energy for humanity. However, for this to take place there must be a total renewal of habits and customs that characterize [humanity] now..." She next received a message, "from a young girl from Serbia who had channelled 'Estella from Constellation *Grui*' since age twelve." Anya tells the amazing story, "She found me on the internet and handed me texts as Estella advised her. I read it, found it very interesting and set it aside. That year she gave me the same text *again*, guided by Estella."

Through these messages Anya was led to the realization, she was to assist with human evolution by using Tesla energy from the *Field* surrounding us, to bring the body into "perfect Light balance." Based on healing insights transmitted to her by Nikola Tesla, Anya calls this reactivation of Light in the body, "Tesla Metamorphosis." Clients report speedy, often miraculous recovery. She is attracting Attention from science, as "incurables" such as HIV, cancer, coma, spinal injuries and deformities resolve. In her work and teaching, hands act as a Tesla coil, activating Light in the Body, triggering DNA to Reconstruct.

She teaches that Consciousness Evolution is essential currently on Earth. "We must advance ourselves to become multidimensional Beings; go beyond the logical mind, open to our extrasensory ability, so we can evolve with Earth and Cosmic changes." She tells us, "there are no such things as miracles; these already exist in nature. *The miracle is what we are willing to open our minds to, accept and understand.*"

> ...the miracle entails a sudden shift from horizontal to vertical perception. ...giver and receiver...emerge farther along in time... The miracle thus has the unique property of abolishing time to the extent that it renders the...time it spans unnecessary...it substitutes for learning that might have taken thousands of years.
>
> *A Course In Miracles*
> *Page 8, Chapter 1:2-6*

After *Tesla Metamorphosis* sessions clients report seeing people, angels, or landscapes different from planet Earth, feel a physical touch, or similar observations during the session. It seems that those healing frequencies open communication with other dimensions and parallel planes of existence. Throughout the sessions, purple violet Light has been recorded transmitting through Anya and participants. Even one year later participants still have the violet color surrounding them, as is shown in special images. Anya says, "There are significant changes happening in the electro-magnetic field of our planet Earth in this period of time. The consciousness evolution of the human race is of crucial importance and a prerequisite to undergo this transition."

At this key moment in Earth's history Lightworkers are emerging, bringing through healing, restorative energies from other dimensions. We will be led to those by whom we are ignited to Evolve, as a result of being with them. This is where it is important to attune to our own intuition, and follow through when directed.

Thousands of generations of history in the blame-fear-hostility paradigm, is Now like an old shoe we are ready to kick off for the last time. Freeing ourselves from these shadows, we awake to our *Essence*, to bring Greater Unity to Collective Conscious of humanity. Are you stepping into *Essence* to Live from the Heart?

The powerful grid system of Light in the energy matrix of Earth is raising by the many holding LOVE and Light on the Planet today. These new frequencies are influencing thought patterns of everyone on Earth. Its power and influence is growing and expanding as millions Now join in. Each person "waking up" has a natural ability to attune to this network and add to its effectiveness. The more "waking up" add to exponential change.

Life is a transformational journey. The more we open ourselves to possibilities that go beyond what we've always believed in the old paradigm explanation of our World, the more we open ourselves to experiencing the miraculous. We are like little ones just learning to walk. We are being reborn from old ways, developing new skills and a new experience base. It's good to try it out and *laugh at ourselves.* There are always tumbles before little ones take their first steps. And then there are those who just stand up one day and walk! Shifting energies Now activate us, to step into Beyond where we've ever been.

Healing Cary's Broken Arm In 6 Hours

Experience gives confidence to move forward and test it out again and again, until we strengthen our muscles with practice, courage, inspiration and commitment. We were blessed to have miraculous happenings decades ago under tutelage of Dr. John Ray. In fact, before we ever went to class with him, we used his teachings to experience a miracle of a broken arm healing in a matter of six hours!

I (Cary) was co-directing a wheatgrass institute in southern Michigan in 1980-81. A young couple came from Bloomington, Indiana, handed me 6 audio cassettes, and told me I must listen to them! Little did I know at the time what "angels" they were! I never saw them again, so I hope if they read this they will contact me. Of course, curious, I listened to the tapes. Somewhere right around that time Teddi visited the Institute, then called Hippocrates, (later changed to Creative Health) where we met for the first time.

During this visit Teddi and her then husband Lou connected with me, and we became fast friends, "Soul family," who had already known each other for aeons... so of course, I shared the tapes with them. On suggestion from these amazing tapes by Dr. John Whitman Ray, we ordered a case of strange-tasting liquid minerals "to get our electrical potential up." We tasted them, and immediately said, "ugh!" there is no way we'll drink that "nasty tasting stuff," (so they sat in a corner at Teddi and Lou's farm).

Shortly thereafter I met Bill who I would eventually be married to for 12 years, and had much of my own "issues" begin to surface from past relationships, and as a "result" fell ice skating, breaking my arm. One friend encouraged me to go to the hospital, based on the suggestion that if we wanted to fix it, we needed to know if it was broken. Sure enough, X-rays showed 2 fractures in upper and lower arm; doctors wanted to immediately do surgery and put two pins in. My arm was in a sling, and as I looked at the x-rays I made a life-changing decision, to leave the hospital and use Body Electronics to fix it. I signed multiple release forms to get out of the hospital and went home. I talked to my group of friends, and convinced them we should heal my arm with Body Electronics.

The next day Teddi, Lou, Bill, Jamie (co-director of the wheatgrass institute) and his then wife agreed to "hold points" on me. We called one of Dr. Ray's students, Robert Stevens, who was practicing in a city an hour away. He explained the methodology to us: hold STO points at base of skull, glandular reflex points on feet, and hold points as close to the break as possible, on the opposite side of the break from the heart. We chugged down minerals (that had been sitting in the corner), I lay on a massage table, everyone positioned around me to hold points.

Lou was at the base of my skull, and every time I'd process a thought into consciousness, by "going into the pain" and releasing unconscious content connected with it, his fingers would burn and he'd give me feedback, "Whatever you're doing, keep doing it." This was a several hour process through which my friends kept their fingers faithfully glued to points that were now giving off searing-burning heat. I kept going into the pain, allowing emotions connected with the pain to rise to conscious awareness, till each emotion moved up the Emotional Tone Scale to LOVE, transmuting them all one by one.

After a couple of hours of fingers faithfully 'mashed" into points, through numbing, burning layers, something amazing happened...suddenly a searing burning heat began to go through my arm, Jamie's fingers followed it up along the break, as the intensity increased and increased. We could literally hear bones click back into place, black and blue patches cleared, muscles that had been hanging and out of place moved back to where they belonged, and as if it had never been broken, my arm was restored! The searing burning current going through my arm dissolved and it was whole! We held points on it for a little while the next day with additional help from friend Len, for residual cleanup while riding in a van on the way to Manitowish Waters, Wisconsin, to go to class with Dr. John Ray. Tiny pieces of bone clicked back into place, and my arm has been fine ever since! ♥ Cary

This amazing experience of a broken arm healing in a matter of hours, reflected several things. There was a great deal of True Connection with Source happening in Hearts and Minds of those in our group. Most were deeply committed to individual spiritual paths, meditation, high frequency nutrition, with faith and vision that such things were possible. There was a high level of personal and group dedication and integrity of purpose among us - and even so - it was a deeply miraculous experience.

It was as if we reversed the break "through spacetime," and still had the "experience," a very en-Light-ening and educational practical phenomenon, for each of us to carry forward into our lives. We taught Body Electronics groups for several years thereafter, with miraculous healings a relatively common occurrence.

A few years later Teddi was on a "wheatgrass cleanse" at the same institute, and with her was her 5 year old daughter Micah. They were there with dr. michael ryce, his friend and son Michael J. who was 7. One day there was a screech of tires, and a dog cried out. Micah 5 and Michael J. ran to the spot and pulled the dog out of harm's way. They held his hips which had been hit, and after a few minutes the dog jumped up and ran away. Micah and Michael J. had grown up with the idea that anything was possible. They never doubted, and just "acted as if!"

We realized over the years that it didn't take a point holding table, or even a group of people to do this type of work. It became a representative experience, that taught us how to assist ourselves and others to go "into the pain" and (guess what) - clear our unconscious content that (Vibrationally) caused the issue in the first place. This essence has carried into many areas of life, and offered foundational principles still valid today.

I (Cary) was with a partner on a wilderness river trip who blew out a shoulder in a rapid. He had heard me share these stories enough that he had a good understanding of the process. He also had excellent powers of concentration. I held points on him in the tent that night, and he went through his own inner journey "into the pain." He went into all the places the pain took him, to clear old crystalized thought-emotion, some even into a "past life." By the next day, his sling was off and he had oars in hand again navigating the rapids!

Revealed: Consciousness A Form of Matter!

Masaru Emoto, introduced amazing discoveries in the past couple of decades about how thought literally shapes water molecules, that show up as beautiful when associated with kind, Loving thoughts, and dis-integrative when exposed to Not of LOVE thought.

Water records energetic resonance and forms either coherent and beautiful or jagged, incoherent crystal patterns, based on thought held around it. His groundbreaking book, *The Hidden Messages in Water,* crosses boundaries between hard and soft science, with visible demonstrations of how thought-emotion Creates. His water crystals show resonance recorded in rivers, oceans, and even our bodies, or our "water vehicle" 75%-90% water.

Mr. Emoto reports conducting an experiment with chlorinated tap water at his office in Tokyo, when making crystals by his usual methods with just a few people placing thought around it was not working. He asked for the help of 500 people throughout Japan. On the appointed day and time, they all successfully sent positive thoughts to the water on his desk, with the message "Thank You." Mr. Emoto's observations on the results fortify understanding of how thoughts shift our World.

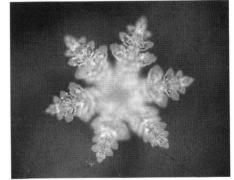

> As expected, the water changed and was able to form beautiful crystals. The chlorinated water from the tap had changed to pure water.
>
> How could this happen? I think you know the answer. Thoughts and words of 500 people reached the water without regard to borders of time and space.
>
> And in the very same way, the Vibration of your thought at this very moment is having a certain effect on the world. If you understand this, then you can also understand that you are already holding in your hands all the keys you need to change your Life.
>
> *Masaru Emoto*
> *The Secret Life of Water*

View images of Mr. Emoto's water crystals either online or in his books. They are a stupendous visual demonstration of how powerful we are as Observer-Creators.

RESTRUCTURING WATER WITH THOUGHT: Apply thought-emotion "signs" to filter or dispenser, such as LOVE, Peace, Compassion, Gratitude, Thank You, Joy, Dance, Play. Become aware of focusing your Attention on these thoughts whenever you notice your labels on the water. Enjoy drinking this water imbued with good thought-feelings of LOVE;

it often tastes sweeter. Relate to water, food, everything in Life, prayerfully, with Gratitude. Great for kids! Show them Emoto's water crystals online or in his books..

LESSON: This is an example of how thoughts affect Life. If an unkind comment occurs, it's a nice reference point to ask if they are making a not-pretty water crystal with their words, and they can change it, because they have a "picture" of what their energy is creating.

Neuroscientists and theoretical physicists Now reveal *Consciousness* is a form of matter! Giulio Tononi, U. of Wisconsin and Max Tegmark of MIT, differentiate Consciousness from other types of matter (solids, liquids, gases) with mathematically sound principles.

> ...we may finally have found a way of analyzing the mysterious, metaphysical realm of *consciousness* in a scientific manner. Latest breakthrough in this new field, published by Max Tegmark of MIT, postulates consciousness is actually a state of matter. "Just as there are many types of liquids, there are many types of consciousness," he says. With this new model, Tegmark says that consciousness can be described in terms of quantum mechanics and information theory, allowing us to *scientifically* tackle murky topics such as self awareness, and why we perceive the world in classical three-dimensional terms, rather than infinite objective realities offered by the many-worlds interpretation of quantum mechanics.
>
> ...consciousness results from a system that can store and retrieve vast amounts of information efficiently..."the most general substance that feels subjectively self-aware." This substance can not only store and retrieve data, but it's also indivisible and unified...

> *Sebastian Anthony, Extreme Tech*
> *Human Consciousness Is Simply a State of Matter*

Magically, our Attention on the *Field* affects Creation surrounding us. Miracles occur when we connect with Heart, *Essence* and Infinite possibilities, clearing ourselves of "old resonance." *21st Century Superhuman* lives in Quantum awareness that thoughts, words and emotions imprint in our "reality." "Reality" is not static, continuously flowing into New form around and through us. We are Self-Aware, and Live with Response-Ability.

We move into Living more from the Heart, expressing *Essence*. We dedicate habits of Thought and Action to the Greater Good; transitioning from service to Self to service for ALL! "There is no 'out there' out there." Ultimately, it is up to us: how we Think, Live, Eat and Play forms our Well-Being and our World. We enter Heaven here and Now, integrating with family, children, pets and Community of LOVE.

Modern medicine is not "all bad," neither is the modern World. Many incredible inventions and abilities will lead us to more amazing things. Synchronistically, our future survival as a species depends on harmonizing with nature, Earth Mother Gaia, Pachamama and her elementals, and the ever creative *Field* flowing from Source. Our greatest Achievements, Joy, Well-Being and Abundance arrive, as we enter *LOVE, Compassion, Gratitude, to Live from the Heart with True Authenticity, called En-Light-enment.* ♥ ♥ ♥

Epilogue

These are guideposts along the path to Awakening during this powerful *Shift of the Ages*. 21st Century Superhuman continues to be published as one complete book; and for ease of handling we have ALDO divided the book into 4 Parts. If you choose the route of the smaller books, please read all 4 as each contains essential "pieces to the puzzle" The exact same material is in the complete single book *21st Century Superhuman Quantum Lifestyle.*

We invite you to Journey with us on YouTube and our Festy-Workshops and invite your friends. This miraculous journey of En-Light-enment means Living Authentically from the Heart, clearing ALL "Not of LOVE," to access and restore our Infinite True Design, LOVE. New perspectives Now unfolding allow us to live beyond the "norm," discovering our own Higher expression, to manifest our greatest dreams, desires and aspirations.

Always Question "Reality," and grow in Wisdom of your Heart and *Essence*. As Richard Feynman, Nobel Laureate Quantum physicist, said, *"If you thought that science was certain - well, that is just an error on your part,"* pointing out in ultimate wisdom -

The highest forms of understanding we can achieve
are laughter and human compassion.

Richard P. Feynman (1918-1988)
Albert Einstein Award, Nobel Prize in Physics

The "breadcrumb trail" in this guide is designed to share YOUR unique gifts with the World. Remember to as Leonard Orr says, *"Speak the Truth Quicker and Have More Fun Per Hour!"* Breathing and Smiling all the way...

Inlakesh - I am another yourself

Aloha, Many Blessings and Namaste

We bow to the Divine within You

See you "on the path!"

♥ *Cary and Teddi* ♥

LOVE

♥ ♥ ♥

Contributor

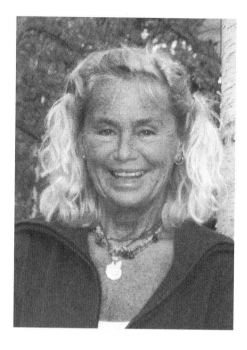

THEODORA SUSAN MULDER, PHD, CRA

Gifted with the ability to see Energy *Fields* at a young age, Teddi was drawn to metaphysical and holistic practices, opening doors for exploration of many dimensions on her Earth-Walk. She focuses on our "Grand Design."

Teddi's background and training: biofeedback Menninger Foundation; Spiritual Midwifery - The Farm Tennessee; Dr. Christopher Hill - Herbalism, Kirlian photography, cellular biology University of the Trees; Permaculture with Founder of Findhorn Peter Kaddy. She is an active meditator, initiated in Kriya Yoga, which was brought to the West by Parmahansa Yogananda. Initiated into shamanic realms she apprenticed with Sun Bear, Native American Medicine Man; mysteries of ancient Tibetan point holding with Dr. John Whitman Ray; and rebirthing techniques with Leonard Orr, Florida School of Massage. Teddi studied Cellular Biology with Dr. Bruce Lipton in Madison, Wisconsin. She completed two internships with Dr. D. A. Versendaal (founder of C.R.A. Contact Reflex Analysis), over eight years, for which she earned a PhD based in research of Clinical Nutrition, specializing in *Health of Women and Children*. Teddi has performed client services for over 30 years.

Mother of four and currently grandmother of eleven (last count); she is LOVED as an embodiment of the nurturing qualities of Mother Earth, and as one who represents the Deeper Science of Life, LOVE and Universal principles. Teddi often goes by her Soul Name, Nivana. She offers support for clarity and balance of each individual's lifestream, essential to our Future on Planet Earth and Beyond.

Her collaborative work with Cary over many years, producing classes, retreats, materials and manuals for Conscious Living, has these days moved into "midwifery" toward development of global communities through *Virtual Earth Village dot com* and **21st Century Superhuman**. She is dedicated to offering tools and resources of these visions, bringing forth our greater possibilities through implementing **Quantum Lifestyle** habits and wise Living practices.

Raising four children and many beautiful grandchildren has been the greatest learning curve of my Life - allowing each one to be who they are, supporting their individuality and their well being, to let their Lights shine in the World. Teddi ♥

Author

CARY DIANE ELLIS DD

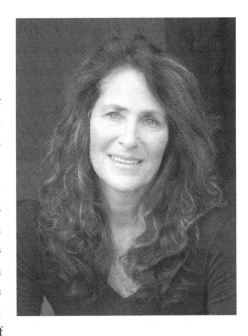

Cary's Innate Ability to assimilate languages of Light and LOVE into practical everyday tools is like having the gentle hand of a friend on your shoulder, guiding you into greater Awareness.

Introducing transformation into mainstream culture for decades in the human potentials movement, she assisted thousands in breakthrough workshops: putting Tony Robbins on stage with Firewalking and Fear into Power in the 1980s; miraculous healing of her own broken arm in a matter of 6 hours when doctors wanted to do surgery and put in 2 pins; co-founder of Dolphin Camp she entered transcendental states while swimming with wild dolphins; has experienced age reversal and rejuvenation with wheatgrass, living foods and more.

Cary's wealth of knowledge comes from hands on experience as: Co-Director Hippocrates Health Institute (later Creative Health), with Lifestyle learning programs filled to capacity, exceptional organic gardens, permaculture, wheatgrass and living foods. She was Educator with Gerson Cancer Therapy Institute in Mexico, did rounds with Charlotte Gerson, experiencing "miraculous recoveries" firsthand. She trained with Dr. John Whitman Ray in revolutionary Health and Human Mind and Body Electronics and Iridology. She is also well versed in Human Design and Astrology.

Passion for the outdoors lead Cary to live remotely in high mountains of the American West, with many years of outdoor adventure, snowboarding, mountain biking, river rafting, hiking and horseback riding with her dogs and a large outdoor community. She also assisted with colloquiums for Earth-friendly building. Her lifework has been dedicated to user-friendly knowledge, easily applied to harmonious, Earth-friendly Living.

Curiosity and a sense of adventure inspired Cary to venture into unknown territories for knowledge useful, practical and necessary in our Evolutionary Leap toward a wise, ecological future. Her innate vision of Higher Dimensions, offers Light and LOVE on the Path for those seeking Wisdom for Humanity's current Evolutionary Leap. Honored for her Life-work as a Doctor of Divinity by the *Church of Tzaddi*, Cary is involved in developing cutting edge "New Earth" Communities, and is often called by her Soul Name, Kirastar.

With their current project VirtualEarthVillage.com, Cary and Teddi offer cutting edge tools to align with millions Now around the Planet ushering in communities founded in LOVE, amplifying this Current Evolutionary Wave on Planet Earth called the Shift of the Ages. ♥

Front Cover Art

FRANZI TALLEY - FRONT COVER - Earth Mother Gaia aligns with the resonance of Oneness and Harmonious living on Planet Earth, brought forth in the Ninth Wave of the Mayan Calendar, as humanity rides this wave into their own transformation through LOVE.

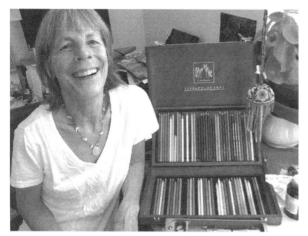

FRANZI TALLEY

I came from a family where creativity was always encouraged and I was, more often than not, surrounded by the sounds of classical music and a feeling of great freedom. Our neighborhood, in Bienne, a small town in the north of Switzerland. perched on the side of a deep green forest. The woods called to me daily and I answered that call.

I spent much of my time in nature, in the abundant beauty and wilderness of my country. There, I was able to ignore the over-clean, controlled, organized side of my homeland's culture. As a child I made sure to take ample advantage of delicious goods offered by numerous bakeries dotting towns, and colorful harvests in the open-air markets.

At sixteen, I began a four-year graphic design program. A few years later I moved to the US, met my husband and started a family. For the next twenty-four years we raised our children happily in Asheville, NC, as my husband worked to establish Natural Food stores all over North Carolina. During that time I was an illustrator and graphic designer for numerous projects in the Natural Foods industry. As my free time increased with the maturing of our children, I have been able to bring forth ideas and projects, carried deep inside of me for many years.

As a child I had been touched by the glory of nature and by the medieval towns of Europe with their small churches and cloisters. Their stone walls were alive with ancient art, simple and yet full of meaning. Those walls carried many stories as did the trees and the old mountain trails. The forests, lakes and valleys held within the booming mountains, are for me some of the most holy places in Creation. I have carried all of them, deep in my mind and heart for a Lifetime and to this day they provide a fertile reservoir of ideas for my work. I draw for my own enjoyment, and in the hope that my offerings will surprise, delight, amuse, and uplift others. ♥ *Franzi* ♥

NOTE: *Earth Mother Gaia image on cover of this book, brought forth by artist, Franzi Talley, is aligned with the resonance of Oneness and Harmonious living on Planet Earth, and our return to LOVE activated by our transit throught the Cosmos with the Ninth Wave of the Mayan Calendar.* ♥

Back Cover Art

*ENDRE BALOGH - BACK COVER - Sacred Geometry aligns with the resonance of Oneness and fractals of Creation, as we **Arc the Hologram** to transform our World with our True Design LOVE.*

ENDRE BALOGH - Violinist, Photographer, Artist

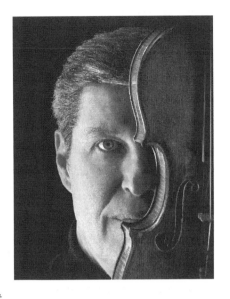

Endre's interest in spirituality has led him to Create hundreds of "Sacred Geometry" designs, the basis for his contribution to this book. Endre's extraordinary visionary work in the realms of Sound, Light and Color bring transformation to his audiences.

He is an internationally acclaimed concert violinist and soloist, who has performed for over thirty years with renowned orchestras, conductors, chamber music and productions internationally throughout Europe, Canada and the US. *"We were under the spell of a formidably brilliant artist."* (London Times) *"Poise and assurance, technical precision, tonal refinement and personal charm."* (new York Times) *"Dazzling technique and great gusts of temperament...eloquent master of his instrument."* (Los Angeles Times)

In 2004, curtailing his concert schedule to spend more time with his children, Endre honed his passion for photography and design. He won top awards in contests with unique aesthetic vision that earned him an enviable reputation among photographic colleagues. His photos are displayed in the collections of connoisseurs of fine photographic arts, and he has had prominent gallery showings. His photo "Egg On Glass" was chosen from nearly 3000 entries from 40 countries displayed with 87 others in the prestigious "Art of Digital" International Exhibition 2007. Endre is a highly sought after headshot photographer and graphic artist, having designed covers for numerous books. *Shutterbug* Magazine's annual publication "Expert Photo Techniques Guide" showcased his article with his cover shot and six more images inside. He was "Photographer Of the Year - 2012."

Endre's diverse work can be seen and purchased in many formats EndreBalogh.ArtistWebsites dot com Main website: EndresPhotos dot com

THANKS TO BRANDON LAVERGNE anime & manga artist, for Mediation Drawings. He can be found on Facebook as Brandon Indigo Starseed.

Bibliography

PART 1 - SHIFT OF THE AGES: Cosmic Light & Ancient Texts
SECTION 1 - COSMIC EVENTS
Chapter 1 Great Change, Quantum "Reality"
David R Hawkins, *MD PhD, Power VS Force, The Hidden Determinants of Human Behavior,* (Hay House 2002)
   148
Chapter 2 Mayan Calendar Ends
Carl Johan Calleman,Seattle, WA, *Ninth Wave Mayan Calendar: World Oneness Revolution*
   (mayanprophecy2012.blogspot.com/2011/11/9th-wave-mayan-calendar-world-oneness.html and interview
   with Lilou's Juicy Living Tour, Friday November 18, 2011 Youtube)
Ac Tah, *The Night of the Last Katún 2012 Maya,* (Printed in Mexico 2012) 31
Chapter 3 Earth's Magnetics and Consciousness
Imagine Do You, The 'Overlooked' Van Allen Belt & Its Relationship to the Photon Band, imaginedoyou.com/
   2012/06/the-overlooked-van-allen-belt-its-relationship-to-the-photon-band/
Gregg Braden, *Awakening to Zero Point* ((Radio Book Store Press 1997) amazon.com book description
NASA Science - Science News, (Online - science1.nasa.gov/science-News/science-at-nasa/
   2003/29dec_magneticfield/ December 29, 2003)
Raymond Trevor Bradley, The Psychology of Intuition: A Quantum-Holographic Theory of Nonlocal
   Communication (Institute for Whole Social Science, Carmel, California, USA; Institute of HeartMath,
   California, USA; e~Motion Institute, Auckland, new Zealand; Routledge, Taylor and Francis Group 2006)
   spiritualscientific.com/yahoo_site_admin/assets/docs/
   Intuition_Psychophysiology_and_Quantum_Holography.153141247.pdf
Dr. Rollin McCraty, Earth Rhythms (Global Coherence Initiative,
http://www.glCoherence.org/monitoring-system/earth-rhythms.html)
Dr. Rollin McCraty, Establishing the new Paradigm 2013 and Ongoing Global Earth Changes, (Global Coherence
   Initiative, http://www.glCoherence.org/monitoring-system/commentaries.html)
Jeffrey Mishlove Ph.D. interview with Jean Houston, Possible Human, Possible World Part I with Jean Houston,
   Ph.D. (The Intuition Network, A Thinking Allowed Television Underwriter, presents the following transcript
   from the series Thinking Allowed, Conversations On the Leading Edge of Knowledge and Discovery, with Dr.
   Jeffrey Mishlove. ntuition.org/txt/houston1.htm)
Chapter 4 Pineal Gland & DMT Spirit Molecule
Supermassive Galactic Plasma Ray (redlotus888, Youtube Video April 20, 2013) youtube.com/watch?
   v=klSQzBgFRoY Based on *Solar (R)Evolution* (excerpts from full length documentary by renowned German
   biophysicist, Dieter Broers)
Ac Tah, *The Night of the Last Katún 2012 Maya,* (Printed in Mexico 2012) 33
Supermassive Galactic Plasma Ray (redlotus888, Youtube Video April 20, 2013) youtube.com/watch?
   v=klSQzBgFRoY Based on *Solar (R)Evolution* (excerpts from full length documentary by renowned German
   biophysicist, Dieter Broers)
Meg Benedictine, Entering the Galactic Photon Belt, (Newearthevolution.com/library/Newsletters/431-entering-the-
   galactic-photon-belt
Dieter Broers, Solar Revolution (North Atlantic Books, Ecover Editions 2009) 8-10
Chapter 5 Adapting to Solar Changes
Aluna Joy Yaxk'in *Solar Flares Assist in Our Ascension* Blog Post Copyright © 2012 - Permission is granted to
   copy and redistribute this article on the condition that the content remains complete, full credit is given to the
   author(s), and that it is distributed freely. Aluna Joy Yaxk'in, PO Box 1988 Sedona, AZ 86339 USA Web:
   AlunaJoy.com Email: aluna@alunajoy.com
Tom Kenyon, Hathors, www.tomkenyon.com/hathors-archives
SECTION 2 HOW QUANTUM "REALITY" OPERATES
Chapter 6 When The World is Flat & the Double Slit Experiment
Lynne McTaggart, *The Field, The Quest for the Secret Force of the Universe* (Harper Collins Publishers, Great
   Britain 2001) 120-121
Chapter 7 Quantum Threads in Ancient Tradition
Drunvalao Melchezedek, The Great White Pyramid of Tibet, One Vibration: Egyptian and Atlantean Origins
   http://one-vibration.com/group/egyptianandatlantianorigins/forum/topics/the-great-white-pyramid-of?
   commentId=2127676%3AComment%3A426305&groupId=2127676%3AGroup%3A404113#.U06y4eZdUuo
Chapter 8 The *Field* Awaits Our Command
Winifred Gallagher, NY Times Bestseller, *Rapt, Attention and the Focused Life* (Penguin Books 2009)
SECTION 3 MAKING THE LEAP

Chapter 10 Beyond Time 4-5 D

Penny Kelly, *Consciousness and Energy, Volume 1: Multi-Dimensionality and A Theory of Consciousness* (Lily Hill Publishing. 32260 - 88th Ave, Lawton, MI 49065) 222-223

Lynne McTaggart, *The Field, The Quest for the Secret Force of the Universe* (Harper Collins Publishers, Great Britain 2001) 120-121

Jeffrey Mishlove Ph.D. interview with Jean Houston, *Possible Human, Possible World Part I with Jean Houston, Ph.D.* (The Intuition Network, A Thinking Allowed Television Underwriter, presents the following transcript from the series Thinking Allowed, Conversations On the Leading Edge of Knowledge and Discovery, with Dr. Jeffrey Mishlove. ntuition.org/txt/houston1.htm)

Bill Ballard, The Great Awakening, (edited and pub.Gillian C Grannum shiftfrequencies.com) Download Ebook Free at shiftfrequency.com/bill-ballard-official-release-of-my-ebook-the-great-awakening Donations greatly appreciated via Paypal pearls2u@hotmail.com

Discover Magazine, *Newsflash: Time May Not Exist, Not to mention the question of which way it goes...* (online: discovermagazine.com/2007/jun/in-no-time#.UczozD44Vdh June 2007)

Dieter Broers, Solar Revolution, Why Mankind is on the Cusp of an Evolutionary Leap, Creating a new Form of Consciousness & Harmony (North Atlantic Books, Evolver Editions, Berkeley, CA 2012) 126

Chris Griscom, *Time Is An Illusion* (Fireside; First Edition edition (July 15, 1988) 103

Chapter 11 Dimensional Doorways

Ken Carey, Starseed Transmissions (First Harper Collins Paperback Edition 1991)

Bill Ballard, The Great Awakening, (edited and pub.Gillian C Grannum shiftfrequencies.com) Download Ebook Free at shiftfrequency.com/bill-ballard-official-release-of-my-ebook-the-great-awakening Donations greatly appreciated via Paypal pearls2u@hotmail.com

Kelly La ShaLiquid Mirror Blog (liquidmirror.org/wp1/)

A Course In Miracles, Electronic Version, Chapter 1 (Copyright© 1975,1985,1992,1996 by the Foundation for Inner Peace) 12

Nellie B. Cain, *Exploring the Mysteries of Life, 30 Years Research* (self-published, 740 Hubbard St. N.E., Grand Rapids, Michigan 49505,1972) 265

Chapter 12 Phase-Shifting

Dieter Broers, Solar Revolution, Why Mankind is on the Cusp of an Evolutionary Leap - Creating a new Form of Consciousness and Harmony (N. Atlantic Books Evolver Editions, Berkeley, CA 2012) XXII

Chapter 13 Change is Afoot

Nellie B. Cain, *Exploring the Mysteries of Life, 30 Years Research* (self-published, 740 Hubbard St. N.E., Grand Rapids, Michigan 49505,1972) 265 Walter Cruttenden, *Lost Star of Myth and Time* (St. Lynn's Press 2005) description

Ovotron, The Photon Belt Story - *bibliotecapleyades.net* (Feb-Mar 1991 Nexus, Australia)

Sri Yukteswar Giri, *The Holy Science* (Atul Chondra Chowdhary, Secretary Sadhusaba) 1920

The Galactic Center → → The Eye of Horus??davidicke.com/forum/showthread.php?t=187477

Jeffrey Mishlove Ph.D. interview with Jean Houston, *Possible Human, Possible World Part I with Jean Houston, Ph.D.* (The Intuition Network, A Thinking Allowed Television Underwriter, presents the following transcript from the series Thinking

Patricia Cota-Robles, *The Violet Flame*, eraofpeace.com

Chapter 14 There Is No 'Out There' Out There

Danielle Graham, *Interview with Dr. Bruce Lipton, Genetics, Epigenetics and Destiny* (superconsciousness.com/topics/science/interview-dr-bruce-lipton Sept.2008)

Teal Swan, Spiritual Bypassing (YouTube) https://www.youtube.com/watch?v=0ErlTinKrQw

Barbara Marciniak, *Bringers of the Dawn* (Bear and Company, Santa Fe, NM 1992) 53

Stephen Davis, *Butterflies Are Free to Fly* (download free at butterfliesfree.com) *A new and Radical Approach to Spiritual Evolution* (Smashwords Edition, 2010 by L & G Productions, LLC) 77-78

Nellie B. Cain, Exploring the Mysteries of Life, 30 Years Research

Chapter 15 What Is The Dream?

A Course In Miracles, Electronic Version, Chapter 1 (Copyright© 1975,1985,1992,1996 by the Foundation for Inner Peace) 13

Chapter 17 Restoring Our True Design LOVE

Nellie B. Cain, Exploring the Mysteries of Life, 30 Years Research

APPENDIX: Universal Laws

The Three Initiates, *The Kybalion* (1908 public domain)

Dr. Wayne W. Dyer, Excuses Begone, How to Change Lifelong, Self-Defeating Thinking Habits, (Hay House, Inc. 2009) 15-16

Marc Gamma, *Archangel Michael Looking for the Special Key* (soul4free.wordpress.com/2013/09/25/looking-for-the-special-key-it-is-hidden-in-your-hearts-archangel-michael-through-marc-gamma-25-09-2013/)

PART 2 - MIND: The BEST Secret Formula to Manifest LOVE, Health, Abundance
SECTION 1 - 21ST CENTURY SUPERHUMAN A NEW FRONTIER
Ervin Lazlo, Akashic Think... World Changing (*huffingtonpost.com/ervin-laszlo/akasha-think_b_1654078.html*)
Ervin Lazlo, ervinlazlo.org
Chapter 1 Meditation & Inner Stillness
John Hagelin, Biographical Information, sourcewatch.org/index.php/John_Hagelin
Georgi Stankov, *General Theory of the Universal Law* stankovuniversallaw.com/2013/11/finally-elohim-confirm-surprising-message-mpr-progressing-smoothly-opening-megaportal-11-11-occur-weeks-november-23-25/
Dennis Elwell, *"Cosmic Loom, The new Science of Astrology,"* (The Wessex Astrologer, 4A Woodside Rd., Bournemouth, BH5 2AZ *wessexastrologer.com* 2008) 41
Robert Brumet, *"Finding Yourself in Transition, Using Life's Changes for Spiritual Awakening,"* (Unity House, Unity Village, Missouri 2006) 20-21
Chapter 2 *Being* Prayer
Wikipedia, Holonomic Brain Theory
Gregg Braden *Secret Ancient Knowledge:The Divine Matrix* (YouTube)
Gregg Braden *Cancer Cured in 3 Minutes - Awesome Presentation by Gregg Braden* (YouTube)
Chapter 3 Response-Ability
Matthew 7:1-5 Biblegateway (online)
Nellie B. Cain, *Exploring the Mysteries of Life, 30 Years Research* (self-published, 740 Hubbard St. N.E., Grand Rapids, Michigan 49505,1972) 60-61
Annie Payson Call, *How to live Quietly* (Little, Brown and Company, Boston, September, 1914)
Chapter 4 *Effluvia:* Letting Go Our "Story"
Gregg Braden, *The Divine Matrix* (Hay House, Inc. Carlsbad, CA 2007) 39, 3-4
Amit Goswami, amitgoswami.org/
Gregg Braden, *The Divine Matrix* (Hay House, Inc. Carlsbad, CA 2007) 39, 3-4
SECTION 2 - OUR TRUE DESIGN LOVE
Gregg Braden, *The Divine Matrix, Bridging Time, Space, Miracles and Belief* (Hay House 2007) 206-207
Chapter 5 Loving
dr. michael ryce, Mindshifter Radio Show (whyagain.org Mindshifter Radio Aug. 28, 2013)
Gregg Braden, *The Divine Matrix, Bridging Time, Space, Miracles and Belief* (Hay House 2007) 206-207
Chapter 6 Our True Power Supply
Ervin Laszlo, The Quantum Brain, Spirituality and the Mind of God, Huffington Post, Religion (huffingtonpost.com/ervin-laszlo/the-Quantum-brain-spiritu_b_510843.html)
Dieter Broers, Solar Revolution, Why Mankind is on the Cusp of an Evolutionary Leap - Creating a new Form of Consciousness and Harmony (N. Atlantic Books, Evolver Editions, Berkeley, CA 2012) 114
Chapter 7 The LOVE Channel
Marianne Williamson, *A Return to LOVE: Reflections on the Principles of A Course in Miracles* (Harper Collins 1992) Wiki
Dieter Broers, Solar Revolution, Why Mankind is on the Cusp of an Evolutionary Leap - Creating a new Form of Consciousness & Harmony (N Atlantic Books, Evolver Editions, Berkeley, CA 2012) 118-120
His Holiness The Dalai Lama, *The Dalai Lama's Little Book of Wisdom* (Barnes and Noble, 1995, 1997, 2000) 156
Jeffrey Mishlove Ph.D. interview with Jean Houston, *Possible Human, Possible World Part I with Jean Houston, Ph.D.* (The Intuition Network, A Thinking Allowed Television Underwriter, presents the following transcript from the series Thinking Allowed, Conversations On the Leading Edge of Knowledge and Discovery, with Dr. Jeffrey Mishlove. ntuition.org/txt/houston1.htm)
Dieter Broers, Solar Revolution, Why Mankind is on the Cusp of an Evolutionary Leap - Creating a new Form of Consciousness and Harmony (N. Atlantic Books, Evolver Editions, Berkeley, CA 2012)
Chapter 9 A Fairy Tale For Our Newborn
Jeffrey Mishlove Ph.D. interview with Jean Houston, *Possible Human, Possible World Part I with Jean Houston, Ph.D.* (The Intuition Network, A Thinking Allowed Television Underwriter, presents the following transcript from the series Thinking Allowed, Conversations On the Leading Edge of Knowledge and Discovery, with Dr. Jeffrey Mishlove. ntuition.org/txt/houston1.htm)
SECTION 3 - CLEARING THE TEMPLE
Chapter 11 Aramaic Filters: Rakhma - Khooba, Rookha d'Koodsha
Rocco A. Erico, www.roccoaerrico.com
Dr. Michael Ryce, Kabouris, whyagain.org
Dr. Michael Ryce, Reality Management Worksheet, No Fault Empowerment Tool (11 Step) (Download free at whyagain.org/Start Here)
dr. michael ryce, FAQ whyagain.org Question: *Explain Rakhma or Khooba LOVE from the Aramaic (whyagain.org)*
Dr. Candace Pert *"Discovered Opiate Receptors; "Your Body Is Your Unconscious Mind"* Audio

Chapter 12 Tuning Up Our DNA: LOVE Is Freedom
(x3)Michael Tellinger, *Slave Species of the Gods, The Secret History of the Anunnaki and Their Mission on Earth,* (Bear and Company, One Bear St. Rochester, VT 05767 2012) 22-23, 50

Patricia Diane Cota-Robles, *Who Am I? Why Am I Here?* (New Age Study of Humanity's Purpose, PO Box 41883, Tucson, AZ 85717 2010, www.eraofpeace.org) 86

Dieter Broers, *Solar Revolution,* (N. Atlantic Books, Evolver Editions, Berkeley, CA 2012) 62

Nicholas Roerich, *Altai-Himalaya,* (roerich.org/roerich-writings-altai-himalaya.php 1929)

Chapter 14 Reclaiming Our Power
Dr. Michael Ryce - Please live, share, teach and support this work freely. COPY ONLY IF this notice is included on all copies and adaptations. www.whyagain.com for 10x13 parchment copies send 3.00 ea., 2 for 5.00, 5 for 10.00 2 Hr. Video or 4 Hr. Audio Tapes– 40.00 (+ 5.00 S&H) Please send exchange or a POSTAL money order to: dr. michael ryce, C/O HC3 Box 3280, Theodosia, Missouri 65761 (417) 273-4838 From the workshop "Empowered To Heal" ®1993, 2006, 2011 whyagain.org

SECTION 4 - WAKEUP CALL FROM THE HEART
Business Insider Oct. 2011, *"Facts About Military Spending that Will Blow Your Mind:"* businessinsider.com/military-spending-budget-defense-cuts-2011-10?op=1

Michael Tellinger, *Slave Species of the Gods* (Bear and Company, Rochester VT 2012) back cover

David Wilcock, Source Field Investigations and The Synchronicity Key (Dutton Adult Aug. 20, 2013)

Chapter 15 Brain And Heart Team Up
Gregg Braden, *The Role of the Heart in the Law of Attraction* (Youtube youtube.com/watch?v=ElW4-IuT3K4 Aug. 1, 2010)

Ralph and Marsha Ring: Antigravity and Conscious Awareness in Aether Technology bluestarenterprise.com http://www.youtube.com/watch?v=8v3Bsh1E_8Y#t=760

Chapter 16 Success with Heart Coherence
Susan Barber interview with Howard Martin, *HeartMath™ When LOVE Is Not An Emotion,* (Published in Drunvalo Melchizedek's online *Spiritual Community Magazine - Spirit of Ma'at - The Secret Space in the Heart* - Vol. 4 No. 1 Aug. 12, 2013) http://www.spiritofmaat.com/archive/aug4/martin.htm

PART 3: SPIRIT: Live Your Dreams: Success, Passion, Relationship, Community
SECTION 1 WE ARE ENERGY BEINGS
Chapter 1 Co-Creating This Shift Of The Ages
Barbara Marx Hubbard, *Birth 2012 and Beyond, Humanity's Great Shift to the Age of Conscious Evolution* (Shift Books, shiftmovement.com)75

Carolanne Wright, Guest Waking Times, Y*ou Really Can Change Your DNA* (wakingtimes.com/2013/09/24/really-can-change-dna-heres/ Sept. 24, 2013)

Chapter 2 Emotional Tone Scale & Healing Crisis
Deepak Chopra MD, *"Synchrodestiny: Harnessing the Infinite Power of Coincidence to Create Miracles,"* (Published in 2003 by Rider, an imprint of Edbury Press, Random House, 20 Vauxhall Bridge Road, London SWV SA 2005)

Chapter 3 Our Chakra System
Barbara Marciniak, *Bringers of the Dawn* (Bear and Company, Santa Fe, NM 1992) 65

Michael Mirdad, Sacred Sexuality, a Mantra for Living Bliss http://www.spiritualtantra.net/

Chapter 4 You're A Shining Star
Barbara Marciniak, *Bringers of the Dawn* (Bear and Company, Santa Fe, NM 1992) 52, 154-155

Dr. Michael Ryce, Commitment to Myself, Please live, share, teach and support this work freely. COPY ONLY IF this notice is included on all copies and adaptations. whyagain.org for 10x13 parchment copies send 3.00 ea., 2 for 5.00, 5 for 10.00 2 Hr. Video or 4 Hr. Audio Tapes– 40.00 (+ 5.00 S&H) Please send exchange or a POSTAL money order to: dr. michael ryce, C/O HC3 Box 3280, Theodosia, Missouri 65761 (417) 273-4838 From workshop "Empowered To Heal" ®1993, 2006, 2011

SECTION 2: LIVING LIVES WE LOVE
Allen Smith, Rainbow Didge Music

Chapter 5 Creative Genius - Following Your Bliss
Barbara Marx Hubbard http://barbaramarxhubbard.com/

Eckhart Tolle - http://www.eckharttolle.com/

TealScott, http://www.thespiritualcatalyst.com/teachings

A Course In Miracles, Chapter 20, The Vision of Holiness p 433

Dr. Richard Bartlett, Matrix Energetics http://www.matrixenergetics.com/

Chapter 6 Living From *Essence*
Steve Jobs, Secrets of Life video, 1994, (youtube.com/watch?v=kYfNvmF0Bqw)

Lynne McTaggart, *The Field, The Quest for the Secret Force of the Universe* (Harper Collins Publishers, Great Britain 2001)

Godfé Ray King, *Original Unveiled Mysteries* (Saint Germain Press, 1120 Stonehedge Drive, Schaumburg, Illinois 60194 1982) 58

Sierra Goodman, *Oceans of Inspiration* (oceansofinspiration.com/)

Chapter 8 Manifestation of Abundance

Edgar Cayce and John Van Auken, Toward a Deeper Meditation (A.R.E. Press 2007), referred from In5D.com article "*Time and No-Time*"

Chapter 9 Changing Timelines

Michael Tellinger, *Slave Species of the Gods* (Bear and Company, Rochester VT 2012) 61

HeartMath Institute, The Heart's Intuitive Intelligence: A Path to Personal, Social and Global Coherence, www.heartmath.org

Amit Goswami, PhD, amitgoswami.org

SECTION 3: A NEW CIVILIZATION BASED IN LOVE

Alexander Del Sol, *We Went Against The Story*, June 30, 2014 https://waverider1.wordpress.com/2014/06/30/we-went-against-the-story/

Chapter 10 - Spirit of Community

Kamala Everett and Sharon Rose, Saint Germain and Lady Portia WalkTheEarthAsALivingMaster.com

Michel Bauwens, Reality Sandwich, The Next Buddha Will Be a Collective http://realitysandwich.com/1207/next_buddha_will_be_a_collective/

Chapter 62 Article, "Time and No-Time" at In5D.com, excerpt John Van Auken's book Toward a Deeper Meditation. http://www.in5d.com/edgar-cayce-time-and-no-time.html

HeartMath Institute, Global Coherence Project http://www.glcoherence.org/

Nassim Haramein, The Resonance Project, http://resonance.is/

Chapter 12 - Family, Children, Pets

Lee Carroll & Jan Tober (1999) *The Indigo Children* (Hay House Inc. PO Box 5100 Carlsbad, CA 92018-5100) 134, 124-125

Kirpal Singh (1974), World Conference on the Unity of Man http://www.kirpalsingh-teachings.org/en/

Chapter 13 One With Mother Earth Gaia

Jose Arguelles, The Mayan Factor (Bear and Company 1987)

Arjun Walia, Lucid dreaming: a state of consciousness with features of both waking and non-luciddreaming (PubMed September 2009 by JW, Goethe University in Frankfort Germany)

Gregg Braden *The Key to True Harmony* YouTube https://www.youtube.com/watch?v=pr0QpwNSaVo#t=128

Chapter 14 Death The Great Mystery

Alexander III M.D., Eben (2012-10-23). Proof of Heaven: A Neurosurgeon's Journey into the Afterlife (Kindle Locations 916-919). Simon & Schuster. Kindle Edition.

Chapter 63 Amen - Namasté

Garret John LoPorto, Wayseer Manifesto http://www.wayseermanifesto.com/

Galactic Free Press http://soundofheart.org/galacticfreepress/content/researchers-finally-show-how-mindfulness-and-your-thoughts-can-induce-specific-molecular

Galactic Free Press http://soundofheart.org/galacticfreepress/content/researchers-finally-show-how-mindfulness-and-your-thoughts-can-induce-specific-molecular

Great Invocation: ww.lucistrust.org/en/service_activities/e_mantrams/the_great_invocation

PART 4: BODY - Rejuvenation & Growing Younger with Healthy Eating, Cleanse & Detox

SECTION 1 - BACK TO THE GARDEN

Darksunblade, Review at amazon.com *Survival Into The 21st Century*

Viktoras Kulvinskas, *Survival Into The 21st Century - Planetary Healers Manual* (Omangod Press, PO Box 255, Wethersfield, CT 06109

Chapter 1 - Choosing Your Approach to Wellness

John Robbins, The Food Revolution: How Your Diet Can Help Save Your Life and Our World, (Kindle, Conari Press 2010)

Chapter 2 How Thought Affects the Body

Marco Torres, Scientist Finally Present Evidence On Expanding DNA Strands, http://preventdisease.com/news/13/012313_Scientists-Present-Evidence-on-Expanding-DNA-Strands.shtml

Chapter 3 What Is Ideal Nutrition

Dr. Caldwell Esselstyn, Prevent and Reverse Heart Dis-Ease (Avery Trade; January 31, 2008) 4-5, 84, 38

John Robbins, *Diet for a New America* (quotes online)

John Robbins, *Diet for a New World* (AVON BOOKS, A Division of The Hearst Corporation, 1350 Avenue of the Americas, New York, NY 10019 Copyright John Robbins and Jia Patton 1992) 27-28

Chapter 4 Superior Supplements: Superfoods

John D. Haymaker & Donald Weaver, The Survival Of Civilization: Carbon Dioxide, Investment Money, Population – Three Problems Threatening Our Existence http://remineralize.ning.com/profiles/blogs/hello-and-update-from-don-weaver-co-author-of-the-survival-of

Kailash Kokopelli *Walking Tree* "trust in the song of your heart" (INNER World MUSIC) Sing-dance along: http://www.kailash-kokopelli.com/songdances_kk.html www.kailash-kokopelli.com

SECTION 2 - HOW TO CLEANSE & DETOX

Chapter 6 "7 Days" To A New YOU!

Interview by Diane with Drunvalo Melchizdek, By Enoch Tan, new Earth Daily #1 Source for Positive News

Chapter 7 Cleanse And Detox - 3-7-30 Day Cleanses

drpielet.com/3-things-you-can-do-today-to-start-losing-weight/

Chapter 9 Supportive Modalities

NAET, naet.com

SECTION 3 - DIS-EASE THE ILLUSION

Chapter 10 Toxemia The Cause of Dis-Ease

Kiera Butler, Mother Jones, *The Scary Truth About Antibiotic Overprescription* (motherjones.com/blue-marble/2013/10/scary-truth-about-antibiotic-overprescription)

Chapter 11 The Curse Causeless Shall Not Come

A Course In Miracles, Electronic Version, Chapter 2 (Copyright© 1975,1985,1992,1996 by the Foundation for Inner Peace) 16-17

Wes Annac, Aquarius Paradigm, DL Zeta: Upgrading our Lens of Perception Shifts us to Fifth-Dimensional Timelines (aquariusparadigm.com/2013/10/12/dl-zeta-upgrading-our-lens-of-perception-shifts-us-to-fifth-dimensional-timelines/ Oct. 12, 2013,)

Chapter 12 Enviro Toxins

HSPH - Harvard School of Public Health News, Impact of fluoride on neurological development in children http://www.hsph.harvard.edu/news/features/fluoride-childrens-health-grandjean-choi/

Global Healing Center's blog, Natural Health and Organic Living, Chlorine, Cancer and Heart Disease http://www.globalhealingcenter.com/natural-health/toxic-chemical-health-dangers-chlorine/

Chapter 13 Miraculous Tales

Deepak Chopra M, The Way of the Wizard: Twenty Spiritual Lessons for Creating the Life You Want (Kindle, Harmony, Random House 2009)

Edward Bach M.D. and F.J. Wheeler M.D., *The Bach Flower Remedies* (Keats Publishing Inc. New Canaan Connecticut www.keats.com 1977 The Edward Bach Center) 40-41

Energy Scientists and Developer of Vogel Crystals www.treeofLifetech.com on Dr. Marcel Vogel

Masaru Emoto, The Secret Life of Water (Kindle, Atria Books, Simon and Schuster Inc. Digital Sales 2009)

Extreme Tech, *Human consciousness is simply a state of matter, like a solid or liquid – but quantum* http://www.extremetech.com/extreme/181284-human-consciousness-is-simply-a-state-of-matter-like-a-solid-or-liquid-but-quantum

Useful Resources

Activate your DNA, put *21st Century Superhuman Quantum Lifestyle* tips and tools to work in your Life and accelerate your progress. Your personal Awakening affects the entire hologram. Express your Life with greater authenticity, empowerment and LOVE. Shift yourself. Shift the entire Hologram! *Arc the Hologram Now with LOVE!*

Keep posted at our website for more books, tools, playshops, retreats, gatherings.

If this book is in your hands, there is a special reason. It is a tool for one of the most powerful activations in human history, as we enter an Evolutionary Leap called by many *The Shift of the Ages.* This is an amazing moment in which to be participating! See You there!

SUGGESTED READING - VIEWING

Dieter Broers - *Solar Revolution*

Gregg Braden - *The Divine Matrix*

Michael Tellinger - *Slave Species of the Gods*

Graham Hancock - *Fingerprints of the Gods*

Nassim Haramein - *Youtube and theresonanceproject.org*

Bruce Lipton and Steve Bhaerman - *Spontaneous Evolution*

dr. michael ryce - *http://www.whyagain.org*

Ervin Laszlo - *New Thinking ervinlaszlo.com*

HeartMath.org HeartMath.com - *Heart Coherence Practices*

Ram Dass • Foster Gamble • David Wilcock • i-uv.com

Lynn McTaggart - *The Field and The Intention Experiment*

Sacred Sounds - Mirabai Ceiba • Deva Premal • Krishna Das
Rainbow Didge • Kailash Kokopelli

Where To Find Us

21st Century Superhuman
Quantum Lifestyle

by Cary Ellis with Theodora Mulder PhD

Amazon

Kindle

Nook

iBooks

Audio

more

Follow Us - and Share with Friends
Facebook - *21t Century Superhuman*
Youtube - *21st Century Superhuman*
Twitter.com / caryellis

www.21stcenturysuperhuman.com

~ All in progress - thank you for your patience ~
If you have skills to offer let us know - web, promo, admin
Contact us at our website or message us at Facebook.
~ *Thank you!* ~

A Virtual Earth Village Publication
VirtualEarthVillage dot com

VOLUME DISCOUNTS *check our website for details*

Made in the USA
San Bernardino, CA
19 February 2015